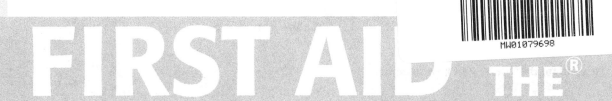

FIRST AID THE®

NBDE PART I

Third Edition

DEREK M. STEINBACHER, DMD, MD, FAAP
Assistant Professor
Plastic and Reconstructive Surgery
Director of Craniofacial Surgery
Yale University School of Medicine
New Haven, Connecticut

STEVEN R. SIERAKOWSKI, DMD, MDSc
Diplomate, American Board of Periodontology
Private practice
Philadelphia, Pennsylvania

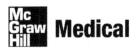 **Medical**

New York / Chicago / San Francisco / Lisbon / London / Madrid / Mexico City
Milan / New Delhi / San Juan / Seoul / Singapore / Sydney / Toronto

First Aid for the® NBDE Part I, Third Edition

1 2 3 4 5 6 7 8 9 0   QDB/QDB   17 16 15 14 13 12

ISBN 978-0-07-176904-4
MHID 0-07-176904-8
ISSN 1931-2407

NOTICE

Medicine is an ever-changing science. As new research and clinical experience broaden our knowledge, changes in treatment and drug therapy are required. The authors and the publisher of this work have checked with sources believed to be reliable in their efforts to provide information that is complete and generally in accord with the standards accepted at the time of publication. However, in view of the possibility of human error or changes in medical sciences, neither the authors nor the publisher nor any other party who has been involved in the preparation or publication of this work warrants that the information contained herein is in every respect accurate or complete, and they disclaim all responsibility for any errors or omissions or for the results obtained from use of the information contained in this work. Readers are encouraged to confirm the information contained herein with other sources. For example and in particular, readers are advised to check the product information sheet included in the package of each drug they plan to administer to be certain that the information contained in this work is accurate and that changes have not been made in the recommended dose or in the contraindications for administration. This recommendation is of particular importance in connection with new or infrequently used drugs.

This book was set in Palatino by Cenveo Publisher Services.
The editors were Catherine A. Johnson and Peter J. Boyle.
The production supervisor was Catherine H. Saggese.
Project management was provided by Sapna Rastogi, Cenveo Publisher Services.

To our families and loved ones who supported us through this endeavor,

and

To those mentors who sparked our enthusiasm for learning.

Derek M. Steinbacher, DMD, MD, FAAP
Steven R. Sierakowski, DMD, MDSc

CONTENTS

CONTRIBUTING AUTHORS

Jordan Bower
Temple University Kornberg School of Dentistry, Class of 2013

Tommy Burk
Harvard School of Dental Medicine, Class of 2013

Austin Eckard
Harvard School of Dental Medicine, Class of 2013

Raha Ghafurian, DMD, MSEd
University of Pennsylvania School of Dental Medicine, 2010
Yale Pediatric Dental Fellow

Virginia Hogsett
Harvard School of Dental Medicine, Class of 2013

Grace Kim
Harvard School of Dental Medicine, Class of 2013

Sarah Krygowski
Harvard School of Dental Medicine, Class of 2013

Katie McCafferty
Harvard School of Dental Medicine, Class of 2013

Veronica Mitko
Harvard School of Dental Medicine, Class of 2013

Marc D. Thomas, DDS
UCLA School of Dentistry, 2008
Yale Pediatric Dental Fellow

Janelle Tonn, DDS
Loma Linda School of Dentistry, 2010
Yale Pediatric Dental Fellow

ACKNOWLEDGMENTS

Thanks to our publisher, McGraw-Hill, for making this third edition a reality. We extend sincere gratitude to our editor, Catherine Johnson, for her continued support and guidance. Thanks also to Peter Boyle for supervising the production process and to the graphics team for their excellent rendering of anatomic illustrations.

Derek M. Steinbacher, DMD, MD, FAAP
Steven R. Sierakowski, DMD, MDSc

HOW TO CONTRIBUTE

We welcome your comments, suggestions, ideas, corrections, or other submissions to help with this and future editions of *First Aid for the NBDE Part I*. What information can you contribute?

- Test-taking tips and study strategies for the exam
- Suggestions for mnemonics, diagrams, figures, and tables
- Critiques related to the content or arrangement of facts contained herein
- Other sources of study material you find useful

Contributions used will result in a personal acknowledgment in the next edition of this book.

If you wish to contribute, e-mail your entries or suggestions to the following address:

nbde_firstaid@yahoo.com

Please include your name, address, e-mail address, and school affiliation.

NOTE TO CONTRIBUTORS

All contributions become property of the authors and are subject to editorial manipulation. In the event that similar or duplicate entries are received, only the first entry received will be used. Please include a reference to a standard textbook to verify the factual data.

HOW TO USE THIS BOOK

We feel that this book is an organized and resourceful guide to help you prepare for the NBDE Part I.

It is recommended that you use this book as early as possible, preferably in conjunction with your basic science and dental anatomy curriculum. The information contained within this book highlights the major facts and concepts commonly used in the NBDE Part I. Determine your own study strategy using not only this book, but also the materials you find most appropriate: concise review texts, the Internet, or your own class notes.

First Aid for the NBDE Part I is not meant to be a comprehensive review text; nor is it meant to be used as a substitute for a lack of studying during the first two years of dental school. As you study each topic, refer to the corresponding section in this book for a concise review or self-test. You may even want to make your own notes in the margins or highlight particular facts.

Some of the information found in the NBDE Part I is repeated in different sections. Many of the Key Facts in this book will guide you in cross-referencing a particular topic to another section. Use this to test yourself and integrate these facts into your body of knowledge.

During the last week before the exam, review the topics about which you feel the most unsure. The tables and figures in this book will help you keep the heavily-tested information fresh in your memory.

As soon as possible after you take the exam, we recommend that you review the book to help us create an even better fourth edition. Tell us what information should be revised, included, or removed. You may even send in your own annotated book.

INTRODUCTION

The National Board Dental Examination (NBDE) Part I is the first of two national standardized examinations administered by the Joint Commission on National Dental Examinations. Its purpose is to provide state dental licensing boards an objective method of evaluating the qualifications of prospective applicants. The NBDE Part I is intended to assess competency in the preclinical dental and basic biomedical sciences.

WHY DO WELL ON THE EXAM?

Achieving a passing score is a necessary requisite for both graduation from a dental school accredited by the Commission on Dental Accreditation, and for obtaining dental licensure in the United States. Although each state reserves the authority to use the scores from the NBDE as a requisite to fulfill its written examination requirement, all 50 states, the District of Columbia, Puerto Rico, and the Virgin Islands use the NBDE for their licensing protocol. Additionally, each jurisdiction may have its own minimum NBDE Part I score requirement in order to obtain a dental license. It is essential that the future dentist be aware of the licensure requirements for each state in which he or she wishes to practice. A score of 85 or above is adequate in every state.

The NBDE Part I scores are also a major criterion used to gauge the quality of students applying to post-doctoral training programs. Since this examination is usually taken after the second year of dental school, it is often the only objective method of comparing soon-to-be graduates for such programs. Performing well on the NBDE Part I gives the student more bargaining potential when applying for these programs, as well as positions in academic, military, or private practice settings. In short, it behooves you to earn a good score on the NBDE Part I. Much diligence and a targeted study strategy, using materials like this book, will help you accomplish this goal.

STRUCTURE OF THE EXAMINATION

The NBDE Part I is administered at Prometric Test Centers throughout the United States, its territories, and Canada. Once your application has been approved by the Joint Commission office, you will be notified by mail to contact Prometric to register for the examination. You have 12 months after application approval to take the examination. A list of test centers can be found at www.prometric.com. The fee for the exam is $260.

The exam consists of two test sections of 200 questions each, for a total of 400 questions. The questions are in the form of multiple-choice test items, each with four to five possible answer choices. Approximately 80% of the questions are individual discipline-based items, while 20% are testlet questions based on a patient-centered scenario. All of the test items are evenly distributed in four broad categories:

- Anatomic Sciences
- Microbiology and Pathology
- Biochemistry and Physiology
- Dental Anatomy and Occlusion

The total testing time is seven hours, allowing 3.5 hours per section with an optional one-hour (maximum) break between sections. There is a 15-minute tutorial at the start of the exam and a post-examination survey to complete when you are finished.

SCORING OF THE EXAMINATION

The NBDE Part I is scored on a scale of 49 to 99. Scores are graded against a predetermined standard and are not based on a curve. The total number of questions you answered correctly (your raw score) determines your scaled score. There is no penalty for answering a question incorrectly. Furthermore, up to 15% of the questions may be discarded, as they may be used for other evaluation purposes. A scaled score of 75 for each section is considered the minimum passing score for the NBDE Part I.

Your score report will be mailed approximately three to four weeks after the examination. You will receive a total of five scores: the overall standard score and the raw scores (total number correct answers out of the total number of questions) for each of the four subject areas. The report also gives the national averages for each of the scores. The dean of your dental school will also receive a copy of your scores. Requesting additional copies of score reports is possible upon written request and is necessary for both postdoctoral program and state licensure applications.

REGISTERING FOR THE EXAM

An active or former dental student is eligible for the NBDE Part I after his or her dental school certifies, either by signature or electronic approval, that the student has successfully completed all subjects included in Part I. For US and Canadian students, the signature of the dean or school designee is the only requirement. For graduates of international dental schools, Educational Credential Evaluators, Inc. (ECE) must verify their official dental school transcripts.

You can request an application in writing, by telephone, or online. For more information, or to request a Candidate's Guide, contact the address below:

The Joint Commission on National Dental Examinations
American Dental Association
211 East Chicago Avenue, 6th Floor
Chicago, IL 60611
(312) 440-2678
www.ada.org

PREPARATION FOR THE EXAMINATION

The best preparation for the NBDE Part I is, of course, performing as well as possible in your preclinical dental school courses. The examination will address each of the subjects you have encountered during years one and two of dental school, although sometimes more or less depending on the specifics of your curriculum. Make a concerted effort to master the material when it is initially presented at your school. Be organized. Keep your notes for each course and have them arranged by topic or theme. Be aware of the subjects covered on NBDE Part I and create your study sheets accordingly. Use this book as an outline or an umbrella under which you can incorporate the pertinent details of each individual dental school course. For instance, when taking dental school microbiology in first year, cross-reference the subject matter with the outlines and material presented here in *First Aid*. In this way you will create organized study materials that will be easy to reference when you go back to study for the NBDE Part I.

If you are now just a few months away from taking the NBDE Part I and have not prepared in the manner just mentioned over the past two years, do not fret. The major obstacle is the disparate location of information. There is a lot of material to cover, but what is most important is that all facts are compiled in one place. Choose your study materials and then cross-reference and combine information pertaining to each topic in one location. Try to decide on a study method that has worked for you. This could be note cards, subject outlines, or categorical maps. The process of organizing the information in one place will force you to learn it. A combination approach that we find helpful is looking at the broad categories of topics with study sheets or maps and focusing on the particular details with note cards or lists. For example, when studying microbiology it is useful to first divide bacteria generally into classes based, say, on Gram stain (outline this on one sheet), then prepare flashcards with more specifics, e.g., organism names on one side and pertinent descriptive details on the other.

If you are only days or weeks away from the exam you need to do some self-reflection. Now that the exam is computerized you can postpone the date of the exam with relative ease. If, for some reason, you cannot push back the exam you must focus on quickly hammering out the high-yield facts. Recognition and recall are essential for last-minute cramming. Go through lists of buzzwords. Try to organize these in different categories if possible. Visualize their interrelationships. If you are in a private place, it may help to talk aloud. The mantra is: "repetition to create recognition and recall."

STUDY TACTICS

It is ideal to plan well ahead and orchestrate your exam date at a convenient time. You should allow for ample time to address all subject areas and review thoroughly. As mentioned, the best situation is to concurrently use the *First Aid* book as a study aid while taking each preclinical course. You will want to commit to memory all of the topic headings and buzzwords. This is made more tangible by linking concepts to associations and looking at the interrelationships of different ideas.

Set up a schedule at least one to two months ahead of time. The laxity of the schedule depends on your circumstances. If you are very busy during the spring semester of your second year, you may want to arrange for a longer study phase with less information covered each day. Alternatively, your school may set aside dedicated NBDE study time. You can plan to complete most of your rigorous studying during this period and concentrate on your dental school classes up until then. If you know you are weak in a particular subject area, it would be prudent to spend some extra time reviewing that topic earlier in the semester.

Do not jeopardize a healthy lifestyle at the expense of studying. It is important to eat well, exercise regularly, and get ample sleep each night. All of these things will allow you to be maximally efficient during your studying. Feeling good and maintaining yourself personally will help your mind absorb all of the meticulous information required. When studying, take regular breaks. Some advocate a breather every 45 minutes or so. You should take a 15-minute break at least every hour-and-a-half to two hours. Get up and stretch. Have a snack. Take a power nap. Do something to distract yourself from preclinical dental and basic science courses.

An important tenet to follow is to start your studying with areas that you find most difficult or that will require the most time to master. Set your schedule with time allotted for each subject and goals you want to achieve with each session. You may want to allow two weeks to study pathology and each night you will cover a subset thereof—e.g., cellular injury. At the end of each session it is a good idea to test yourself; either with released test questions or with questions you derive on your own during the course of studying. Equally important is taking time to review. Before each new study session, take 15–20 minutes to review the material you have learned last time. Your study timeline should allow for one to two weeks prior to the exam for a comprehensive review. You can use your cross-referenced summary study sheets or lists and take old examinations. Taking loads of old exams the last week is very helpful. For one, you get into the groove of taking eight hours worth of questions in a single day. Second, you will gain familiarity with the writing style of NBDE questions. Lastly, you will be able to witness your deficiencies and take time to work them out.

Lore has it that the day prior to the exam should be reserved for leisurely activity and getting a good night's rest. True, you should engage in some stress-relieving activity and be sure to go to bed early. However, it is completely reasonable to review material for a few hours that day. This may mean reading over your review sheets for each subject, listing aloud high-yield buzzwords, or going through the practice questions that you got wrong. Do not try to learn brand new material or complete a rigorous study session during these final hours!

In the end, try to relax. It is only an exam and, if anything happens to go wrong, it is not the end of the world. The vast majority of students pass on their first try. If you have a bad day—and we all have had one—the exam will be there for you to take again. It may set you back some money, but spend some time preparing and you will make it through dental school perfectly fine and go into the field you have always imagined.

DAY OF THE EXAM

Be sure to set your alarm with plenty of time allowed. You need to perform your morning routine in an unhurried fashion. Do some light stretching and eat a healthy breakfast. Plan on arriving at the test site with 10–15 minutes to spare. Bring ample snacks with you. We would advise that you take a break between at least every other section. Use this time to go to the restroom, eat a banana, or breathe some fresh air. Save time to take at least a 25-minute lunch break.

During the exam, relax. Read each question carefully from start to finish. Do not jump to the answer choices until you have read the entire question. As you process the question in your mind you should be thinking about the possible answers. Try and deduce what the answer should be and see if it matches with the available choices. If you look at the answer choices prior to fully processing the question, you are apt to be swayed by the "trap answers." Go with your first instinct. If you are not sure about the correct answer do not worry. Mark the question so you can return to it later. Do not get bogged down and spend 10 minutes on a single question. Move on to the next question and continue until you have gone through all the items for a single pass. Then you can return to the questions you have marked. Pay attention to the clock. You want to divide your marked questions by the available time. Go through with your best choice or best guess and be done. By all means, answer every question—there is no penalty for wrong answers.

You have studied hard and prepared well. This book will help guide your studying. Good luck.

Anatomic Sciences

- Gross Anatomy
- General Histology
- Oral Histology
- Developmental Biology

CHAPTER 1

Gross Anatomy

There are four unpaired bones of the neurocranium: ethmoid, sphenoid, frontal, occipital.

Bones of the viscerocranium (except the mandibular condyle) form by intramembranous growth.

Cranium

■ The neurocranium encloses the brain and the viscerocranium comprises the face.

Neurocranium	Viscerocranium
Frontal bone	Maxillae (2, then fuse)
Parietal bones (2)	Nasal bones (2)
Temporal bones (2)	Zygomatic bones (2)
Occipital bone	Palatine bones (2)
Sphenoid bone	Lacrimal bones (2)
Ethmoid bone	Inferior conchae (2)
	Vomer
	Mandible
	Hyoid

ANTERIOR SKULL

See Figure 1–1 for the anterior aspect of the skull.

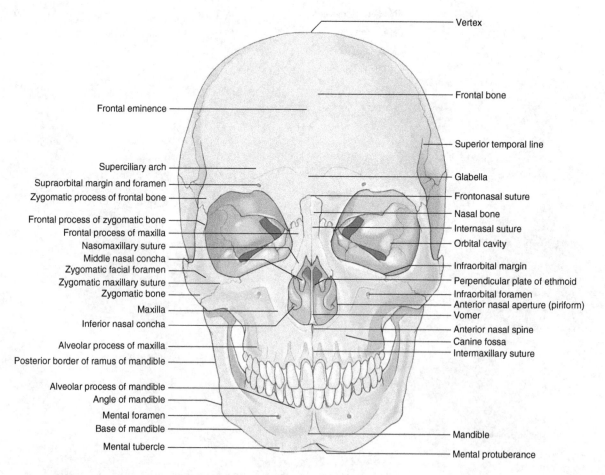

FIGURE 1–1. **Anterior aspect of the skull.**

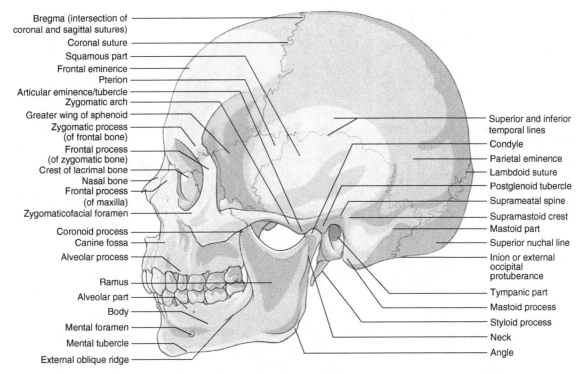

Bregma (intersection of coronal and sagittal sutures)
Coronal suture
Squamous part
Frontal eminence
Pterion
Articular eminence/tubercle
Zygomatic arch
Greater wing of sphenoid
Zygomatic process (of frontal bone)
Frontal process (of zygomatic bone)
Crest of lacrimal bone
Nasal bone
Frontal process (of maxilla)
Zygomaticofacial foramen
Coronoid process
Canine fossa
Alveolar process
Ramus
Alveolar part
Body
Mental foramen
Mental tubercle
External oblique ridge

Superior and inferior temporal lines
Condyle
Parietal eminence
Lambdoid suture
Postglenoid tubercle
Suprameatal spine
Supramastoid crest
Mastoid part
Superior nuchal line
Inion or external occipital protuberance
Tympanic part
Mastoid process
Styloid process
Neck
Angle

FIGURE 1–2. **Lateral aspect of the skull.**

LATERAL SKULL

See Figure 1–2 for the lateral aspect of the skull.

POSTERIOR SKULL

See Figure 1–3 for the posterior aspect of the skull.

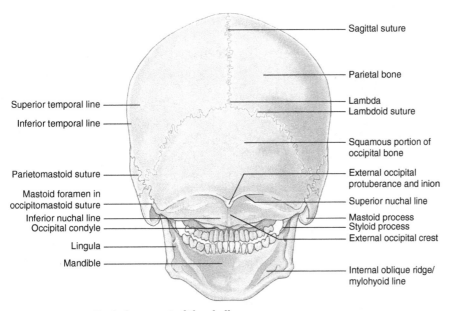

Sagittal suture
Parietal bone
Lambda
Lambdoid suture
Squamous portion of occipital bone
External occipital protuberance and inion
Superior nuchal line
Mastoid process
Styloid process
External occipital crest
Internal oblique ridge/ mylohyoid line

Superior temporal line
Inferior temporal line
Parietomastoid suture
Mastoid foramen in occipitomastoid suture
Inferior nuchal line
Occipital condyle
Lingula
Mandible

FIGURE 1–3. **Posterior aspect of the skull.**

The pterion is considered the weakest part of the skull. Deep to the pterion runs the middle meningeal, which may be damaged with trauma to the pterion.

Petrous temporal bone forms the floor of the middle cranial fossa and separates middle and posterior cranial fossae.

Middle meningeal artery is located in middle cranial fossa (exits foramen spinosum).

Cranial Fossae

See Figure 1–4.

	Anterior Cranial Fossa	Middle Cranial Fossa	Posterior Cranial Fossa
Formed by (bones)	Orbital plates of the frontal bone, cribriform plates of the ethmoid bone, and small wings of the sphenoid bone	Greater wings of the sphenoid bone and petrous and squamous portions of the temporal bones	Squamous and mastoid portion of temporal bones and occipital bone
Contents	Frontal lobes Cribriform plate Foramen cecum Crista galli	Temporal lobes Pituitary Optic foramen Superior orbital fissure Carotid canal Trigeminal ganglion Foramen rotundum Foramen ovale Foramen spinosum	Occipital lobes Brain stem Cerebellum Internal acoustic meatus Jugular foramen Foramen magnum Hypoglossal canal

See Figures 1–4 and 1–5.

Important Cranial Foramina

Foramina	Bone(s)	Contents Passed
Foramen cecum	Frontal and ethmoid	Emissary vein
Greater palatine foramen	Palatine	Greater palatine nerve, artery, vein
Lesser palatine foramen	Palatine	Lesser palatine nerve, artery, vein
Incisive canal	Maxilla	Nasopalatine nerve
Supraorbital foramen	Frontal	Supraorbital nerve, artery, vein
Infraorbital foramen	Sphenoid and maxilla	Infraorbital nerve (V2), artery, and vein
Optic canal	Sphenoid	Optic nerve (II) and ophthalmic artery
Superior orbital fissure	Sphenoid (between greater and lesser wings)	Oculomotor (III), trochlear (IV), abducens (VI), trigeminal (V1–lacrimal, frontal, and nasociliary nerves), and superior ophthalmic vein
Inferior orbital fissure (leads to infraorbital foramen)	Sphenoid, maxilla	V2, infraorbital vessels, ascending branches of sphenopalatine ganglion
Foramen rotundum	Sphenoid	V2
Foramen ovale	Sphenoid	V3, parasympathetic fibers from CN IX via lesser petrosal nerve, accessory meningeal artery
Foramen spinosum	Sphenoid	Middle meningeal artery and vein
Petrotympanic fissure	Temporal	Chorda tympani, anterior tympanic artery
Foramen lacerum	Temporal and sphenoid	Greater and deep petrosal nerve and parasympathetic fibers from CN VII via nervus intermedius
Internal acoustic meatus	Temporal (petrous)	VII and VIII
Stylomastoid foramen	Temporal	Facial nerve (VII)
Jugular foramen	Temporal and occipital	IJV, glossopharyngeal (IX), vagus (X), and spinal accessory (XI) nerves
Foramen magnum	Occipital	Medulla oblongata/spinal cord, vertebral arteries, spinal accessory nerve
Mandibular foramen	Mandible	Inferior alveolar nerve, artery, vein
Mental foramen	Mandible	Mental nerve, artery, and vein

INTERNAL SKULL

See Figure 1–4 for the internal skull base.

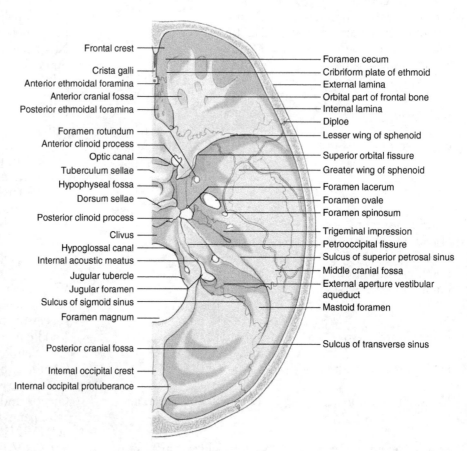

FIGURE 1–4. **Internal skull.**

CRANIAL BASE

See Figure 1–5 for the cranial base.

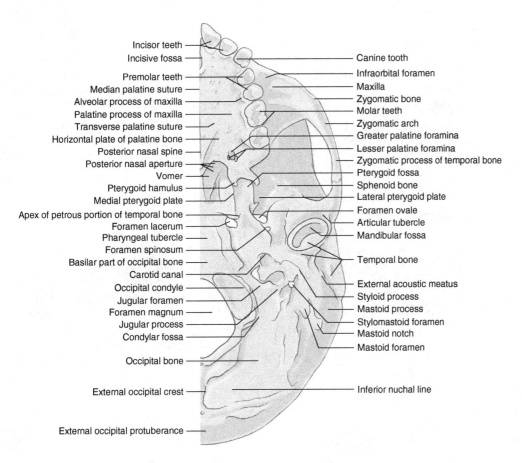

FIGURE 1–5. Cranial base.

ETHMOID AND SPHENOID BONES

- Single (unpaired) midline, bilaterally symmetric bones.
- Contribute both to the neurocranium and viscerocranium.

The inferior nasal conchae is its own bone.

The greater wing of sphenoid contains three foramina: rotundum, ovale, spinosum (middle cranial fossa).

	Component	Function
Ethmoid	Cribriform plate	Olfactory foramina.
	Crista galli	Attaches to falx cerebri.
	Lateral plates	Contain ethmoid sinuses, lamina papyracea, superior and middle nasal conchae.
	Perpendicular plate	Superior part of nasal septum.
Sphenoid	Hollow body	Sella turcica and sphenoidal sinuses.
	Greater wings	Lateral orbital wall and roof of infratemporal fossa.
	Lesser wings	Optic canal, superior orbital fissue, anterior clinoid process
	Medial and lateral pterygoid plates	Lateral pterygoid plate is attachment for both medial and lateral pterygoid muscles; medial pterygoid plate ends as a hamulus (tensor veli palatine muscle hooks around this).

The ophthalmic artery (a branch of the internal carotid artery, ICA) is the major blood supply to the orbit and eye. It enters the orbit with the optic nerve via the optic canal.

Face and Viscerocranium

BONES OF THE ORBIT

The orbit comprises seven bones (Figure 1–6):

- Frontal
- Maxilla
- Zygoma
- Ethmoid
- Sphenoid
- Lacrimal
- Palatine

See the chart Important Cranial Foramina (p. 9).

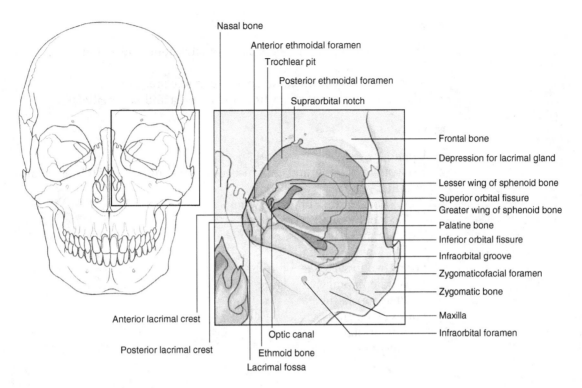

Nasal bone
Anterior ethmoidal foramen
Trochlear pit
Posterior ethmoidal foramen
Supraorbital notch

Frontal bone
Depression for lacrimal gland
Lesser wing of sphenoid bone
Superior orbital fissure
Greater wing of sphenoid bone
Palatine bone
Inferior orbital fissure
Infraorbital groove
Zygomaticofacial foramen
Zygomatic bone
Maxilla
Infraorbital foramen

Anterior lacrimal crest
Posterior lacrimal crest
Optic canal
Ethmoid bone
Lacrimal fossa

FIGURE 1-6. The orbit, frontal view.

ORBITAL CONTENTS (FIGURE 1-7)

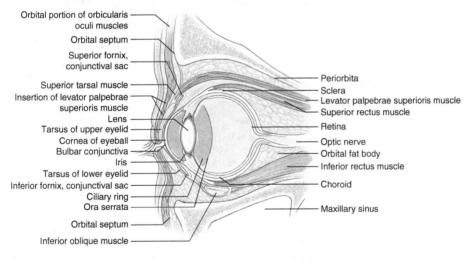

Orbital portion of orbicularis oculi muscles
Orbital septum
Superior fornix, conjunctival sac
Superior tarsal muscle
Insertion of levator palpebrae superioris muscle
Lens
Tarsus of upper eyelid
Cornea of eyeball
Bulbar conjunctiva
Iris
Tarsus of lower eyelid
Inferior fornix, conjunctival sac
Ciliary ring
Ora serrata
Orbital septum
Inferior oblique muscle

Periorbita
Sclera
Levator palpebrae superioris muscle
Superior rectus muscle
Retina
Optic nerve
Orbital fat body
Inferior rectus muscle
Choroid
Maxillary sinus

FIGURE 1-7. The orbit, sagittal view.

The upper orbital septum is continuous with the levator palpebrae superioris and the lower orbital septum is continuous with the tarsal plate.

ZYGOMA

The zygomatic bone is also referred to as the malar bone or cheekbone.

- Located in the upper and lateral part of the face.
- Prominence of the cheek.
- Part of the lateral wall and floor of the orbit.
- Parts of the temporal and infratemporal fossae.
- Articulates with the maxilla (anteriorly), temporal bone (posteriorly), and frontal bone (superiorly).

ZYGOMATIC ARCH

- Formed by temporal process of zygomatic bone and zygomatic process of temporal bone.
- Temporalis muscle passes deep to zygomatic arch.
- Masseter muscle originates from the zygoma and zygomatic arch.

MAXILLA

- Upper jaw.
- Consists of a body and four processes: zygomatic, frontal, alveolar, and palatine.
- Forms boundaries of three cavities.
    - Roof of the mouth (palate).
    - Floor and lateral wall of the nose.
    - Floor of the orbit.
- Forms two fossae (See Table 1–1).
    - Infratemporal (See Figure 1–8).
    - Pterygopalatine.
- Forms two fissures.
    - Infraorbital.
    - Pterygomaxillary.

TABLE 1-1.   Infratemporal and Pterygopalatine Fossae

Fossa	Anterior	Posterior	Medial	Lateral	Roof	Floor	Contents
		BOUNDARIES					
Infratemporal fossa	Posterior maxilla	Temporal bone (articular tubercle) and spenoidal spine of the spenoid bone	Lateral pterygoid plate (sphenoid)	Mandibular ramus	Greater wing of sphenoid (with foramen ovale →CN V3)	Medial pterygoid muscle (superior surface where inserts into mandible)	Temporalis and pterygoid muscles Maxillary artery (and branches, eg, middle meningeal) Pterygoid plexus of veins Mandibular nerve (V3) Chorda tympani (VII) Otic ganglion (IX)
Pterygopalatine fossa	Maxilla	Pterygoid plates	Nasal fossa	Infratemporal fossa	Greater wing of sphenoid; opens into inferior orbital fissure	Pyramidal process of palatine bone; inferior end contains palatine canals	Pterygopalatine (3rd) part of maxillary artery and its branches Maxillary nerve (V2) Nerve of pterygoid canal Pterygopalatine ganglion and branches[a]

[a]For pterygopalatine ganglion, see the parasympathetic ganglia chart.

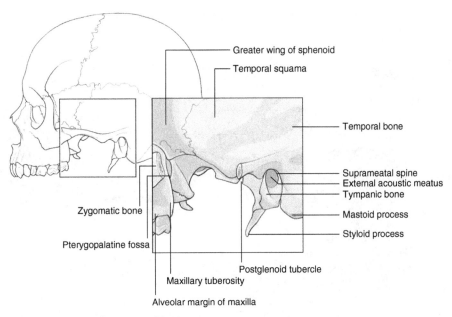

FIGURE 1–8. Infratemporal fossa.

Pterygopalatine Fossa Major Communications

Direction	Passageway	Contents Passing	Space
Lateral	Pterygomaxillary fissure	Posterior superior alveolar NAV, maxillary artery	Infratemporal fossa
Anterosuperior	Inferior orbital fissure	CN V2	Orbit
Posterosuperior	Foramen rotundum and pterygoid canal	CN V2; nerve of pterygoid canal (formed by deep and greater petrosal nerves)	Middle cranial fossa
Medial	Sphenopalatine foramen	Sphenopalatine artery and vein, nasopalatine nerve	Nasal cavity
Inferior	Palatine canals	Greater and lesser palatine NAVs	Oral cavity

See Figure 1–9 for lateral scheme of the pterygopalatine fossa.

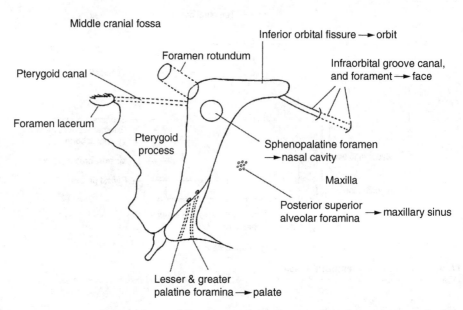

FIGURE 1–9. **Lateral scheme of the pterygopalatine fossa to show the entrances and exits.**

Reproduced, with permission, from Liebgott B. *The Anatomical Basis of Dentistry.* Toronto: BC Decker, 1986.

HARD PALATE

The palate forms the roof of the oral cavity and the floor of the nasal cavity.

- Maxilla are palatal processes (anterior two-thirds).
- Palatine bones are horizontal palates (posterior one-third).
- Pterygoid plates of the sphenoid articulate with the maxillary tuberosity (posterior palate).

Palatal Foramen

- Incisive foramen (Scarpa, midline; Stenson, lateral)—descending palatine vessels and the nasopalatine nerves (of V2)—anterior palatal block.
- Greater and lesser palatine foramen—descending palatine vessels and anterior palatine nerve (of V2)—site of palatal anesthetic block.

Nasal Cavity

Boundary	Contributing Structures
Floor	Hard palate (maxilla and palatine bones)
Roof	Cribriform plate of ethmoid, anterior body of sphenoid, nasal spine of frontal bone, nasal bones, lateral nasal cartilages
Lateral wall	Nasal, ethmoid, sphenoid, maxilla, palatine, and inferior conchal bones
Medial wall	Nasal septum
External nose	Two nasal bones, nasal cartilages

NASAL CAVITY

See Figure 1–10.

- Sensory innervation is from branches of V2.
  - Nasopalatine
  - Infraorbital
  - Greater palatine
- Some sensory branches are from V1 (ophthalmic division).
  - Anterior ethmoidal nerve
- Parasympathetic to secretory glands supplied by branches of the pterygopalatine ganglion.
- Olfactory epithelium (roof of the nasal cavity) is innervated by the olfactory nerve (I).
- Blood supply—sphenopalatine branch of maxillary artery, anterior ethmoidal branch of ophthalmic artery, and septal branch of superior labial branch of facial artery.
- Superior nasal conchae and upper third of septum contain yellowish olfactory mucosa.

CN I (olfactory nerve) projects to the primary olfactory cortex (pyriform cortex).

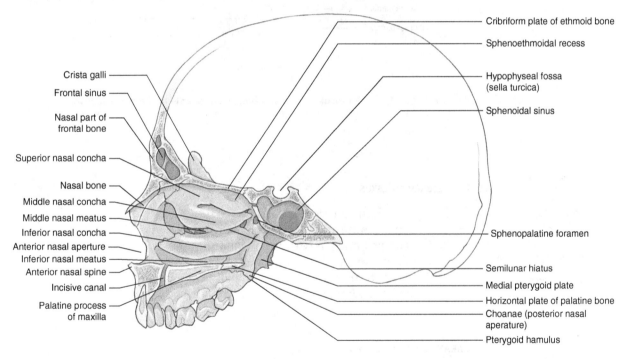

FIGURE 1–10.   Lateral nasal cavity and hard palate.

Conchae	Meatuses
Superior and middle (ethmoid bone) inferior (its own bone)	Areas below each conchae are the superior, middle, and inferior meatuses, respectively
Increase air turbulence for warming, filtering, olfaction	Drainage points for sinuses and nasolacrimal apparatus

NASAL SEPTUM

The nasal septum comprises five bones and one cartilage (See Figure 1–11).

- Vertical plate of ethmoid
- Vomer
- Nasal crest of maxilla and palatine bones
- Nasal crest of sphenoid bones
- Septal cartilage

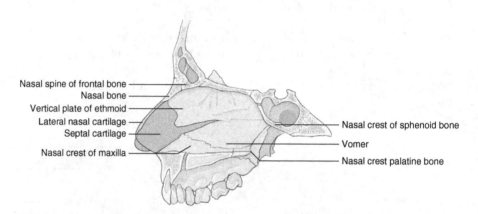

Nasal spine of frontal bone —
Nasal bone —
Vertical plate of ethmoid —
Lateral nasal cartilage —
Septal cartilage —
Nasal crest of maxilla —

— Nasal crest of sphenoid bone
— Vomer
— Nasal crest palatine bone

FIGURE 1–11. The cartilaginous and bony components of the nasal septum.

KIESSELBACH'S PLEXUS

Most cases of epistaxis arise from this area.

- This plexus is the anastomosis of five arteries:
    - Sphenopalatine artery (from maxillary artery)
    - Greater palatine artery (from maxillary artery)
    - Superior labial artery (from facial artery)
    - Anterior ethmoid artery (from opthalmic artery)
    - Lateral nasal branches from facial artery

PARANASAL SINUSES (FIGURE 1–12)

The maxillary sinus is lined by the Schneiderian membrane which is pseudo-stratified columnar epithelium.

- Frontal
- Maxillary
- Ethmoid
- Sphenoid

System	Location of Drainage
Nasolacrimal apparatus	Inferior meatus (below inferior concha)
Frontal sinuses	**Middle meatus:** Hiatus semilunaris (below middle concha)
Maxillary sinuses	**Middle meatus:** Ostium (below middle concha) (within hiatus semilunaris)
Ethmoid sinuses: ▫ Anterior ▫ Middle ▫ Posterior	**Middle meatus** Hiatus semilunaris Ethmoidal bullae Superior meatus
Sphenoid sinuses	Sphenoethmoidal recess of nasal cavity

A surgical approach to pituitary gland is via the sphenoid sinus.

The middle meatus contains openings for the frontal sinus, anterior and middle ethmoidal sinuses, and maxillary sinuses.

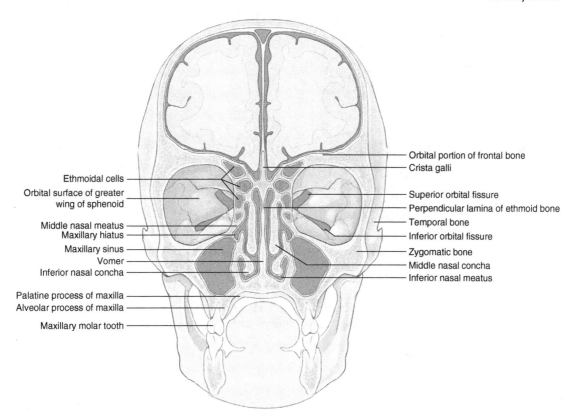

FIGURE 1–12. Paranasal sinuses.

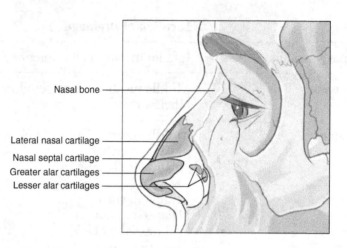

Nasal bone

Lateral nasal cartilage
Nasal septal cartilage
Greater alar cartilages
Lesser alar cartilages

FIGURE 1–13. The nose.

EXTERNAL NOSE (FIGURE 1–13)

Cartilage of the external

nose is hyaline.

- Nasal bones
- Septal cartilages
- Lateral cartilages
- Alar cartilages

MANDIBLE

- Largest and strongest bone of the face.
- Lower jaw: houses lower teeth.
- Consists of:
  - Body (curved, horizontal).
  - Rami (two perpendicular portions).
    - Body and rami unite at angle (nearly 90 degrees).
  - Coronoid process (attachment of temporalis muscle).
  - Condyle.

See Section Mastication and TMJ of this chapter for information on temporo-mandibular joints and the muscles of mastication.

FORAMINA

Mandibular Foramen

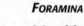

The mandibular canal

traverses the mandibular

body and opens anteriorly at

the mental foramen.

- Is located on the medial side of the ramus (just below lingula), midway between anterior and posterior borders of the ramus.
- It passes
  - Inferior alveolar nerve (IAN) (of V3).
  - Inferior alveolar artery and vein.

Mental Foramen

- Is located below the second premolar on each side.
- It passes
  - Mental nerve; the inferior alveolar nerve exits as the mental nerve. It supplies skin and mucous membrane of the mental region.
  - Incisive branch, which supplies the pulp chambers of the anterior teeth and adjacent mucous membrane.

The lingula is a tongue-shaped projection above the mandibular foramen where the sphenomandibular ligament attaches.

Scalp (Figure 1–14)

A mnemonic device to remember the components of the scalp is:

- Skin
- Connective tissue
- Aponeurosis (galea aponeurotica, epicranial aponeurosis)
- Loose connective tissue
- Periosteum

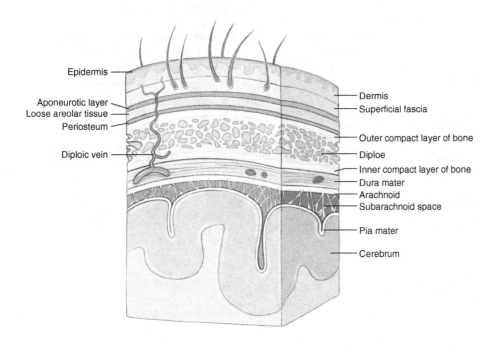

Epidermis
Aponeurotic layer
Loose areolar tissue
Periosteum
Diploic vein

Dermis
Superficial fascia
Outer compact layer of bone
Diploe
Inner compact layer of bone
Dura mater
Arachnoid
Subarachnoid space
Pia mater
Cerebrum

FIGURE 1–14. The scalp.

Meningitis is inflammation of the meninges. For more information, see "Systemic Pathology," Chapter 22.

Blood surrounds the meninges in the following ways:

- **Epidural hematoma** involves the middle meningeal artery.
- **Subdural hematoma** involves a bridging vein.
- **Subarachnoid hemorrhage** often involves a ruptured aneurysm (eg, anterior communicating artery).

Meninges

Meninge	Space	Description
	Epidural space	Potential space between periosteum of inner surface of skull and dura; middle meningeal artery is in this location.
Dura mater		Tough membranous, outermost layer, continuous with the periosteum within the skull; forms the venous sinuses in the cranial cavity. Endosteal layer is continuous with cranial periosteum. Meningeal layer folds between brain.
	Subdural space	Between dura and arachnoid; bridging veins and cranial venous sinuses are located here.
Arachnoid		Weblike (spiderlike) lattices interposed between dura and pia; does not follow the sulci; bridges them.
	Subarachnoid space	Between arachnoid and pia; is filled with CSF; cerebral circulation is here (circle of Willis). This is the space entered with a lumbar puncture ("spinal tap").
Pia mater		Layer adherent to the brain; spinal cord follows the sulci.

DURAL FOLDS

See Figure 1–15 for the folds of the dura mater.

Fold	Description
Vertical	
Falx cerebri	Vertical, midline. Separates the cerebral hemispheres. Forms the superior and inferior sagittal sinuses.
Falx cerebelli	Separates cerebellar hemispheres. Contains occipital sinus.
Horizontal	
Tentorium cerebelli	Separates cerebral hemispheres (occipital lobes) from cerebellum below. Contains straight, transverse, and superior petrosal sinuses. **Uncus** (medial parahippocampal gyrus); amygdala lies beneath; herniates below tentorium.
Diaphragma sella	Roof of the sella turcica. Small hole allows passage of the pituitary stalk.

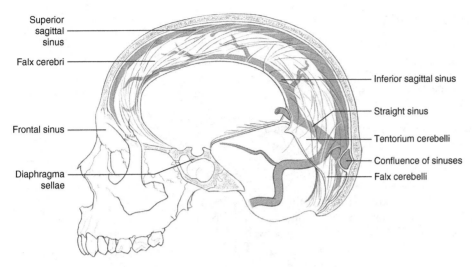

FIGURE 1–15. The folds of the dura mater.

*Lumbar puncture
(from outside to in):*
- Skin
- Subcutaneous tissue
- Supraspinous ligament
- Interspinous ligament
- Ligamentum flavum
  (if not midline)
- Epidural space
  (fat, venous plexus)
- (Subdural space–
  potential space)
- Subarachnoid space
  with cerebrospinal
  fluid (CSF)

VENOUS SINUSES (FIGURE 1–16)

The **dural sinuses** are:

- Superior sagittal sinus
- Inferior sagittal sinus
- Straight sinus
- Cavernous sinus (2)
- Superior petrosal sinus (2)
- Inferior petrosal sinus (2)
- Occipital sinus
- Transverse sinus (2)
- Confluence of sinuses (torcular of herophile)
- Sigmoid

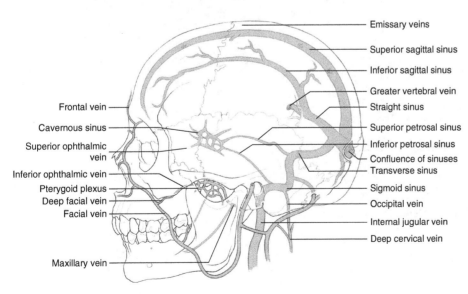

FIGURE 1–16. The venous sinuses.

Drainage of the head/brain is via the internal jugular vein (IJV).

*IJV forms from the inferior petrosal and sigmoid sinuses.

Ophthalmic veins (superior and inferior) can communicate with the cavernous sinus. Because there are no valves, retrograde flow occurs.

Tributaries of Dural Sinuses

Emissary veins	Drain scalp into dural sinuses.
Diploic veins	Drain the diploe of the skull into dural sinuses.
Meningeal veins	Drain meninges into dural sinuses.

CAVERNOUS SINUS (FIGURES 1–17 AND 1–18)

Location	Connections	Contents	Description
Middle cranial fossa (on either side of sella turcica)	**Anterior:** Superior and inferior ophthalmic veins, pterygoid plexus of veins (via facial vein)	Lateral wall: CNs III, IV, V1, V2	Route of infection to brain (eg, zygomycosis)
	Posterior: Superior and inferior petrosal, intercavernous sinus	Running through cavernous sinus: CN VI ICA	Cavernous sinus thrombosis (see Chapter 22, Systemic Pathology)

The superior petrosal sinus connects the cavernous and sigmoid sinuses.

CN VI is the smallest and most medial nerve in the cavernous sinus and will be the first nerve affected by an infection.

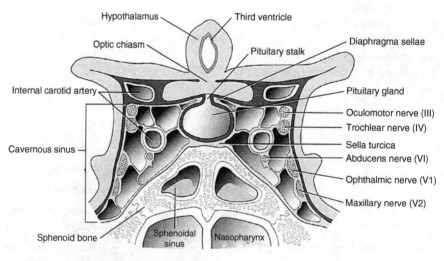

FIGURE 1–17. Cavernous sinus.

Reproduced, with permission, from Bhushan V, et al. *First Aid for the USMLE Step 1*. New York: McGraw-Hill, 2003. Adapted from Stobo J, et al. *The Principles and Practice of Medicine*, 23rd ed. Stamford, CT: Appleton & Lange, 1996:277.

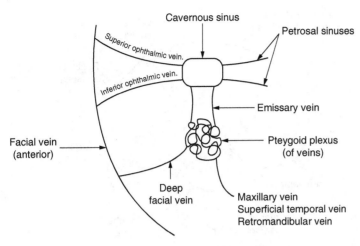

FIGURE 1-18. **Cavernous sinus and its communications.**

The abducens nerve is most likely affected from a laterally expanding pituitary tumor because it is medially located within the cavernous sinus.

Pterygoid Plexus of Veins

Location	Receives	Drains
Located in the infratemporal fossa Surrounds the maxillary artery Associated with the pterygoid muscles	Venous branches corresponding with those of the maxillary artery	Maxillary vein posteriorly Deep facial vein into the facial vein anteriorly

The deep facial vein connects the anterior facial vein and pterygoid plexus.

Ventricular System

This system is lined with ependymal cells. It consists of these parts: lateral ventricle, interventricular foramen, third ventricle, cerebral aqueduct, fourth ventricle (releases CSF into subarachnoid space). See Figure 1–19.

The choroid plexus and ventricular system regulate intracranial pressure.

Ventricle	Nearby Anatomical Structure
Lateral ventricle	Caudate nucleus
Lateral ventricle (inferior horn)	Hippocampus
Third ventricle	Hypothalamus
Floor of fourth ventricle	Pons

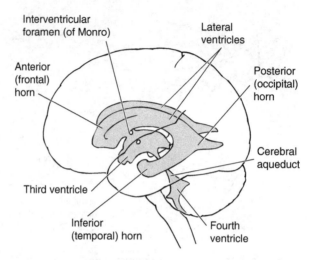

FIGURE 1–19. The ventricular system.

Reproduced, with permission, from Waxman SG. *Clinical Neuroanatomy*, 25th ed. New York: McGraw-Hill, 2003.

Ependymal cells can also produce CSF.

*Foramina of **L**uschka are **L**ateral aperatures*

*Foramina of **M**agendie are **M**edial aperatures.*

CSF CIRCULATION

- The CSF flows from lateral ventricles (produced in choroids plexus) through the ventricular system to the subarachnoid space, where it enters the venous circulation.

- *Pathway*

Lateral ventricles

↓

Foramen of Monro

↓

Third ventricle

↓

Cerebral aqueduct

↓

Fourth ventricle

↓

Foramina of Magendie and Luschka (exits ventricular system into subarachnoid space)

↓

Bathes the cisterns in the subarachnoid space

↓

Arachnoid granulations protrude into the superior sagittal sinus and empty CSF into the venous circulation.

Blood-Brain Barrier

The blood-brain barrier (BBB) consists of three parts:

Blood-CSF Barrier	Vascular-Endothelial Barrier	Arachnoid Barrier
CSF produced in choroid plexus in ventricles. Choroid plexus epithelial cells are joined by tight junctions, allowing selective passage.	Tight junctions between endothelial cells	Arachnoid cells form a barrier, preventing substances from dural vessel from diffusing in toward brain.

Intracranial Circulation

▨ Blood is supplied to the brain via many arteries.

CIRCLE OF WILLIS

See Figures 1–20 and 1–21.

▨ Contents:
  ▨ Posterior cerebral artery
  ▨ Posterior communicating artery
  ▨ Internal carotid artery
  ▨ Anterior cerebral artery
  ▨ Anterior communicating artery
▨ Four arteries contribute: vertebral arteries (2) and carotid arteries (2)

Blood-brain barrier is absent in hypothalamus, pineal gland, area postrema (of fourth ventricle), and areas near third ventricle.

Circle of Willis

Feeder Arteries	Branches	Supplies
Right and left internal carotid arteries	1. Anterior cerebral artery (branch from right and left ICAs and communicate via anterior communicating artery).	Medial aspect of frontal and parietal lobes.
	2. Middle cerebral artery (continuation of ICA).	Anterior temporal lobes and cortex of insula.
Basilar artery which arises from convergence of right and left vertebral arteries.	Posterior cerebral artery (connects to middle cerebral artery via the posterior communicating artery).	Occipital cortex (visual area).

Vertebral arteries are branches of the subclavian artery.

The ICA has no branches in the neck.

The ophthalmic artery is a branch of the ICA (follows optic nerve through optic foramen into orbit); it gives off the anterior ethmoidal branch that supplies the nasal cavity.

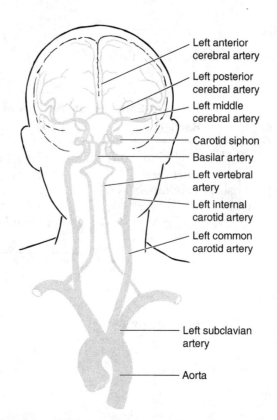

FIGURE 1–20.   Major cerebral arteries.

Reproduced, with permission, from Waxman SG. *Clinical Neuroanatomy*, 25th ed. New York: McGraw-Hill, 2003.

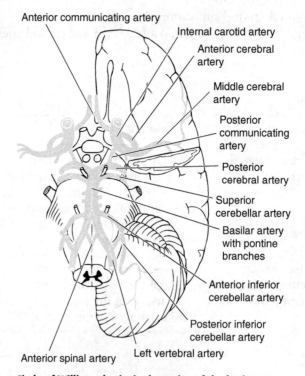

FIGURE 1–21.   Circle of Willis and principal arteries of the brain stem.

Reproduced, with permission, from Waxman SG. *Clinical Neuroanatomy*, 25th ed. New York: McGraw-Hill, 2003.

MIDDLE CEREBRAL ARTERY

- Largest branch of the ICA.
- If blocked, it causes the most ischemic injury.
- Leticulostriate arteries, branches of the MCA, are often involved in stroke, are thin-walled, and can rupture.

▶ ORAL CAVITY AND PHARYNX

Oral Cavity (Figure 1–22)

Components	Description
Oral vestibule	Slitlike space between lips and cheeks and the facial surfaces of teeth and gingivae.
Oral cavity proper	Space posterior and medial to dental arches (deep to lingual surfaces of teeth). Posterior termination is palatoglossal arch. Roof is the palate. Tongue occupies this space at rest with mouth closed.

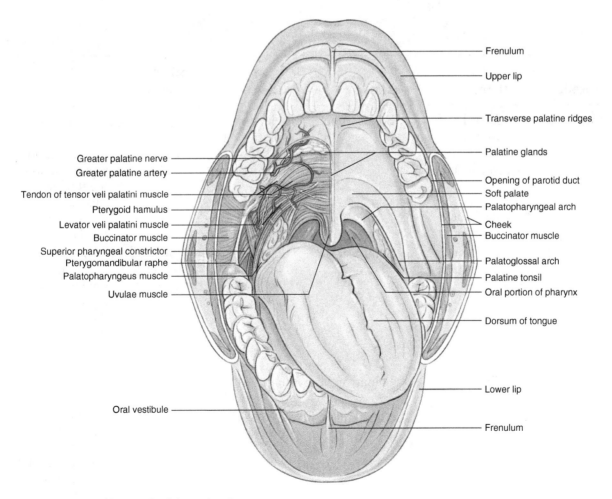

FIGURE 1-22. The mouth of the oral cavity.

Damage to right or left CN XII will cause the tongue to deviate to the side of the lesion.

Tongue

Function	Innervation
Motor	CN XII
Sensation	CN V3, IX, X
Taste	CN VII, IX, X

The tongue is derived from the first four pharyngeal arches and is innervated by associated nerves of those arches: arch 1 (V), arch 2 (VII), arch 3 (IX), and arch 4 (X).

GENERAL SENSATION OF THE TONGUE

See Figure 1–23 for the innervation of the tongue, which is mediated by these cranial nerves (CNs):

- V3
- IX
- X

TASTE SENSATION OF THE TONGUE

The sense of taste is mediated by the following CNs:

- VII
- IX
- X

Location	Nerve	Pathway	Brain stem Nucleus	Thalamic Nucleus	
Anterior 2/3	CN VII Chorda tympani nerve travels via lingual nerve (of V3) to the geniculate ganglion	Solitary tract	Nucleus of solitary tract (gustatory nucleus)	VPM	Gustatory cortex next to the somatosensory representation of the tongue (frontal-parietal operculum, insula)
Posterior 1/3	CN IX	Solitary tract	Nucleus of solitary tract (gustatory nucleus)	VPM	Gustatory cortex next to the somatosensory representation of the tongue (frontal-parietal operculum, insula
Epiglottis	CN X	Solitary tract	Nucleus of solitary tract (gustatory nucleus)	VPM	Gustatory cortex next to the somatosensory representation of the tongue (frontal-parietal operculum, insula)

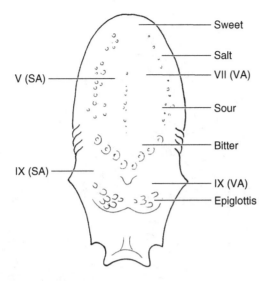

FIGURE 1-23. **Sensory innervation of the tongue.**

Reproduced, with permission, from Waxman SG. *Clinical Neuroanatomy*, 25th ed. New York: McGraw-Hill, 2003.

CHORDA TYMPANI NERVE

- This nerve is part of the structure of the facial nerve (CN VII).

COURSE

- Nucleus of solitary tract (accepts taste fibers).
- Superior salivatory nucleus (parasympathetic to submandibular, sublingual glands).
- Chorda tympani nerve arises from the geniculate ganglion.
- Emerges from petrotympanic fissure.
- Crosses the medial surface of the tympanic membrane.
- Joins the lingual nerve (of V3) in the infratemporal fossa.

COMPONENTS

- Taste (pathway): See Figure 1–24.
  - Anterior two-thirds of tastebuds.
  - Chorda tympani (travels with lingual nerve).
  - Cell bodies are located in the geniculate ganglion (within facial canal or petrous temporal).
- **Preganglionic parasympathetic**
  - Synapse in submandibular ganglion.

INFERIOR SURFACE OF THE TONGUE

- Lingual frenulum: vertical fold in the midline.
- Plica fimbriata: fold of mucous membrane, lateral to the frenulum.
- Wharton's and Rivian ducts: openings of the submandibular and sublingual glands.
- (Blood supply of the tongue: see external carotid artery.)

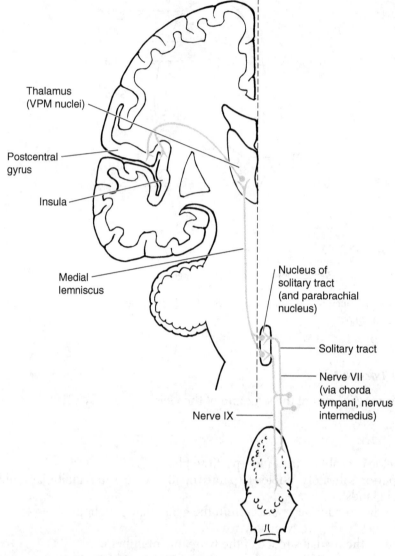

Thalamus
(VPM nuclei)

Postcentral
gyrus

Insula

Medial
lemniscus

Nucleus of
solitary tract
(and parabrachial
nucleus)

Solitary tract

Nerve VII
(via chorda
tympani, nervus
intermedius)

Nerve IX

*All tastebuds except filiform
are vascular.*

FIGURE 1–24.   Diagram of taste pathways.

Reproduced, with permission, from Waxman SG. *Clinical Neuroanatomy*, 25th ed. New York:
McGraw-Hill, 2003.

TASTEBUDS

Tastebud Type[a]	Description
Filiform papillae	Rough texture of tongue; found in rows; avascular; most numerous papillae of tongue; do not contain tastebuds.
Fungiform papillae	Mushroom-shaped; scattered among filiform papillae; *usually* contain tastebuds.
Circumvallate papillae	Seven to nine large circular structures *with tastebuds*; serous-only salivary glands within (von Ebner's glands).
Foliate papillae	On lateral surface of tongue in ridges; rudimentary and nonfunctional.

[a]Listed from smallest to largest.

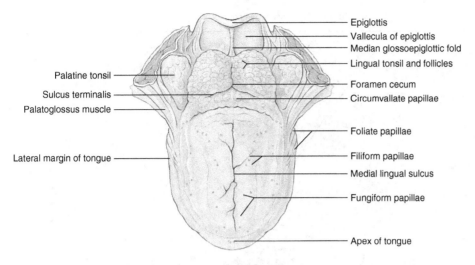

Labels (clockwise from top right):
Epiglottis
Vallecula of epiglottis
Median glossoepiglottic fold
Lingual tonsil and follicles
Foramen cecum
Circumvallate papillae
Foliate papillae
Filiform papillae
Medial lingual sulcus
Fungiform papillae
Apex of tongue
Palatine tonsil
Sulcus terminalis
Palatoglossus muscle
Lateral margin of tongue

FIGURE 1–25. **The tongue, dorsal view.**

OTHER SURFACE COMPONENTS OF THE TONGUE

See Figure 1–25 for the dorsal view of the tongue.

- Foramen cecum
  - Upper part of thyroglossal duct
- Sulcus terminalis
- Lingual tonsils (See the section "Waldeyer's Ring.")
- Glands
  - Mucous (back, front, and sides)
  - Serous (posteriorly)
  - Anterior lingual glands (mixed seromucous glands)

LYMPHATIC DRAINAGE OF THE TONGUE

See Figure 1–26 for an illustration of the lymph nodes of the tongue. Also see lymphatic drainage of head and neck.

MUSCLES CONTROLLING THE TONGUE (FIGURE 1–27)

Bony Attachments

- Genial tubercles
- Styloid process
- Hyoid bone

All tongue muscles, except palatoglossus, are innervated by CN XII.

The muscles attaching to genial tubercles are the genioglossus and the geniohyoid.

The tongue's blood supply is via lingual artery; veins drain into IJV.

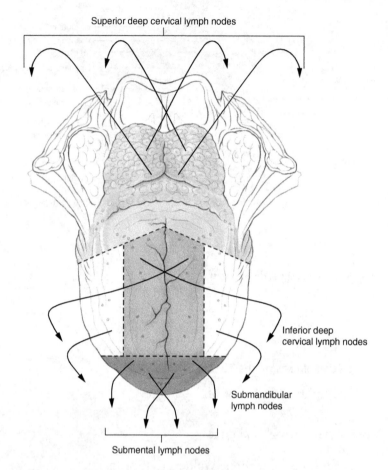

FIGURE 1–26. **Lymph drainage of the tongue.**

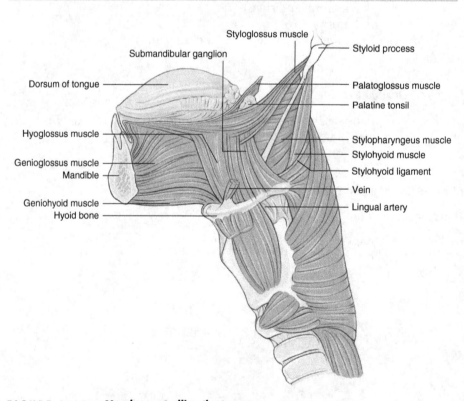

FIGURE 1–27. **Muscles controlling the tongue.**

EXTRINSIC MUSCLES

Muscle	Origin	Insertion	Action	Innervation
Genioglossus	Genial tubercles	**Inferior:** Hyoid **Superior:** Tongue	Protrude tongue	XII
Hyoglossus	Hyoid (body, greater cornu)	Side of tongue, medial to styloglossus	Depress tongue, pull down sides (retracts)	XII
Styloglossus	Styloid process	Side of tongue	Pull tongue up and back	XII
Palatoglossus	Anterior soft palate	Side and dorsum of tongue	Pull tongue up and back (toward palate)	X (pharyngeal plexus)

INTRINSIC MUSCLES

These muscles lie within the tongue itself.

Longitudinals (superior and inferior)	Underneath mucosa; shorten the tongue (both); make dorsum concave (superior); make dorsum convex (inferior).
Transversus	Arise from median fibrous septum and pass laterally; narrows and elongates the tongue.
Verticalis	Flattens and broadens the tongue.

SPEAKING SOUNDS

- "La-la" CN XII moves tongue against roof of mouth.
- "Mi-mi" CN VII moves lips.
- "Kuh-kuh" CN X raises the palate.

RELATIONSHIP OF LINGUAL ARTERY, VEIN, AND SUBMANDIBULAR DUCT

The relationships to the hyoglossus muscle are:

- Medial to the hyoglossus.
  - Lingual artery
- Lateral to the hyoglossus.
  - Lingual vein
  - Lingual nerve
  - Submandibular duct
  - Hypoglossal nerve

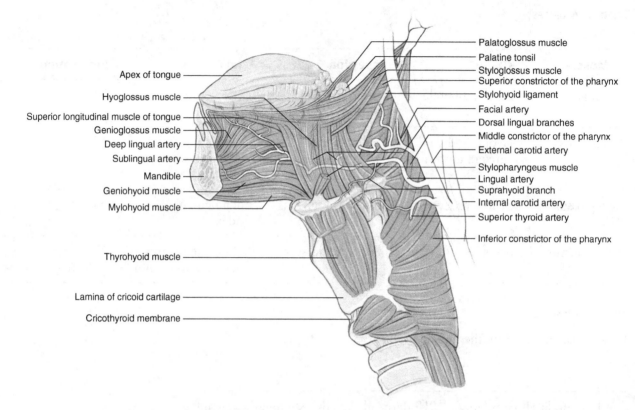

FIGURE 1–28. **Branches of the lingual artery.**

See Figure 1–28 for branches of the lingual tongue.

Palate

- Roof of oral cavity, floor of nasal cavity.

INNERVATION

- Motor
  - Pharyngeal plexus (except tensor veli palatine, CN V3).
- Sensory
  - CN V2
    - Greater palatine nerve is located posteriorly; it travels anteriorly.
    - Nasopalatine nerves are located anteriorly; they join the greater palatine posteriorly.

The palatal salivary glands are mostly mucous, located beneath the mucous membrane of hard and soft palates, and contribute to oral fluid.

BLOOD SUPPLY

- Third part of the maxillary artery (branch of ECA).
  - Greater palatine artery travels with nerve and vein from the greater and lesser palatine foramina.
  - Sphenopalatine vessels travel with nasopalatine nerves from the incisive foramen.

Hard Palate	Soft Palate (Muscles)
Maxillary bone (palatine processes)	Palatopharyngeus
	Palatoglossus
Palatine bones (horizontal plates)	Levator veli palatini
	Tensor veli palatini
	Uvular
Covered by keratinized mucosa (with rugae anteriorly)	Covered by nonkeratinized mucosa
	Submucosa
Palatal salivary glands (beneath mucosa)	Anterior zone of palatal submucosa contains fat
	Posterior zone contains mucous glands
	Palatal aponeurosis: Fibrous connective tissue of soft palate (muscles beneath)

The soft palate attaches to the tongue by the glossopalatine (palatoglossal) arches and to the pharynx by the palatopharyngeal arches.

Uvula

- Suspended from soft palate.
- Bifid uvula results from incomplete fusion of palatine shelves.
- Unilateral damaged pharyngeal plexus causes uvula to deviate to contralateral side. Contraction on intact side pulls it to functional side.

Fauces

- The fauces are between anterior and posterior pillars, and they house the palatine tonsils.

Remember: Most muscles of the soft palate attach to the palatal aponeurosis.

Pillar	Muscle	Muscle Function
Anterior pillar	Palatoglossus (palatoglossal fold)	Draws tongue and soft palate closer together (with swallowing)
		Narrows isthmus of fauces
Posterior pillar	Palatopharyngeus (palatopharyngeal fold)	Elevates pharynx
		Helps close the nasopharynx
		Aids in swallowing

Tonsils

Tonsil	Location	Description
Pharyngeal tonsils (adenoids)	Nasopharynx (posterior wall and roof)	**No lymph, sinuses, nor crypts**
		Surrounded in part by connective tissue and in part by epithelium
Palatine tonsils	In isthmus of fauces (between palatoglossal and palatopharyngeal folds) on either side of the posterior oropharynx	Reach maximum size during childhood then diminish
		Contain **crypts and lymphoid follicles** (No sinuses)
		Covered partly by connective tissue, partly by epithelium
Lingual tonsils	Dorsum of tongue (posteriorly)	**Lymphoid follicles**, each with a **single crypt**

(See Peyers patches in GI section).

The tensor and levator veli palatini muscles prevent food from entering the nasopharynx. (See Figure 1–29 for parasagittal view of the soft palate and pharynx).

WALDEYER'S RING

Ring of lymphoid tissue

- Lingual tonsil (inferiorly)
- Palatine tonsils (faucial tonsils) (laterally)
- Nasopharyngeal tonsils (adenoids) (superiorly)

Tensor versus Levator Veli Palatini

Muscle	Origin	Insertion	Action	Innervation
Tensor veli palatini	Greater wing of sphenoid (scaphoid fossa), lateral cartilage of auditory tube	Wraps around pterygoid hamulus to insert onto midline palatal aponeurosis (with contralateral fibers)	Tenses palate, opens auditory tube with mouth opening	CN V3
Levator veli palatini	Inferior petrous temporal bone, medial auditory tube	Palatine aponeurosis	Elevates/raises palate (during swallowing)	CN X

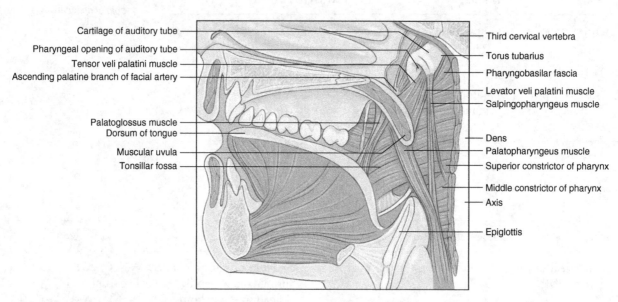

FIGURE 1-29. **Parasagittal view of soft palate and pharynx.**

Cartilage of auditory tube
Pharyngeal opening of auditory tube
Tensor veli palatini muscle
Ascending palatine branch of facial artery
Palatoglossus muscle
Dorsum of tongue
Muscular uvula
Tonsillar fossa

Third cervical vertebra
Torus tubarius
Pharyngobasilar fascia
Levator veli palatini muscle
Salpingopharyngeus muscle
Dens
Palatopharyngeus muscle
Superior constrictor of pharynx
Middle constrictor of pharynx
Axis
Epiglottis

Pharynx

See Figures 1–30 and 1–31 for views of the throat and Table 1–2 for locations and descriptions.

- Pharynx is behind nasal and oral cavities.
- Pharynx shares conduit to larynx and esophagus.

The pterygomandibular raphe is the meeting point of the buccinator muscle and the superior pharyngeal constrictor.

PHARYNGEAL MUSCLES

Muscle	Origin	Insertion	Action	Innervation
Constrictors				
Superior	Pterygomandibular raphe and pharyngeal tubercle; mylohyoid line of mandible.	Midline pharyngeal raphe (posteriorly); pharyngeal tubercle.	Contract in waves (to propel food).	**Sensory:** CN X **Motor:** CN XI (via X)
Middle	Hyoid bone (greater and lesser horns).	Midline pharyngeal raphe (posteriorly).	Contract in waves (to propel food).	**Sensory:** CN X **Motor:** CN XI (via X)
Inferior	Thyroid and cricoid cartilages.	Midline pharyngeal raphe.	Contract in waves (to propel food).	**Sensory:** CN X **Motor:** CN XI (via X)
Cricopharyngeus	Lower fibers of inferior constrictor.	Midline raphe.	Constant contraction (serves as UES).	**Sensory:** CN X **Motor:** CN XI (via X)
Longitudinal muscles				
Palatopharyngeus	Palatal aponeurosis.	Posterolateral pharynx.	Raise pharynx and larynx during swallowing.	CN XI (via X) (pharyngeal plexus)
Salpingopharyngeus	Cartilage of eustachian tube.	Palatopharyngeus muscle.	Elevate nasopharynx, open auditory tube, equalize pressure between pharynx and auditory canal.	CN XI (via X) (pharyngeal plexus)
Stylopharyngeus	Styloid process.	Pass between superior and middle constrictors; blend with palatopharyngeus.	Raise pharynx and larynx during swallowing.	CN IX

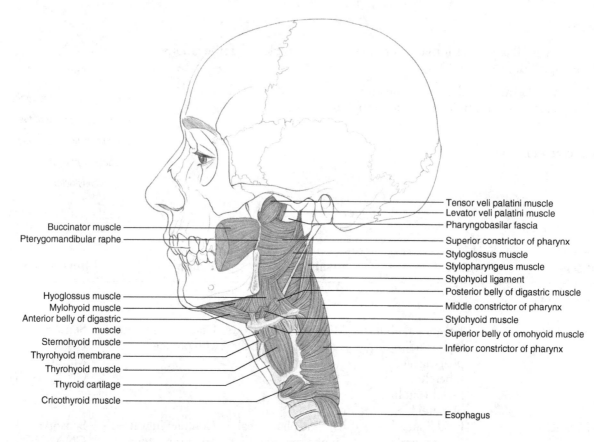

Tensor veli palatini muscle
Levator veli palatini muscle
Pharyngobasilar fascia
Buccinator muscle
Pterygomandibular raphe
Superior constrictor of pharynx
Styloglossus muscle
Stylopharyngeus muscle
Stylohyoid ligament
Posterior belly of digastric muscle
Hyoglossus muscle
Mylohyoid muscle
Middle constrictor of pharynx
Anterior belly of digastric
muscle
Stylohyoid muscle
Superior belly of omohyoid muscle
Sternohyoid muscle
Inferior constrictor of pharynx
Thyrohyoid membrane
Thyrohyoid muscle
Thyroid cartilage
Cricothyroid muscle
Esophagus

FIGURE 1–30. **External view of the pharynx.**

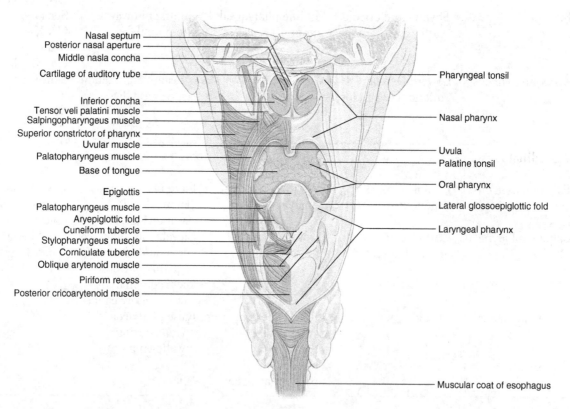

Nasal septum
Posterior nasal aperture
Middle nasla concha
Cartilage of auditory tube
Pharyngeal tonsil
Inferior concha
Tensor veli palatini muscle
Salpingopharyngeus muscle
Nasal pharynx
Superior constrictor of pharynx
Uvular muscle
Uvula
Palatopharyngeus muscle
Palatine tonsil
Base of tongue
Epiglottis
Oral pharynx
Palatopharyngeus muscle
Lateral glossoepiglottic fold
Aryepiglottic fold
Cuneiform tubercle
Laryngeal pharynx
Stylopharyngeus muscle
Corniculate tubercle
Oblique arytenoid muscle
Piriform recess
Posterior cricoarytenoid muscle
Muscular coat of esophagus

FIGURE 1–31. **Posterior view of the soft palate and pharynx.**

TABLE 1-2. **Pharynx**

	LOCATION	DESCRIPTION
Nasopharynx	Above the soft palate; continuous with nasal passages; soft palate and uvula form anterior wall.	Auditory tube connects nasopharynx with middle ear.
Oropharynx	Extends from anterior pillars to larynx.	Communicates with oral cavity via fauces; food and air from mouth; air and sinus drainage from nasopharynx; contains palatine and lingual tonsils.
Laryngopharynx	Area inferior to oropharynx containing entrance to both larynx and esophagus.	Allows food into esophagus; air into larynx.

Pharyngeal plexus = CNs IX, X, XI. Provides innervation to constrictors, palatoglossus, palatopharyngeus, and cricopharyngeus.

Stylopharyngeus muscle is the only muscle supplied by CN IX. This muscle is a landmark for finding the nerve.

SWALLOWING (THREE PHASES)

Oral Phase

- Moisten food
- Masticate food (CN V)
- Tongue assumes trough shape (CN XII)
- Voluntary posterior movement of food bolus

Food can get caught in the vallecula or pyriform recesses.

Pharygeal Phase

- Close Nasopharynx
  - Tense vensor veli palatini (CN V)
  - Raise velum: palatoglossal, levator veli palatini (CN X)
- Elevate pharynx and hyoid
  - Stylopharyngeus, salpingopharyngeus, palatopharyngeus (CN IX, X)
- Close pharynx
- Retroversion of the epiglottis, adduction of vocal cords
- Bolus passes through pharynx
  - Wavelike contraction of superior, middle, and inferior pharyngeal constrictor muscles (CN X, XI)
  - Relaxation of cricopharyngeus

Sensory information goes to the swallowing center (nucleus ambiguous in medulla oblongata). Nucleus ambiguous sends motor information (SVE), via CNs IX, X, XI, XII, to facilitate swallowing.

Esophageal Phase

- Esophageal peristalsis (CN X)
- Relaxation phase
  - Larynx, pharynx, and hyoid return to initial position

*Lymphatic drainage:
Parotid gland, through parotid
nodes, then superior deep
cervical lymph nodes.
Submandibular and
sublingual glands, through
submandibular and deep
cervical nodes.*

*The external carotid artery
supplies blood to all salivary
glands.*

See Figure 1–32.

- **Lacrimal gland**
  - Located in the lacrimal sulcus in the superolateral aspect of the orbit.
  - Produces tears that wash across the globe superolateral to inferomedially.
- **Lacrimal puncta** collects tears and drains into the
- **Lacrimal canals** (superior and inferior), which join the
- **Lacrimal sac**, which drains down the
- **Nasolacrimal duct** to empty underneath the inferior nasal concha in the
- **Inferior meatus.**

Lacrimal Gland

- Paired serous glands.
- Involved in tear production.
- Parasympathetic innervation.
  - **Superior salivatory nucleus** (brain stem)
  - **Greater petrosal nerve** (of CN–VII) (preganglionic synapses at pterygopalatine ganglion)
  - **Lacrimal nerve** (of V1) (postganglionic parasympathetics from pterygopalatine ganglion)

*Postganglionic nerves from
the pterygopalatine ganglion
exit via the inferior orbital
fissure and join the lacrimal
nerve (of V1) to supply the
lacrimal gland.*

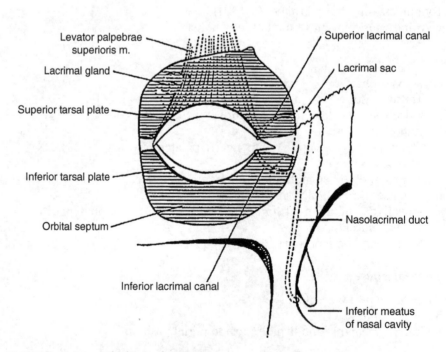

FIGURE 1–32. **The lacrimal apparatus.**

Reproduced, with permission, from Liebgott B. *The Anatomical Basis of Dentistry.* Toronto: BC Decker, 1986.

*The lingual artery and facial
artery are both branches of the
external carotid artery (ECA).*

Gland	Location	Secretion	Duct	Innervation	Blood Supply
Parotid gland (See Figure 1–33.)	Parotid region, between posterior border of mandibular ramus and anterior border of SCM. (Below and anterior to ear.)	Serous	Stenson's (parotid duct) goes anterior along lateral masseter, rolls over anterior border of masseter and pierces cheek, buccinator muscle; empties next to maxillary second molar.	**Preganglionic:** Lesser petrosal nerve (of CN IX). **Synapse:** Otic ganglion. **Postganglionic:** Leaves otic ganglion, travels with auriculotemporal nerve (of V3) to parotid.	Glandular branches of superficial temporal artery and transverse facial artery.
Submandibular gland (See Figure 1–34.)	**Superficial portion** Between lateral aspect of mylohyoid muscle and submandibular fossa of mandible (submandibular triangle). **Deep portion:** In floor of mouth between base of tongue and sublingual gland (between mylohyoid and hyoglossus)	Serous and mucous	Wharton's (submandibular duct) continues forward from deep portion of gland, crosses lingual nerve (near the sublingual gland), and empties into oral cavity at the sublingual caruncle (papilla) (next to sublingual frenulum; behind lower central incisors).	**Preganglionic:** Chorda tympani (of VII). **Synapse:** Submandibular ganglion. **Postganglionic:** Leaves ganglion and passes to gland.	Glandular branches of the facial artery.
Sublingual gland (See Figure 1–35.)	Floor of mouth medial to sublingual fossa of mandible (above mylohyoid muscle).	Mucous	Sublingual (Rivian) ducts open directly into oral cavity through openings in sublingual fold; anterior ducts open medially into submandibular duct (the single Bartholin's duct empties into submandibular duct at sublingual papilla).	**Preganglionic:** Chorda tympani (of VII). **Synapse:** Submandibular ganglion. **Postganglionic:** Leaves ganglion and passes to gland.	Glandular branches of lingual artery (sublingual artery).

(Adapted, with permission, from Liebgott B. *The Anatomical Basis of Dentistry*. Toronto: BC Decker, 1986:346.)

The submandibular gland emits the highest volume of salivary fluid per day. The parotid gland is second in volume to submandibular gland.

Going from largest to smallest, the major salivary glands go from serous to mixed to mostly mucous (parotid, submandibular, and sublingual, respectively).

MINOR SALIVARY GLANDS

Gland	Location	Secretion
Labial and buccal minor salivary glands	Labial and buccal mucosa	Mucous only
von Ebner's glands	At base of circumvallate papillae (rinse food away from papilla)	Serous only saliva
Glands of Blandin-Nuhn (anterior lingual glands)	Anterior lingual	Mixed serous-mucous

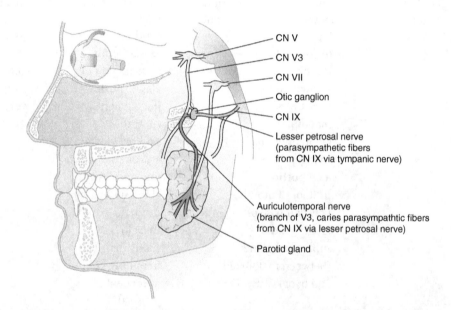

FIGURE 1–33. **Schematic of the innervation of the parotid gland by the glossopharyngeal nerve.**

Light gray: Preganglionic parasympathetic nerves leave the brain stem with the glosopharyngeal nerve (CN IX) and run with the lesser petrosal nerve to the otic ganglion.

Dark gray: Postganglionic parasympathetic nerves travel with the auriculotemporal branch of CN V3 and then the facial nerve to reach the parotid gland. (Reproduced, with permission, from Lalwani AK (ed). *Current Diagnosis & Treatment in Otolaryngology–Head & Neck Surgery.* New York: Lange Medical Books/McGraw-Hill, 2004.)

Parotid and von Ebner's glands are the only glands to secrete serous-only saliva.

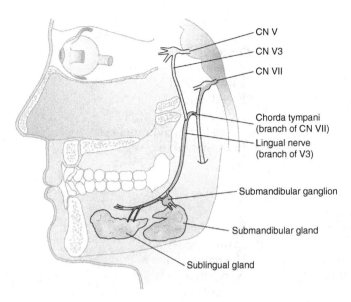

FIGURE 1-34. Schematic of the innervation of the submandibular and sublingual glands by the facial nerve.

Light gray: Preganglionic parasympathetic nerves leave the brain stem with the facial nerve (CN VII) and run with the chorda tympani and the lingual branch of CN V3 to the submandibular ganglion.

Dark gray: Postganglionic parasympathetic nerves travel either directly to the submandibular gland or back to the lingual branch of CN V3 to the sublingual gland. (Reproduced, with permission, from Lalwani, AK (ed). *Current Diagnosis & Treatment in Otolaryngology–Head & Neck Surgery.* New York: Lange Medical Books/McGraw-Hill, 2004.)

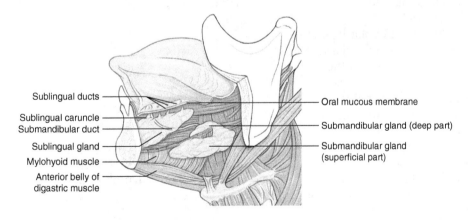

FIGURE 1-35. The sublingual gland.

Fascial Spaces (see Figure 1–36)

Space	Boundaries	Contents
Parotid	**Superficial:** Skin. **Deep:** Styloid process. **Superior and inferior:** Parotid capsule. **Posterior:** Sternocleidomastoid. **Anterior:** Posterior mandibular ramus, stylomandibular ligament.	Parotid gland Facial nerve External carotid artery (and terminal branches) Retromandibular vein
Submandibular	**Lateral:** Superficial fascia, body of mandible. **Medial:** Mylohyoid muscle. **Superior:** Mylohyoid line. **Inferior:** Hyoid bone.	Submandibular gland Lymph nodes Hypoglossal nerve Nerve to mylohyoid Facial artery
Sublingual	**Lateral:** Mandibular body. **Medial:** Base of tongue. **Superior:** Floor of mouth mucosa. **Inferior:** Mylohyoid.	Sublingual gland Deep submandibular gland and duct Lingual nerve (and submandibular ganglion) Lingual artery Hypoglossal nerve
Tonsillar	**Anterior:** Palatoglossus. **Posterior:** Palatopharyngeus. **Lateral:** Pharyngobasilar fascia. **Medial:** Oropharyngeal mucosa.	Palatine tonsil Glossopharyngeal nerve Tonsillar and ascending palatine branches of the facial artery
Masticator	**Lateral:** Lateral side of cervical fascia, masseter fascia, and temporalis fascia (all blend) to superior temporal line. **Medial:** Deep fascia—deep to mandibular ramus and medial pterygoid. **Posterior:** Stylomandibular ligament. **Anterior:** Anterior mandibular ramus, temporalis tendon (part of the fascia blends with buccopharyngeal fascia of buccinator). **Superior:** Limited by roof of infratemporal fossa and superior aspect of temporalis muscle.	Mandibular ramus and TMJ Muscles of mastication Mandibular nerve Maxillary artery Pterygoid plexus of veins Chorda tympani nerve
Parapharyngeal	**Anterior:** Neck viscera. **Posterior:** Vertebral column. **Lateral:** Sternocleidomastoid muscle.	Carotid sheath Deep cervical chain of lymph nodes
Retropharyngeal space	Posterior aspect of parapharyngeal space. Extends from the skull base to the superior mediastinum component.	

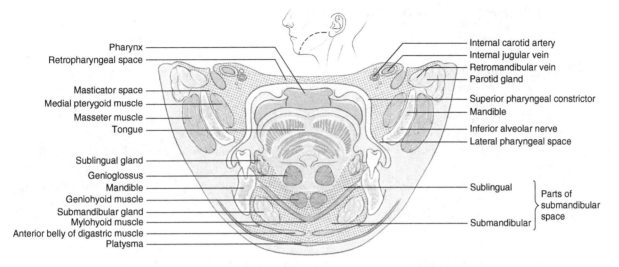

FIGURE 1–36. Buccal, masticator, temporal, and pterygomandibular spaces, space of body of the mandible, and parotid, submaxillary, submental, submandibular, and sublingual spaces of the face and jaws.

▶ **MASTICATION AND TMJ**

Mastication

- Mastication is the process of biting and chewing food to make it soft enough to swallow.
- Muscles of mastication, which are all controlled by CN V3:
  - Masseter
  - Temporalis
  - Medial and lateral pterygoids
- Accessory muscles of mastication include the supra- and infrahyoids.
- Tongue and buccinator are essential for controlling the food bolus and propelling it posteriorly for swallowing (CNs XII, VII, respectively).

The lateral pterygoid muscles protrude the mandible and move it toward the contralateral side. For example, a left subcondylar fracture will deviate the mandible to the left because only the right lateral pterygoid is functional.

Muscles of Mastication (Figures 1–37, 1–38, and 1–39)

Muscle	Origin	Insertion	Action
Masseter	**Superficial:** Zygomatic process of maxilla, anterior 2/3 zygomatic arch.	**Superficial:** Angle of mandible.	Elevation Retrusion (deep and posterior fibers)
	Deep: Zygomatic arch (inner posterior 1/3).	**Deep:** Lateral ramus.	Ipsilateral excursion
Temporalis	Curvilinear lower temporal line. Temporal fossa. Temporal fascia.	Medial coronoid, anterior ramus (passing deep to zygomatic arch).	Elevation (anterior and superior fibers) Retrusion (posterior fibers) Ipsilateral excursion
Medial pterygoid	Medial side of lateral pterygoid plate.	Medial side of mandibular angle.	Elevation Protrusion Contralateral excursion
Lateral pterygoid	**Superior:** Greater wing of the sphenoid.	**Superior:** Articular capsule and disc.	Protrusion Depression
	Inferior: Lateral side of lateral pterygoid plate.	**Inferior:** Anterior condylar neck.	Contralateral excursion

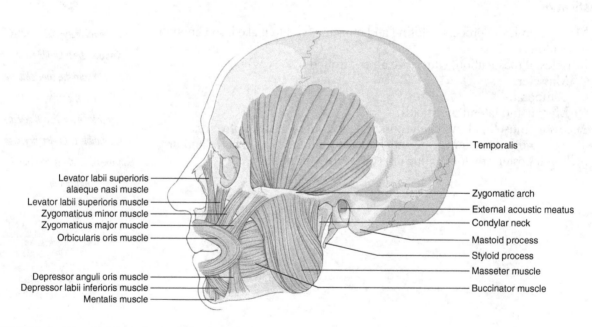

FIGURE 1–37.   The masseter muscle.

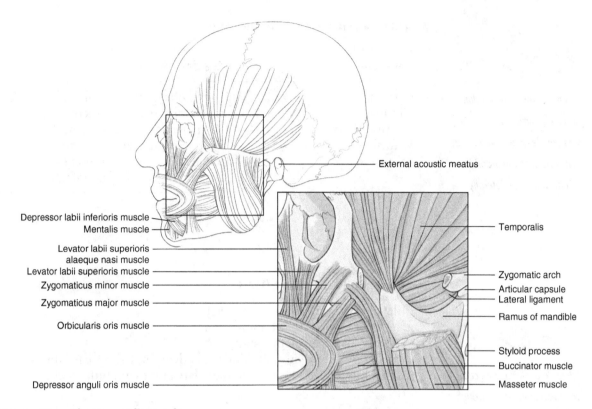

Depressor labii inferioris muscle
Mentalis muscle
Levator labii superioris alaeque nasi muscle
Levator labii superioris muscle
Zygomaticus minor muscle
Zygomaticus major muscle
Orbicularis oris muscle
Depressor anguli oris muscle

External acoustic meatus
Temporalis
Zygomatic arch
Articular capsule
Lateral ligament
Ramus of mandible
Styloid process
Buccinator muscle
Masseter muscle

FIGURE 1–38.   **The temporalis muscle.**

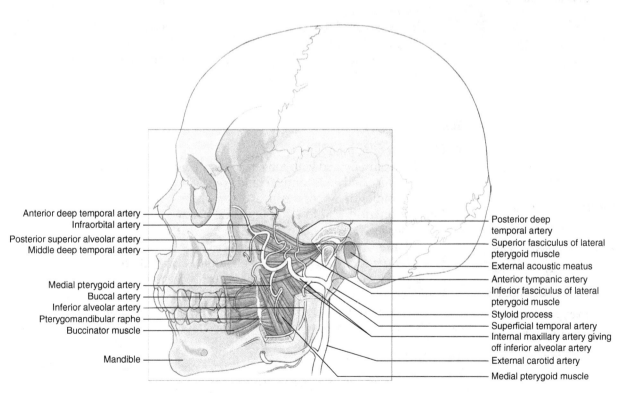

Anterior deep temporal artery
Infraorbital artery
Posterior superior alveolar artery
Middle deep temporal artery
Medial pterygoid artery
Buccal artery
Inferior alveolar artery
Pterygomandibular raphe
Buccinator muscle
Mandible

Posterior deep temporal artery
Superior fasciculus of lateral pterygoid muscle
External acoustic meatus
Anterior tympanic artery
Inferior fasciculus of lateral pterygoid muscle
Styloid process
Superficial temporal artery
Internal maxillary artery giving off inferior alveolar artery
External carotid artery
Medial pterygoid muscle

FIGURE 1–39.   **Lateral and medial pterygoid muscles.**

The masseter and medial pterygoid muscles form a sling at the angle of mandible; both elevate/close the mandible and stabilize it laterally.

MANDIBULAR FUNCTIONS FOR MASTICATION

Function	Muscles Involved
Opening	Lateral pterygoids, suprahyoids, infrahyoids
Closing	Temporalis, masseter, medial pterygoids
Protrusion	Pterygoids (medial and lateral)
Retrusion	Temporalis, masseters (deep)
Excursion	Ipsilateral masseter, temporalis; contralateral pterygoids (medial and lateral)

Palpate posterior aspect of mandibular condyle through external auditory meatus and lateral aspect in front of the external auditory meatus (anterior to the tragus).

Temporomandibular Joint (TMJ)

- Bilateral synovial joint (diarthrodial).
  - Upper compartment: translation
  - Lower compartment: rotation
- Articulation between mandibular condyles and skull base on both sides. (Other articulation is between maxillary and mandibular teeth.)

COMPONENTS

- Moving from superior to inferior:
  - Glenoid/mandibular fossa (of temporal bone)
  - Articular cartilage
  - Disc/meniscus
  - Condylar cartilage cap
  - Condyle of mandible
- Articular capsule surrounds joint, with synovium internally.
  - Ligaments stabilize.

The lateral pterygoid attaches to neck of the condyle, capsule, and articular disc of TMJ.
Damage to the disc, where the lateral pterygoid inserts, can render the lateral pterygoid nonfunctional on that side. (The mandible will deviate to the damaged side)

BONY COMPONENTS

- **Condyle** of the mandible
  - Elliptically shaped with long axis oriented mediolaterally.
  - Posterior condyle is rounded and convex.
  - Anteroinferior aspect is concave.
- **Glenoid/mandibular fossa** (of temporal bone)
  - Concave.
- **Articular eminence**
  - Anterior part of glenoid fossa (squamous temporal bone).
  - Articular eminence (tubercle) is convex.
- Articular sufaces
  - Glenoid fossa and condyle are lined with dense fibrocartilage.
  - **Not** hyaline cartilage like most synovial joints.

Articular Disc (Meniscus)

- Fibrocartilaginous biconcave disc.
- Lies between articular surfaces of condyle and mandibular fossa.

- Divides disc space into superior and inferior compartments.
- Attaches peripherally to the capsule and anteriorly to the lateral pterygoid muscle.
- Attaches to medial and lateral poles of the condyle via collateral ligaments.
- Regions
  - Thin intermediate zone.
  - Thick anterior and posterior bands.
  - Posterior band is contiguous with the posterior attachment tissues (bilaminar zone).
  - Bilaminar zone is vascular, innervated tissue (role in allowing condyle to move forward).

Articular Capsule

- Fibrous capsule that surrounds the TMJ.
- Attaches superiorly to the glenoid fossa (tubercle of articular eminence).
- Attaches inferiorly to the condylar neck.
- **Synovium**
  - Lines the internal surface of the joint capsule.
  - Secretes synovial fluid for joint lubrication.
  - Does **not** cover the articular surfaces or articular disc.

TMJ IMAGING

Bony Structures of TMJ

- Panorex x-ray
- CT scan
- Plain films

Soft Tissue of TMJ

- MRI (magnetic resonance imaging)
  - Especially the position of the articular disc

MRI uses a magnetic field to alter energy levels of water in tissues. The advantage of MRI is the lack of x-ray radiation exposure, with no harmful effects being shown.

NERVES OF THE TMJ

TMJ receives only **sensory** innervation (motor is to the muscles).

- **Auriculotemporal nerve** (of V3) conducts primary innervation to the TMJ.
  - Transmits pain in capsule and periphery of disc.
  - Also provides parasympathetics to the parotid gland via lesser petrosal nerve (CN IX).
- **Nerve to masseter** (of V3)
  - A few sensory fibers to anterior part of TMJ.
- **Posterior deep temporal nerve** (of V3)
  - Also supplies anterior part of TMJ.

51

LIGAMENTS OF THE **TMJ**

- TMJ ligaments stabilize the mandible.

Ligament	Description
Temporomandibular ligament (lateral ligament)	This ligament has two parts: the outer oblique portion (prevents posterior and inferior displacement) and the inner horizontal portion (prevents lateral or mesial displacement).
Accessory ligaments	
Sphenomandibular ligament	Remnant of Meckel's cartilage. Thickened fibrous band connecting spine of sphenoid with lingula of mandible.
Stylomandibular ligament	Connects styloid process to mandibular angle.

To reduce luxated TMJ, apply pressure inferiorly and posteriorly.
Stand behind patient; thumbs on patient's occlusal surfaces, fingers below chin; press thumbs inferiorly while fingers close the mandible; condylar head then slides back into articular fossa.

TMJ DISLOCATION

- TMJ can be dislocated anteriorly only (known as "lockjaw").
  - Luxation: requires assistance for reduction.
  - Subluxation: auto-reduces.

TMJ DISC PLACEMENT

- Usually occurs anteromedially.
- Collateral ligaments loosen or tear, allowing the lateral pterygoid to pull the disc anteromedially.

TMJ Noises

Noise	Description
Click	With anterior disc displacement: First click **Opening:** The disc clicks over the anteriorly moving condyle (condyle clicks past the thick posterior band of articular disc). Second click **Closing:** Condyle moves posteriorly past the disc. Can also hear this click with lateral excursion to the contralateral side (as the disc is anteromedially located and the condyle is moving medially).
Crepitus	Associated with osteoarthritis of the condyle (degenerative disease).
Dull thud	With self-reducing subluxation of the condyle.

TMJ MOVEMENTS

- Six mandibular movements:
  - Protrusion
  - Retrusion
  - Opening
  - Closing
  - Medial and lateral excursions
- Normal mandibular range of motion (ROM) is 50 mm opening, 10 mm protrusively and laterally.
- See Posselt's envelope of motion.

Hinge-Type Rotation

- With small movements (lower compartment).

Translation

- With larger movements (upper compartment).
- Slides forward out of the mandibular fossa.

See Figure 1–40 for mandibular condyle and meniscus.
See Figure 1–41 for mandibular capsule, temporomandibular ligament, and sphenomandibular ligament.

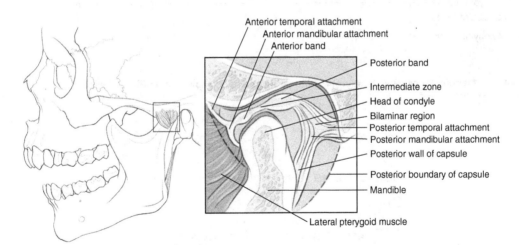

FIGURE 1–40. The mandibular condyle and meniscus.

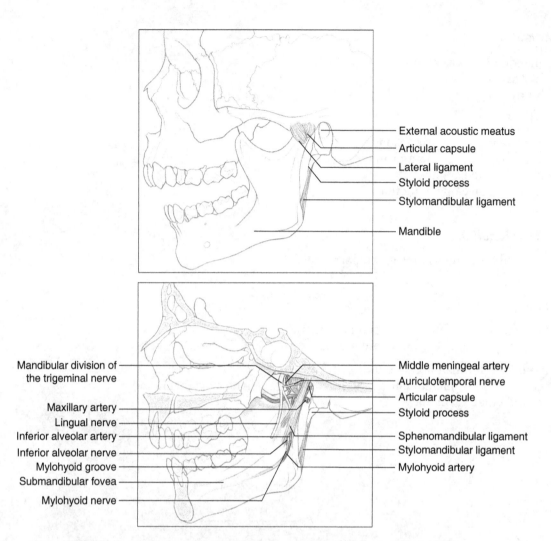

External acoustic meatus
Articular capsule
Lateral ligament
Styloid process
Stylomandibular ligament
Mandible

Mandibular division of
the trigeminal nerve
Maxillary artery
Lingual nerve
Inferior alveolar artery
Inferior alveolar nerve
Mylohyoid groove
Submandibular fovea
Mylohyoid nerve

Middle meningeal artery
Auriculotemporal nerve
Articular capsule
Styloid process
Sphenomandibular ligament
Stylomandibular ligament
Mylohyoid artery

FIGURE 1–41. Mandibular capsule, temporomandibular ligament, and sphenomandibular ligament.

▶ **NECK ANATOMY**

Cervical Vertebrae

- C1–C7
  - C1 atlas (no vertebral body)
  - C2 axis (dens or odontoid process)
- Transverse foramen allow passage of the vertebral artery (from subclavian; forms basilar).

ATLANTO-OCCIPITAL JOINT

- Articulation between C1 (atlas) superior facets and the occipital condyles of the skull.
  - Allows to nod head *yes* (flexion and extension).

ATLANTO-AXIAL JOINT

- Articulation between C1 vertebrae (atlas) inferior facets and the C2 vertebrae (axis) superior facets.
  - Allows to shake head *no* (pivot).

Layers and Fascia of the Neck

Layer	Contents
Skin	
Subcutaneous tissue (superficial cervical fascia).	Cutaneous nerves, blood and lymphatic vessels, fat, platysma (anterolaterally).
Deep cervical fascia (muscular fascia)	
▧ Investing	Sternocleidomastoid and trapezius muscles and submandibular and parotid glands
▧ Pretracheal	Thyroid gland, larynx, pharynx, and esophagus
▧ Prevertebral	Vertebrae and deep cervical muscles

PLATYSMA MUSCLE

See Figure 1–42.

▧ Innervated by cervical branch of CN VII; blends with orbicularis oris.
▧ Superficial to the deep cervical fascia.

Investing Layer of Deep Cervical Fascia

| Description | Attachments | |
	Superiorly	Inferiorly
The most superficial deep fascial layer.	Superior nuchal line (occipital bone)	Manubrium (sternum)
Splits into superficial and deep layers to invest the SCM and trapezius.	Mastoid process (temporal bone) Zygomatic arches Inferior border of mandible	Clavicles Acromions and spines of scapula
Splits to enclose submandibular gland.	Hyoid bone Spinous processes of cervical vertebrae	
Splits to form fibrous capsule of parotid gland.		

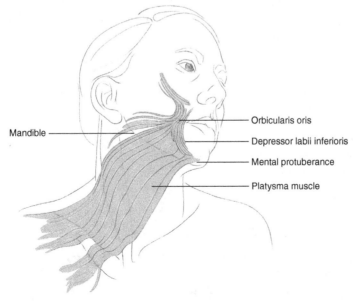

Mandible

Orbicularis oris

Depressor labii inferioris

Mental protuberance

Platysma muscle

FIGURE 1–42. The platysma muscle.

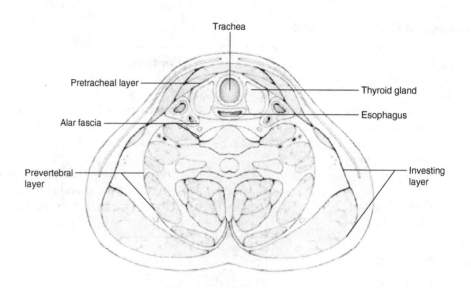

FIGURE 1–43. **The pretracheal layer.**

Modified, with permission, from White JS. *USMLE Road Map Gross Anatomy.* New York: McGraw-Hill, 2003.

The prevertebral layer of deep cervical fascia is why the thyroid moves with laryngeal movements.

PRETRACHEAL LAYER (OF DEEP CERVICAL FASCIA)

See Figure 1–43.

- Extends from hyoid bone to thorax (blends with fibrous pericardium).
- Has a thin muscular layer enveloping infrahyoid muscles.
- Visceral layer encloses thyroid gland, trachea, esophagus.
    - Visceral layer is continuous with buccopharyngeal fascia.
- Blends laterally with carotid sheaths.

CAROTID SHEATH

See Figure 1–44.

- Extends from base of cranium to root of neck.
- Blends with investing and pretracheal fascia anteriorly.
- Blends with prevertebral fascia posteriorly.

Contents

- Common carotid artery
- Internal jugular vein
- CN X
- Also associated with:
    - Lymph nodes
    - Carotid sinus nerve
    - Sympathetic nerves

PREVERTEBRAL LAYER (OF DEEP CERVICAL FASCIA)

- Runs from investing layers in both sides of the lateral neck; splits to enclose the thyroid.
- **Superiorly:** Attaches to laryngeal cartilages.

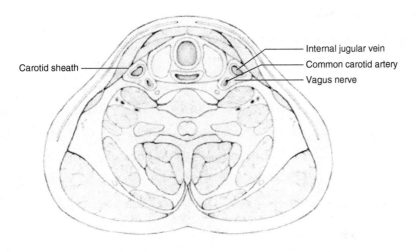

FIGURE 1–44. The carotid sheath.

Modified, with permission, from White JS. *USMLE Road Map Gross Anatomy*. New York: McGraw-Hill, 2003.

- **Inferiorly:** Fuses with perichondrium
- **Posteriorly:** Fuses with anterior longitudinal ligament

RETROPHARYNGEAL SPACE

See Figure 1–45.

- Between pharynx (buccopharyngeal fascia) and prevertebral fascia
- Communicates with mediastimum (concern for infection spread, Ludwig's angina)

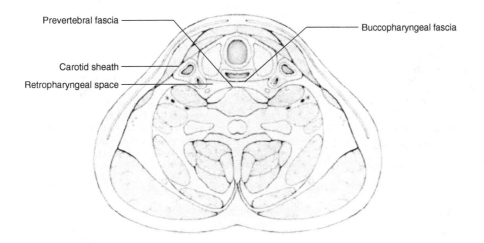

FIGURE 1–45. The retropharyngeal space.

Modified, with permission, from White JS. *USMLE Road Map Gross Anatomy*. New York: McGraw-Hill, 2003.

Triangles of the Neck

See Figure 1–46 for regions of the neck.

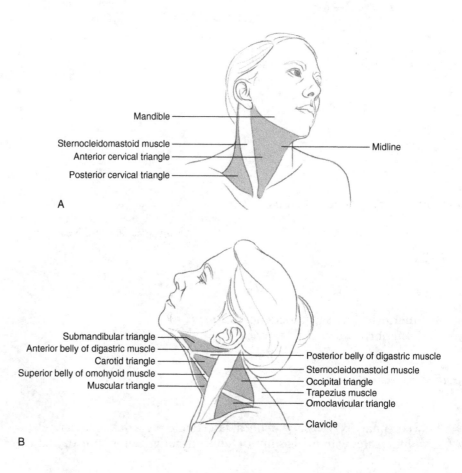

A

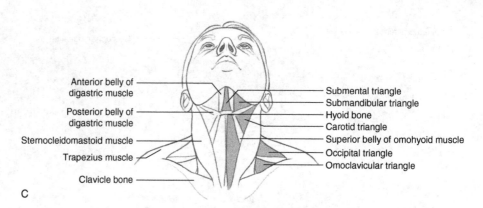

B

C

FIGURE 1–46. **Topographic anatomy: regions of the neck.**

POSTERIOR TRIANGLE

Boundaries					
Anterior	**Posterior**	**Inferior**	**Floor**	**Roof**	**Contents**
SCM (post border)	Trapezius (anterior border)	Clavicle (middle 1/3)	Splenius capitus Levator scapulae Scalene muscles	Skin Superficial fascia, platysma, Deep investing fascia of neck	Exterior jugular vein Cervical plexus, lesser occipital nerve, great auricular nerve; CN XI, phrenic nerve Subclavian vein, artery, brachial plexus

ANTERIOR TRIANGLE

Boundaries					
Anterior	**Posterior**	**Inferior**	**Floor**	**Roof**	**Contents**
Neck midline	SCM (anterior border)	Inferior border of mandible	Pharynx, larynx, thyroid	Skin Superficial fascia Platysma Deep investing fascia	Infrahyoid, suprahyoid muscles Common, internal, external carotid arteries Internal, external jugular vein Retromandibular vein CNs X, XI, XII, cervical plexus

SUBSETS OF THE ANTERIOR TRIANGLE

Submandibular Triangle (see Figure 1–47)

Boundaries				
Inferior	**Superior**	**Floor**	**Roof**	**Contents**
Bellies of digastric	Inferior border of mandible	Mylohyoid Hyoglossus	Skin Superficial fascia Platysma Deep fascia	Submandibular gland (Figure 1–48) Submandibular lymph nodes Hypoglossal nerve Mylohyoid nerve Lingual and facial arteries and veins

Submandibular triangle contains two glands (or nodes), two nerves, two arteries, and two veins.

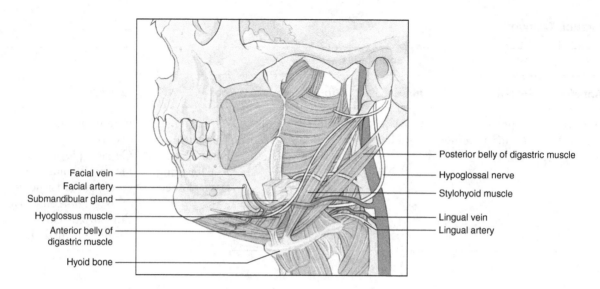

Facial vein
Facial artery
Submandibular gland
Hyoglossus muscle
Anterior belly of
digastric muscle
Hyoid bone

Posterior belly of digastric muscle
Hypoglossal nerve
Stylohyoid muscle
Lingual vein
Lingual artery

FIGURE 1–47. **The submandibular triangle.**

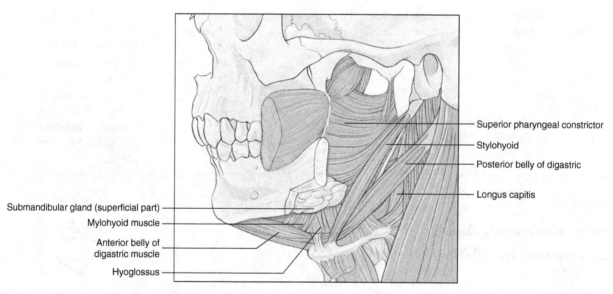

Submandibular gland (superficial part)
Mylohyoid muscle
Anterior belly of
digastric muscle
Hyoglossus

Superior pharyngeal constrictor
Stylohyoid
Posterior belly of digastric
Longus capitis

FIGURE 1–48. **The submandibular gland.**

Muscular Triangle

Boundaries	Superior belly of omohyoid, SCM, midline of neck
Contents	Infrahyoid strap muscles

Carotid Triangle

Boundaries	Superior belly of omohyoid, posterior belly of digastric, SCM
Contents	Common carotid artery, internal jugular vein, CNs X, XI, XII, cervical plexus

Submental Triangle

Boundaries	Right and left anterior bellies of the digastric, body of hyoid
Contents	Mylohyoid muscle (midline raphe)

Three infrahyoid muscles innervated by ansa cervicalis: sternohyoid, sternothyroid, omohyoid (SOS). Thyrohyoid innervated by C1 via CXII.

SCM, Trapezius Muscles

	Origin	Insertion	Action	Innervation
SCM	Manubrium, medial one-third clavicle	Mastoid process, superior nuchal line (lateral)	**Bilateral:** Flexes neck. **Unilateral:** Pulls head to shoulder, turns head to opposite side.	CN XI
Trapezius	Thoracic and cervical spines Ligamentum nucha Superior nuchal line	Scapula (spine and acromion) Lateral one-third clavicle	**Bilateral:** Extends head. **Unilateral:** Chin up to opposite side; elevate acromion (rotates, elevates scapula and clavicle).	CN XI

With damage to CN XI (spinal accessory), in the posterior triangle, you cannot raise an arm above horizontal and cannot shrug shoulder (because of the trapezius).

Hyoid Bone

- U-shaped floating bone (from second and third branchial arches).
- Composed of body, greater and lesser horns (cornua).

Torticollis (head tilts to affected side) results from injury to SCM.

Connections to styloid process (of temporal bone):

- Stylomandibular ligament
- Stylopharyngeus muscle
- Stylohyoid muscle
- Styloglossus muscle

Hyoid Attachments

Ligaments	Muscles (Innervation)
Stylohyoid ligament	Mylohyoid (V3)
Hypoepiglottic ligament	Anterior digastric (V3)
	Posterior digastric (VII)
	Stylohyoid (VII)
	Hypoglossus (XII)
	Geniohyoid (C1 fibers via CN XII)
	Omohyoid (ansa cervicalis)
	Sternohyoid (ansa cervicalis)
	Thyrohyoid (C1 fibers via CN XII)

Supra- and Infrahyoid Muscles (see Figure 1–49)

Supra- and Infrahyoid Muscles

Muscle	Origin	Insertion	Action	Innervation
Suprahyoids				
Digastric (anterior)	Intermediate tendon	Anterior mandible (digastric fossa)	Raises hyoid	CN V3 (nerve to mylohyoid)
Digastric (posterior)	Temporal bone (digastric notch)	Intermediate tendon	Raises hyoid	CN VII
Mylohyoid	Medial mandible (mylohyoid line)	Median raphe; body of hyoid	Raises hyoid, base of tongue, floor of mouth	CN V3 (nerve to mylohyoid)
Geniohyoid	Genial tubercles (mandible)	Body of hyoid	Raises hyoid (pulls hyoid forward to open pharynx)	C1 fibers via CN XII
Stylohyoid	Styloid process	Hyoid (greater horn)	Raises hyoid	CN VII
Infrahyoids				
Omohyoid	**Superior belly:** Intermediate tendon	**Superior belly:** Hyoid (body, lower surface)	Depresses hyoid and larynx	Ansa cervicalis
	Inferior belly: Superior scapula	**Superior belly:** Intermediate tendon		
Sternohyoid	Manubrium of sternum	Hyoid (lower surface)	Depresses hyoid and larynx	Ansa cervicalis
Sternothyroid	Manubrium of sternum	Thyroid cartilage (oblique line)	Depresses larynx	Ansa cervicalis
Thyrohyoid	Thyroid cartilage (oblique line)	Hyoid (body and greater horn)	Depresses hyoid and larynx	C1 fibers via CN XII

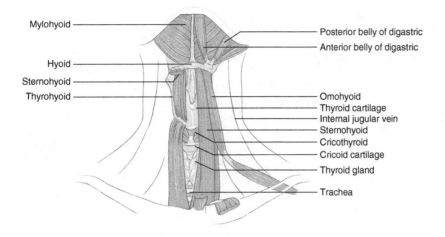

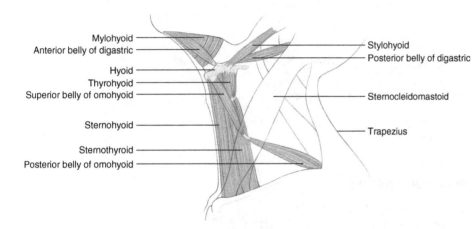

FIGURE 1-49. Infrahyoid muscles.

The mylohyoid is the muscle that makes it difficult to place lower, posterior periapical films in the mouth when it is not relaxed.

Cervical Plexus (of nerves)

See Figure 1–50.

Cervical Plexus

- C1 through C4
- Positioned deeply in the neck (lateral to first four cervical vertebra).
- **Cutaneous innervation** to:
    - Skin of neck.
    - Shoulder.
    - Anterior upper chest wall.
- **Motor** to:
    - Infrahyoid muscles.
    - Geniohyoid.
- **Phrenic nerve** (C3, C4, and C5) is contributed to, in part, by ansa cervicalis.
- **Supraclavicular nerves** innervate skin over the shoulder.
- **Transverse cervical nerve** carries sensory innervation to anterior and lateral neck.

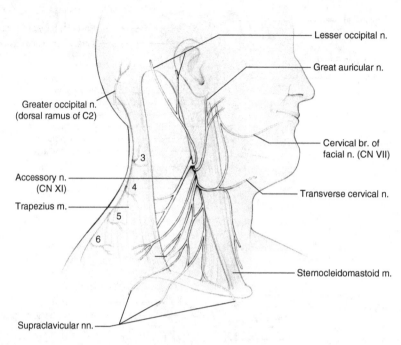

FIGURE 1-50. The cervical plexus.

Reproduced, with permission, from White JS. *USMLE Road Map Gross Anatomy*. New York: McGraw-Hill, 2003.

See innervation of external ear. Remember, four nerves are involved.

ANSA CERVICALIS (MOTOR)

- Motor division of cervical plexus.
- Comes from C1 (runs with CN XII), C2, C3.
- Innervates:
  - Infrahyoids (except thyrohyoid, which is innervated by C1).
  - Geniohyoid (moves hyoid anteriorly to hold open the pharynx).

Branches of C2, C3 Loop (Sensory)

Nerve	Supplies
Lesser occipital nerve (C2)	Skin of neck and scalp (posterosuperior to auricle)
Great auricular nerve (C2, C3)	Skin over parotid gland, posterior aspect of auricle, area from angle of mandible to mastoid
Transverse cervical nerve (C2, C3)	Skin of anterior triangle

The terminal branches of the ECA are the maxillary and superficial temporal arteries.

Phrenic Nerve

- C3, C4, C5 "keeps the diaphragm alive."
- Contains motor, sensory, and sympathetic nerve fibers.
- Sole motor innervation to the diaphragm.

Blood Supply to Face

See Figure 1–51 for arteries of the head and neck.

- Blood is supplied to the face via the external carotid branches.

External Carotid Artery

Course

- Branches from the common carotid artery at the level of the upper border of thyroid cartilage.
- Gives off branches and continues to the substance of the parotid gland where it ends as:
  - Maxillary artery.
  - Superficial temporal branch (superiorly).

In addition to the lingual artery, the tongue receives some blood supply from the tonsillar branch of the facial artery and the ascending pharyngeal artery.

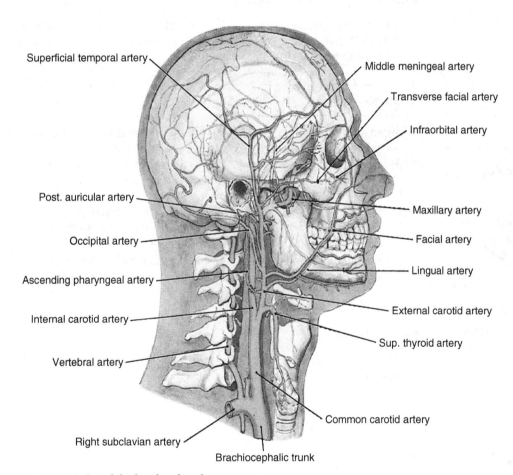

FIGURE 1–51. **Arteries of the head and neck.**

Reproduced, with permission, from Langman J, Woerdeman MW. *Atlas of Medical Anatomy.* Philadelphia: WB Saunders Company, 1978.

Supply

- Supplies most of head and neck (**except** the brain).
  - Face
  - Thyroid
  - Salivary glands
  - Tongue
  - Jaws
  - Teeth
- Carotid sinus (baroreception for blood pressure).
  - At the common carotid bifurcation.
- Carotid body (chemoreception including O_2, CO_2, pH, and temperature).
  - Posterior to the bifurcation of the CCA.

See also the Physiology section in Chapter 12.

BRANCHES OF THE EXTERNAL CAROTID

- The mnemonic to remember the branches of the external carotid artery is **SALFOPSM**: Some Anatomists Like Football, Others Prefer Soccer Matches.

Branch	Supplies
Superior thyroid	Thyroid gland, gives off SCM branch and the superior laryngeal artery
Ascending palatine	Soft palate, eustachian tube, palatine tonsils, levator veli palatini muscle
Lingual	Tongue
Facial	Face and submandibular gland
Occipital	Pharynx and suboccipital triangle
Posterior auricular	Posterior scalp
Superficial temporal	Parotid gland, auricle, temple, scalp
Maxillary	Infratemporal fossa, nasal cavity

LINGUAL ARTERY

- Originates from the ECA at the greater horn of hyoid bone (in the carotid triangle).
- Supplies:
  - Tongue.
  - Sublingual gland.
  - Floor of mouth.
- Branches:
  - Dorsal lingual.
  - Suprahyoid.
  - Sublingual arteries (to sublingual gland).
- Ends as the deep lingual artery
  - Between the genioglossus and hyoglossus muscles.
- Passes deep to hyoglossus muscle, then supplies tongue

FACIAL ARTERY

- The facial artery is considered in two portions.

Portion	Branches	Supplies
Cervical	Tonsillar Ascending palatine Glandular Submental	Tonsils Pharyngeal wall Submandibular gland Beneath chin
Facial	Inferior labial Superior labial Lateral nasal Angular	Lower lip Upper lip, anterior nose Lateral wall of nose Medial eye; anastomose with ophthalmic artery (of ICA)

MAXILLARY ARTERY

- Divided into three parts by the lateral pterygoid muscle.
- Branches from the ECA at the posterior border of the mandibular ramus.
- Supplies:
  - Muscles of mastication.
  - Maxillary and mandibular teeth.
  - Palate.
  - Most of the nasal cavity.

The greater palatine artery (via greater palatine foramen) supplies the hard palate (posterior to the maxillary canines).

The lesser palatine artery (via lesser palatine foramen) supplies the soft palate and tonsils.

The middle meningeal artery is a branch of the maxillary artery.

Maxillary Artery

Portion	Branches	Supplies
Mandibular	Deep auricular Anterior tympanic Middle meningeal Accessory meningeal Inferior alveolar	External auditory meatus Eardrum Middle cranial fossa Cranial cavity Chin, lower teeth
Pterygoid	Anterior and posterior deep temporal Pterygoid (medial and lateral branches) Masseteric Buccal	Temporalis muscle Pterygoid muscles Masseter muscle Buccinator muscle
Pterygopalatine	Posteriosuperior alveolar (PSA) Infraorbital becomes anterior superior alveolar Descending palatine Artery of pterygoid canal Pharyngeal Sphenopalatine	Maxillary molars and premolars Maxillary canines and incisors Greater and lesser palatine arteries to posterior palate Oropharynx Pharynx Terminal branch of maxillary artery; gives rise to nasopalatine artery (out incisive foramen to anterior palate and anastomoses with palatine vessels)

Venous Drainage from the Face

See Figure 1–52.

FACIAL VENOUS DRAINAGE

See Figure 1–53.

Remember: The scalp can drain superficially (via superficial temporal and posterior auricular veins) or deeply (via emissary veins).

SUPERFICIAL TEMPORAL VEIN

- Drains scalp and side of head.
- Merges with maxillary vein and plunges into parotid gland.

MAXILLARY VEIN

- Forms from the pterygoid plexus of veins, which is the connection of deep system with superficial venous drainage.

RETROMANDIBULAR VEIN

- Formed by the superficial temporal and maxillary veins.
- Divides at the angle of the mandible into anterior and posterior branches.

EXTERNAL JUGULAR VEIN

- Formed by the posterior auricular and retromandibular veins.
- Crosses the SCM.
- Drains the

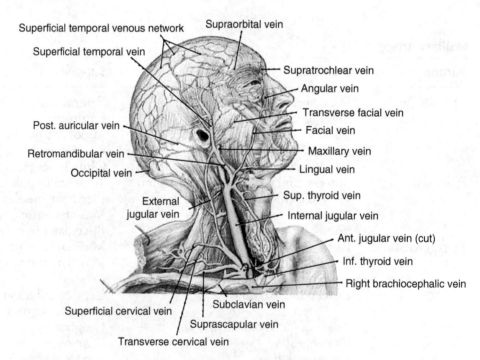

FIGURE 1–52. Veins of the head and neck.

Reproduced, with permission, from Langman J, Woerdeman MW. *Atlas of Medical Anatomy.* Philadelphia: WB Saunders Company, 1978.

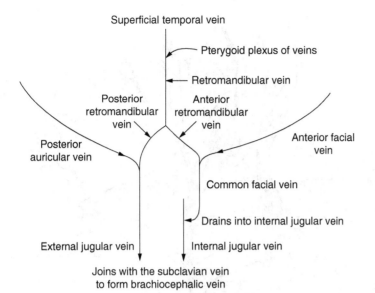

FIGURE 1–53. **Facial venous drainage.**

- Skin.
- Parotid gland.
- Muscles of the face and neck.
- Empties into the subclavian vein.

FACIAL VEIN (ANTERIOR FACIAL VEIN)

- Forms from the angular vein (which itself forms from the supraorbital and supratrochlear veins).
- Receives infraorbital and deep facial veins.
- Enters into the IJV (directly or by way of the common facial vein).

COMMON FACIAL VEIN

- Formed by the anterior facial and retromandibular veins.

INTERNAL JUGULAR VEIN

- Arises from the sigmoid and inferior petrosal sinuses.
- Drains the dural venous sinuses.
- Exits the skull via the jugular foramen (along with CNs XI, X, IX).
- Descends the neck in the carotid sheath.
- Merges with the subclavian vein to form:
    - Large brachiocephalic vein (behind the sternoclavicular joint).
    - Left and right brachiocephalic veins form the superior vena cava.

DANGER TRIANGLE OF THE FACE

- Area where superficial facial veins communicate with deep system (dural sinuses).
    - **Base:** Upper lip/anterior maxilla.
    - **Apex:** Infraorbital region.

Lymph Nodes in the Face

See Figures 1–54 and 1–55.
See the section "Tongue" for illustration of tongue lymph drainage.

Important:

Veins of the head and neck contain no valves.

Because there are no valves, retrograde flow can allow infection to spread via the deep facial vein, pterygoid plexus, and ophthalmic veins to the cavernous sinus.

The deep cervical nodes form the jugular lymph trunk (along IJV).

The jugular lymph trunk
empties into either

- The thoracic duct
  (on left) or the right
  lymphatic duct (which
  then empties into the
  brachiocephalic vein).
- Example:
- Infection of lower lip
  - Enters blood
    stream at right
    brachiocephalic
    vein.
  - Infection of abdomen
    - Enters at left
      brachiocephalic
      vein.

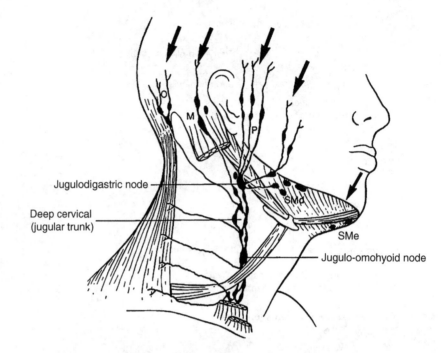

FIGURE 1–54. Lymphatic drainage of the face. M, mastoid nodes: O, occipital nodes; P, parotid nodes; SMd, submandibular nodes; SMe, submental nodes.

Reproduced, with permission, from Liebgott B. *The Anatomical Basis of Dentistry*. Toronto: BC Decker, 1986.

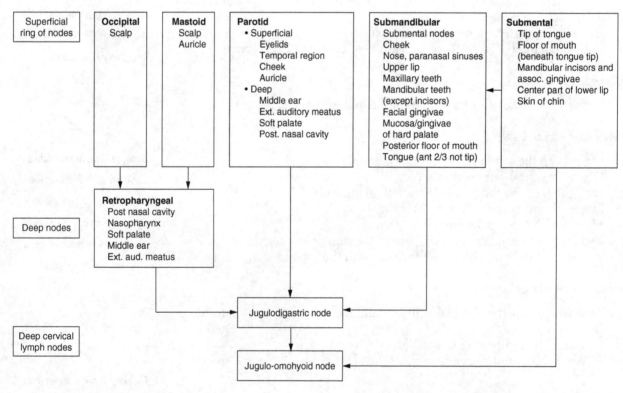

FIGURE 1–55. Lymph nodes in the face.

Thyroid

See Figure 1–56.

- ▩ H-shaped gland at laryngotracheal junction at anterior neck.
- ▩ Two lobes (right and left) joined by isthmus.
- ▩ Largest endocrine gland.
- ▩ Produces/secretes
  - ▩ Thyroid hormone.
  - ▩ Calcitonin.

T3 is about 20 times more potent than T4 at increasing cellular metabolism.

Calcitonin acts to "tone down" blood calcium levels.

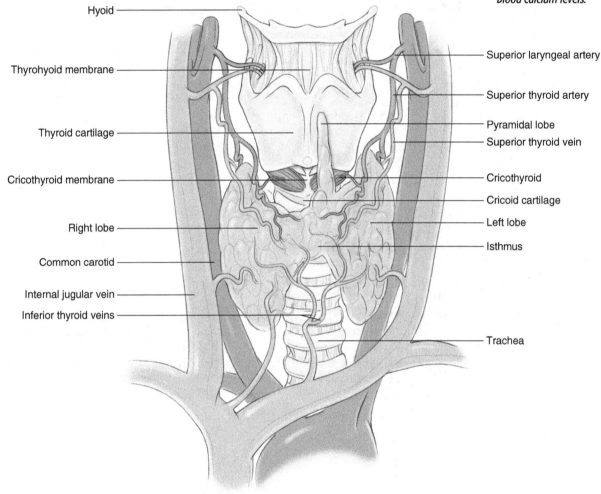

Hyoid

Thyrohyoid membrane

Thyroid cartilage

Cricothyroid membrane

Right lobe

Common carotid

Internal jugular vein

Inferior thyroid veins

Superior laryngeal artery

Superior thyroid artery

Pyramidal lobe

Superior thyroid vein

Cricothyroid

Cricoid cartilage

Left lobe

Isthmus

Trachea

FIGURE 1–56. Thyroid gland.

- ▩ **Blood supply:** See the following chart.
- ▩ **Nerve supply**
  - ▩ Glandular branches of cervical ganglia of sympathetic trunk.

Follicular Cells

- ▩ Produce thyroglobulin (tyrosine-containing).
  - ▩ Stored in colloid.
  - ▩ Precursor to T3 (triiodothyronine) and T4 (thyroxine) (involved in basal metabolic rate).

*Important: There is **no** middle thyroid artery; however, up to 10% of the population also receives a blood supply via the thyroid ima artery.*

Parafollicular (C) Cells

- Produce calcitonin.
  - Lower blood calcium and phosphate.

Thyroglossal Duct

- Connects thyroid gland to tongue development.
- Foramen cecum at base of tongue is proximal remnant.

THYROID BLOOD SUPPLY AND DRAINAGE

Artery	Branch of	Vein	Drains to
Superior thyroid artery	ECA	Superior thyroid vein	IJV
—	—	Middle thyroid vein	IJV
Inferior thyroid artery	Thyrocervical trunk	Inferior thyroid vein	Brachiocephalic vein

Parathyroid Glands

- Small pea-shaped organs.
- Two superior parathyroids develop from the 4th pharyngeal pouch.
- Two inferior parathyroids develop from the 3rd pharyngeal pouch.
- Encased in the posterior surface of the thyroid.
- **Blood supply**
  - Superior thyroid artery (from ECA) (to superior part of gland).
  - Inferior thyroid artery (from thyrocervical trunk) (to inferior part of gland).
- **Innervation**
  - Postganglionic sympathetic fibers of superior cervical ganglion.
- Produces parathyroid hormone (PTH).
  - Regulates calcium and phosphate metabolism.
  - Deficiency of PTH $\rightarrow$ decrease Ca^{2+} can cause tetany.

The vocal cords attach anteriorly at the lamina of thyroid cartilage and posteriorly at the vocal process of arytenoid cartilages.

Larynx

- The larynx is responsible for voice production.

LARYNGEAL SKELETON

- Nine cartilages (three single, three paired)

Cartilage	Description
Thyroid	Largest; forms the laryngeal prominence ("Adam's apple"); superior thyroid notch; superior surface is attached to hyoid by thyrohyoid membrane
Cricoid	Only laryngeal cartilage to form a complete ring around the airway.
Epiglottic	Fibrocartilage; gives flexibility to epiglottis.
Arytenoid (2)	Vocal cord attaches posteriorly.
Corniculate (2)	
Cuneiform (2)	

The cricothyroid membrane is incised at the midline for an emergent cricothyroidotomy/ tracheotomy. The cricothyroid space is entered (inferior to rima glottis where aspirated objects are often lodged or laryngospasm is occurring).

EPIGLOTTIS

- Thin leaf-shaped cartilage, covered with mucous membrane, at the root of the tongue.
- Flap closing over the larynx when swallowing.
- Median glossoepiglottic fold (1).
- Lateral glossoepiglottic folds (2).
- Valecullae (2) (lie between the glossoepiglottic folds).
- Taste buds (CN X) are located on superior surface of epiglottis.

VESTIBULAR FOLDS

- False vocal folds.
- **No** role in vocalization.
- Protective.

VOCAL FOLDS

- True vocal cords.
- Composed of vocal ligament and vocalis muscle.
- Involved in sound production.
- Sphincter of respiratory tract.

GLOTTIS

- Composed of vocal fold and rima glottis.
- Rima glottis is the opening between vocal folds.

LARYNGEAL MUSCLES

EXTRINSIC MUSCLES

Muscle Group	Function
Suprahyoids and stylopharyngeus muscle	Raise larynx.
Infrahyoids	Depress larynx.

*All intrinsic laryngeal muscles are supplied by the recurrent laryngeal nerve **except** the cricothyroid muscle, which is innervated by the external laryngeal nerve (a branch of the superior laryngeal nerve).*

INTRINSIC MUSCLES

Muscle	Origin	Insertion	Action	Innervation
Cricothyroid	Anterolateral cricoid cartilage	Thyroid cartilage (inferior margin and inferior horn)	Stretches and tenses vocal fold	External laryngeal nerve
Posterior cricoarytenoid	Cricoid cartilage (posterior laminae)	Muscular process of arytenoid cartilage	Abducts vocal fold	Recurrent laryngeal nerve
Lateral cricoarytenoid	Cricoid cartilage (arch)	Muscular process of arytenoid cartilage	Adducts vocal fold	Same as above
Thyroarytenoid	Thyroid cartilage (posterior surface)	Muscular process of arytenoid cartilage	Relaxes vocal fold	Same as above
Transverse and oblique arytenoids	Arytenoid cartilage	Opposite arytenoids cartilage	Closes rima glottides	Same as above
Vocalis	Depression between laminae of thyroid cartilage	Vocal ligament and vocal process of arytenoids cartilage	Relaxes posterior vocal ligament Tenses anterior vocal ligament Antagonist of cricothyroid muscle	Same as above

LARYNGEAL NERVES

See also Vagus.

RECURRENT LARYNGEAL NERVE

See Figure 1–57.

Injured nerves (eg, after thyroid or neck surgery) cause hoarseness.

- Is a branch of the vagus nerve (CN X).
- Comes off the vagus in the mediastinum and ascends to the larynx in the tracheoesophageal groove.

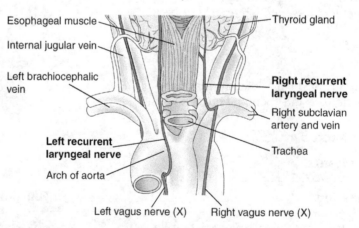

View from posterior

Esophageal muscle

Internal jugular vein

Left brachiocephalic vein

Left recurrent laryngeal nerve

Arch of aorta

Left vagus nerve (X)

Thyroid gland

Right recurrent laryngeal nerve

Right subclavian artery and vein

Trachea

Right vagus nerve (X)

FIGURE 1–57. Course of the recurrent laryngeal nerve (posterior view).

Reproduced, with permission, from Bhushan V, et al. *First Aid for the USMLE Step 1.* New York: McGraw-Hill, 2003.

- Has close association with thyroid gland and inferior thyroid artery.
- **Left recurrent laryngeal nerve** wraps around aortic arch (ligamentum arteriosum).
- **Right recurrent laryngeal nerve** wraps around right subclavian.
- **Motor innervation:** Involves all intrinsic muscles of larynx (via the inferior laryngeal branch) except cricothyroid.
- **Sensory innervation:** Involves laryngeal mucosa below vocal folds and upper trachea.

SUPERIOR LARYNGEAL NERVE

- Branch of the vagus nerve arising just after exit from jugular foramen.
- Passes through thyrohyoid membrane.
- **External branch:** Innervates cricothyroid muscle (tenses vocal cords, increasing pitch).
- **Internal branch:** Provides sensory information to laryngeal mucosa above the vocal folds.

Respiratory System

- Nasal cavity
- Pharynx
- Larynx
- Trachea
- Bronchi
- Bronchioles
- Alveoli

TRACHEA

- Air tube lined by C-shaped tracheal rings.
- Lined with respiratory epithelium.
- Formed from hyaline cartilage.
- ~10 cm long.
- ~2.5 cm diameter.
- Extends from:
  - C5–C6 level (base of larynx—starts as ligamentous attachment to cricoid) to Sternal angle (of Louis) T4/5 level (second rib level).
- Branches into left and right mainstem bronchi (at Carina).

Branching Pattern

Trachea
↓
Primary bronchi: two mainstem bronchi (one per lung)
↓
Secondary bronchi: five lobar bronchi (three in right lung; two in left lung)
↓
Tertiary bronchi
↓
Terminal bronchioles
↓
Respiratory bronchioles
↓
Alveoli

Axilla

Boundaries

Medial	Upper 4–5 ribs
	Intercostal muscles
	Serratus anterior muscle
Lateral	Humerus
	Coracobrachialis and biceps muscles
	Within intertubercular groove
Posterior	Subscapularis
	Teres major
	Latissimus dorsi
Anterior	Pectoralis major and minor
	Subclavius muscles
Base	Axillary fascia
	Skin

The subclavian arteries supply the upper extremities.

Contents

- Axillary vessels
- Brachial plexus
- Biceps brachii (both heads)
- Coracobrachialis

AXILLARY ARTERY

- Continuation of subclavian artery.
    - Named axillary artery as it passes lateral border of first rib.
- Travels close with the medial cord of the brachial plexus.
    - Aneurysm can compress the medial cord.
- Passes posterior to pectoralis minor muscle.
- Becomes brachial artery.
    - As it passes inferior border of teres major and enters the arm.

BRACHIAL ARTERY

- Continuation of axillary artery in the arm.
- Immediately medial to tendon of biceps brachii at elbow.

Profunda brachii artery arises from brachial artery in proximal arm.

AXILLARY VEIN

- Formed from the brachial veins and the basilic vein at the inferior border of teres major.
- Changes name to subclavian vein at the lateral border of the first rib.

CEPHALIC VEIN

- Drains into the axillary vein.
- Found in deltopectoral groove.
    - Located between deltoid and pectoralis major.
- Drains superficial arm.
    - Drains blood from the radial side of arm.

Brachial and basilic veins merge to form the axillary vein.

BRACHIAL VEIN

- Drains blood from the deep arm.

BASILIC VEIN

- Drains blood from the superficial arm.

SCALENE MUSCLES

- There are three scalene muscles per side:
  - Anterior
  - Middle
  - Posterior
- Phrenic nerve and subclavian vein pass on the surface of the anterior scalene.
- Brachial plexus and subclavian artery pass between the anterior and middle scalene.

See Figure 1–58 for the dorsal scapular artery.

Thoracic outlet syndrome results from compression of the lower trunk of the brachial plexus and the subclavian artery between the anterior and middle scalene.

Brachial Plexus

- The brachial plexus innervates the shoulder girdle and upper limb (ventral rami C5–T1).

OTHER BRANCHES OF THE BRACHIAL PLEXUS

See Figure 1–59.

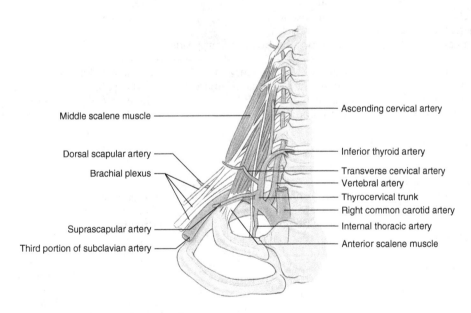

FIGURE 1–58. **Scalene muscles.**

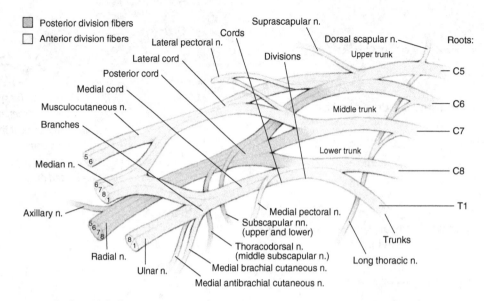

Posterior division fibers
Anterior division fibers

FIGURE 1-59.   The brachial plexus.

Reproduced, with permission, from White JS. *USMLE Road Map Gross Anatomy*. New York: McGraw-Hill, 2003.

Major Terminal Nerves of the Brachial Plexus

Nerve	Course	Motor	Sensory
Median (C5–T1) (from lateral and medial cords)	Lateral and medial cords Passes between two heads of pronator teres Enters carpal tunnel in wrist between: Palmaris longus Flexor carpi radialis	Forearm flexors: Flexor carpi radialis Palmaris longus Pronators Digital flexors Thenar muscles Lateral two lumbricals (thumb side)	Anterior arm Lateral palm (radial 2/3; thumb side) Lateral 3$^{1}/_{2}$ digits (thumb, 2, 3, including nailbeds)
Ulnar (C8–T1)	Medial cord Behind medial epicondyle (elbow) Between flexor carpi ulnaris and flexor digitorum profundus (wrist) Superficial to flexor retinaculum in wrist	Flexors of wrist and fingers (including flexor carpi ulnaris) Ulnar two lumbricals Interosseous muscles	Medial arm/forearm Medial palm Medial 1$^{1}/_{2}$ digit (pinky)
Radial (C6–C8)	Posterior cord Musculospiral groove (posterior humerus) Passes between brachioradialis and brachialis muscles	Extensors of arm/forearm: ▪ Triceps ▪ Brachioradialis ▪ Extensor carpi radialis ▪ Extensor carpi ulnaris ▪ Extensors of wrist/fingers ▪ Adductor pollicus ▪ Supinator ▪ Triceps brachii (medial and lateral head) [BEAST]	Posterior arm Forearm hand (not fingers)
Axillary	Comes off in axilla	Deltoid, teres minor, triceps brachii (long head)	Skin of lower $^{1}/_{2}$ of deltoid
Musculocutaneous (C5–C7)		Arm flexors ▪ Biceps brachii ▪ Coracobrachialis ▪ Brachialis	Anterolateral arm Forearm

Summary of Brachial Plexus Actions by Roots

Root(s)	Action(s)
C5	Shoulder
	Flexion
	Abduction
	Lateral rotation
	Elbow
	Flexion
C5, C6	Elbow
	▨ Extension
C6, C7	Wrist
	▨ Flexion
C7, C8	Shoulder
	▨ Extension
	Elbow
	▨ Pronation
	Fingers
	▨ Extension

Nerve	Supplies
Dorsal scapular (C4–C5)	Rhomboids
Upper/lower subscapular (C5–C6)	Subscapularis, teres major
Long thoracic (C5–C7)	Serratus anterior
Suprascapular (C4–C6)	Supraspinatus
Thoracodorsal (C6–C8)	Infraspinatus
	Glenohumeral joint
	Latissimus dorsi

Limb Muscles and Functions by Joint

MOVEMENT OF THE ARM AT THE SHOULDER

▨ This movement involves the glenohumeral joint.

Muscle(s)	Movement
Pectoralis major	Flexion
Deltoid	
Biceps	
Coracobrachialis	
Triceps	Extension
Teres major	
Pectoralis major	
Deltoid	
Latissimus dorsi	
Deltoid	Abduction
Supraspinatus	

The thenar (thumb) region of the hand and nailbeds of thumb, index, and middle fingers (and half of ring finger) are supplied by palmar digital nerves of the median nerve.

The hypothenar (pinky) region of the palm is supplied by the ulnar nerve.

The posterior cord gives rise to the radial and axillary nerves.

The radial nerve is the "great extensor nerve." It is motor to all muscles of the posterior arm. It is the most often injured nerve in a mid-humeral shaft fracture because it runs in the radial (spiral) groove of the humerus. Radial nerve deficit includes wrist drop, inability to make a tight fist, and sensory deficit to the radial hand and lower part of thumb and digits 2 and 3 (and half of 4).

Muscle(s)	Movement
Pectoralis major Latissimus dorsi Teres major Triceps Coracobrachialis	Adduction
Teres major Pectoralis major Latissimus dorsi Subscapularis Deltoid	Medial rotation
Infraspinatus Teres minor Deltoid	Lateral rotation

Axillary nerves are often injured by falling on an outstretched arm when the glenohumeral joint is dislocated because the nerve runs immediately inferior to the glenohumeral joint.

MOVEMENT OF THE ARM AT THE ELBOW

- This movement involves the humeroulnar joint.

Muscle(s)	Movement
Biceps Brachialis Coracobrachialis	Flexion
Triceps Anconeus	Extension

One can damage the lower part of the brachial plexus if the arm is abruptly extended above the head (eg, when grabbing a fixed object to slow a fall, as with a skier grabbing a tree).

MOVEMENT OF THE HAND AT THE ELBOW

- This movement involves the radioulnar joint.

Muscle(s)	Movement
Pronator quadratus, pronator teres	Pronation
Supinator, biceps	Supination

The long thoracic (nerve of Bell) supplies the serratus anterior (C5, C6, C7, or "wings of heaven").

The interosseous membrane holds radius and ulna together.

Rotator Cuff

- **Supraspinatus:** Abduction of arm at shoulder.
- **Infraspinatus:** External roation of arm at shoulder.
- **Teres minor:** External rotation of arm at shoulder.
- **Subscapularis:** Internal rotation of arm at shoulder.

The mnemonic for the muscles of the rotator cuff is SITS.

> ▶ **EXTERNAL THORAX AND ABDOMEN**

Sternum

- Anterior rib articulation (upper seven ribs articulate directly with sternum).
- Three parts (from superior to inferior):
    - Manubrium (articulates with clavicles and first ribs).
    - Body (articulates with ribs 2–7).
    - Xiphoid process.
- Jugular notch (suprasternal notch).
    - Superior border of manubrium.
- Angle of Louis (sternal angle).
    - Articulation of manubrium and body at second rib.

If one stabs the fourth intercostal space near sternal border, the right ventricle is injured.
If one fractures the tenth and eleventh ribs, the spleen is injured.

Clavicle

- S-shaped bone.
- Articulates with:
    - Acromion of scapula (laterally).
    - Manubrium of sternum (medially).
- Posterior dislocation at sternoclavicular joint can damage:
    - Trachea.
    - Subclavian vessels.
    - Nerves to arm (brachial plexus).
- Subclavius muscle helps prevent fractured clavicle from doing this damage.
- Clavicle forms by membranous bone formation.

Ribs

- Twelve total:
    - Ribs 1–7 are true: Attach directly to sternum (via costal cartilage).
    - Ribs 8–10 are false: Attach indirectly to sternum (via costal cartilage of rib above).
    - Ribs 11–12 are floating: Do not attach to sternum at all.

Intercostal Space

- The intercostal NVB runs on the inferior surface of the rib.
- Going from the closest undersurface of the rib inferiorly:
    - **Vein**
        - Intercoastal vein drains into the hemiazygos and azygos veins.
    - **Artery**
        - Anterior intercostal artery arises from internal thoracic artery.
        - Posterior intercostals arteries arise from thoracic aorta.
    - **Nerve**
        - Nerve is most exposed; least protected by costal groove.
        - Nerve at angle of rib is at inferior surface in costal groove, so you can anesthetize here.
- Intercostals muscles are involved in respiration.

Muscles of Respiration

- Diaphragm.
- Intercostals.
- Accessory muscles.

DIAPHRAGM

- Main muscle for breathing.
- Flat, domelike muscle.
- Muscular tent divides thoracic and abdominal cavities.
- Upper surface contacts heart, lungs.
- Lower surface contacts liver, stomach, spleen.
- Contraction (inspiration)
  - Flattens; moves inferiorly into abdomen.
  - Creates negative intrathoracic pressure/vacuum.
- Relaxes (exhalation/expiration).
  - Forms dome; moves up.
  - Positive intraabdominal pressure pushes it up.
  - Contract abdominal muscles for forceful exhalation.
- Openings and passageways:
  - **Aortic opening** (at level of T12)
    - Aorta (passes through two crura).
    - Thoracic duct (passes through with aorta).
    - Azygos and hemiazygos veins.
  - **Caval opening** (at level of T8)
    - Inferior vena cava.
  - **Esophageal opening** (at level of T10)
    - Esophagus.
  - Other things that pass:
    - Posterior and anterior vagal trunks.
    - Splanchnic nerves.
    - Sympathetic trunk.
    - Superior epigastric artery.
- Innervation
  - Phrenic nerve (C3, C4, C5).
- Blood supply to diagphragm and lower anterior intercostals spaces.
- Musculophrenic artery.

INTERCOSTAL MUSCLES

- All are innervated by the intercostals nerves.

The phrenic nerve travels through the thorax between pericardium and pleura.

Muscle	Orientation
External intercostal	Run from rib to rib in "hands-in-pocket" direction (homologous to external obliques).
Internal intercostal	Run from rib to rib 90 degrees from external intercostals; continue toward vertebral column *as* posterior intercostal membrane.
(NVB lies here) Innermost intercostal	Same direction as internal intercostals but the intercostal NVB lies in between.

- Sternocleidomastoid.
- Scalenes.
- Subcostals.
- Transversus thoracis.
- These latter two are innervated by intercostals nerves.

Muscles of the Thorax

Muscle	Origin	Insertion	Action	Innervation
Pectoralis major	Medial half of clavicle; sternum and costal cartilages 1–6	Greater tubercular crest (crest leading downward from greater tubercle)	Medially rotates, flexes, and adducts humerus	Lateral and medial pectoral nerves (C6–C8 and T1)
Pectoralis minor	Anterior ends of ribs 3–5	Coracoid process	Protracts and depresses glenoid of scapula	Lateral and medial pectoral nerves (C8 and T1)
Subclavius	Anterior end of rib 1	Underside of clavicle	Protracts and depresses clavicle	Nerve to subclavius (C5–C6)

MUSCLES OF THE PECTORAL GIRDLE

- Serratus anterior
- Pectoralis minor
- Subclavius
- Trapezius
- Levator scapulae
- Rhomboideus major
- Rhomboideus minor

Abdominal Regions

- **Umbilical:** Central around the umbilicus.
- **Lumbar:** Right and left of umbilical region.
- **Epigastric:** Midline region above umbilicus (subxiphoid, area of stomach).
- **Hypochondriac:** Left and right of epigastric regions (beneath rib cage).
- **Hypogastric (pubic):** Midline below umbilicus.
- **Iliac (inguinal):** Right and left of hypogastric region.

Abdominal Muscles

Muscle	Origin	Insertion	Action	Innervation
External oblique	Superficial aspect of lower 8 ribs	Iliac crest, linea alba	Increases abdominal pressure	Lower intercostal nerves
Internal oblique	Lumbodorsal fascia, iliac crest, inguinal ligament	Costal cartilages of last 3 ribs, linea alba	Same as above	Lower intercostals, iliohypogastric, ilioinguinal nerves
Transversus abdominis	Internal surface of lower 6 costal cartilages, lumbodorsal fascia, iliac crest, inguinal ligament	Linea alba	Same as above	Lower intercostals, iliohypogastric, and ilioinguinal nerves
Rectus abdominis	Pubic symphysis	External surface xiphoid process, external surface costal cartilages 5–7	Increases abdominal pressure, flex vertebral column	Lower intercostal nerves

POINTS

- **External oblique fibers** (like external intercostals)
  - Run in a "hands-in-pocket" fashion.
  - Obliquely; lateral to medial going superior to inferior.
- **Internal oblique fibers** (like internal intercostals fibers)
  - Run opposite (perpendicular) to external oblique fibers.
  - Obliquely from lateral to medial going inferior to superior.
- **Cremaster muscle**
  - Derived from internal oblique muscle.

Rectus Sheath

- Aponeurotic sheath covering the rectus muscle.
- **Anterior rectus sheath**
  - Formed from the tendinous continuations of the external oblique and internal oblique.
- **Posterior rectus sheath**
  - Formed from the aponeurosis from the internal oblique and tranverse abdominis.
- **Linea alba**
  - Midline fusion of the anterior and posterior rectus sheath.
  - At the midline of two bellies of the rectus.

Fascia

- Covers muscles.
- Attaches to nearby bones by blending with covering periosteum.

Breast

- Mammary glands.
- Modified sweat glands.
- Lie in superficial fascia.

- Myoepithelial cells (star-shaped)
  - Encircle some of the secretory cells.
  - Force secretion toward the ducts.
- Suspensory ligaments (Cooper's ligaments)
  - Strong fibrous processes.
  - Run from dermis to deep layer of superficial fascia through breast.
  - Support the breasts.
  - Can cause dimpling of overlying skin and nipple retraction in breast cancer.
- Innervation:
  - Fourth intercostal nerve (T4) (to the nipple).
- Blood supply:
  - Lateral thoracic (branch of axillary).
  - Internal thoracic arteries.
- Lymph drainage.
- To lymph nodes (LNs) in axilla.

Dermatomes

See Figure 1–60. A dermatome is an area of skin supplied by a single nerve.

- CN V: Head and face.
- CN V, VII, IX, X: Ear.
- C1: **Does not** supply a dermatome.
- C2 (greater occipital nerve): Posterior scalp (posterior half of skull cap).
- C3: Neck.
- C4: Low collar.
- T4: Nipple
- T7: Xiphoid.
- T10: Umbilicus.
- L1: Inguinal ligament.
- L4: Knee caps.
- S2, S3, S4: Erection, sensation of penile and anal zones.

> *Cranial nerve dermatomes **do not** overlap.*
>
> - Spinal nerve dermatomes overlap by as much as 50%.
> - May require loss of three spinal nerves to produce anesthesia in middle dermatome.
> - For example, lesion to dorsal root of T7, T8, and T9 to produce numbness of T8 dermatomal distribution.

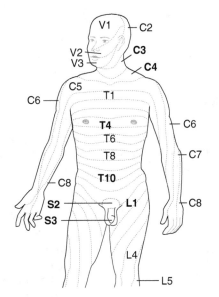

FIGURE 1–60. Areas of skin supplied by a single nerve.

Reproduced, with permission, from Bhushan V, et al. *First Aid for the USMLE Step 1*. New York: McGraw-Hill, 2003.

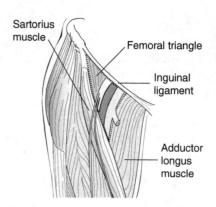

FIGURE 1–61.   Femoral triangle.

Reproduced, with permission, from Bhushan V, et al. *First Aid for the USMLE Step 1*. New York: McGraw-Hill, 2003.

Reflexes

- C5, C6: Biceps
- C7: Triceps
- L4: Patella
- S1: Achilles

Femoral Triangle

See Figure 1–61. The femoral triangle has the following boundaries:

- **Lateral:** Sartorius.
- **Medial:** Adductor longus.
- **Superior:** Inguinal ligament.
- **Floor:** Iliopsoas and pectineus.
- **Femoral:** NVB.
- **From lateral to medial:** Nerve, artery, vein.

► **THORACIC AND ABDOMINAL VISCERA**

Body Cavities

Posterior	Anterior
Cranial: Contains brain. **Spinal:** - Contains spinal cord. - These two cavities communicate via foramen magnum. - Lined by meninges. - Bathed in CSF.	**Thoracic** **Pericardial cavity:** Surrounds heart **Pleural** (right and left) - Surrounds each lung. - Mediastinum lies between two pleural cavities. **Abdominopelvic abdominal** - Stomach - Spleen - Liver - Gallbladder - Pancreas - Small and large intestines **Pelvic cavity** - Rectum - Urinary bladder

Lung

See Figure 1–62.

- Housed in left and right pleural cavities.
- **Visceral pleura:** Covers the lungs.
- **Parietal pleura:** Covers the thoracic cavity.
- Pleural cavity.
  - Between the two layers of pleura.
  - Filled with serous fluid.

Right Lung	Left Lung
Three lobes	Two lobes
▪ Superior	▪ Superior
▪ Middle	▪ Inferior
▪ Inferior	Lingula
Three lobar bronchi (secondary bronchi)	▪ Tongue-shaped part of superior lobe corresponding to middle lobe of right lung
Ten bronchial segments (tertiary bronchi)	Two lobar bronchi (secondary bronchi)
One bronchial artery	Eight bronchial segments (tertiary bronchi)
Larger capacity than left lung	Cardiac notch
	▪ Medial side of the superior lobe of left lung
	Two bronchial arteries

LUNG HILUM (ROOT)

- Pulmonary artery
- Pulmonary vein
- Bronchus

OTHER STRUCTURES PASSING INTO THE HILUM

Bronchial Arteries

- Supply the lung tissues with oxygen.
- Also pass into the hilum.
- Follow the bronchial tree.

Describes where the pulmonary artery sits in relation to the bronchus:

RALS

Right
Anterior
Left
Superior

Aspiration occurs more often in the right lung (apical aspect of right lower lobe) because the right mainstem bronchus is straighter, shorter, and larger than the left. The left mainstem takes a more acute angle.

See the "Physiology" section in Chapter 13 for Hering-Breuer and cough reflexes.

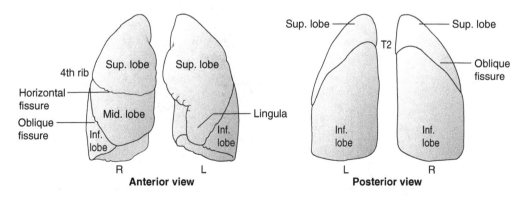

FIGURE 1–62. **Anterior and posterior view of the lungs.**

Reproduced, with permission, from Bhushan V, et al. *First Aid for the USMLE Step 1.* New York: McGraw-Hill, 2003.

The superior lobe of the left lung has a lingula.

Branches of the Vagus Nerve

- Also pass into the root of the lung.

Heart and Great Vessels

See Figure 1–63.

	From Body (Deoxy)	From Lungs (Oxy)
Chamber	Right atrium	Left atrium
Valve	Tricuspid valve	Mitral valve
Chamber	Right ventricle	Left ventricle
Valve	Pulmonic valve	Aortic valve
	To lungs	To body

VALVES

SEMILUNAR

- Each has three semilunar cusps.
- No chordae tendineae or papillary muscles are associated with semiluar valves.
- **Pulmonic valve**
    - Right ventricle (RV) to pulmonary arteries.
    - At left sternal border, second intercostal space.
- **Aortic valve**
    - Left ventricle (LV) to aorta.
    - Over right sternal border, second intercostal space.

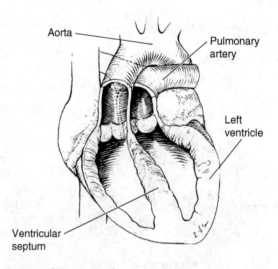

FIGURE 1-63. Heart and great vessels.

Reproduced, with permission, from Way LW, Doherty GM (eds). *Current Surgical Diagnosis and Treatment*, 11th ed. New York: McGraw-Hill, 2002.

Atrioventricular

- **Tricuspid valve**
  - Right atrium (RA) to right ventricle (RV).
  - Over left sternal border, fifth intercostal space.
- **Mitral valve**
  - Left atrium (LA) to left ventricle (LV).
  - Over fifth intercostal space, midclavicular line.

Atria

Right Atrium

- Incoming deoxygenated blood from vena cavae.

- **Fossa ovalis**
  - Depression remnant of the foramen ovale.
  - Lies on atrial septum (interatrial); dividing the left and right atria.
  - Anulis ovalis is the upper margin of the fossa.
- **Crista terminalis**
  - Vertical ridge between vena cavae orifices.
  - Sinoatrial (SA) node is located here.
  - Junction of sinus venosus and the heart in the developing embryo.
- **Sulcus terminalis**
  - Vertical groove on external heart represents crista terminalis (internally).
- **Pectinate muscles**
  - Radiate from crista terminalis to atrial appendage.
- **Right auricle**
  - Appendage of right atrium.
- **Conduction system**
  - SA node.
  - AV node.
  - Both nodes innervated by parasympathetic fibers from CN X and sympathetic fibers from T1–T4.

Left Atrium

- Incoming blood from pulmonary veins.

Ventricles

Right Ventricle

- Responsible for the pulmonic circulation.
  - Pumps deoxygenated blood through the pulmonic valve to pulmonary artery and lungs for oxygenation.
- Trabeculae carnae.
  - Ridges of cardiac muscle in the ventricles.
- Chordae tendinae.
  - Thin tendinous cords passing from valve cusps to papillary muscles.
- Papillary muscles.
  - Anchor chordae tendinae to heart wall.

Left Ventricle

- Apex of the heart.
  - Auscultate fifth intercostals space at midclavicular line.
- Responsible for the systemic circulation.

The chordae tendinae and papillary muscles do **not** help the AV valves close. They prevent the valve from everting back into the atria.

See the "Pathology" section in Chapter 19. Heart strain and hypertrophy secondary to increased resistance to flow:

- Left heart
  - Coarctation of the aorta
  - Systemic hypertension
  - Right heart
  - Pulmonary hypertension

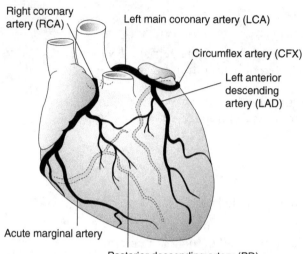

FIGURE 1–64.   Coronary arteries.

Reproduced, with permission, from Bhushan V, et al. *First Aid of the USMLE Step 1*. New York: McGraw-Hill, 2003; Adapted from *Ganong WF. Review of Medical Physiology*, 19th ed. Stamford CT: Appleton & Lange, 1999.

The pericardial cavity lies between the two layers of pericardium.

- Receives oxygenated blood from the lungs and pumps it out to the rest of the body.
- Out the aortic valve to aorta.
- Thicker than RV because of higher afterload from systemic circulation.
- Same internal features as RV.

PERICARDIUM

- Tough, double-walled covering of the heart
- Innervated by the phrenic nerve
- **Parietal pericardium:** Outer fibrous
- **Visceral pericardium:** Inner serous

CORONARY ARTERIES

See Figure 1–64.

- First branches of the aorta.
  - Coronary ostia located within aortic valve leaflets.
  - Drain to coronary sinus which drains back to RA.
- Coronary arteries fill during diastole.
- Blockage; thrombus on disrupted plaque can lead to:
  - Ischemia (angina).
  - Infarction (heart attack).

Vessel	Area Supplied
Left circumflex	LV lateral wall
Left anterior descending artery (LAD)	Anterior wall LV
	Interventricular septum
Right coronary artery (RCA)	Right ventricle
	AV node
	Posterior, inferior walls of LV

Veins of the Heart

- Cardiac veins lie superficial to the arteries.
- **Coronary sinus**
  - Continuation of **great cardiac vein.**
  - Opens into the right atrium between the IVC and the tricuspid orifice.
  - All veins drain into the coronary sinus **except** the **anterior cardiac veins** (drain directly into the right atrium).

Mediastinum

- The mediastinum is the area medial to lungs in the thorax.

Mediastinum	Location	Contents
Anterior	Anterior to pericardium	Thymus Connective tissue Lymph nodes Branches of internal thoracic artery
Middle	Within pericardium	Pericardium Heart Roots of great vessels Phrenic nerve
Posterior	Posterior to pericardium	Thoracic duct Descending aorta Azygous vein Hemiazygous vein Esophagus Vagus nerves Splanchnic nerves Lymph nodes
Superior	Above manubriosternal junction (T4)	Thoracic duct Ascending aorta Aortic arch Branches of aortic arch Descending aorta SVC Brachiocephalic veins Thymus Trachea Esophagus Cardiac nerve Left recurrent laryngeal nerve

The superior vena cava (SVC), the inferior vena cava (IVC), and coronary sinus all empty deoxygenated blood into the RA.

The thymus is located in both the anterior and superior mediastinum.

The inferior mediastinum is split into anterior, middle, and posterior.

Zinc is the most important element for immunity (involved in almost all aspects of immunity).

The thymus has no afferent lymphatics or lymphatic nodules.

Thymus

FUNCTION

- A primary lymphoid organ.
  - Along with spleen, tonsils, lymph nodes, Peyer's patches.
- Master organ of immunogenesis in young.
  - Proliferation and maturation of T cells (cell-mediated immunity).
- Releases factors important in development of immune system:
  - Thymopoietin.
  - Thymosin.
  - Thymic humoral factor.
  - Thymic factor.
- Zinc, vitamin B_6, vitamin C are important for thymic hormones.

ANATOMY

- Located inferior to thyroid, ventral/anterior to heart.
- Deep to sternum in **superior mediastinum.**
- Two lobes (soft, pinkish).
- Inner medulla
  - Lymphocytes.
  - Hassall's corpuscles (epithelial vestiges with unknown function).
- Blood supply
  - Internal thoracic artery.
  - Inferior thyroid arteries.
- Nerve supply
  - Vagus nerve.
  - Phrenic nerve.

Thymoma is associated with myasthenia gravis.

Aorta

See Figure 1–65.

- Descending thoracic aorta extends from T4 to T12.
- Descending abdominal aorta extends from T12 to L4.

Remember: *The ligamentum arteriosum connects the aortic arch to the pulmonary trunk and is a vestige of the ductus arteriosis.*

Remember: *There is one brachiocephalic artery, two brachiocephalic veins.*

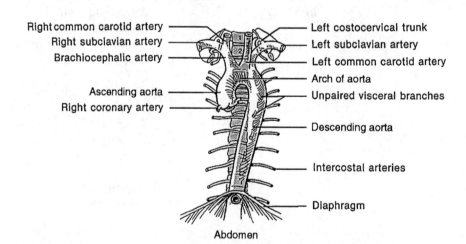

FIGURE 1–65. **The thoracic aorta and its branches.**

Reproduced, with permission, from Liebgott B. *The Anatomical Basis of Dentistry.* Toronto: BC Decker, 1986.

■ Aorta terminates around L4 when it divides into left and right common iliac arteries (supplying lower limbs and pelvic viscera).

Parts	Major Branches	Supplies
Ascending	Right and left coronary arteries	Heart
Aortic arch	Brachiocephalic artery Left common carotid Left subclavian	Head, neck, upper limbs
Descending thoracic aorta	Posterior intercostals	Posterior thorax, diaphragm
Descending abdominal aorta	**Unpaired:** Celiac trunk SMA IMA **Paired:** Renal Gonadal	Abdominal viscera

Remember: The right renal artery is longer than the left renal artery and the left common carotid is longer than the right common carotid.

COMMON CAROTID

■ Supplies head and neck.
■ Bifurcates into external and internal carotid arteries at superior border of the thyroid cartilage.

See the "Neck" section for branches.

SUBCLAVIAN ARTERY

■ Supplies the upper extremity.
■ Continues as the axillary artery past the inferior margin of the first rib.

BRANCHES OF SUBCLAVIAN ARTERY

■ Vertebral (forms basilar—circle of Willis)
■ Thyrocervical
■ Internal thoracic
■ Costocervical

INTERNAL THORACIC ARTERY

■ Runs underneath the sternum.
■ Gives off anterior intercostals (meets posterior intercostals off the aorta).
■ Extends inferiorly as superior epigastric artery.

SUPERIOR EPIGASTRIC ARTERY

■ Continuation of the internal thoracic artery.
■ Enters rectus sheath and supplies rectus muscle.
■ Anastomoses with inferior epigastric artery (branch of the external iliac artery) near the umbilicus.

If the celiac trunk is blocked, blood can still reach the foregut by way of anastomoses between the superior pancreaticoduodenal artery (a branch of the gastroduodenal) and the inferior pancreaticoduodenal (a branch of the SMA).

The third part of duodenum passes anterior to the IMA.

ABDOMINAL AORTA

Midline Branches

Branch	Branches	Structures Supplied
Celiac	Common hepatic, splenic, left gastric	Foregut: Stomach, liver, spleen, and upper half of pancreas/duodenum
SMA	Inferior pancreaticoduodenal, intestinal (ileal, jejunal), right and middle colic arteries	Midgut: Head of pancreas, lower duodenum, rest of small intestine, ascending and transverse colon
IMA	Superior rectal, sigmoid, left colic arteries	Hindgut: Descending and sigmoid colon and upper 2/3rd of rectum

Azygous System

See Figure 1–66.

- The azygous system drains the thoracic wall.

Remember:

The right superior intercostal vein drains into the azygos vein.

The left superior intercostal vein drains into left brachiocephalic vein.

Anatomy	Formed by	Drains to
Ascends through aortic orifice of diaphragm Lies within posterior mediastinum Leaves a notch in the right lung as it passes over the hilum	Right ascending lumbar vein Right subcostal vein	Empties into the superior vena cava (SVC)

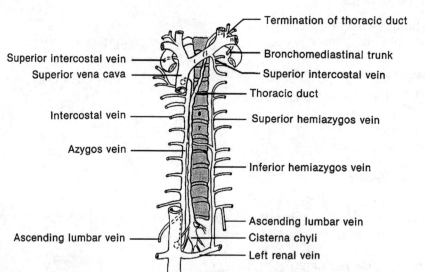

FIGURE 1-66. **The azygous system of veins and the thoracic duct.**

Reproduced, with permission, with Liebgott B. *The Anatomical Basis of Dentistry*. Toronto: BC Decker, 1986.

Hemiazygos Vein (Left) (Inferior Hemiazygos Vein)	Accessory Hemiazygos Vein (Right) (Superior Hemiazygos Vein)
Formed by: ▫ Left ascending lumbar vein ▫ Left subcostal vein ▫ Empties into the azygos vein	Formed by: ▫ 4th to 8th intercostal veins ▫ Empties into the azygos vein

Splanchnic Nerves

▫ Sympathetic nerves to the abdominal viscera.
  ▫ Counteract vagal/parasympathetic inputs.
▫ Arise from thoracic ganglia
  ▫ T5–T12.
  ▫ All pass through the diaphragm.
▫ Preganglionic sympathetic fibers pass through ganglia of the sympathetic trunk **without** synapsing.
  ▫ This is the exception to the short preganglionic, long postganglionic.
  ▫ They synapse with small ganglia in the tissues/effector organs which give off short postganglionics.
▫ Distribute to smooth muscle and glands of viscera.

Nerve	Components	Innervates
Greater splanchnic nerve	T5–T9	Synapse at cervical plexus (foregut)
Lesser splanchnic nerve	T10, T11	Synapse with superior mesenteric plexus; aorticorenal ganglion (midgut)
Least splanchnic nerve	T12	Inferior mesenteric plexus/renal plexus (hindgut)

Superior Vena Cava

▫ Drains the
  ▫ Head.
  ▫ Neck.
  ▫ Upper extremities.
  ▫ Upper chest.
▫ No valve.
▫ Formed by left and right brachiocephalic veins (merging in the superior mediastinum).
▫ Brachiocephalic veins are formed from
  ▫ Internal jugular vein.
  ▫ Subclavian vein.
▫ Azygos vein empties into SVC.
▫ SVC empties into RA.

SVC Syndrome

▫ Example: Compression of SVC with lung cancer
▫ Dyspnea
▫ Facial swelling and flushing
▫ Jugular venous distention
▫ Mental status changes

Remember: *The left gonadal vein drains into left renal vein. The right gonadal vein empties directly into the IVC.*

The left renal vein is longer than the right and the right renal artery is longer than the left. This is due to the positions of the vena cava and aorta, respectively.

A pelvic kidney may be supplied by the common iliac artery.

Remember: *There is a celiac artery but **no** celiac vein.*

Inferior Vena Cava

- Larger than SVC.
- Rudimentary, nonfunctioning valve.
- Drains
  - Thorax.
  - Abdomen.
  - Lower extremities.
- Receives blood from the hepatic veins.
- Empties into RA.

PAIRED BRANCHES OF THE IVC

Branch	Structures Supplied
Suprarenal	Adrenal glands
Renal	Kidneys
Gonadal	Testes/ovaries
Lumbar	Lumbar epaxial muscles

Portal Vein (Figure 1–67)

- Transmits venous blood from the abdominal viscera (with absorbed substances) to the liver and, via the portal system, to the heart.

Portal vein → hepatic sinusoids → central vein → hepatic veins → IVC. **The portal vein arises from:**

- Splenic vein
  - Drains:
    - Spleen.
    - Stomach (L and R gastroepiploic veins, R and L gastric veins).
    - Pancreas (pancreatic vein).
    - Gallbladder (cystic vein).

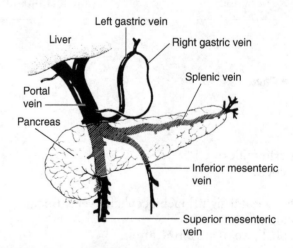

FIGURE 1–67. **Anatomic relationship of portal vein and branches.**

Reproduced, with permission, from Way LW, Doherty, GM (eds). *Current Surgical Diagnosis and Treatment*, 11th ed. New York: McGraw-Hill, 2002.

- **Superior mesenteric vein**
  - Drains
    - Small intestine.
    - Cecum.
    - Ascending and transverse colon.
- **Inferior mesenteric vein**
  - Enters into the splenic vein, the SMV, or crotch of the two.
  - Drains:
    - Transverse colon distal to L colic flexure (splenic flexure).
    - Descending colon.
    - Rectum.

Portal Triad

- Consists of:
  - Portal vein.
  - Hepatic artery.
  - Bile duct.
- Lies on free edge of lesser omentum (anterior to epiploic foramen of Winslow).
- Portal vein is posterior while hepatic artery and bile duct are anterior.
- Portal vein carries twice as much blood as the hepatic artery.

VENOUS ANASTOMOSES

See Figure 1–68.

Portal blood can also get to the IVC by the azygos and hemiazygos veins.

Portocaval shunt can be created by anastomosing the splenic vein and renal vein (a portal component and a systemic venous component).

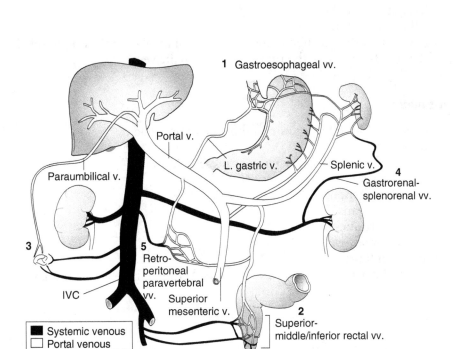

1 Gastroesophageal vv.

Portal v.

L. gastric v.

Paraumbilical v.

Splenic v.

4 Gastrorenal-splenorenal vv.

3

5 Retro-peritoneal paravertebral vv.

IVC

Superior mesenteric v.

2 Superior-middle/inferior rectal vv.

■ Systemic venous
□ Portal venous

FIGURE 1–68. Portal systemic anastomoses.

Reproduced, with permission, from Bhushan V, et al. *First Aid for the USMLE Step 1*. New York: McGraw-Hill, 2003.

*Occlusion of lymph supply
(eg, cancer) leads to
intractable edema.*

*Aside from the right arm,
chest, and right head, the
rest of the body—including the
right leg—is drained by the
thoracic duct.*

Important: *The diaphragm
divides the thoracic cavity and
abdominal cavity.*

*Pleura is the analog to
peritoneum in the pleural
cavity.*

*The **pericardioperitoneal
canal** embryologically
connects the thoracic and
peritoneal cavities.*

Lymphatic System

CISTERNA CHYLI

- Located in the para-aortic region below the diaphragm at level of T12.
- Drains lymph from
  - Abdomen.
  - Pelvis.
  - Inguinal region.
  - Lower extremities.
- Continuous superiorly with the thoracic duct.

THORACIC DUCT

- Continuation of the dilated cisterna chyli.
- Located in posterior and superior mediastinum.
- Drains lymph from
  - Lower limbs.
  - Abdomen.
  - Chest wall.
- Empties into venous system at junction of the subclavian and internal jugular vein (on the left side only).

RIGHT LYMPHATIC DUCT

- Drains
  - Right arm.
  - Right side of chest.
  - Right side of head.
- Empties into the junction of the right internal jugular vein and right subclavian veins (formation of the right brachiocephalic vein).

Peritoneum

- Membrane lining the interior of the abdominopelvic cavity.
- Consists of:
  - Single layer of simple squamous mesothelium.
  - Thin layer of irregular connective tissue.
- **Visceral peritoneum**
  - Covers organs.
- **Parietal peritoneum**
  - Covers body walls.
- **Peritoneal fluid**
  - Fills the peritoneal space/cavity (space between these two serous layers).

Mesentery

- Double-layer fold of peritoneum pushed into peritoneal cavity.
- Suspends most organs of abdominoperitoneal cavity (holds them in place).
- Allows path for blood vessels and nerves.

Embryonic Mesentery	Adult Mesentery
Dorsal mesogastrium	Greater omentum
	Omental bursa
Dorsal mesoduodenum	Disappears (duodenum lies retroperitoneal)
Pleuropericardial membrane	Pericardium
	Contribution to diaphragm
Ventral mesentery	Falciform ligament
	Ligamentum teres
	Lesser omentum (hepatogastric, hepatoduodenal ligaments)

*The **greater omentum** begins at its attachment to the greater curvature of the stomach, drapes over (apronlike) the small and large intestines, and loops back to insert on the transverse colon.*

Peritoneal Ligaments

- Either a mesentery or omentum.
- Named double fold of the peritoneum and connects
  - Two organs or
  - Organ to the abdominal wall.
- Are associated with the stomach, jejunum, ileum, appendix, transverse colon, sigmoid colon, spleen, liver, and gallbladder.

Ligament	Description
Splenorenal ligament	Connects spleen to posterior abdominal wall.
	Contains splenic artery, vein, and tail of pancreas.
	Passes from spleen to parietal peritoneum on the anterior surface of the kidney.
	Separates the greater peritoneal sac from the left portion of the lesser peritoneal sac.
Gastrosplenic ligament	Part of dorsal mesogastrium between greater curve of stomach and spleen.
	Separates greater peritoneal sac from left portion of lesser peritoneal sac.
	Incise to gain access to left side of lesser peritoneal sac.
Gastrocolic ligament	Part of greater omentum, between greater curvature of stomach and transverse colon.
	Contains gastroepiploic arteries.
Gastroduodenal ligament	Between lesser curve of stomach and duodenum.
Gastrohepatic ligament	**Part of lesser omentum** between liver and lesser curvature.
	Separates greater peritoneal sac and right part of lesser peritoneal sac.
	Contains no significant blood vessels (so may be incised for access).
Hepatoduodenal ligament	**Part of lesser omentum**
	Connects liver to first part of duodenum.
	Contains common bile duct, proper hepatic artery (with brachial cystic artery), and portal vein.
	Separates greater peritoneal sac from right part of lesser peritoneal sac.
	Forms anterior portion of epiploic foramen.
Falciform ligament	Connects liver to anterior abdominal wall.
	Contains ligamentum teres (remnant of umbilical vein).

Epiploic Foramen of Winslow

- Inlet to lesser sac.
- Posterior to the free edge of the lesser omentum (hepatoduodenal ligament).
- Portal triad is located over top (anteriorly).

See histology for the myenteric nervous system.

Gastrointestinal Tract

See Figure 1–69 for the cross section of the gastrointestinal tract.

GI Segment	Derivatives	Arterial Supply	Innervation
Foregut	Esophagus Stomach Duodenum (1st part) Liver Gallbladder Pancreas	Celiac trunk	Vagal parasympathetics Thoracic nerve Greater splanchnic sympathetics
Midgut	Duodenum (2nd–4th parts) Jejunum Ileum Appedix Ascending colon Transverse colon (to splenic flexure)	Superior mesenteric artery	Vagal parasympathetics Thoracic splanchnic sympathetic nerve
Hindgut	Transverse colon (distal to splenic flexure) Descending colon Sigmoid colon Rectum	Inferior mesenteric artery	Pelvic splanchnic nerve (S2–S4) parasympathetic Lumbar splanchnic sympathetic nerve

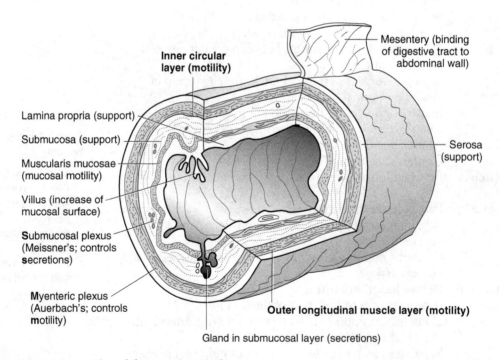

FIGURE 1–69. Cross section of the gastrointestinal tract.

Reproduced, with permission, from Bhushan V, et al. *First Aid for the USMLE Step 1.* New York: McGraw-Hill, 2003. Adapted from McPhee S, et al. *Pathophysiology of Disease: An Introduction to Clinical Medicine,* 3rd ed. New York: McGraw-Hill, 2000.

ESOPHAGUS

Description	Blood Supply	Innervation
10-inch muscular tube Peristalsis Food propelled from pharynx to stomach (pierces diaphragm at cardiac orifice) Posterior to trachea Travels through the mediastinum (superior and posterior) Upper 1/3 skeletal muscle Middle 1/3 skeletal and smooth muscle Lower 1/3 smooth muscle	Inferior thyroid artery Descending thoracic aorta (direct branches) Left gastric artery	**Parasympathetic:** Vagus (esophageal branches) **Sympathetic:** Esophageal plexus **Motor:** Recurrent laryngeal nerve (of vagus)

Stomach

See Figure 1–70 for the anatomy of the stomach.

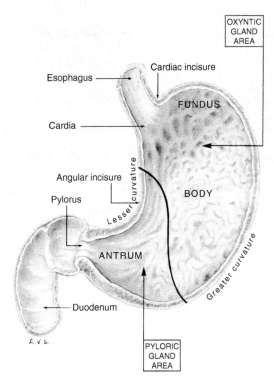

Cardiac glands mainly produce mucus. Oxyntic glands mainly produce pepsinogen, histamine, and HCl. Pyloric glands mainly produce mucus and gastrin.

FIGURE 1–70. **The stomach.**

The line drawn from the lesser to the greater curvature depicts the approximate boundary between the oxyntic gland area and the pyloric gland area. No prominent landmark exists to distinguish between antrum and body (corpus). The fundus is the portion craniad to the esophagogastric junction. (Reproduced, with permission, from Way LW, Doherty GM (eds). *Current Surgical Diagnosis and Treatment*, 11th ed. New York: McGraw-Hill, 2002.)

Pyloric stenosis in children causes violent, nonbilious projectile vomiting.

SPHINCTERS OF THE STOMACH

- **Cardiac/lower esophageal sphincter**
- Composed of:
- Internal esophageal sphincter (intrinsic esophageal muscle).
- External sphincter (crura of diaphragm).
- **Pyloric sphincter**
- Outlet of stomach into duodenum.

BLOOD SUPPLY TO STOMACH (FIGURE 1–71)

Artery	Description
Splenic artery	Direct branch of celiac trunk Supplies: ◦ Spleen ◦ Stomach Branches: ◦ Short gastrics to fundus ◦ Left gastroepiploic to left greater curvature
Left gastric artery	Direct branch of celiac trunk. Supplies: ◦ Left lesser curvature of stomach ◦ Inferior esophagus
Right gastric artery	Branch of gastroduodenal (a branch of the hepatic artery proper off the celiac trunk) Supplies: ◦ Right lesser curvature of the stomach
Right gastroepiploic	Branch of gastroduodenal Supplies: ◦ Right 1/2 greater curvature of stomach ◦ Gastric ulcer likely bleeds from this

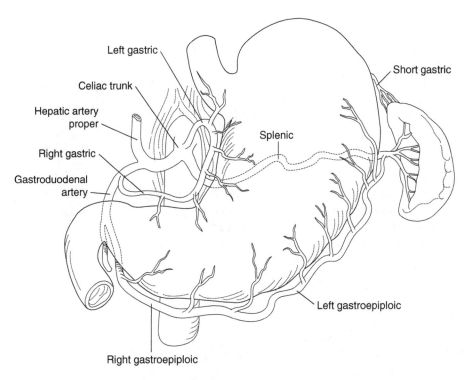

Left gastric

Celiac trunk

Hepatic artery
proper

Right gastric

Gastroduodenal
artery

Short gastric

Splenic

Left gastroepiploic

Right gastroepiploic

FIGURE 1–71. **Blood supply to the stomach.**

Reproduced, with permission, from Bhushan V, et al. *First Aid for the USMLE Step 1.* New York: McGraw-Hill, 2003.

Liver

Function	Anatomy	Blood Flow
Metabolic Produces bile. Involved in cholesterol metabolism. Urea cycle. Produces proteins. Clotting factors. Enzymes. **Detoxification** Liver enzymes. Receives substances from portal blood. **Phagocytosis** **Kupffer cells** (phagocytic); line sinusoids. Filter bacteria and other particles.	Lies under right diaphragm. Two lobes (large right, small left). **Falciform ligament** Attaches to anterior body wall. **Coronary ligaments** Attach liver to diaphragm. **Hepatic sinusoids** With fenestrated endothelial cells. Permit flow of serum across. **Portal triad** Structural unit.	**Arterial supply** Hepatic artery. From common hepatic artery (branch of the celiac trunk). Oxygenated blood to keep liver viable. **Portal venous blood** Drains intestines. Filtering. Detoxification of newly absorbed substances. All blood (hepatic artery and portal blood) is emptied into the same **sinusoids.** Sinusoids empty into **common central vein.** Central vein empties into hepatic veins. **Hepatic veins** empty into **IVC.**

Spleen

- Develops from mesenchymal cells (of the mesentery attached to primitive stomach).
  - **Does not** develop from the primitive gut (ie, forgut, midgut, hindgut).
- Lies in the left hypochondrium (of the abdominal cavity).
  - Between the stomach and diaphragm.
- Ovoid organ.
- Size of a fist.
- Functions:
  - Blood reservoir.
  - Phagocytosis (foreign particles and red blood cell [RBC] senescence).
  - Production of mononuclear leukocytes.
- Blood supply: Splenic artery (from celiac trunk).
- Venous drainage: Splenic vein (part of portal system).
- Innervation: From celiac plexus.
- Histology.
  - White pulp.
    - Lymphocytes located around splenic artery branches.
  - Red pulp.
  - Blood-filled sinusoids.
  - Phagocytic cells (macrophages, monocytes).
  - Lymphocytes.
  - Plasma cells.

*The gallbladder **does not** contain a submucosa (the stomach and small and large bowel do).*

Bile is composed of bile salts, pigments, cholesterol, and lecithin. Bile serves to emulsify fats, and fat-soluble vitamins (A, D, E, K).

Gallbladder

- Pouch on inferior surface of liver.
- Stores and concentrates bile.
- Bile is produced by the liver.
- **Common bile duct** formed by:
  - Cystic duct (from gallbladder).
  - Hepatic duct (from liver).
- Common bile duct empties into duodenum.
- Sphincter of Oddi (ampulla of Vater) (on duodenal papilla).
  - Relaxes:
    - Cholecystokinin; fat into intestine.
    - Gallbladder contracts
    - Bile released into duodenum for fat emulsion.
  - Contracts:
    - No cholecystokinin; intestine is empty.
    - Forcing bile up the cystic duct to the gallbladder for storage.
- Blood supply: Cystic artery (branch of right hepatic).
- Innervation: Vagal fibers (celiac plexus).
- Lymph drains into cystic lymph node, then hepatic nodes, then celiac nodes.

Small Intestine

Segment	Blood Supply	Description
Duodenum	Superior pancreaticoduodenal artery (indirect Celiac branch) Inferior pancreaticoduodenal artery (of SMA)	C-shaped. Surrounds pancreas. Shortest and widest part of small intestine. Part of it is retroperitoneal. Connects stomach to jejunum. Common bile duct and pancreatic duct empty into duodenum at duodenal papilla. Contains Brunners glands (submucosal glands) secreting mucous.
Jejunum	SMA—intestinal branches	Valves of Kerckring (plicae circulares). Most villi (for greatest absorption). Thickest muscular wall (of any small intestine segment; for peristalsis).
Ileum	SMA—intestinal branches and ileocolic branch	Peyer's patches. Vitamin B_{12} and bile salt absorption. More goblet cells and mesenteric fat than jejunum. **No** plicae circulares in lower lieum.

> *Enzymes present in intestinal villi:*
>
> - Carbohydrate
>   - Maltase
>   - Sucrase
>   - Lactase
> - Protein
> - Aminopeptidase
> - Dipeptidase
> - Activating pancreatic enzymes
>   - Enterokinase
>   - Converts trypsinogen to trypsin.
>   - Trypsin activates other pancreatic enzymes.

Large Intestine

- Extends from ileocecal valve to anus.
- Site of fluid and electrolyte reabsorption.
- Lack villi (unlike small intestine).
- **Does not** secrete enzymes or have enzymes along brush border (unlike small intestine).
- Has goblet cells, absorptive cells, microvilli (see Chapter 2).

Descending and sigmoid colon, rectum, and anus are part of the hindgut, so they are supplied by the pelvic splanchnic nerves rather than the vagus.

Segment	Blood Supply	Description
Cecum	SMA; cecal branches, appendicular artery (to appendix)	"Blind sac" Ileocecal valve enters Vermiform appendix Lymphoid tissue
Colon ▫ Ascending ▫ Transverse ▫ Descending ▫ Sigmoid	SMA—Ileocolic, right colic SMA—Middle colic IMA—Left colic IMA—Sigmoid	1/4 length of small intestine Larger diameter than small intestine **Teniae coli** (3 smooth muscle bands) **Haustra** (pouches created by teniae) **Epiploic appendages** (fat globules on serosal surface) Ascending and descending colon are retroperitoneal
Rectum	IMA—Superior rectal artery ▫ Middle rectal arteries (of hypogastric)	From sigmoid to anus Straight Located with in pelvic cavity **No** teniae **No** Haustra **No** epiploic appendages
Anal canal	Internal iliac— ▫ Inferior rectal (of internal pudendal)	Last 3–4 cm of rectum Internal sphincter (involuntary) External sphincter (volunatary)

> *Each part of the colon alternates between retroperitoneal and intraperitoneal.*
>
> ▫ Ascending colon (retroperitoneal)
> ▫ Transverse colon (intraperitoneal)
> ▫ Descending colon (retroperitoneal)
> ▫ Sigmoid (intraperitoneal)
> ▫ Rectum (retroperitoneal)

PEYER'S PATCHES

▫ Subepithelial, nonencapsulated lymphoid tissue (like tonsils).
▫ Located in ileum (small intestine).
▫ Limit numbers of harmful bacteria.

Retroperitoneal Structures (Figure 1–72)

▫ **Not** suspended from mesenteries.
▫ Plastered against posterior body wall, behind the peritoneum.

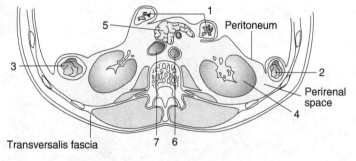

1. Duodenum (2nd, 3rd, 4th parts)
2. Descending colon
3. Ascending colon
4. Kidney and ureters
5. Pancreas (except tail)
3. Aorta
7. IVC
Adrenal glands and rectum (not shown in diagram)

FIGURE 1-72. **Retroperitoneal structures.**

Reproduced, with permission, from Bhushan V, et al. *First Aid for the USMLE Step 1*. New York: McGraw-Hill, 2003.

Posterior Abdominal Muscles

Muscle	Innervation
Psoas major and minor	Lumbar plexus
Quadratus lumborum	Lumbar plexus
Iliacus	Femoral nerve

Pancreas

- Lobulated gland.
- Extends from curve of duodenum to spleen.
- Retroperitoneal (except for small portion of tail).
- **Head** (from ventral bud)
  - Lies in the C (concavity) of the duodenum.
  - Located to right of midline (anterior to origin of SMA).
  - Extends from L1–3.
- **Body:** Extends across; splenic vein lies underneath.
- **Tail:** Abuts spleen hilum (intraperitoneal, covered by lienorenal ligament).

PANCREATIC DUCTS

- **Duct of Wirsung** (main pancreatic duct)
  - Begins at tail and joins common bile duct to form ampulla of Vater (hepatopancreatic ampulla), where it empties into duodenum.
- **Santorini's duct** (accessory pancreatic duct)
  - Opens separately into duodenum (when present).

Adrenal Gland

- Triangular glands.
- Located in adipose tissue on superior aspect of kidneys.

ADRENAL CORTEX

- Develops from mesoderm (**unlike** medulla).

ADRENAL MEDULLA

- Modified nervous tissue (like postganglionic sympathetic cells).
- Develops from neuroectoderm.
  - Neural crest cells differentiate into medullary cells (chromaffin cells).
- Releases
  - Epinephrine.
  - Norepinephrine.
- Same effect as direct sympathetic stimulation but lasts longer.
- **Can** live without adrenal medulla because postganglionic cells provide same function and will compensate for the loss.

Retroperitoneal pneumonic:

RAKE A CUPID

Rectum

Aorta

Kidneys

Esophagus

Adrenal glands

Colon (ascending/descending)

Ureters

Pancreas

Inf. vena cava

Duodenum (distal 3/4th)

Bile and pancreatic enzymes are released at ampulla of Vater into the second part of duodenum.

Urinary System

- Consists of:
  - Kidneys (2).
  - Ureters (2).
  - Urinary bladder.
  - Urethra.
- Lined with transitional epithelium.
- Parasympathetic fibers from pelvic splanchnic nerve.
- Kidneys, ureters, and bladder are all retroperitoneal.

As ureter enters pelvic cavity it crosses over the top of the common iliac artery (at its point of bifurcation) and dives deep into the pelvis.

Kidney

See Figure 1–73.

- Retroperitoneal.
- Upper portion protected by ribs 11 and 12.
- Left kidney attached to the spleen by the lienorenal ligament.

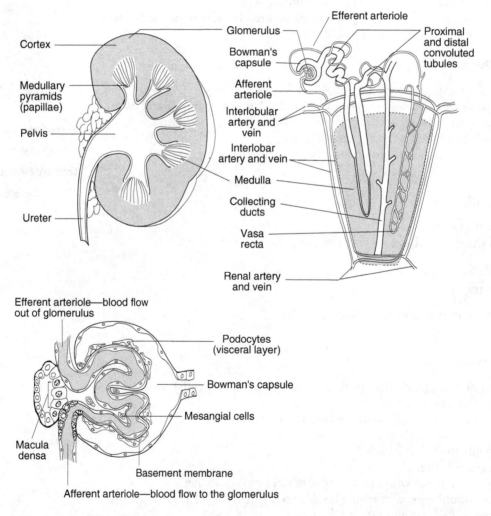

FIGURE 1–73. Structure of the kidney.

Reproduced, with permission, from Bhushan V, et al. *First Aid for the USMLE Step 1.* New York: McGraw-Hill, 2003. (Adapted from McPhee S, et al. *Pathophysiology of Disease: An Introduction to Clinical Medicine,* 3rd ed. New York, McGraw-Hill, 2000.)

URETER

- Long slender muscular tubes (peristalse).
- Transports urine from kidney to urinary bladder.
- Travels in retroperitoneal location.

Females are more prone to urinary infections because of the shorter urethra.

URETHRA

- Passes urine from bladder to outside.
- Female: 4 cm; opens into vestibule (between clitoris and vagina).
- Male: 20 cm; travels through penis; also conveys semen.

URINARY BLADDER

- Distensible sac in pelvic cavity; posterior to pubic symphysis.
- Holds urine.

Pelvic Cavity

- From anterior to posterior:
  - Bladder
  - Uterus
  - Rectum
- **Females:** Paired ovaries and single uterus
  - Vesicouterine pouch
    - Between bladder and uterus
  - Rectouterine pouch
  - Between rectum and uterus
- **Males:** Paired ductus deferens and seminal vesicles, and single prostate
  - Rectovesicle pouch
    - Between rectum and bladder

Inguinal Canal

- **Females:** Round ligament of the uterus.
  - Fibromuscular band attached to the uterus extending from fallopian tube, through inguinal canal to labia majora.
- **Males:** Spermatic cord.
  - Suspends the testes within the scrotum.

The inguinal canal is larger in males than females.

SPERMATIC CORD

Layers	Contents
External spermatic fascia	Ductus deferens
Cremaster muscle	Testicular artery
Internal spermatic fascia	Pampiniform plexus
Loose areolar tissue	Vessels and nerves of ductus deferens
Remnants of the processus vaginalis	

Remember: SEVEN-UP

Seminiferous tubules

Epididymis

Vas deferens

Ejaculatory duct

(Nothing)

Urethra

Penis

- **Ductus (Vas) deferens:** Conveys epididymis from testis to ejaculatory duct.
- **Ejaculatory duct** (ductus deferens + seminal vesicle ducts): Empties into prostatic urethra.
- **Pampiniform plexus:** Form the testicular vein.
  - Left testicular vein drains into left renal vein.
  - Right testicular vein drains into the IVC.

DEFECATION

- Mediated by pelvic and pudendal nerves.
- Internal sphincter relaxes
  - Pelvic nerve (senses distention then reflexively relaxes internal sphincter).
- External anal sphincter contracts
  - Pudendal nerve.
- Conscious urge to defecate is sensed.

▶ NEUROANATOMY

Nervous System

- Peripheral nervous system = Somatic.
- Autonomic system = Visceral.
- Myenteric nervous system = GI, intrinsic.

Central nervous system =

Brain + spinal cord.

Brain

See the "Embryology" section in Chapter 4 for derivation.

CEREBRUM

See Figure 1–74 for functions of the cerebral cortex.

- Is 80% of brain mass.
- Has four paired lobes within two cerebral hemispheres.
- Commands higher function.
- See also the section "Homunculus" in Chapter 10.

Component	Description
Cerebral cortex	Gray matter externally (6 layers)
Cerebral medulla	Internal white matter (myelinated)
Corpus callosum	White matter tracts; connect the two hemispheres

Area	Function
Frontal lobe (precentral gyrus: 4)	Primary motor area
Frontal lobe	Frontal association areas; executive function
Parietal lobe (postcentral gyrus: 3, 1, 2)	Primary sensory area
Parietal lobe	Taste (tongue distribution on homunculus)
Parietal lobe	Integration and interpretation areas
Temporal lobe	Olfaction
	Hearing/auditory cortex
Occipital	Visual cortex (17)

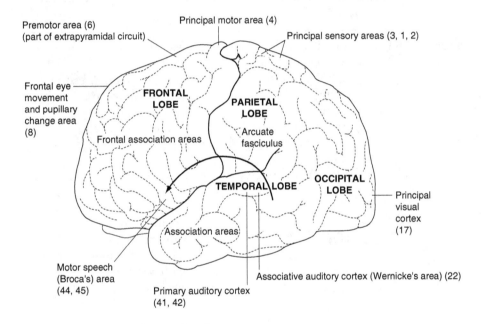

FIGURE 1–74. Cerebral cortex functions.

Reproduced, with permission, from Bhushan V, et al. *First Aid for the USMLE Step 1.* New York: McGraw-Hill, 2003.

Remember: Diencephalon contributes to Rathke's pouch (forming part of posterior pituitary).

- **Basal nuclei** modulate motor activity first initiated from area 4: precentral gyrus of frontal lobe.

DIENCEPHALON

The diencephalon consists of:

- Thalamus.
- Hypothalamus.
- Epithalamus.
    - Pineal gland is located within epithalamus.
        - Releases melatonin (as does hypothalamus); plays a role in:
            - Circadian rhythms/sleep—wake cycle.
            - Body temperature regulation.
            - Appetite.
- Pituitary gland (See Chapters 2 and 17).

	General	Nuclei	Functions
Thalamus	Sensory relay station	Lateral geniculate	Visual
		Medial geniculate	Auditory
		Ventral posterior lateral (VPL)	Proprioception, pressure, touch, vibration
		Ventral posterior medial (VPM)	**Facial sensation (including pain)**
		Vental anterior/ventral lateral	Motor
Hypothalamus	Body homeostasis	Ventromedial nucleus	Satiety center (hyperphagia with bilateral destruction; decreases urge to eat with stimulation)
		Lateral nucleus	Hunger center (starvation with destruction; increase eating with stimulation)
		Septal nucleus	Aggressive behavior
		Suprachiasmatic nucleus	Circadian rhythms; input from retina
		Supraoptic nucleus	Water balance; ADH, oxytocin production

CEREBELLUM

Function	Components
Coordinates muscle movement Maintains equilibrium and posture Receives proprioceptive inputs and position sense (eg, dorsal columns)	**Purkinje cells:** Project to deep cerebellar nuclei (which then project out of cerebellum) **Climbing fibers:** Afferents to cerebellum **Golgi cell bodies** **Granule cells** **Mossy fibers:** All afferents to cerebellum (except climbing fibers)

BRAIN STEM

See Figure 1–75 for a ventral view of the brain stem.

- Connects cerebrum and spinal cord (fiber tracts to and from spinal cord pass).
- Embryologically is the midbrain + hindbrain.
- Cranial nerves (3–12) originate from brain stem.
- Basic life functions:
  - Respiration.
  - Swallowing.
  - Heart rate.
  - Arousal.

Segment	Comments
Midbrain	Auditory and visual reflex
Pons	Relay station
	Respiratory center
Medulla oblongata	Relay station
	Respiratory, cardiac, vasomotor centers
	Reflexes: coughing, gagging, swallowing, vomiting

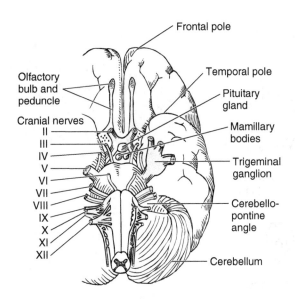

FIGURE 1–75. Ventral view of the brain stem with cranial verves.

All cranial nerves (except I and II) originate from the brain stem.

Tracts: Olfactory, Optic; no nuclei for CNs I and II.

Reproduced, with permission, from Waxman SG. *Clinical Neuroanatomy.* 25th ed. McGraw-Hill, 2003.

All cranial nerve motor nuclei have unilateral corticonuclear connections except:

- *CN VII: Upper third muscles of facial expression have bilateral innervation.*
- *CN XII: Genioglossus muscles have bilateral motor innervation.*

All cranial nerve sensory nuclei have unilateral representation except hearing. Hearing is bilateral; you can't go deaf in one ear from a stroke to the unilateral temporal area.

The mnemonic for the cranial nerves is: On Old Olympus' Towering Top a Finely Vested German Viewed A Hawk.

Remember: *Taste to the anterior 2/3 of the tongue is CN VII via the chorda tympani and the posterior 1/3 by CN IX. CN X caries taste fibers from the palate.*

IMPORTANT BRAIN STEM NUCLEI

		Nuclei (CN)	Function
Efferent (motor/ parasympathetic)	Receive higher levels information (eg, cortical) then project efferent neurons to end organs (via ganglia in the case of parasympathetics).	**Superior salivatory nucleus** (VII)	Salivation (submandibular, sublingual glands), Glandular secretion
		Inferior salivatory nuclei (IX)	Salivation (parotid)
		Nucleus ambiguous (IX, X)	Swallowing
Afferent (sensory)	Receives sensory information and relays this to the thalamus and cortex.	**Nucleus of the solitary tract (VII, IX, X)**	Taste

Cranial Nerves

- Olfactory (I)
- Optic (II)
- Oculomotor (III)
- Troclear (IV)
- Trigeminal (V)
- Abducens (VI)
- Facial (VII)
- Vestibulocochlear/auditory (VIII)
- Glossopharyngeal (IX)
- Vagus (X)
- Spinal accessory (XI)
- Hypoglossal (XII)

CRANIAL NERVE COMPONENTS

See Table 1–3 for a complete chart of the cranial nerves.

- **Sensory:** I, II, VIII
- **Motor:** III, IV, VI, XI, XII
- **Sensory and motor:** V, VII, IX, X

Characteristic		Cranial Nerves
General afferent	Sensory	V, VII, IX, X
	Proprioceptive	V, VII
Special afferent (*special sense*)		I, II, VII, VIII, IX, XI
Voluntary efferent (*motor to skeletal muscle*)		III, IV, V, VI, VII, IX, X, XI, XII
Involuntary efferent (*parasympathetic to smooth muscle or glands*)		III, VII, IX, X

Preganglionic parasympathetics are provided by CNS III (ciliary ganglion), VII (pterygomandibular and submandibular ganglia), IX (otic ganglion), and X (small terminal ganglia).

PARASYMPATHETIC GANGLIA (AND CRANIAL NERVES)

Ganglion	Location	Parasympathetic Root	Sympathetic Root	Distribution
Ciliary	Lateral to optic nerve	CN III	Internal carotid plexus	Ciliary muscle Spincter pupillae Dilator Pupillae Tarsal muscles
Pterygopalatine	Pterygopalatine fossa (on branch of V2)	Greater petrosal (CN VII) N. of pterygoid canal	Internal carotid plexus	Lacrimal gland Glands in palate and nose
Otic	Just distal to Foramen ovale (on trunk of V3)	Lesser petrosal (CN IX) (and tympanic branch of CN IX)	Plexus associated with middle meningeal artery	Parotid gland
Submandibular	On Hyoglossus muscle (on Lingual n. of V3)	Chorda tympani (CN VII) by way of lingual nerve	Plexus on facial artery	Submandibular Sublingual small salivary glands

SYMPATHETIC GANGLIA OF THE HEAD AND NECK

Ganglia	Location	Comments
Superior cervical ganglia	Lies between ICA and IJV at level of T1–T2.	Largest and responsible for most sympathetic fibers to head and neck (cell bodies of postganglionics are here); these postganglionics give rise to the plexuses in the parasympathetic ganglia chart.
Middle cervical ganglia	At level of cricoid cartilage.	Related to loop of inferior thyroid artery.
Inferior cervical ganglia	C7 vertebral level.	Fused to first thoracic sympathetic ganglion to forma stellate ganglion.

Preganglionics come from the T1–2 (ciliospinal center of Budge) where they have descended from the brain stem.

115

TABLE 1–3.   Cranial Nerve Chart

CRANIAL NERVE	(DIVISION)	TO/FROM SKULL	TYPE	ORIGIN OF CELL BODIES	FUNCTION	INNERVATED STRUCTURES	
						AFFERENT	EFFERENT
I-Olfactory		Cribriform plate	SVA	Bipolar cells	Smell	Nasal mucosa	
II-Optic		Optic foramen	SSA	Retinal ganglion cells	Vision, pupillary light reflexes (with CN III)	Retina	
III-Oculomotor		Superior orbital fissure	GSE	Oculomotor nucleus (rostral midbrain)	Ocular movements		Levator palpebrae, all extraocular muscles, except lateral rectus, superior oblique, pupillary constrictor (ciliary ganglion), ciliary muscle (ciliary ganglion)
			GVE	Edinger-Westphal nucleus (rostral midbrain) (ciliary ganglion)	Miosis, convergence, accommodation		
IV-Troclear		SOF	GSE	Trochlear nucleus (caudal midbrain)	Turns eye down and laterally		Superior oblique
VI-Abducens		SOF	GSE	Abducent nucleus (caudal pons)	Turns eye laterally		Lateral rectus
V-Trigeminal	V1 (Ophthalmic)	SOF	GSA	Trigeminal ganglion and mesencephalic nucleus of CN V	Facial sensation	Upper eyelid, globe, lacrimal gland, paranasal sinus mucous membrane, forehead skin	

(Continued)

CRANIAL NERVE	(DIVISION)	TO/FROM SKULL	TYPE	ORIGIN OF CELL BODIES	FUNCTION	INNERVATED STRUCTURES	
						AFFERENT	EFFERENT
	V2 (Maxillary)	Foramen rotundum	GSA		Sensation	Lower eyelid, mid-face skin, upper lip, nasopharynx, maxillary sinus, soft palate, tonsils, hard palate, upper teeth	
	V3 (Mandibular)	Foramen ovale	GSA		Sensation	Anterior 2/3rd of tongue (general not taste sensation!), temporoauricular skin, lower face, lower teeth	
			SVE	Motor nucleus CN V (mid pons)	Chewing, opening, swallowing		Muscles of mastication, tensor veli palatini, tensor tympani
VII-Facial		Internal acoustic meatus, stylomastoid foramen	GSA	Geniculate ganglion (facial canal of temporal bone)	Sensation	External ear, soft palate, auditory tube	
			SVA	Geniculate ganglion (facial canal)	Taste	Anterior 2/3rd tongue	
			SVE	Facial nucleus (caudal pons)	Facial expression		Ms. Facial expression, stylohyoid, postdigastric, stapedius

(Continued)

117

TABLE 1-3. **Cranial Nerve Chart (Continued)**

CRANIAL NERVE	(DIVISION)	TO/FROM SKULL	TYPE	ORIGIN OF CELL BODIES	FUNCTION	INNERVATED STRUCTURES	
						AFFERENT	EFFERENT
			GVE	Superior salivatory nucleus (caudal pons)	Secretomotor		Lacrimal gland, glands of nasopharynx and sinuses (pterygopalatine ganglion)
							Submandibular and sublingual glands (submandibular ganglion)
VIII-Vestibulo-cochlear (auditory)		Internal acoustic meatus	SSA	Spiral ganglion (modiolus)	Hearing	Organ of corti (cochlea)	
				Vestibular ganglion (int. auditory meatus)	Balance	Semicircular canals (vestibular)	
IX-Glossophar-yngeal		Jugular foramen	GSA	Superior ganglion (jugular foramen)	Sensation	Auricle	
			GVA	Inferior petrosal ganglion (jugular foramen)	Sensation	Posterior 1/3 tongue, pharynx, middle ear	
			GVA	Inferior petrosal ganglion (jugular foramen)	Chemoreception, baroreception	Carotid body, carotid sinus	
			SVA	Inferior petrosal ganglion (jugular foramen)	Taste	Post 1/3 tongue	

(Continued)

TABLE 1–3. **Cranial Nerve Chart (Continued)**

CRANIAL NERVE	(DIVISION)	TO/FROM SKULL	TYPE	ORIGIN OF CELL BODIES	FUNCTION	INNERVATED STRUCTURES	
						AFFERENT	EFFERENT
			SVE	Nucleus ambiguus (rostral medulla)	Motor for swallowing		Stylopharyngeus
			GVE	Inferior salivatory nucleus (rostral medulla)	Secretomotor		Parotid gland (via otic ganglion and aurioculotemporal branch of V3), parasympathetic path of pharynx, larynx
X-Vagus		Jugular foramen	GSA	Superior ganglion (jugular foramen)	Sensation	Posterior meninges, external ear	
			GVA	Nodose ganglion (jugular foramen)	Sensation	Viscera of pharynx, larynx, thoracic and abdominal viscera (to left colic flexure)	
			SVA	Nodose ganglion (jugular foramen)	Taste	Laryngeal additus and epiglottis	
			SVE	Nucleus ambiguus (medulla)	Motor		Pharyngeal constrictors, palatopharyngeus, levator palatini, palatoglossus, laryngeal ms

(Continued)

TABLE 1-3.   Cranial Nerve Chart (Continued)

CRANIAL NERVE	(DIVISION)	TO/FROM SKULL	TYPE	ORIGIN OF CELL BODIES	FUNCTION	INNERVATED STRUCTURES	
						AFFERENT	EFFERENT
			GVE	Dorsal nucleus of CN X (medulla)	Secretomotor		Viscera of neck, thoracic and abdominal cavities (to left colic flexure)
XI-Spinal accessory	Cranial	Jugular foramen	SVE	Nucleus ambiguus (medulla)	Motor		Cranial-ms larynx, pharynx, esophagus
	Spinal	Foramen magnum		Ventral horn C1–C6			Spinal—SCM, trapezius
XI-Hypoglossal		Hypoglossal canal	GVE	Hypoglossal nucleus (medulla)	Motor		All intrinsic and extrinsic muscle of tongue (not palatoglossus)

CN II–Optic Nerve

See Figure 1–76 and Table 1–3.
See also the "Neurophysiology" section in Chapter 10 for lesions involving the optic nerve.

Course

- Ganglion cells of retina (converge at optic disc to form optic nerve).
- Leaves orbit via optic foramen/canal (sphenoid).
- Optic chiasm (two optic nerves unite at floor of diencephalons; anterior to pituitary stalk).
- Optic tracts.
- Lateral geniculate nuclei (thalamus).
- Geniculocalcarine fibers (optic radiations).
- Calcarine sulcus in the primary visual cortex (area 17) of the occipital lobe.

Important

- Nasal side fibers (most medial) decussate and go with contralateral optic tract.
- Temporal hemiretina fibers stay ipsilateral.
- Left visual field = right optic tract.
- Right visual field = left optic tract (right visual field is interpreted on left brain).

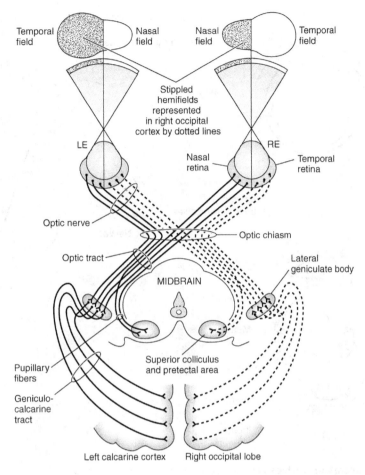

FIGURE 1-76. **The optic pathway.**

The dotted lines represent nerve fibers that carry visual and papillary afferent impulses from the left half of the visual field. (Reproduced, with permission, from Riordan-Eva P, Hoyt WF. *Vaughan and Asbury's General Ophthalmology*, 17th ed. New York: McGraw-Hill, 2008.)

CNs III, IV, VI—Oculomotor, Trochlear, Abducens

See Figure 1–77.

▪ **Oculomotor nerve:** Controls most of the extraocular muscles, the levator palpebrae superioris, and carries parasympathetic and sympathetic control to the pupil.
▪ **Trochlear nerve:** Is the smallest cranial nerve and the only cranial nerve that exits from the posterior surface of the brain stem.

Extraocular Movements

Muscle	Nerve	Movement
Medial rectus	CN III	Adduction (in)
Superior rectus	CN III	Elevation and adduction
Inferior rectus	CN III	Depression and adduction
Inferior oblique	CN III	Elevation and abduction
Superior oblique	CN IV	Depression and abduction
Lateral rectus	CN VI	Abduction (out)

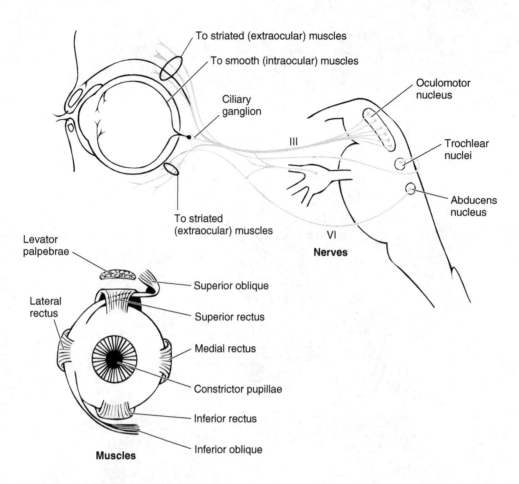

FIGURE 1–77. The occulomotor, trochlear, and abducens nverves; ocular muscles.

Reproduced, with permission, from Waxman SG. *Clinical Neuroanatomy*, 25th ed. New York: McGraw-Hill, 2003.

EYE ELEVATORS

See Figure 1–78 for a diagram of the eye muscle action.

- **Superior rectus:** Adducts and elevates (only muscle that elevates from abducted position).
- **Inferior oblique:** Abducts and elevates (only muscle to elevate from adducted position).

Pupillary Light Reflex

- Direct and consensual papillary responses.
- Does **not** involve cortex.
- Shine light into one eye that eye (direct) pupil constricts as does the pupil of the contralateral eye (consensual).

Response	Afferent	Efferent
Direct response	Optic nerve of eye tested (ipsilateral)	CN III to the eye tested (ipsilateral)
Consensual response	Optic nerve of eye tested (ipsilateral)	CN III of opposite eye (contralateral)

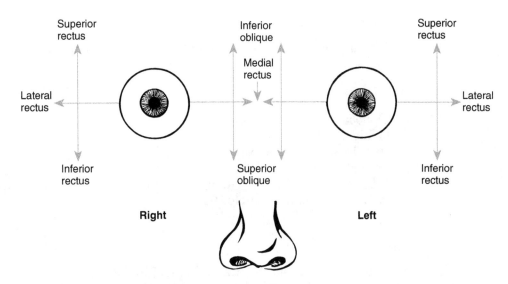

FIGURE 1–78. Diagram of eye muscle action.

Reproduced, with permission, from Waxman SG. *Clinical Neuroanatomy*, 25th ed. New York: McGraw-Hill, 2003.

Pathway/Reflex Arc

See Figure 1–79.

- Optic nerve
- Edinger-Westphal nucleus (midbrain) bilaterally
- Ciliary ganglia
- Short ciliary nerve (postganglionic)
- Constrictor pupillae muscle

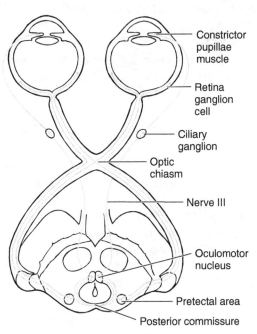

FIGURE 1–79. The path of the papillary light reflex.

Reproduced, with permission, from Waxman SG. *Clinical Neuroanatomy*. 25th ed. New York: McGraw-Hill, 2003.

ACCOMMODATION AND CONVERGENCE

- Gazing from distant to near, pupils constrict (accommodate), eyes move midline (converge), lenses become more convex.

Pathway

- Optic nerve
- Geniculate body
- Visual association cortex
- Frontal eye fields
- Edinger-Westphal nuclei and main oculomotor nuclei (both in midbrain)
- Constrictor pupillae muscle and medial recti, respectively

LESION

- Blurred vision with a lesion to any of CN III, IV, VI.
- Ptosis (drooping eyelid) and dilated pupil with CN III injury (levator palpebrae superioris and sphincter pupillae muscle).
- Lesion CN VI eye persistently directed toward nose (because of lateral rectus).
- See Table 1–4.

TABLE 1–4. Common Lesions to CN III, IV, and VI

LESION	DESCRIPTION
Ophthalmoplegia	Internal: EOMs spared, selective loss of autonomically innervated sphincter and ciliary muscles (because parasympathetic fibers are more peripheral, can be compressed). External: Paralysis of all EOMs (except superior oblique, rectus); sphincter and ciliary muscles spared (as with DM neuropathy).
Internuclear ophthalmoplegia	Lesion within the medial longitudinal fasciculus—lose connection III, IV, VI. If lesion on right—look laterally to the right, both eyes move look laterally to left, only left eye moves (right eye medial rectus does not pull it medially); however with accommodation, both medial recti work.
Relative afferent (Marcus-Gunn) pupil	Lesion in optic nerve (afferent limb of papillary light relflex, eg, MS optic neuritis). Swinging flashlight test—both pupils constrict when shine light in good eye; quickly swing to contralateral eye and both pupils dilate.
Horner's syndrome	Lesion of oculosympathic pathway (sympathetics don't come from CNs but run with them; come from superior cervical ganglion, ciliospinal center of Budge); miosis, ptosis, hemianhidrosis, apparent enophthalmos.
Argyll Robertson pupil (pupillary light-near dissociation)	Think prostitute's pupil—accommodates but does not react; also associated with syphilis. No miosis (papillary constriction) with either direct or consensual light; does constrict with near stimulus (accommodation-convergence). Occurs in syphilis and diabetes.

CN V—Trigeminal Nerve

- Largest cranial nerve.
- Trigeminal or gasserian ganglion—in the middle cranial fossa.
- Three divisions leave through foramina in the sphenoid bone.
- **Sensory (GSA):** Facial sensation (light touch; pain and temperature; proprioception)
  - Divisions V1, V2, V3.
- **Efferent (SVE):** Motor to muscles of mastication, tensor veli palatini, tensor tympani.
  - Division V3.
- **No** parasympathetic fibers are contained with the trigeminal nerve at its origin; other nerves distribute parasympathetic preganglionics by way of trigeminal branches.
  - Oculomotor (III).
  - Facial nerve (VII).
  - Glossopharyngeal nerve (IX).

V1 and V2 are purely sensory; V3 is both sensory and motor.

Remember: The buccal nerve of V3 provides sensation to the cheek; whereas the buccal branch of CN VII is motor to the buccinator muscle.

TRIGEMINAL NERVE DIVISIONS

See Figure 1–80 for the trigeminal nerve and its branches.

Division	Sensory	Motor
Ophthalmic (V1)	Upper eyelid, cornea, conjunctiva, frontal sinus, upper nasal mucosa, forehead	N/A
Maxillary (V2)	Lower eyelid, upper cheek, lip, gums, palate, nose, tonsils, hard palate, upper teeth	N/A
Mandibular (V3)	Tongue (general), temporoauricular skin, lower face, lower teeth	Muscles of mastication, tensor tympani, mylohyoid, anterior belly of digastric, tensor veli palatini

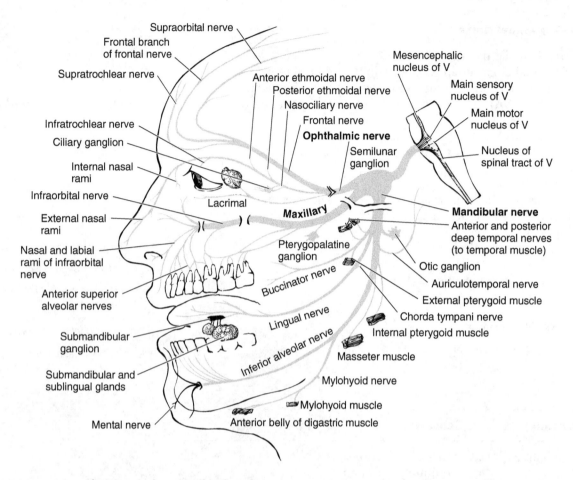

FIGURE 1-80. The trigeminal nerve and its branches.

Reproduced, with permission, from Waxman SG. *Clinical Neuroanatomy*, 25th ed. New York: McGraw-Hill, 2003.

IMPORTANT BRANCHES OF V3

Nerve	Distribution
Lingual nerve	**General sensation:** Anterior 2/3rd of tongue, floor of mouth, and mandibular lingual gingival. *Carries* (from chorda tympani [VII]): **Taste sensation:** Anterior 2/3rd tongue. **Preganglionic parasympathetics:** To submandibular ganglion.
Auriculotemporal nerve	**Sensory:** Front of ear, TMJ. **Postganglionic parasympathetic:** To parotid gland.
Inferior alveolar nerve	Gives off nerve to mylohyoid and inferior dental plexus; terminates as mental nerve. **Motor** to mylohyoid. **Sensory** to teeth, skin of chin, lower lip.
Mental nerve	Termination of inferior alveolar nerve. **Sensory** to skin of chin, skin, and mucous membrane of lower lip.
Motor branches	**Motor to** muscles of mastication, anterior digastric, and so on.

INFERIOR ALVEOLAR NERVE BLOCK

- Anesthetize the mandibular teeth.
- Block this branch of V3 as it enters the mandibular foramen.

Needle Course (See Figure 1–81)

- Pierces:
  - Buccinator (between palatoglossal and palatopharyngeal folds).
  - Lies lateral to medial pterygoid at the mandibular foramen.
- If the needle penetrates too far posteriorly can hit parotid gland and CN VII:
  - Ipsilateral facial paralysis.

*The lingual nerve is found in the pterygomandibular space with the inferior alveolar nerve, artery, and vein. The lingual artery does **not** run with the lingual nerve. The lingual artery is medial to the hyoglossus muscle, whereas the lingual vein and nerve are lateral to the hyoglossus (as is the submandibular duct and hypoglossal nerve [XII]).*

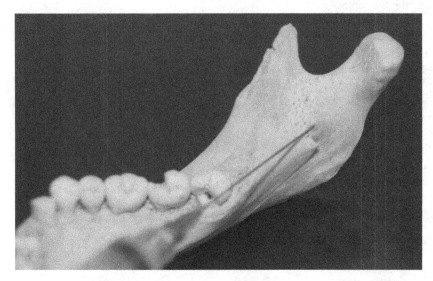

FIGURE 1–81. Needle course.

The submandibular duct is crossed twice by the lingual nerve.

*If the lingual nerve is cut after the chorda tympani joins, you lose **both** taste and tactile sensation.*

The lingual nerve can be damaged with third molar extraction because it lies close to the mandibular ramus in the vicinity of the third molar.

LINGUAL NERVE

Course	Information	Chorda Tympani (VII) Component
Lies deep to the lateral pterygoid muscle, anteromedial to the inferior alveolar nerve (chorda tympani (from VII) joins here). Runs between the medial pterygoid and the mandibular ramus to enter the side of the tongue obliquely. Continues forward between the hyoglossus and deep part of the submandibular gland. Submandibular ganglion hangs from lingual nerve on top of hyoglossus muscle. Finally, it runs across the submandibular duct to lie at the tongue tip (beneath the mucous membrane).	**General sensation:** Anterior 2/3rd of tongue, floor of mouth, and mandibular lingual gingiva.	Chorda tympani (of VII) contributes: <ul><li>Preganglionic parasympathetic fibers to submandibular ganglion.</li><li>Taste fibers to anterior 2/3rd of tongue.</li></ul>

TRIGEMINAL NUCLEI

- There are four paired nuclei (both motor and sensory).

Nuclei	Location	Comments
Motor (masticatory) nucleus	Lateral pons	Motor information originates in the motor (area 4) and premotor (area 6) cortices. This information is modulated by the basal ganglia and striatal motor systems then: Descends as corticobulbar tracts to the: Motor nucleus of the trigeminal where: LMNs then project past the trigeminal ganglion (without synapse) to the: Respective effector muscles.
Sensory nucleus	Pons	All sensory information from the face is relayed through **VPM nucleus of thalamus** (VPL for the body). From here information relays to the: **Somatosensory cortex** (areas 3, 1, 2). <ul><li>The facial segment of the sensory homunculus comprises a large area of the lateral parietal lobe.</li></ul>
Spinal trigeminal nucleus	Midpons to cervical cord	Pain/temperature from the face travel to the spinal trigeminal nucleus (pain/temperature from body travel in the spinothalamic tract).
Mesencephalic nucleus	Upper pons, midbrain border	Proprioceptive inputs are **not** located within the trigeminal ganglia (all other afferent cell bodies are). Proprioceptive inputs synapse in the mesencephalic nucleus.

Proprioceptive fibers from muscles and TMJ are found only in the mandibular division (V3).

FACIAL SENSATION

CN V

- All sensory information from the face is relayed through VPM nucleus of thalamus; sensory information from the rest of the body is through the VPL.
- From the thalamic nuclei (VPM or VPL), information relays to the somatosensory cortex (areas 3, 1, 2); the facial segment of the sensory homunculus comprises a large area of the lateral parietal lobe.
- Remember, parts of CNs VII and IX travel with trigeminospinal tract.
- All CN V afferent cell bodies are located within trigeminal ganglion **except** proprioceptive inputs.
- Mesencephalic nucleus of CN V is the only case where primary sensory cell bodies are located within the CNS, rather than in ganglia.

Modality	Fiber Type	Tract	1st-Order Neuron	2nd-Order Neuron	3rd-Order Neuron
Touch and pressure	A-beta fibers	Dorsal trigeminothalamic tract (via Meissner's and Pacini's corpuscles)	Trigeminal ganglion, (principal sensory nucleus of CN V).	Principal sensory nucleus of CN V projects to ipsilateral VPM (doesn't cross over).	VPM projects through posterior internal capsule to the face area of somatosensory cortex.
Pain and temperature	A-delta C-fibers	Ventral trigeminothalamic tract	Trigeminal ganglion; then axons descend in the spinal trigeminal tract and synapse with the spinal trigeminal nucleus.	From the spinal trigeminal nucleus, ascend and **cross over** to the contralateral VPM.	From VPM, project via posterior limb of posterior capsule to the face area of somatosensory cortex.
Proprioception	A-alpha fibers (stretch and tendon receptors in muscles of mastication)	Spinocerebellar tract	Afferents pass the trigeminal ganglia (without synapse).	Mesencephalic nucleus (within the CNS). Motor nucleus (many central fibers from mesencephalic nucleus synapse here to create reflex arc).	Cerebellum

Sensation in teeth can be misinterpreted in ear (because of the cross innervation).

Herpes zoster often affects V1 division. Trigeminal neuralgia (tic douloureux) can affect V2 and V3.

SENSORY INFORMATION IN THE FACE VERSUS BODY

	Face	Body
Touch and pressure	Trigeminal main sensory nucleus	Gracile and cuneate nuclei
		Dorsal columns
	Dorsal trigeminothalamic tract	Medial lemniscus
	VPM	VPL
Pain and temperature	Spinal trigeminal nucleus	Dorsal root ganglion
	Ventral trigeminothalamic tract	Lissauer's tract
		Spinothalamic tract
	VPM, periaqueductal grey, reticular formation	VPL, periaqueductal grey, reticular formation
Proprioception	Mesencephalic nucleus	Clarke's nucleus
	Spinocerebellar tract	Spinocerebellar tract
	Cerebellum	Cerebellum

FACIAL SENSATION

See Figure 1–82 for areas of facial sensation.
See Figure 1–83 for cutaneous innervation of the face, scalp, and uricle.
See Figure 1–84 for innervation of the external ear.

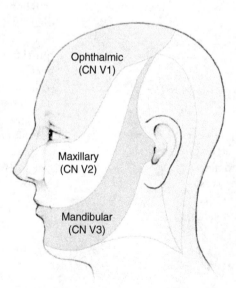

FIGURE 1–82. **Sensory distribution of CN V.**

Reproduced, with permission, from White JS. *USMLE Road Map Gross Anatomy.* New York: McGraw-Hill, 2003.

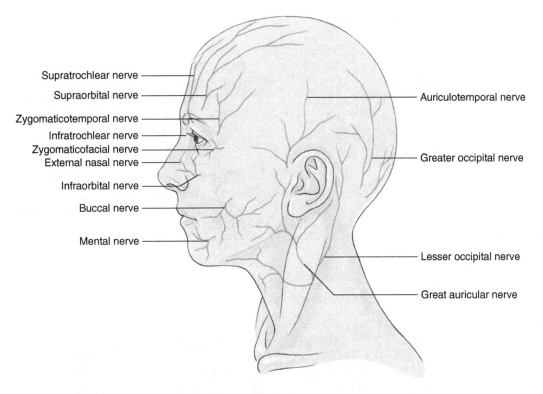

FIGURE 1–83. Cutaneous innervation of the face, scalp, and auricle.

SENSATION OF EXTERNAL EAR

Nerve	Distribution
Auriculotemporal nerve (V3)	Anterior half of external ear canal and facial surface of upper part of auricle
Auricular branch of vagus (CN X)	Posterior half of external ear canal (so stimulation can cause reflex symptoms: eg, fainting, coughing, gagging).
Greater auricular nerve (C2, C3)	Inferior auricle (anterior and posterior)
Lesser occipital nerve (C2, C3)	Cranial surface of upper auricle

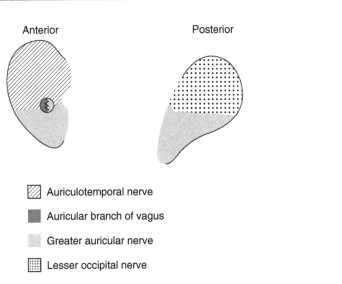

Corneal reflex: *If stimulating right eye:*

- Lesion R V1 neither eye blinks.
- Lesion L V1 bilateral blink.
- Lesion R VII only left eye blinks (indirect).
- Lesion L VII only right eye blinks (direct).

- Levator palpebrae superioris (CN III) keeps the eyelid open; lesion results in ptosis.
- Orbicularis oculi (CN VII) closes eyelid; lesion results in inability to close, no corneal reflex.

FIGURE 1–84. Innervation of the external ear.

131

TRIGEMINAL LESIONS

Type	Location	Finding
Sensory	Division V1, 2, 3	Deficits along distribution (pain, temperature, touch, pressure, proprioception)
Motor	Division V3 only	Temporalis and masseter muscles ▪ Ipsilateral weakness of jaw closure ▪ Ipsilateral open bite Pterygoid muscle ▪ Weakness of jaw opening ▪ Deviation to ipsilateral side on opening Diminished/loss of reflexes

Facial Reflexes (Involving CN V)

Reflex	Description	Afferent	Efferent	Comments
Corneal reflex	Touch cornea with cotton causes both eyes to close	V1	CN VII (orbicularis oculi)	**Pathway** ▪ Cornea (V1) ▪ Main sensory nucleus of trigeminal ▪ Medial longitudinal fasciculus ▪ Main motor nucleus of facial nerve (CN VII) ▪ Orbicularis oculi muscle ▪ Causes ipsilateral (**direct**) and contralateral (**indirect**) eye blinking
Jaw jerk reflex	Mouth open and relaxed; tap chin lightly to get contraction/mouth closure	V3 — proprioceptive	V3 — motor	Reflex is lost only with bilateral CN V lesions (uncommon)

CN VII-Facial Nerve

See Figure 1–85.

Facial Nerve Branches

Mnemonic: To Zanzibar By

Motor Car

Temporal

Zygomatic

Buccal

Marginal Mandibular

Cervical

Course

- Originates in pons.
- Enters internal acoustic meatus.
- Passes through facial canal.
- Exits skull via stylomastoid foramen.
- Courses through the parotid gland (inadvertent deposition of anesthetic into parotid can result in facial paresis).
- Motor branches.

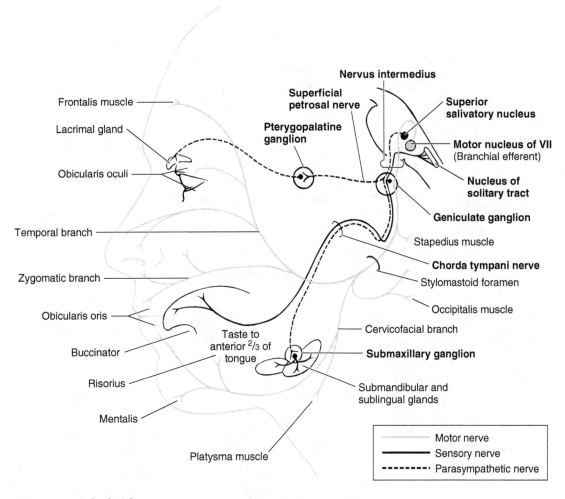

FIGURE 1-85. **The facial nerve.**

Reproduced, with permission, from Waxman SG. *Clinical Neuroanatomy*, 25th ed. New York: McGraw-Hill, 2003.

Components

- Motor
- Sensory
- Secretomotor (parasympathetic):
  - Lacrimal gland
  - Submandibular gland
  - Sublingual gland
- Special sense
  - Taste anterior two-thirds of tongue, floor of mouth, palate

CN VII NUCLEI

Nuclei	Comments
Main motor nucleus	Upper face receives bilateral innervation; lower face receives unilateral innervation. Muscles of facial expression, posterior belly of digastric, stylohyoid muscle, stapedius.
Superior salivatory nucleus	Submandibular and sublingual glands.
Nucleus of the solitary tract (gustatory nucleus)	Mediates taste.

FACIAL EXPRESSION

See Figure 1–86 for facial musculature.

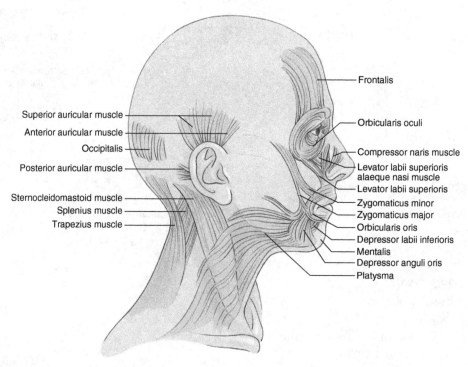

FIGURE 1–86. Facial musculature.

IMPORTANT MUSCLES OF FACIAL EXPRESSION (ALL CONTROLLED BY CN VII)

Muscle	Origin	Insertion	Action
Orbicularis oris	Circumoral muscles, maxilla, mandible	Lips and skin of lip	**Whistle** Pulls lips against teeth, protrudes lips
Depressor anguli oris	Mandibular oblique line	Angle of mouth	**Frown** Pulls down angle of mouth
Zygomaticus major	Zygomatic bone	Angle of mouth	**Smile** Pulls angle of mouth up and back
Risorius	Parotid and masseteric fascia	Angle of mouth	**Smile** Pulls angle of mouth laterally
Orbicularis oculi	Upper medial orbit, medial palpebral ligament, lacrimal bone	Encircle orbit; insert on medial palpebral, ligament medial side of lids, laterally in raphe	**Closes eye**

OTHER MUSCLES CONTROLLED BY CN VII

Muscle	Origin	Insertion	Action	Paralysis
Buccinator	Alveolar process of maxilla and mandible Pterygomandibular raphe	Orbicularis oris	Holds food on occlusal table (accessory muscle of mastication); tenses cheek (blowing, whistling)	Food/saliva fall between teeth and cheek
Stapedius		Neck of stapes	Decreases vibration of the stapes (decreases perception of sound)	Hyperacusis

CN VII LESIONS

Lesion	Clinical Finding	Comments
Lower motor neuron lesion	Ipsilateral paralysis/weakness of upper and lower face; loss of corneal reflex (efferent limb). (**Bell's palsy:** Acute 7th nerve palsy.)	If lesion proximal to greater petrosal and chorda tympani take off, patient experiences: ▪ Decreased taste (anterior 2/3rd). ▪ Hyperacusis (due to stapedius muscle paralysis). ▪ Decreased salivation on affected side (though not clinically apparent if other salivary glands intact).
Upper motor neuron lesion	Contralateral lower face weakness only.	With a central lesion to the facial motor nucleus (eg, stroke), one can still raise eyebrows on affected side (the side opposite the central lesion) because of bilateral innervation to muscles of upper face.

Stroke is an example of an upper motor neuron lesion. Bell's palsy is an example of a lower motor neuron lesion.

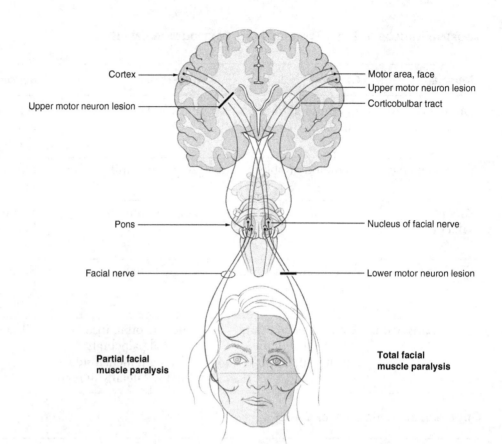

FIGURE 1–87. **Corticobulbar innervation of lower motor neurons in the facial nucleus.**

Reproduced, with permission, from White JS. *USMLE Road Map Neuroscience*, 2nd ed. New York: McGraw-Hill, 2008.

See Figure 1–87 for total and partial facial paralysis.

GREATER PETROSAL NERVE

Course

- Cell body is at superior salivatory nucleus.
- Nerve arises at geniculate ganglion.
- Joins deep petrosal nerve (bringing sympathetic fibers from superior cervical ganglion).
- Exits cranium via foramen lacerum.
- Enters pterygoid canal (as nerve of the pterygoid canal).
- Nerve of pterygoid canal synapses in pterygopalatine ganglion (within the pterygopalatine fossa) (gives fibers to branches of V1 or V2 to supply structures).

Components

- Autonomic to:
  - Lacrimal gland.
  - Glands of mucous membrane of nasal cavity, pharynx, palate.
- **Parasympathetic** preganglionics
  - Synapse at geniculate ganglion (cell bodies in geniculate ganglion).

Facial and maxillary arteries supply blood to the buccinator.

- **Sympathetics** (postganglionic)
  - Pass through geniculate without synapsing.
- **Taste**
  - From palate via palatine nerves.
  - Taste fibers pass through pterygopalatine ganglion and travel with nerve of pterygoid canal.
  - It reaches the greater petrosal nerve (the tractus solitarius and nucleus of solitary tract in pons).

Greater petrosal nerve is the parasympathetic root of the pterygopalatine ganglion.

CN VIII—Vestibulocochlear

See Figure 1–88.

Course

- Located within temporal bone, innervates:
  - Cochlea (hearing).
  - Semicircular canals and maculae (balance).
- Passes internal acoustic meatus.
- Into brain stem at the junction pons and medulla, fibers terminate in:
  - Cochlear nucleus.
  - Vestibular nuclear complex (near floor of fourth ventricle).

EAR ANATOMY

See Figure 1–89.

- **External ear**—Receives sound waves
  - Auricle
  - External auditory canal
- **Middle ear**—tympanic cavity
  - Three ossicles:
    - Malleus (hammer)
    - Incus (anvil)
    - Stapes (stirrup)
  - Two muscles:
    - Stapedius (VII)
    - Tensor tympani (V3)

The stapedius is the smallest skeletal muscle in the body.

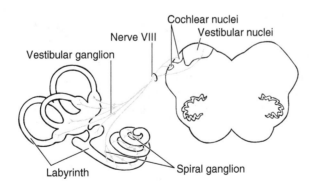

FIGURE 1–88. The vestibulocochlear nerve.

Reproduced, with permission, from Waxman SG. *Clinical Neuroanatomy*, 25th ed. New York: McGraw-Hill, 2003.

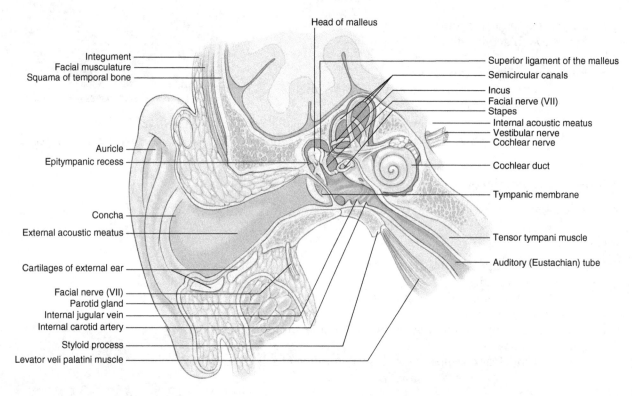

Head of malleus
Integument
Facial musculature
Squama of temporal bone
Superior ligament of the malleus
Semicircular canals
Incus
Facial nerve (VII)
Stapes
Internal acoustic meatus
Vestibular nerve
Cochlear nerve
Auricle
Epitympanic recess
Cochlear duct
Tympanic membrane
Concha
External acoustic meatus
Cartilages of external ear
Tensor tympani muscle
Auditory (Eustachian) tube
Facial nerve (VII)
Parotid gland
Internal jugular vein
Internal carotid artery
Styloid process
Levator veli palatini muscle

FIGURE 1–89. **External, middle, and internal ear.**

Middle ear communicates posteriorly with the mastoid cells and the mastoid antrum via the aditus ad antrum.

- **Inner ear**—composed of membranous and bony labyrinth
  - Acoustic apparatus
  - Vestibular apparatus
  - Semicircular canals

MUSCLES IN MIDDLE EAR

- The muscles in the middle dampen sounds; paralysis results in hyperacusis.

Muscle	Innervation
Tensor tympani	V3
Stapedius	VII

Otitis media: *Middle ear infections; can extend to both mastoid and nasopharynx via eustachian tube.*

Otitis externa: *Infection of ear canal (past external auditory meatus).*

EUSTACHIAN (AUDITORY) TUBE

- Also called the pharyngotympanic tube.
- Connection between middle ear and pharynx.
- Equalizes air pressure between the tympanic cavity and nasopharynx.

CN VIII LESIONS

HEARING LOSS

Presbycusis

- Loss occurring gradually with aging because of changes in the inner or middle ear.

- **Conductive loss:** Thickening and stiffening of cochlear basilar membrane.
- **Sensorineural loss:** Loss of hair and/or nerve cells.

(See also hearing under special sense area.)

NYSTAGMUS

- Involuntary rapid and repetitive movement of the eyes.
- Results from irritation to
  - Labyrinth.
  - Vestibular nerve or nuclei.
  - Cerebellum.
  - Visual system.
  - Cerebral cortex.
- Rhythmic oscillations are slow to one side rapid to the opposite side.
- Defined by the direction of the rapid reflex movement.
- Usually horizontal, occasionally vertical or rotatory.

Cold Caloric Test

- Instill water to the external auditory meatus stimulates nystagmus.
- Cool water fast component to side opposite.
- Warm water fast component toward stimulated side.

Central hearing connections are bilateral, so a central lesion will not cause deafness in either ear.

Caloric test is testing the vestibulo-ocular reflex.

COWS

Cold
Opposite
Warm
Same

CN IX—Glossopharyngeal

See Figure 1–90.

Course

- Originates in anterior surface of medulla oblongata (with X and XI).
- Passes laterally in the posterior cranial fossa.
- Leaves skull via jugular foramen.

Components

- **Motor:** Stylopharyngeus muscle.
- **General sensory:** Sensory cell bodies are within superior and inferior ganglia of CN IX.
- Mucosa of pharynx.
  - Posterior third of the tongue.
- **Visceral sensory:**
  - Taste perceived on posterior third of the tongue.
  - Gag reflex (afferent limb) (fauces).
  - Chemo-, baroreception (afferent limb)—carotid body, carotid sinus.
- **Parasympathetic/secretomotor:** Parotid via otic ganglion
  - Preganglionics.
    - Leave glossopharyngeal nerve as the tympanic nerve.
    - Enter middle ear cavity.
    - Contribute to tympanic plexus.
    - Re-form as the lesser petrosal nerve.
    - Leave cranial cavity via foramen ovale.
    - Enter otic ganglion.
  - Postganglionics.
    - Carried by the auriculotemporal nerve (V3) to the parotid.

The gag reflex is mediated by CN IX (afferent-unilateral) and CN X (efferent-bilateral).

Chemoreception: *Carotid body; oxygen tension measurement.*
Baroreception: *Carotid sinus; blood pressure changes. Mediated CN IX (afferent) and CN X (efferent).*

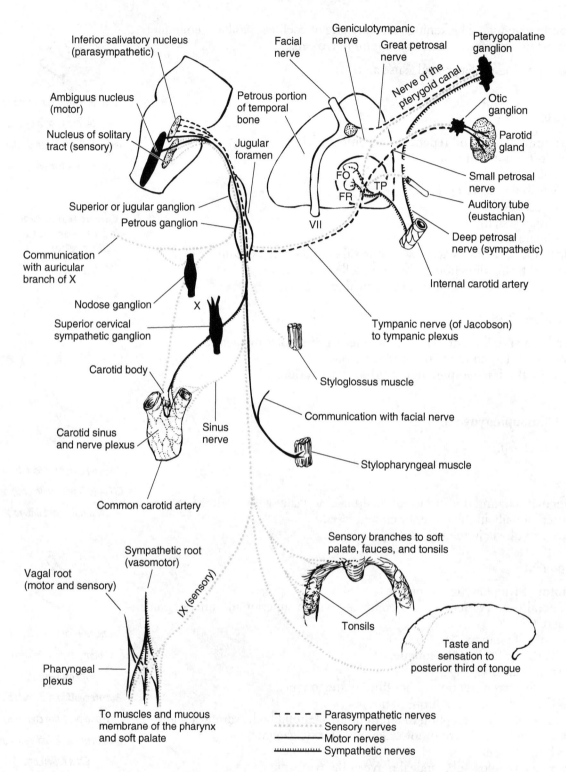

FIGURE 1-90. The glossopharyngeal nerve. TP, tympanum plexus; FR, foramen rotundum; FO, foramen ovale.

Reproduced, with permission, from Waxman SG. *Clinical Neuroanatomy*, 25th ed. New York: McGraw-Hill, 2003.

CN X—Vagus

- Cranial nerve with the widest distribution.
- Supplies the viscera of neck, thorax, and abdomen to left colic flexure.
- Course:
  - Leaves the medulla.
  - Passes out jugular foramen.
  - Descends neck in carotid sheath (behind internal and common carotid arteries, and IJV).
  - Posterior mediastinum (travels on the esophagus).
  - Enters abdominal cavity with the esophagus.

Vagus nerves lose their identity in the esophageal plexus. The anterior gastric nerve can be cut (vagotomy) to reduce gastric secretion.

Right Vagus Nerve	Left Vagus Nerve
Crosses anterior surface of right subclavian artery.	Enters thorax in front of left subclavian artery, behind left brachiocephalic vein.
Enters the thorax posterolateral to the brachiocephalic trunk, lateral to the trachea, and medial to the azygos vein.	Crosses the left side of the aortic arch (and is itself crossed by left phrenic nerve).
Passes posterior to the root of the right lung (contributing to the pulmonary plexus).	Passes behind left lung (contributing to the pulmonary plexus).
Travels with the esophagus (contributes to the esophageal plexus).	Travels with the esophagus (contributes to esophageal plexus).
Enters the abdomen behind the esophagus (via esophageal hiatus of diaphragm).	Enters abdomen in front of esophagus (via the esophageal hiatus of the diaphragm).
Branches of esophageal plexus unite:	Branches of esophageal plexus unite:
Posterior vagal trunk (*posterior gastric nerve*—reaches posterior surface of stomach).	**Anterior vagal trunk** (*anterior gastric nerve*—reaches anterior surface of stomach).

BRANCHES OF THE VAGUS IN THE HEAD AND NECK

See Figure 1–91 and Table 1–3.

Branch	Description
Meningeal	To dura.
Auricular	To auricle, posterior 1/2 of external auditory meatus.
Pharyngeal	Forms pharyngeal plexus.
	Supplies:
	■ Muscles of pharynx (except stylopharyngeus [innervated by CN IX]).
	■ All the muscles of the soft palate (except tensor veli palatini, innervated by NC V3).
Superior laryngeal	Travels with superior laryngeal artery.
■ Internal laryngeal	Pierces thyrohyoid membrane.
■ External laryngeal	Supplies mucous membranes of larynx above vocal fold.
	Travels with superior thyroid artery.
	Supplies cricothyroid muscle.

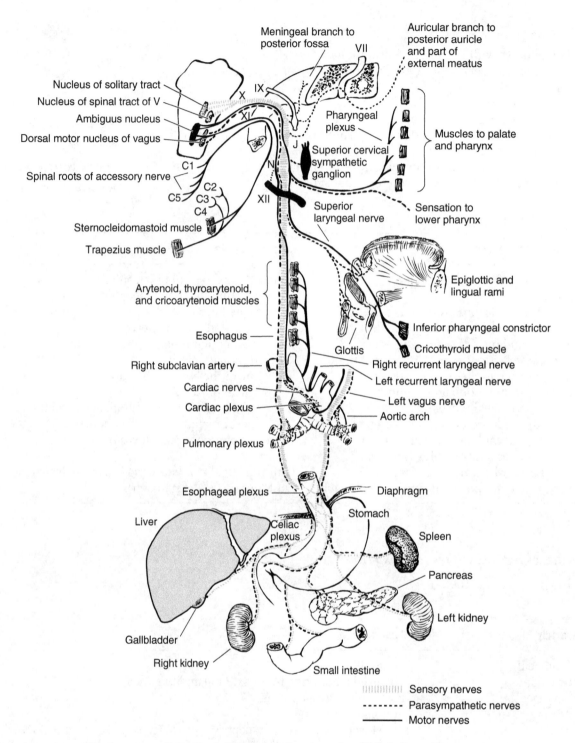

FIGURE 1-91. **The vagus nerve. J, jugular (superior) ganglion; N, nodose (inferior) ganglion.**

Reproduced, with permission, from Waxman SG. *Clinical Neuroanatomy*, 25th ed. New York: McGraw-Hill, 2003.

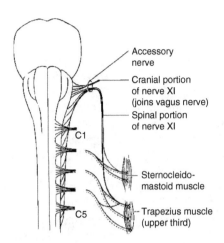

FIGURE 1-92. Schematic illustration of the accessory nerve, viewed from below.

Reproduced, with permission, from Waxman SG. *Clinical Neuroanatomy*, 25th ed. New York: McGraw-Hill, 2003.

CN X LESIONS

- Parasympathetic disturbances
- Loss of gag reflex
- Dysphagia
- Dysphonia

CN XI—Accessory

See Figure 1–92 for a schematic illustration of the accessory nerve.

CN XI LESIONS

- Paralysis of SCM: difficulty turning head to contralateral side.
- Paralysis of trapezius: Shoulder droop.

CN XII—Hypoglossus

See Figure 1–93.

- The hypoglossal nerve is strictly a motor nerve.

Course

- Leaves skull through hypoglossal canal (of the occipital bone) (medial to carotid canal and jugular foramen).
- Joined by C1 fibers from the cervical plexus soon after it leaves skull.
- Passes above hyoid bone on the lateral surface of the hyoglossus muscle (deep to the mylohyoid).
- Loops around occipital artery.
- Passes between ECA and IJV.

The cardiac branches of the vagus (form the cardiac plexus) are preganglionic parasympathetic nerves that synapse with postganglionic parasympathetic nerves in the heart.

The abdominal viscera below the left colic flexure (and genitalia and pelvic viscera) are supplied by pelvic splanchnic nerves (parasympathetic preganglionics).

Also with CN XII paralysis, the tongue tends to fall back and obstruct the airway (genioglossus).

In addition to deviation to the affected side (with damage to CN XII and resultant denervation atrophy), dysarthria (inability to articulate) can be experienced by the patient.

CN XII Lesions

Lesion	Clinical Finding	Description
Lower motor neuron	Tongue deviates toward side of lesion.	Contralateral genioglossus pulls forward because there are ipsilateral fasciculations and atrophy.
Upper motor neuron	Tongue deviates away from side of lesion.	Paralysis without atrophy or fasciculations (corticobulbar fibers are from contralateral hemisphere, so UMN lesion causes weakness of contralateral tongue; eg, left cortical lesion causes deviation of tongue to right (affected side)).

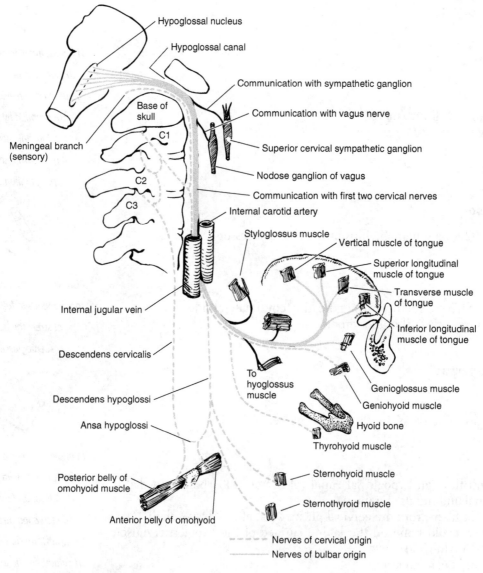

FIGURE 1-93. The hypoglossal nerve.

Reproduced, with permission, from Waxman SG. *Clinical Neuroanatomy*, 25th ed. New York: McGraw-Hill, 2003.

Spinal Cord

- Located in the spinal canal.
- Is 40–45 cm long.
- Continuation of the medulla oblongata.
  - Exits foramen magnum.
- Extends to L1–L2 (L3 in a child).
  - Occupies upper two-thirds of the vertebral canal.
- **Conus medullaris**
  - Spinal cord tapers at L1.
- **Filum terminale**
  - Prolongation of pia matter at apex attaches to coccyx.
  - Where dura and arachnoid fuse at about S2.
- **Cauda equina** ("horse's tail")
  - Nerve roots extending down inferiorly below end of spinal cord.
  - These exit via lumbar and sacral foramina.
- **Meninges** (like brain)
  - Dura
  - Arachnoid (CSF in subarachnoid space)
  - Pia

CSF is located in the subarachnoid space. This space is entered during a lumbar "tap" or puncture.

SPINAL CORD CROSS SECTION

See Figures 1–94 and 1–95.

- Gray matter.
  - Located centrally; H-shaped.
  - Consists of unmyelinated nerve cell bodies.
  - **Anterior/ventral horn**
    - Motor (efferent).
  - **Posterior/dorsal horn**
    - Sensory (afferent).
    - Dorsal root ganglion (cell bodies).
  - **Intermediolateral horn**
    - Autonomic.

In the spinal cord, white matter is peripheral and gray matter is central, the reverse of the cerebral cortex.

The spinal cord is protected by the bony and ligamentous walls of the vertebral canal and CSF.

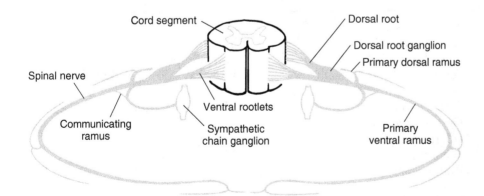

FIGURE 1-94. **Schematic illustration of a cord segment with its roots, ganglia, and branches.**

Reproduced, with permission, from Waxman SG. *Clinical Neuroanatomy*, 25th ed. New York: McGraw-Hill, 2003.

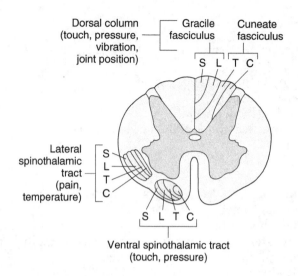

Dorsal column
(touch, pressure,
vibration,
joint position)

Gracile
fasciculus

Cuneate
fasciculus

Lateral
spinothalamic
tract
(pain,
temperature)

Ventral spinothalamic tract
(touch, pressure)

FIGURE 1–95. **Spinal cord cross section.**

Reproduced, with permission, from Ganong WS. *Review of Medical Physiology*, 22nd ed.
New York: McGraw-Hill, 2005.

- White matter.
  - Surrounds the gray matter peripherally.
  - Myelinated axons.
- Central canal.
  - Filled with CSF.

SPINAL CORD TRACTS

See also Chapter 10, "Neurophysiology."

The cell bodies for afferent/sensory nerves are located in the dorsal root ganglion.

Tract	Function
Ascending/sensory	
Anterior spinothalamic	Touch, pressure
Lateral spinothalamic	Pain, temperature
Posterior columns (gracilis and cuneatus)	Proprioception, position sense
Spinocerebellar	Motor coordination, proprioception
Descending/motor	
Corticospinal	Motor
Tectospinal	Movement of head
Rubrospinal	Muscle tone, posture, head, neck, upper extremities
Vestibulospinal	Equilibrium (interface with CN VIII)
Reticulospinal	Muscle tone, sweat gland function

Peripheral Nervous System

- Nerves outside the CNs.
- Consists of:
  - Cranial nerves (12): Leave the brain and pass out the skull foramina.
  - Spinal nerves (31): Leave the spinal cord and pass out via the intervertebral foramina.
    - 8 cervical spinal nerves (only 7 vertebrae).
    - 12 thoracic.
    - 5 lumbar.
    - 5 sacral.
    - 1 coccygeal.
  - Associated plexi and ganglia.
- Divided into
  - Afferent and efferent.
  - Somatic and visceral.
- **Afferent** (sensory)
  - Somatic sensory (afferent).
    - From cutaneous and proprioceptive receptors.
  - Visceral sensory (afferent).
    - From viscera.
- **Efferent** (motor)
  - Somatic motor (efferent).
    - Motor neurons to skeletal muscle.
  - Visceral motor (efferent)
    - Autonomic (parasympathetic > sympathetic) to viscera (eg, smooth and cardiac muscle, glands, GI tract).

SPINAL NERVES

- Comprise dorsal + ventral rami.
- Mixed nerves (motor + sensory).
- After they join as spinal nerve, they split into
  - Dorsal (posterior) rami.
  - Ventral (anterior) rami.
- Supplying both motor and sensory innervation to posterior and anterior body walls.

Spinal Nerve	Root	Location of Cell Body
Motor	Ventral (anterior)	Spinal cord (ventral horn-gray)
Sensory	Dorsal (posterior)	Dorsal root ganglion (outside of cord)

PERIPHERAL NERVE

- Bundle of nerve fibers.
- Formed from 1+ spinal nerve.
- **Example:** Musculocutaneous nerve
  - Formed from three spinal nerves (C5, C6, C7).

Remember histology: epinerium, perinerium, endoneurium.

A peripheral nerve may be a subsegment of a cranial nerve; for example, the lingual nerve is part of the third division of CN V (and it carries taste components from CN VII).

NERVE FIBER TYPES

Fiber	Conduction Velocity (m/s)	Diameter (μm)	Function	Myelin	Local Anesthetic Sensitivity
A Fiber					
A-α	70–120	12–20	Proprioception Motor	Y	Least
A-β	40–70	5–12	Sensory Touch Pressure	Y	
A-γ	10–50	2–5	Muscle spindle	Y	
A-δ	6–30	2–5	Sharp pain Temperature Touch	Y	
B Fiber	3–15	<3	Preganglionic autonomic	Y	
C Fiber	0.5–2	0.4–1.2	Dull pain Temperature Postganglionic autonomic	N	Most

Data from Waxman SG. *Clinical Neuroanatomy*, 25th ed. New York: McGraw-Hill, 2003.

GANGLIA

- Collections of cell bodies.
- Sensory versus autonomic.
- **Sensory:** Dorsal root ganglia.
- **Autonomic:** Sympathetic.
  - Sympathetic chain ganglia.
    - Located on each sympathetic trunk, alongside vertebral column.
    - 3 cervical (superior, middle, inferior).
    - 12 thoracic.
    - 4 lumbar.
    - 4 sacral.
  - Parasympathetic
    - Ciliary.
    - Pterygopalatine.
    - Submandibular.
    - Otic.
    - Celiac.
    - Superior mesenteric.
    - Inferior mesenteric.

Splanchnic nerves are sympathetic nerves to the viscera. They pass through the sympathetic chain ganglia without synapse (exceptions to short preganglionic and long postganglionic) and synapse in the effector.

PLEXUSES

- Interdigitations of nerves (nerves joining neighboring nerves).
- Formed from anterior rami in cervical, brachial, lumbar, and sacral regions.

Four major plexuses:

- Cervical plexus (C1–C4).
- Brachial plexus (C5–T1).

- Lumbar plexus (L1–L4) .
  - Formed in psoas muscle.
  - Supplies lower abdomen and parts of lower limb.
  - Main branches
    - Femoral nerve.
    - Obturator nerve.
- Sacral plexus (L4–L5 and S1–S4)
  - Posterior pelvic wall in front of piriformis.
  - Supplies lower back, pelvis, parts of thigh, leg, and foot.
  - Main branches
    - Sciatic nerve (largest nerve in body).
    - Gluteal nerve.
    - Pelvic splanchnic nerve.

AUTONOMIC NERVOUS SYSTEM

See Figures 1–96 and 1–97 and Chapter 10, "Neurophysiology."

- **Sympathetic**
  - Thoracolumbar
  - "Fight or flight"
- **Parasympathetic**
  - Craniosacral.
  - "Rest and digest."
  - All have afferent and efferent components.
  - Efferent is the major portion.
- **General visceral efferent motor system (GVE)**
  - Involuntary.
  - Controls and regulates smooth muscle, cardiac muscle, and glands.

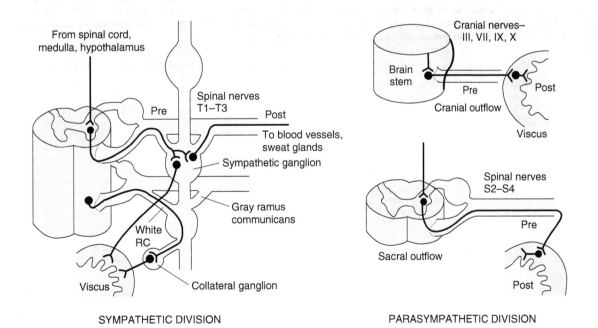

FIGURE 1–96. Autonomic nervous system.

Reproduced, with permission, from Ganong WS. *Review of Medical Physiology*, 22nd ed. New York: McGraw-Hill, 2005.

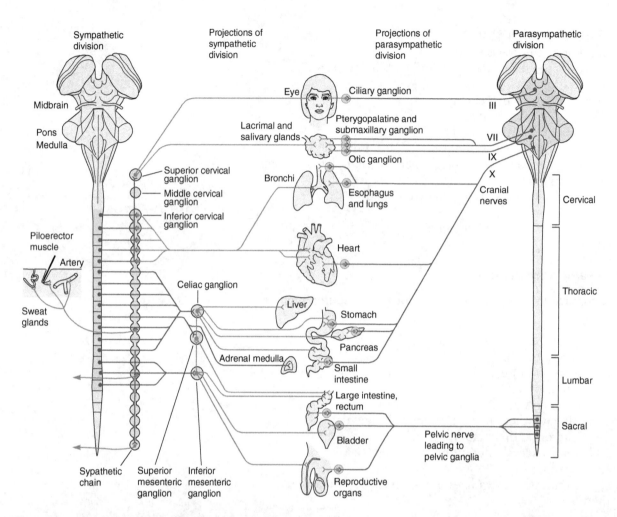

Sympathetic division

Projections of sympathetic division

Projections of parasympathetic division

Parasympathetic division

Midbrain

Pons
Medulla

Eye — Ciliary ganglion

Lacrimal and salivary glands — Pterygopalatine and submaxillary ganglion

Otic ganglion

III

VII

IX

X

Cranial nerves

Superior cervical ganglion

Middle cervical ganglion

Inferior cervical ganglion

Bronchi

Esophagus and lungs

Cervical

Piloerector muscle

Artery

Heart

Thoracic

Sweat glands

Celiac ganglion

Liver

Stomach

Pancreas

Adrenal medulla

Small intestine

Large intestine, rectum

Lumbar

Bladder

Pelvic nerve leading to pelvic ganglia

Sacral

Sympathetic chain

Superior mesenteric ganglion

Inferior mesenteric ganglion

Reproductive organs

FIGURE 1–97. **Sympathetic and parasympathetic divisions of the autonomic nervous system. Sympathetic preganglionic neurons are clustered in ganglia in the sympathetic chain alongside the spinal cord extending from the first thoracic spinal segment to upper lumbar segments. Parasympathetic preganglionic neurons are located within the brain stem and in segments S2–S4 of the spinal cord. The major targets of autonomic control are shown here.**

(Reproduced, with permission, from Kandel ER, Schwartz JH, Jessell TM. *Principles of Neural Science*, 4th ed. New York: McGraw-Hill, 2000:964.)

Pathway

Hypothalamus, reticular formation
↓
Interomediolateral horn (cell body of preganglionic neuron)
↓
Preganglionic neuron (short in sympathetic; long in parasympathetic)
↓
Ganglion (outside of CNS)
↓
Postganglionic neuron (long in sympathetic; short in parasympathetic)
↓
Effector organ

Postganglionic autonomic fibers are unmyelinated C-fibers.

Notes

- Gray rami connect sympathetic trunk to every spinal nerve.
- White rami are limited to spinal cord segments between T1 and L2.
- Cell bodies of the visceral efferent preganglionic fibers (visceral branches of sympathetic trunk) are located in the interomediolateral horn of the spinal cord.
- Cell bodies of visceral afferent fibers are located in the dorsal root ganglia.

ENTERIC NERVOUS SYSTEM

See Chapter 15, "Gastrointestinal Physiology."

CHAPTER 2

General Histology

Plasma (Cell) Membrane

- See also the section "Membranes" in Chapter 9.
- A fluid, selectively permeable barrier consisting of an amphipathic phospholipid bilayer that contains integral and peripheral proteins.

Cytoplasm

- Site of cell-synthesizing activity. Contains the following:
- **Organelles** (See Figure 2–1)
- Cytoplasmic inclusions (metaplasm)
  - Glycogen
  - Pigment granules: lipofuscin, melanin, etc
  - Secretory granules
  - Lipid droplets
- Cytoplasmic matrix (cytosol)
  - Ground substance

Membrane-Bound Organelles

- **Rough endoplasmic reticulum (rER):** Protein synthesis for *export* outside of the cell. Studded with ribosomes.

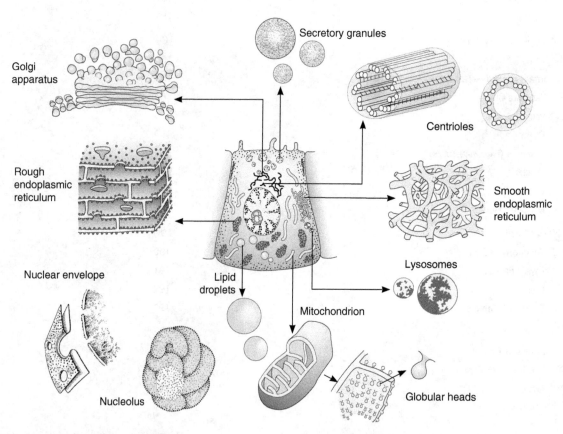

FIGURE 2–1. Major cellular organelles.

Reproduced, with permission, from Ganong WS. *Review of Medical Physiology*, 22nd ed. New York: McGraw-Hill, 2005.

- **Smooth endoplasmic reticulum (sER):** Steroid synthesis (adrenal cortex and testes). Sequesters Ca^{2+} (skeletal and cardiac muscle). Lipid and glycogen metabolism (liver).
- **Golgi apparatus:** Posttranslational modification and packaging of proteins (adds oligosaccharides for glycoproteins, and sulfate groups for proteoglycans). Lysosome production.
- **Mitochondria:** ATP production via the Krebs cycle and oxidative phosphorylation. Have an inner and outer membrane. Contain their own cyclic DNA. Not present in erythrocytes.
- **Lysosomes:** Digestion of microorganisms or other cellular components by various hydrolytic enzymes. Produced by the Golgi apparatus.
- **Peroxisomes:** Elimination of H_2O_2 by various oxidative enzymes (catalase and peroxidase).
- **Endosomes:** Vesicles formed as a result of phagocytosis.

Active cells (fibroblasts, osteoblasts, etc) are characterized by an abundance of rER.

Non Membrane-Bound Organelles

- **Microtubules:** Provide cytoskeletal support, intracellular transport, and cellular movement. Composed of *tubulin*.
    - **Axoneme:** Specialized group of microtubules found in cilia and flagella arranged in a "9 + 2" pattern.
- **Centrioles:** Provide microtubule organization. Form ends of mitotic spindle during mitosis.
- **Filaments**
    - **Microfilaments (actin, myosin, etc):** Important for muscle contraction. Provide cellular movement or anchorage.
    - **Intermediate filaments (vimentin, desmin, cytokeratin, etc):** Provide cytoskeletal support.
- **Basal bodies:** Required for development of cilia. Derived from centrioles.
- **Ribosomes:** Protein synthesis for use *within* the cell. Composed of rRNA and protein.

"9 + 2" pattern: 9 pairs (doublets) of microtubules surrounding 2 central microtubules.

Nucleus

- **Nuclear membrane:** Composed of inner and outer plasma membranes.
- **Nucleoplasm:** Ground substance of the nucleus.
- **Chromatin:** The complex of DNA and proteins (histones).
    - **Euchromatin:** Loosely arranged chromatin. Indicates nuclear activity.
    - **Heterochromatin:** Highly condensed chromatin.
- **Nucleolus:** Site of rRNA synthesis. Nonmembranous.
- **Barr body:** The repressed X chromosome found only in cells of *females*. Appears as a dense chromatin mass adjacent to the nuclear membrane. Its presence (or absence) is used in sex identification.

Microtubules are found in axonemes (of cilia and flagella), basal bodies, centrioles, mitotic spindle, elongating cell processes, and cytoplasm.

Cell Surface Appendages

- **Microvilli:** Fingerlike structures of various lengths located on the apical surface of most epithelial cells. Core composed of microfilaments. Provide increased cell surface area for absorption and transport of fluids.
- **Stereocilia:** Unusually long microvilli located only in the *epididymis* and sensory cells of the *inner ear*.
- **Cilia:** Short, hairlike structures used for locomotion or movement of substances along the cell membrane. Function in a synchronous, coordinated wave motion. Require *basal bodies* for development.
- **Flagella:** Long, whiplike structures used for locomotion. Function in an undulating, snake-like motion. In humans, found only in *spermatozoa*.

The sex of an embryo (via presence/absence of Barr bodies) can be determined by the 8th week.

Protein and RNA syntheses occur in all cell cycle phases except mitosis.

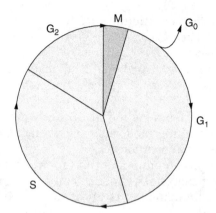

FIGURE 2-2. The cell cycle.

Cell turnover rate

(high → low):

Oral, epidermal, GI epithelial

↓

Smooth muscle, vascular endothelial

↓

Skeletal muscle, cardiac

muscle

↓

Neurons

The Cell Cycle

See Figure 2–2.

- **Mitosis:** Produces two daughter cells with the *same* chromosome number (diploid, $2n$) as the parent cell. All somatic cells except gametes undergo mitosis.
- **Interphase**
  - G_1: First variable period of cellular growth.
    - G_0: Period *outside* of the cell cycle of terminal differentiation.
  - S: Period of DNA synthesis. Takes about 7 hours.
  - G_2: Second variable period of cellular growth.
- **Mitosis (karyokinesis)**
  - **Prophase:** Chromatin coils/condenses within the nucleus. Mitotic spindle forms.
  - **Metaphase:** Nuclear membrane and nucleoli disappear. Chromosomes line up at the equatorial plate of the mitotic spindle.
  - **Anaphase:** Chromosomes split to opposite poles of the cell.
  - **Telophase:** Nuclear membrane forms around the chromosomes at each pole. The chromosomes uncoil and nucleoli reappear. The cytoplasm divides to form two daughter cells (cytokinesis).
- **Meiosis:** Produces four daughter cells with *half* the chromosome number (haploid, n) as the parent cell. Only gametes (spermatozoa and ova) undergo meiosis.

A junctional complex (See Figure 2–3) is a specialized junction commonly found in epithelial tissues consisting of the following (from apical → upper regions):

- *Tight junction*
- *Intermediate junction*
- *Desmosome*

Cell-to-Cell Contacts

See Table 2–1.

- **Tight junction (zonula occludens):** A beltlike junction that completely seals off the intercellular space between adjacent cells.
- **Intermediate junction (zonula adherens):** A beltlike junction that leaves a 15–20 nm wide intercellular space between adjacent cells.
- **Desmosome (macula adherens):** Provides strong but localized adhesion sites between adjacent cells. Composed of an *attachment plaque* on the cytoplasmic side of each adjoining cell surface, to which intermediate filaments are anchored.

TABLE 2-1. Comparison of Cell-to-Cell Contacts

CONTACT TYPE	FUNCTION	AREA OF CONTACT	PRINCIPAL PROTEINS	COMMON LOCATION
Tight junction (zonula occludens)	Occlusion	Cell-cell (band)	Occludins, Claudins	Various epithelium
Intermediate junction (zonula adherens)	Adhesion	Cell-cell (band)	Actin, Cadherins	Various epithelium
Desmosome (macula adherens)	Adhesion	Cell-cell (focal)	Cadherins	Epidermis and other epithelium
Hemidesmosome	Adhesion	Cell-ECM (focal)	Integrins	Epithelium of oral mucosa (JE), skin, esophagus, vagina, and cornea
Gap junction	Communication	Cell-cell (focal)	Connexins	Neurons, smooth and cardiac muscle

▪ **Hemidesmosome:** Provides strong but localized attachment of epithelial cells to connective tissue. Half of a desmosome (the attachment plaque is on the basal surface, facing the basement membrane).

▪ **Gap junction:** Localized areas of free communication between adjacent cells. Enables passage of fluids, ions, and small molecules.

Pemphigus: Autoimmunity against desmosomal attachments.

Pemphigoid: Autoimmunity against hemidesmosomal attachments.

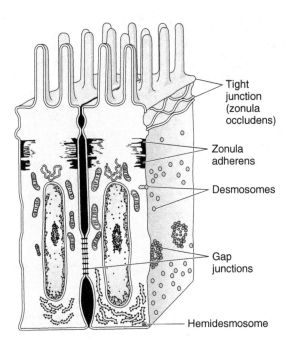

Tight junction (zonula occludens)

Zonula adherens

Desmosomes

Gap junctions

Hemidesmosome

FIGURE 2-3. Epithelial intercellular junctions. Note the relative location of each junction within the cell.

Reproduced, with permission, from Ganong WS. *Review of Medical Physiology,* 22nd ed. New York: McGraw-Hill, 2005.

The thinnest epithelium in the oral cavity is the sublingual mucosa.

Epithelium is classified by cell morphology and arrangement, not by function. See Table 2–2.

▫ Epithelium covers all body surfaces, lines all body cavities, makes up the secretory component of glands, and serves as the receptor in various sensory organs.

Functions of Epithelium

▫ Barrier
▫ Diffusion
▫ Absorption
▫ Secretory
▫ Transport
▫ Sensory

Classification of Epithelium

▫ By number of cell layers.
  ▫ **Simple:** One cell layer thick, all touching the basement membrane.
  ▫ **Stratified:** Two or more cell layers thick, with only the deepest layer touching the basement membrane.
  ▫ **Pesudostratified:** One cell layer thick, all touching the basement membrane, but not all reach the outer surface. Generally columnar.

TABLE 2–2. Comparison of Epithelial Types

EPITHELIUM TYPE	FUNCTION	COMMON LOCATION
Simple squamous	Barrier, diffusion	Endothelium, mesothelium, lung alveoli, Bowman's capsule
Simple cuboidal	Barrier, secretion, apsorption	Small exocrine gland ducts (thyroid follicles), renal tubules, OEE
Simple columnar (often ciliated)	Absorption, secretion, transport	Stomach, small intestine, large intestine, gallbladder, IEE
Pseudostratified columnar (often ciliated)	Absorption, secretion, transport	Trachea, bronchi, nasopharynx, nasal cavity, paranasal sinuses
Stratified squamous	Barrier	Epidermis, oral cavity, gingiva, oropharynx, laryngopharynx, esophagus, anus, vagina
Stratified cuboidal	Barrier, secretion	Medium exocrine gland ducts (sweat glands)
Stratified columnar (often ciliated)	Barrier, transport	Large exocrine gland ducts (salivary glands)
Transitional	Barrier, distension	Urinary bladder, urethra, ureters

- By cell morphology.
  - **Squamous:** Width > height.
  - **Cuboidal:** Width = height.
  - **Columnar:** Height > width.
  - **Transitional:** Ranges from squamous to cuboidal. Distensible.
- By location (almost always simple squamous).
  - **Endothelium:** Lines all blood vessels.
  - **Mesothelium:** Lines all closed body cavities.

▶ BASEMENT MEMBRANE

- Connects the epithelial basal layer to underlying connective tissue.

Functions of Basement Membrane

- Attachment
- Separation
- Filtration
- Scaffolding

Components of Basement Membrane

From epithelium → connective tissue (Figure 2–4)

- **Lamina lucida:** Electron-clear layer
- **Lamina densa (basal lamina):** Product of epithelium
  - *Type IV collagen*
  - Proteoglycans
  - Laminin
  - Fibronectin
  - Anchoring fibrils (type VII collagen)
- **Reticular lamina:** Product of CT
  - Reticular fibers (type III collagen)

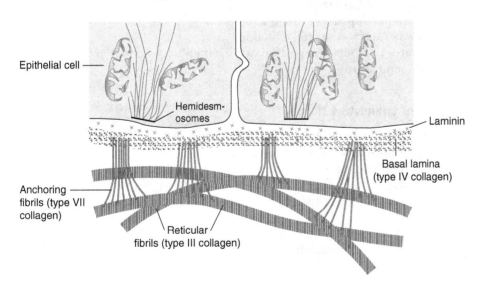

FIGURE 2–4. Components providing attachment between epithelial cells and the underlying connective tissue.

Reproduced, with permission, from Ross MH, Romrell LJ, Kaye GI. *Histology: A Text and Atlas.* 3rd ed. Philadelphia: Williams & Wilkins; 1995.

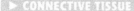

Almost all connective tissues (CT) originate from mesoderm; however, some CTs of the head and neck region derive from neural crest ectoderm.

Classification of Connective Tissue

- Connective tissue proper
  - Loose CT
  - Dense CT
    - Regular
    - Irregular
- Specialized CT
  - Adipose tissue
  - Blood
  - Bone
  - Cartilage
  - Hematopoietic tissue
  - Lymphatic tissue
- Embryonic CT
  - Mesenchyme
  - Mucous CT

Consistency of CT:

- *Soft: Deeper layers of skin, oral mucosa*
- *Firm: Cartilage*
- *Rigid: Bone*
- *Fluid: Blood*

Connective Tissue Proper

- **Loose CT:** Abundant ground substance with sparse fibers and cells. Located under epithelial layers that cover body surfaces and line body cavities.
- **Dense CT:** Greater fiber concentration, which provides structural support.
  - **Irregular:** Irregular arrangement of fibers and cells. Makes up the majority of dense CT. Found in dermis, submucosa of the GI tract, and fibrous capsules.
  - **Regular:** Ordered arrangement of fibers and cells. Found in *tendons, ligaments,* and *aponeuroses.*

Connective Tissue Attachments

- **Ligament:** Connects bone to bone
- **Tendon:** Connects muscle to bone
- **Aponeurosis:** A sheetlike tendon
- **Sharpey's fiber:** The portion of a ligament or tendon that inserts into bone (or cementum)

Cells of Connective Tissue

- Resident cell population
  - **Fibroblasts:** Most common
  - Myofibroblasts
  - Adipocytes
  - Macrophages (histiocytes)
  - Mast cells
  - Mesenchymal cells
- Transient cell population
  - Lymphocytes
  - Neutrophils
  - Monocytes
  - Plasma cells
  - Eosinophils
  - Basophils

Types of Glands

■ There are three major types of glands.

Types of Glands

Gland Type	Function	Examples	Secretions
Exocrine	Secrete products through **ducts**	Sweat, salivary, sebaceous, von Ebner's glands	Sweat, saliva, sebum, digestive enzymes
Endocrine	Secrete products into the **bloodstream** (no ducts)	Pituitary, thyroid, parathyroid, adrenal, gonads, pineal glands	Various **hormones**
Paracrine	Secrete products into **exracellular spaces** that affect other cells within the same epithelium	Gastroenteropancreatic glands	Various peptides

Classification of Exocrine Glands

See Figure 2–5.

Classification	Type	Definition	Examples
Cellularity	Unicellular	Single secretory cells	Goblet cells
	Multicellular	Multiple secretory cells	Gastric pits
Secretion mechanism	Merocrine	Secretory product released from secretory granules	Major salivary glands, pancreatic acinar cells
	Apocrine	Secretory product is released with cytoplasm	Mammary glands, apocrine sweat glands
	Holocrine	Secretory product is released with portion of cell	Sebaceous glands
Duct structure	Simple	Unbranched	Sweat glands
	Compound	Branched	Major salivary glands, pancreas
Secretory unit	Tubular	Secretory portion shaped like a tube	Intestinal glands
	Coiled	Secretory portion shaped like a coiled tube	Eccrine sweat glands
	Acinar	Secretory portion shaped like a saclike dilation	Sebaceous glands, mammary glands, gastric cardiac glands, pancreas
	Tubuloacinar	Combination of tubular and acinar	Major salivary glands
Secretion type	Mucous	Viscous secretion	Sublingual salivary glands, goblet cells
	Serous	Watery secretion	Parotid salivary glands, von Ebner's salivary glands, paneth cells, gastric chief cells
	Mixed	Combination of mucous and serous	Submandibular salivary glands

Simple
tubular

Simple coiled
tubular

Simple
branched tubular

Simple
branched acinar

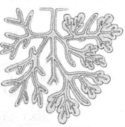 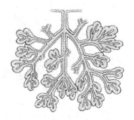

Compound
tubular

Compound
tubuloacinar

Compound
acinar

FIGURE 2-5. Classification of exocrine glands.

Reproduced, with permission, from Ross MH. *Histology*, 3rd ed. Lippincott Williams & Wilkins, 1995. (Based on Weiss L. *Histology*, 4th ed. McGraw-Hill, 1977.)

Serous glands (parotid) have well-developed intercalated and striated ducts that modify their serous secretions. Contrarily, mucous glands (sublingual) have poorly developed intercalated and striated ducts.

Structure of Salivary Glands

- Comprised of lobes subdivided by CT septa.
- Lobe → lobules → terminal secretory units (acini or tubules).
- The structure is variable depending on the type of gland:
    - **Terminal secretory unit:** Contains cells that secrete the glycoprotein and watery elements of saliva. Lined by simple cuboidal epithelium.
        - Serous cells: Secretory
        - Mucous cells: Secretory
        - Myoepithelial (basket) cells: Contractile
    - **Intercalated duct:** Transports saliva to larger ducts. Lined by simple cuboidal epithelium.
    - **Striated duct:** Modifies salivary electrolytes (reabsorption of Na^+/Cl^-; secretion of K^+/HCO_3^-). Numerous elongated mitochondria give the "striated" appearance. Lined by simple low columnar epithelium.
    - **Terminal excretory duct:** Transports saliva to oral cavity. Lined by pseudostratified columnar epithelium.

Hyaline cartilage is the precursor to bones that develop via endochondral ossification.

▶ **CARTILAGE**

- An **avascular** connective tissue. Blood supply comes from perichondrium.
- Composed of **chondrocytes**, which reside in **lacunae**, surrounded by their own specialized extracellular matrix (ECM).
- **Chondroblasts:** The initial cartilagenic cells (prior to extensive matrix formation).

Cartilage Matrix

- Type II collagen
- Ground substance: Extremely hydrophilic
    - Glycosaminoglycans (GAGs)
        - Hyaluronic acid

Cartilage does not contain calcium salts, so it does not appear on radiographs.

- ▨ Chondroitin sulfate
- ▨ Keratin sulfate
- ▨ Proteoglycans

Surface of Cartilage

- ▨ **Perichondrium**
  - ▨ Inner *cellular* layer: Produces chondroblasts
  - ▨ Outer *fibrous* layer: Provides protection

Perichondrium covers all cartilage except:

- ▨ *Fibrocartilage*
- ▨ *Articular cartilage of joints*
- ▨ *Nasal/costal cartilage*

Growth of Cartilage

- ▨ **Appositional growth:** New cartilage forms on the surface of existing cartilage. Must have perichondrium: fibroblastic cells from the inner perichondrium differentiate into chondroblasts, which secrete matrix.
- ▨ **Interstitial growth:** New cartilage forms within existing cartilage. Chondrocytes divide within their lacunae, enabling new matrix to be deposited.

Types of Cartilage

Cartilage	ECM Composition	Perichondrium	Function	Ability to Calcify	Locations
Hyaline	Closely packed, thin collagen fibers	Some	Provides pliability and resilience Precursor to endochondral bone formation	Yes	Nose, trachea, bronchi, larynx, ribs (costal cartilage), articular surfaces of long bones
Elastic	Collagen and elastic fibers	Yes	Provides elastic properties	No	External ear, Eustachian tube, epiglottis
Fibrocartilage	Dense collagen fibers	No	Withstands compression and tension	No	Intervertebral disc, articular disc of TMJ, symphysis pubis, meniscus of knee

▶ BONE

- ▨ A yellowish, mineralized, vascular tissue of varying degrees of density.
- ▨ **Osteoblasts:** Produce **osteoid** (uncalcified bone matrix), which is composed of type I collagen and ground substance. **Mature bone** forms when the osteoid calcifies.
- ▨ During the clacification process, osteoblasts become trapped in spaces within the mineralized matrix called **lacunae.** Here they differentiate into **osteocytes,** which are responsible for maintaining the bone matrix. They maintain nourishment via vascular tunnels within bone called **canaliculi.**

Hydroxyapatite

$[Ca_{10}(PO_4)_6(OH)_3]$ *is the predominant mineral found in bone.*

Functions of Bone

- Support
- Protection
- Movement
- Mineral storage: calcium, phosphorous
- Hematopoiesis: bone marrow

Bone Matrix

Initiation of bone

mineralization:

1. ↑ pores in collagen fibers

2. Osteoblasts secrete matrix

vesicles

3. ↑ alkaline phosphatase

in osteoblasts and matrix

vesicles

4. Degradation of matrix

pyrophosphate, releasing

PO_4^{3-}

- Organic
  - Type I collagen
  - Osteocalcin: Marker of bone formation
  - Osteonectin: Binds Ca^{2+} and collagen
  - Ground substance: GAGs, etc
- Inorganic
  - Hydroxyapatite

Bone Formation

- **Intramembranous ossification:** Mesenchymal cells differentiate into osteo-blasts, which secrete bone matrix within an established locus of loosely arranged **collagen**. This new matrix calcifies, forming immature **woven bone**. Over time, osteoclastic resorption of woven bone occurs, and new osteoblastic matrix is deposited in a more tightly arranged manner. This matrix is then calcified, forming mature bone of a higher strength.
  - Flat bones of skull, maxilla, mandibular body, clavicle.
- **Endochondral ossification:** A subperiosteal bony cuff forms around an already established locus of **hyaline cartilage,** which grows larger and sub-sequently causes the hypertrophy and death of the chondrocytes. The carti-lage matrix then becomes calcified. Over time, osteoclastic resorption of the calcified cartilage occurs, and new osteoblastic matrix is deposited, forming mature bone.
  - Long bones, vertebrae, mandibular condyles.

Bone Growth

Endochondral centers of

ossification:

Primary: Diaphysis

Secondary: Epiphysis

- **Appositional growth:** Occurs in both endochondral and intramembranous bone at any time.
- **Interstitial growth:** Occurs in endochondral bone only until epiphyseal plates close.

Types of Bone

- **Cortical (compact):** Composed of **Haversian systems (osteons),** which are composed of concentric bone matrix **lamellae** surrounding a central **Hav-ersian canal** that contains neurovascular bundles. Canaliculi connect to the central canal, providing nourishment to osteocytes. Osteons are con-nected to each other by **Volkmann's canals.** The space between osteons is composed of previous osteonal lamellae, called **interstitial lamellae.**
- **Cancellous (spongy):** Similar to cortical bone in that it is lamellar, but their configuration and arrangement is less dense. Lamellae are arranged in thin spicules called **trabeculae.** If they are thick enough, they contain osteons. In between the trabeculae are **marrow spaces** of various sizes. Trabeculae follow lines of stress.

Bone Surfaces

- **Periosteum:** A fibrous connective tissue capsule that *surrounds* the outer surface of bone. Contains collagen, fibroblasts, and osteoprogenitor cells.
- **Endosteum:** A one-cell thick layer of mostly osteoprogenitor cells that *lines* the inner surface bone. Contains bone marrow.

Bone Marrow

- **Yellow marrow:** Contains fat cells. The predominant marrow type in the maxilla and mandible.
- **Red marrow:** Contains hematopoietic cells. Found in the mandibular ramus and condyles.

Bone marrow is contained within the medullary spaces of spongy bone.

Bone Remodeling

- Bone constantly remodels, a process involving both osteoclasts (resorption) and osteoblasts (matrix deposition). **Osteoclasts** are multinucleated giant cells that reside in resorption bays known as **Howship's lacunae.** They produce a large number of hydrolytic enzymes from their characteristic ruffled border. The protons lower the pH at the site of resorption, subsequently dissolving the calcified bone matrix. Collagenases and other proteases then digest the decalcified bone matrix.

Mature bone grows only by appositional growth.

Fracture Repair

1. Blood clot formation
2. Bridging callus formation
3. Periosteal callus formation
4. New endochondral bone formation

Calcium Regulation

- **Parathyroid hormone (PTH):** Stimulates osteoclastic bone resorption (blood calcium). Secreted by the parathyroid gland.
- **Calcitonin:** Inhibits osteoclastic bone resorption (↓ blood calcium). Secreted by the parafollicular cells of the thyroid gland.

▶ JOINTS

Classification of Joints

- By motion
    - **Synarthrosis:** Immovable (cranial sutures)
    - **Amphiarthrosis:** Slightly movable (symphysis pubis)
    - **Diarthrosis:** Fully moveable (shoulder, hip, TMJ)
- By connective tissue type
    - **Fibrous:** Joined by fibrous CT
        - **Suture** (cranial sutures)
        - **Syndesmosis** (radius-ulna, tibia-fibula)
        - **Gomphosis** (tooth socket)
    - **Cartilaginous:** Joined by cartilage
        - **Synchondrosis** (epiphyseal plates of long bones)
        - **Symphysis** (symphysis pubis)
    - **Synovial:** Freely movable. Lined by a synovial membrane
        - Majority of joints (shoulder, hip, TMJ)

The TMJ is a synovial, diarthrosis joint.
The alveolar socket is a synarthrosis, gomphosis joint.

The hipbone (os coxa) is formed by the fusion of the ilium, ischium, and pubis. The right and left hipbones articulate anteriorly at the symphysis pubis.

Types of Synovial Joints

- Ball-and-socket: Hip, shoulder
- Gliding: Carpal bones
- Hinge: Elbow, knee
- Pivot: Atlas-axis
- Ellipsoidal: Radius-ulna
- Saddle: Metacarpal bones

Synovial Joint Components

- **Articular capsule (bursa):** Composed of fibrous connective tissue. Surrounds the joint. Lined by synovial membrane.
- **Articular cartilage (meniscus):** Layer of **hyaline** cartilage that covers the articular bone surfaces (**except** the TMJ and knee, which is composed of fibrocartilage).
- **Synovial cavity:** Lies within the articular capsule and contains synovial fluid.
- **Synovial membrane:** Lines the articular capsule. Produces synovial fluid.
- **Synovial fluid:** Lubricates the articular cartilage.

▶ NERVOUS TISSUE

Two Major Divisions of Nervous Tissue

Division	Origin	Location	Cell Body Clusters
CNS	Neural tube ectoderm	Brain and spinal cord	Nuclei
PNS	Neural crest ectoderm	Cranial and spinal nerves, ganglia, and nerve endings	Ganglia

Neurons do not divide.

Neurons

- Nerve cells that conduct electrical impulses (Figure 2–6).
    - **Perikaryon (cell body):** Contains plasma membrane, cytoplasm, nucleus, and **Nissl bodies (rER).**
    - **Axon:** Conducts information *away* from cell body. Only one axon exists per cell body.
    - **Dendrites:** Conducts information *toward* the cell body. The number of dendrites per cell is variable (none to many), depending on the type of neuron.
    - **Cytoskeleton**
        - Actin
        - Microtubules (dendrites)
        - Neurofilaments (axons)

Neuron Classification

- By function
    - Motor (efferent)
    - Sensory (afferent)
    - Mixed (both)

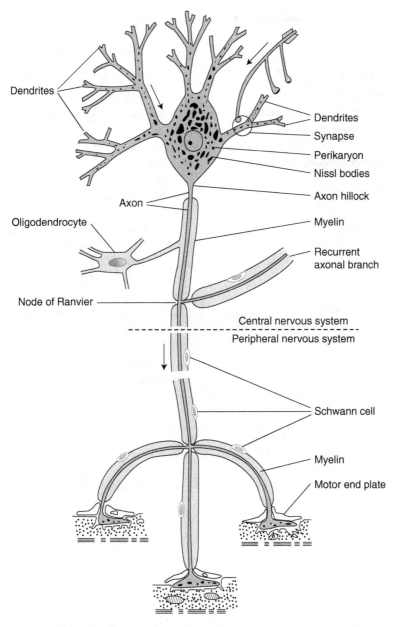

FIGURE 2-6. Schematic diagram of a motor neuron.

Reproduced, with permission, from Junqueira LC, Carneiro J. *Basic Histology: Text & Atlas.*
11th ed. New York: McGraw-Hill; 2005.

- By number of processes
  - **Unipolar:** One process (axon only). Sensory neurons.
  - **Bipolar:** Two processes (one axon and one dendrite). Retina and ganglia of CN VIII.
  - **Multipolar:** Three or more processes (one axon and many dendrites). Motor and mixed neurons.

Synapses

- Junctions that transmit impulses from one neuron to another, or from one neuron to an effector cell.

Interneurons form a communicating network between sensory and motor neurons.

Astrocytes:

▪ *Building blocks of BBB*

▪ *May regulate vasocon-
   striction and vasodilation*

▪ *Communicate via gap
   junctions using calcium*

TABLE 2-3. Supporting Cells of Nervous Tissue

CELL TYPE	FUNCTION
CNS (Glial Cells)	
Astrocytes	Scaffolding of BBB
Protoplasmic: Gray matter	Regulation of metabolites
Fibrous: White matter	
Oligodendrocytes	Myelination
Microglia	Phagocytosis
Ependymal cells	Epithelium of ventricles of brain, spinal cord
Choroidal cells	Secretion of CSF
PNS	
Schwann cells	Myelination
	Surround nerve processes
Satellite cells	Support
	Surround nerve ganglia

▪ Two types of synapses:
  ▪ Electrical: Synaptic cleft is a *gap junction*. Located in smooth and cardiac muscle.
  ▪ Chemical: Synaptic cleft is a 20–30 nm intercellular space.

Supporting Cells

See Table 2–3.

▪ Nonconducting cells that insulate neurons.

Myelination

See Table 2–4.

TABLE 2-4. Myelin-Producing Cells of the Nervous System

CELL TYPE	DIVISION	CELLS/NEURON	MYELIN SHEATH
Oligodendrocyte	CNS	Multiple (as many as 50)	Composed of several internodal tongue-like processes that wrap around the axon
Schwann cell	PNS	1	Composed of multiple layers concentrically wrapped around the axon

- **Myelin sheath:** Lipid-rich layer that surrounds and insulates myelinated axons.
- **Neurilemma (sheath of Schwann):** Layer of myelin cell cytoplasm that is contiguous with the myelin sheath.
- **Node of Ranvier:** *Unmyelinated* junction between two myelin cells.
- Myelin formation begins before birth and during 1st year postnatally (see Babinski reflex).

Not all Schwann cells produce myelin:

A fibers: *Myelinated – have neurilemma and myelin.*

C fibers: *Unmyelinated – only have neurilemma.*

► BLOOD

Functions

- Transportation
- Buffering
- Thermoregulation

Hematocrit *is the percentage of erythrocytes in a blood sample. In males, the average hematocrit is 45%; in females it is 40%.*

Components

See Figure 2–7.

Serum *is blood plasma minus fibrinogen and clotting factors.*

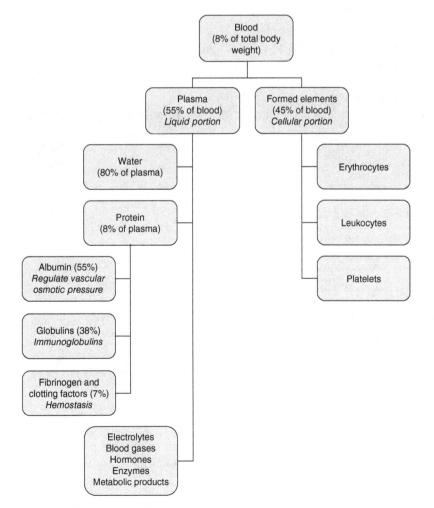

FIGURE 2–7. Components of blood.

Formed Elements

Comparison of Major Blood-Formed Elements

Formed Element	Function	Characteristics	Average Lifespan	Normal Amount Per mm³ Blood
Erythrocytes	Transports O₂ (99%) Transports CO₂ (30%)	Biconcave discs No nucleus No mitochondria Elastic	120 days	4–5 million
Platelets	Hemostasis	Cytoplasmic fragments of **megakaryocytes** No nucleus	5–10 days	200,000–400,000
Leukocytes	Immunoregulation Inflammation Phagocytosis Hypersensitivity	Nucleated, but morphology is variable	Variable	6,000–10,000

Erythrocytes

- Red blood cells.
- Biconcave discs (7–10 μm in diameter).
- Contain hemoglobin.
- No nucleus or mitochondria.
- Function: Transports O_2 (and CO_2).
- Lipid membrane contains lipoproteins and blood group surface markers (A, B, O).
- Amount of bile pigment excreted by liver estimates the amount of erythrocyte destruction per day.

Leukocytes

See Table 2–5.

Monocytes transform into macrophages (histiocytes) once they leave the blood-stream and enter the surrounding connective tissue.

- White blood cells.
- **Granulocytes:** Contain cytoplasmic granules.
    - Neutrophils (60%)
    - Eosinophils (5%)
    - Basophils (1%)
- **Agranulocytes:** Contain few cytoplasmic granules.
    - Lymphocytes (30%)
    - Monocytes (4%)

Hematopoiesis

See Figure 2–8.

- Blood cell formation.
- All blood cells derive from one **pluripotential stem cell.**
- Hormones (erythropoietin, thrombopoietin, etc) and colony stimulating factors (CSFs) regulate hematopoiesis.
- Occurs primarily in **bone marrow,** although some lymphocytes also develop in lymphatic tissues.

TABLE 2-5. Comparison of Leukocytes

LEUKOCYTE	NUCLEAR MORPHOLOGY	CYTOPLASMIC GRANULES	FUNCTION
Neutrophil	3–5 lobes	Specific granules (lysozyme, etc) Azurophilic granules (peroxidases, etc)	Phagocytosis Acute inflammation
Eosinophil	2 lobes	Peroxidase Histaminase Arylsulfatase	Phagocytosis (parasites) Chronic inflammation
Basophil	2–3 lobes, obscured by dense granules	Histamine Seratonin Heparin sulfate	Hypersensitivity (bind IgE)
Lymphocyte	Large, round	Few azurophilic granules	Immunoregulation Chronic inflammation
Monocyte	U-shaped	Few azurophilic granules	Phagocytosis Chronic inflammation

► CARDIOVASCULAR TISSUE

Arrangement of Blood Vessels in Circulation

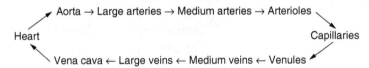

Heart

Aorta → Large arteries → Medium arteries → Arterioles → Capillaries

Vena cava ← Large veins ← Medium veins ← Venules ←

Layers of Blood Vessel Walls

From lumen → outermost layer

- **Tunica intima:** Contains *simple squamous epithelium* (**endothelium**) resting on a basement membrane and subendothelial connective tissue.

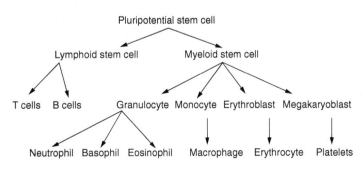

Pluripotential stem cell

Lymphoid stem cell   Myeloid stem cell

T cells   B cells   Granulocyte   Monocyte   Erythroblast   Megakaryoblast

Neutrophil   Basophil   Eosinophil   Macrophage   Erythrocyte   Platelets

FIGURE 2-8. **Hematopoiesis.**

The greatest drop in blood pressure occurs at the transition from arteries to arterioles.

Larger arteries: More elastic fibers.
Smaller arteries: More smooth muscle fibers.

ANATOMIC SCIENCES

GENERAL HISTOLOGY

Present in *all* blood vessels and heart wall. Only arteries have an additional elastic layer here called the **internal elastic membrane.**

- **Tunica media:** Contains *smooth muscle* and *elastic fibers*. Much thicker in arteries.
- **Tunica adventitia:** Connective tissue layer containing *collagen* and *elastic fibers*. Much thicker in veins. Large vessels contain **vasa vasora,** which supply the vessels themselves.

Layers of the Heart

From lumen → outermost layer

- **Endocardium:** Same as tunica intima. Contains a simple squamous endothelium.
- **Myocardium:** Thickest portion of the heart. Contains *cardiac muscle.*
- **Pericardium:** Outer layer of *connective tissue* and *adipose tissue* surrounded by a simple squamous epithelium.

Sinusoids are fenestrated or discontinuous capillaries in the liver, spleen, and endocrine glands. They are larger and more irregularly shaped than capillaries to accommodate phagocytic cells of the reticuloendothelial system.

Major Histologic Differences Among Blood Vessel Types

Blood Vessel	Distinguishing Characteristics
Elastic arteries (aorta, pulmonary arteries, and their main branches)	Thickest tunica media Elastic fibers > smooth muscle Contain vasa vasora
Muscular arteries	Thick tunica media Smooth muscle > elastic fibers Some contain vasa vasora
Arterioles	Thick tunica media Smooth muscle > elastic fibers Directly affect arterial blood pressure
Capillaries	Endothelial layer only One erythrocyte cell wide Slowest velocity of blood flow Enable gas and metabolite exchange via **diffusion**
Venules	Thick tunica adventitia
Veins	Thickest tunica adventitia Some contain valves Some contain vasa vasora

Tachycardia: >100 bpm

Bradycardia: <60 bpm

Cardiac Conduction

- Cardiac muscle maintains its *own* rhythmicity.
- The **sinoatrial (SA) node** is the "pacemaker" of the heart.
- Autonomic nerves only regulate the *rate* of cardiac impulses.
- SA node → AV node → bundle of His → purkinje fibers.
- In sinus rhythm, every P wave is followed by QRS complex.

Lymph

- A yellowish, plasmalike liquid that contains mostly **lymphocytes.**
- Once absorbed in various tissues throughout the body, it is carried through a system of enclosed **lymphatic vessels** and ultimately drains into the venous circulation.
- Lymph is not pumped through its vessels, but relies on valves, gravity, and skeletal muscle contractions for its movement.

Most lymph is returned to the blood at the junction of the left internal jugular and subclavian veins.

Functions of the Lymphatic System

- Transportation of tissue fluid (lymph) to the circulation
- Transportation of fat metabolites to the circulation
- Filtration of foreign agents in lymph nodes
- Provides immunological surveillance against pathogens

Lymph Drainage

- Thoracic duct (drains majority of the body) → left subclavian vein
- Right lymphatic duct (drains upper right body regions) → right subclavian vein

COMPONENTS OF THE LYMPHATIC SYSTEM

- Bone marrow
- Thymus
- Spleen
- Lymph
- Lymphatic vessels
- Lymph nodes
- Lymphatic nodules
  - Tonsils
  - Appendix
  - Peyer's patches of the ileum

Pharyngeal tonsils and Peyer's patches are nonencapsulated and subepithelial.

LYMPH NODES

- Small, fibrous-encapsulated organs that filter lymph (Figure 2–9).
- **Macrophages** and **lymphocytes** process lymph in nodal **cortical and trabecular sinuses.**
- Efferent vessels < afferent vessels.
- Widely distributed throughout the body, but concentrate in the axilla, groin, mesenteries, and neck.
- Consist of:
  - **External capsule:** Trabeculae extend into cortex and medulla.
  - **Outer cortex:** Germinal nodules. Contains **B-cells.**
    - **1° nodules:** Small dormant clusters
    - **2° nodules:** Active germinal centers
  - **Paracortex:** Deeper cortex. Contains **T-cells.**
  - **Inner medulla:** Medullary cords separated by medullary sinuses. Contains **B-cells and macrophages.**

Lymph nodes are the only lymphatic structures with both efferent and afferent vessels.

BONE MARROW

- Site of **B-cell maturation**
- Contains pluripotent stem cells capable of differentiating into lymphocytes or phagocytes

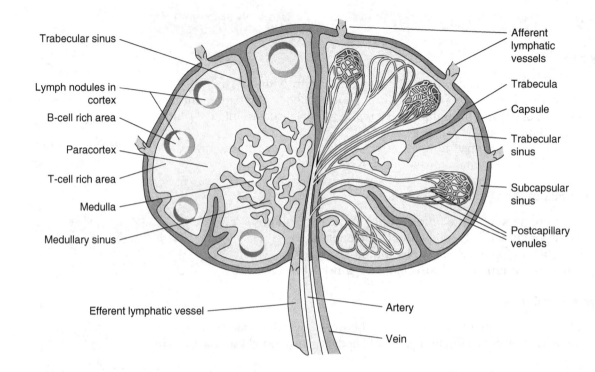

FIGURE 2–9. Schematic diagram of a lymph node.

Reproduced, with permission, from Ross MH, Romrell LJ, Kaye GI. *Histology: A Text and Atlas*. 3rd ed. Philadelphia: Williams & Wilkins; 1995.

THYMUS

- Site of **T-cell maturation**
- Grows in size from birth until puberty, then is reduced and replaced with adipose tissue in adulthood
- Does *not* contain afferent lymphatic vessels
- Consists of:
    - **External capsule:** *Trabeculae* extend into cortex and medulla
    - **Outer cortex:** Contains high concentration of **T-cells**
    - **Inner medulla:** Thymic (Hassall's) corpuscles. Contains **epitheliore-ticular cells**

SPLEEN

- Largest lymphatic organ.
- Does not develop from primitive gut (as do lungs, liver, pancreas, gallbladder, stomach, esophagus, intestines). Instead, it develops from mesenchymal cells of the mesenchyme of the primitive stomach.
- Site of lymphocyte proliferation, scavenging of large antigens and damaged erythrocytes, and fetal erythropoiesis.
- Does *not* contain afferent lymphatic vessels.
- Consists of:
    - **External capsule:** Trabeculae extend into the pulp.
    - **White pulp:** Splenic nodules. Contains **B-cells**.
        - **Periarterial lymphatic sheath (PALS):** Surrounds central artery within white pulp. Contains T-cells.
    - **Red pulp:** Splenic sinuses separated by splenic cords. Contains **erythrocytes, macrophages, and lymphocytes.**

Pituitary Gland (Hypophysis)

See Table 2–6.

- Pea-shaped organ located in the sella turcica of the sphenoid bone.
- Known as the "master endocrine gland." Vital to life.
- Attached to the hypothalamus via infundibulum.
- Provides regulatory feedback to the hypothalamus.
- Blood supply: Inferior and superior hypophyseal arteries (branches in ICA).
- Contains its own *portal system*.
- Composed of two distinct functional compartments:
  - **Adenohypophysis:** Anterior pituitary
  - **Neurohypophysis:** Posterior pituitary

GH is the most abundant of the pituitary hormones. ADH and oxytocin are synthesized in the hypothalamus and stored in the posterior pituitary.

Thyroid Gland

- Bilobed organ located anterolateral to the upper trachea, in the anterior triangle of the neck.
- Surrounded by a connective tissue capsule.
- Numerous **secretory follicles** surround a gel-like **colloid**, which is composed of inactive iodinated thyroglobulin.
- Composed of numerous **secretory follicles** surrounding a gel-like **colloid** (*inactive iodinated thyroglobulin*).
- Active cells stain basophilic; inactive cells stain acidophilic.
- The normal T_4:T_3 ratio is 20:1.

A portal system has two capillary beds. There are three portal systems in the body: hepatic, renal, pituitary.

Major Cellular Components of Thyroid Follicles

Cell Type	Secretory Products	Function
Follicular cells	T_4 (thyroxine) T_3 (triiodothyronine)	Regulate metabolism Regulate metabolism
Parafollicular cells	Calcitonin	↓ blood calcium levels

- Hypothyroidism
  - Cretinism (children)
  - Myxedema (adults)
  - Hashimoto's thyroiditis (autoimmune)
- Hyperthyroidism
  - Grave's disease (toxic goiter)

Parathyroid Glands

See Table 2–7.

- Small, ovoid organs arranged in pairs located in the thyroid connective tissue
- Surrounded by their own connective tissue capsules
- Derive from the third and fourth pharyngeal pouches
- Regulate blood calcium and phosphate
- Innervation: Superior cervical ganglion (postganglionic sympathetic fibers)
- Blood supply: Inferior and superior thyroid arteries

Effects of PTH

- ↑ blood calcium levels (*reciprocal action of calcitonin*)
- Stimulates bone resorption
- ↑renal Ca^{2+} resorption (↓Ca^{2+} excretion)
- ↓renal PO_4^{3-} resorption (↑PO_4^{3-} excretion)
- ↑ intestinal Ca^{2+} absorption

Pineal Gland

- Small, cone-shaped gland located at back of 3rd ventricle of the brain.
- Regulates sleep-wake cycle. Adjusts to sudden changes in day length.
- Contains numerous neurotransmitters, including melatonin.

TABLE 2-6. Functional Components of the Pituitary Gland

FUNCTIONAL COMPONENT	EMBRYONIC DERIVATION	COMPONENTS	SECRETORY PRODUCTS	FUNCTION
Adenohypophysis (anterior pituitary)	Rathke's pouch (oral ectoderm)	Pars distalis	**Somatotropes** Growth hormone (GH, somatotropin)	General growth, AA uptake, protein synthesis, carbohydrate and fat breakdown
			Lactotropes Prolactin (♂)	Mammary gland development
			Gonadotropes Follicle-stimulating hormone (FSH)	Milk production, Ovarian follicle maturation (♀), spermatogenesis (♂)
			Leutinizing hormone (LH)	Stimulates sex steroid secretion, controls ovulation (♀)
			Corticotropes Adrenocorticotropic hormone (ACTH)	Stimulates glucocorticoid (cortisol) secretion
			Thyrotropes Thyroid-stimulating hormone (TSH)	Thyroxine secretion, uptake of iodine
		Pars intermedia	**Lipotropes** Lipotropic hormone (LPH)	No known human function
		Pars tuberalis	**Gonadotropes**	See above
Neurohypophysis (posterior pituitary): ■ Contains unmyelinated nerves	Infundibulum (neurectoderm)	Pars nervosa	Antidiuretic hormone (ADH, vasopressin)	Water reabsorption
			Oxytocin	Uterine contractions, milk ejection
		Infundibulum	None	
		Median eminence	None	

TABLE 2-7. Major Parathyroid Cells

PARATHYROID CELL	CYTOPLASM	FUNCTION
Chief (principal) cell	Clear	Secretes PTH
Oxyphil cell	Granules	Unknown

Adrenal (Suprarenal) Glands

- Triangular organs located just superior to the kidneys.
- Surrounded by a thick connective tissue capsule.
- Provides regulatory feedback to the pituitary and hypothalamus.
- Composed of two regions:
  - Outer cortex
  - Inner medulla

Adrenal Region	Embryologic Derivation	Secretory Zones/Cells	Products	Examples
Outer cortex	Mesoderm	Zona glomerulosa • Thin layer just beneath the capsule	Mineralcorticoids	Aldosterone
		Zona fasiculata • Thick middle layer containing columns of cells	Glucocorticoids	Hydrocortisone Cortisone
		Zona reticularis • Innermost layer containing cells in a network of connected cords	Gonadocorticoids	Sex steroids
Inner medulla	Neural crest ectoderm	Chromaffin cells	Catecholamines	Epinephrine Norepinephrine

Zones of Adrenal Cortex: GFR

- G = Salt
- F = Sugar
- R = Sex

▶ RESPIRATORY SYSTEM

See Table 2-8.

Functions

- Air conduction
- Air filtration
- Gas exchange

TABLE 2-8. Major Respiratory Segments

RESPIRATORY SEGMENT	COMPONENTS	EPITHELIUM
Nasal cavities	Vestibule	Stratified squamous, kertinized
	Respiratory segment	Psuedostratified ciliated columnar
	Olfactory segment	Psuedostratified ciliated columnar
Pharynx	Nasopharynx	Pseudostratified ciliated columnar
	Oropharynx	Stratified squamous, nonkeratinized
Larynx	Vocal folds (true vocal cords)	Stratified squamous, nonkeratinized
	Ventricular folds (false vocal cords)	Pseudostratified ciliated columnar
Trachea	C-shaped hyaline cartilage rings	Pseudostratified ciliated columnar
Bronchi	Primary	Pseudostratified columnar
	Extrapulmonary	Pseudostratified columnar
Bronchioles	Terminal	Simple columnar
	Respiratory	Simple cuboidal
Alveoli	Alveolar ducts	Simple cuboidal
	Alveolar sacs	Simple cuboidal
	Alveolar septa	Simple squamous

Divisions

- Conduction: Warms air, moistens, removes particles
  - Nasal cavities
  - Nasopharynx and oropharynx
  - Larynx
  - Trachea
  - Bronchi
- Respiration: Gas exchange
  - Bronchioles
  - Alveolar ducts
  - Alveolar sacs
  - Alveoli

Alveoli

- Site of gas exchange
- **Alveolar septum:** Separates adjacent alveolar air spaces

ALVEOLAR EPITHELIAL CELL TYPES

Pneumocyte	Alveolar Surface Covered (%)	Function	Characteristic
Type I	95%	Gas exchange	Joined by tight junctions
Type II	5%	Secretion	Produce **surfactant**

Dust cells *are alveolar macrophages.*

▶ UPPER DIGESTIVE SYSTEM

Functions

- Barrier
- Absorption
- Secretion

Layers

From inner → outer (Figure 1–69)

- Mucosa
  - Epithelium: Varies throughout the GI tract
  - Lamina propria: Underlying CT and lymphatic tissue
  - Muscularis mucosae: Smooth muscle
- Submucosa: Dense irregular CT, glands, submucosal plexus of unmyelinated nerves and ganglia
- Muscularis externa: Smooth muscle
  - Circular
  - Longitudinal
- Serosa
  - Mesothelium: Simple squamous epithelium
  - CT: Adipose tissue, vasculature, lymphatics
- Adventitia: Loose CT

Peristalsis *is the waves of smooth muscle contraction of the muscularis externa that propels GI contents along.*

Esophagus

- Function: Transports food from oropharynx → stomach
- Epithelium: Nonkeratinized stratified squamous
- Glands: Mucous
  - Esophageal glands proper: Upper portion
  - Esophageal cardiac glands: Lower portion
  - Innervation: CN X

Stomach

- Function: Mixing and partial digestion of food, producing **chyme**
- Epithelium: Simple columnar, renews every 3–5 days
- Lining
  - **Rugae:** Longitudinal folds along the lumen of the stomach that accommodate expansion
  - **Gastric pits:** Microscopic depressions of the mucosal surface into which the gastric glands empty
- Organization
  - Cardiac: Junction of esophagus

TABLE 2-9. **Major Glands of the Stomach**

GLAND	LOCATION	CELL TYPES	SECRETION	FUNCTION
Cardiac	Cardiac stomach	Cardiac mucosal cells	Mucous	
Fundic (gastric)	Body of stomach	Mucous neck cells	Soluble mucous	
		Chief (zymogenic) cells	Pepsinogen	Converted to pepsin via gastric HCl
		Parietal (oxyntic) cells	HCl Intrinsic factor (a glycoprotein)	↓ stomach pH Essential for vitamin B_{12} absorption
		Enteroendocrine (G) cells	Gastrin	Stimulates HCl secretion from parietal cells
Pyloric	Pyloric stomach	Pyloric mucosal cells	Viscous mucous	

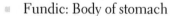

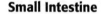

- Fundic: Body of stomach
- Pyloric: Junction of small intestine
- Glands: None are submucosal. See Table 2–9
- Innervation: CN X (regulates emptying)

Small Intestine

See Table 2–10.

- Function: Digestion of chyme and absorption
- Epithelium: Simple columnar, renews every 5–6 days
- Lining
  - **Plicae circulares (valves of Kerckring):** Transverse semilunar folds along the lumen of the small intestine, provide surface area. Most numerous at duodenum-jejunum junction.
  - **Villi:** Fingerlike projections on the plicae.
  - **Microvilli:** Micro fingerlike projections on enterocytes, provide ↑ surface area. Create "brush-border."
- Organization
  - **Duodenum:** Shortest segment (25 cm)
    - Has submucosal glands (Brunner's glands)
  - **Jejunum:** Middle segment (2.5 m)
    - More plicae and villi for increased absorption
  - **Ileum:** Longest segment (3.5 m)
    - Has lymphoid tissue (Peyer's patches)
- Muscularis externa
  - **Myenteric (Auerbach's) plexus:** Located between two layers of smooth muscle
- Muscular contractions
  - Peristalsis
  - Segmentation: Local contractions
- Glands
  - **Intestinal glands (crypts of Lieberkühn):** Throughout small intestine at base of villi
  - **Submucosal glands of Brunner:** Only in *duodenum*

Epithelial cells that line microvilli of "brush border":

- *Enterocytes*
- *Goblet cells*
- *Enteroendocrine (APUD) cells*

TABLE 2-10. **Cells of the Small Intestine**

CELL	LOCATION	SECRETION	FUNCTION
Enterocytes	*Epithelium* throughout small intestine	None Glycoprotein enzymes	Absorption Digestion
Goblet cells	*Epithelium* throughout small intestine (mostly in ileum)	Mucous	
M cells	Peyer's patches (**ileum**)	None	Absorption of antigens to underlying lymphatic tissue
Paneth cells	Intestinal glands throughout small intestine	Lysozyme	Digestion of bacterial cell walls
Enteroendocrine (APUD) cells	Intestinal crypts throughout small intestine (mostly in duodenum)	CCK	↑ pancreatic secretion ↑ increases bile secretion
		Secretin Gastric inhibitory peptide (GIP)	↑ pancreatic HCO_3^- secretion ↓ gastric acid secretion
Mucosal cells	*Submucosal* glands of Brunner (**duodenum**)	HCO_3^-	Neutralizes intestinal pH

Large Intestine

- Function: Reabsorption of water/electrolytes and elimination of waste
- Epithelium: Simple columnar, renews every 5–6 days
  - Goblet cells lubricate dehydrating fecal matter
  - Paneth cells *not* present
- Lining: Smooth surface (no plicae circulares or villi)
- Organization
  - Cecum: Appendix
  - Ascending colon
  - Transverse colon
  - Descending colon
  - Sigmoid colon
  - Rectum: No teniae coli
  - Anal canal
- Muscularis externa
  - **Teniae coli:** Three longitudinal bands of muscle used for peristalsis
  - **Haustra:** Individual segments that allow for independent contraction
- Glands
  - Intestinal glands (crypts of Lieberkühn)
- Innervation
  - CN X to ascending and transverse colon
  - Pelvic splanchnic nerve to descending and sigmoid colon

Epithelial cells that line microvilli of "brush border":

- *Enterocytes*
- *Goblet cells*
- *Enteroendocrine (APUD) cells*

Gut-Associated Lymphatic Tissue (GALT)

- Lamina propria (GI tract)
- Peyer's patches (ileum)
- Lymphoid aggregates (large intestine and appendix)

▶ **LOWER DIGESTIVE SYSTEM**

Liver

- **Exocrine** (via ducts)
  - Bile
- **Endocrine** (via bloodstream)
  - Albumin
  - Lipoproteins
  - α and β globulins
  - Prothrombin
  - Fibronectin

Portal Triad

- Hepatic artery
- Portal vein
- Bile duct

Liver Lobules

- Hexagonal stacks of *hepatocyte cords* separated by anastamosing *sinusoids*
- Surround a *central vein* (into which sinusoids drain)
- *Portal triads* located at each corner

Hepatocytes

- Nuclei: Often bi-nucleate (tetraploid)
- Cytoplasm: Acidophilic
  - Mitochondria
  - Golgi bodies
  - rER
  - sER
  - **Peroxisomes**
    - Catalase
    - Alcohol dehydrogenase
  - Lysosomes
    - Store iron
  - Glycogen deposits
  - Lipid droplets
- Life span: 5 months
- Capable of regeneration

Hepatic Sinusoids

- Lined by a thin, discontinuous epithelium. No basement membrane.
  - Gaps: Between epithelial cells
  - Fenestrae: Within epithelial cells
- Cell types
  - Epithelial cells

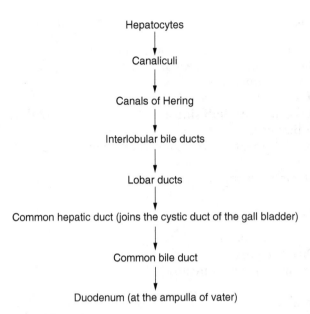

Hepatocytes
↓
Canaliculi
↓
Canals of Hering
↓
Interlobular bile ducts
↓
Lobar ducts
↓
Common hepatic duct (joins the cystic duct of the gall bladder)
↓
Common bile duct
↓
Duodenum (at the ampulla of vater)

FIGURE 2–10. Biliary flow.

Biliary flow is increased primarily by CCK, but also by secretin and gastrin.

- **Kupffer cells:** Mononuclear macrophages
- **Ito cells:** Adipocytes in the space of Disse—store *vitamin A*
- **Perisinusoidal space (space of Disse):** Site of exchange between blood and hepatocytes

Biliary Tree

See Figure 2–10.

- Ductal system that transports bile from hepatocytes → gall bladder (via cystic duct) and duodenum (via common bile duct).
- **Canaliculi:** Small canals formed by grooves in adjacent hepatocytes.
- Bile flow is *opposite* to that of blood flow (central vein → portal canal).
- **Ampulla of Vater:** Opening of common bile duct into the duodenum.
- Sphincters
  - **Sphincter of Boyden:** At common bile duct.
  - **Sphincter of Oddi:** At ampulla of Vater.

Elevated serum bilirubin results in jaundice.

Bile Composition

- Water
- Electrolytes
- Cholesterol
- Lecithin
- Bile salts
  - Glycocholic acid
  - Taurocholic acid
- Bile pigments
  - Bilirubin
  - Biliverdin
  - Glucuronide

Gall Bladder

- Function: Concentrates and stores bile
- Epithelium: Simple columnar
  - Contains microvilli
  - Has lateral plications
  - **Rokitansky-Aschoff sinuses:** Deep diverticula of the mucosa
- **No submucosa**
- Lamina propria: Does *not* contain lymphatic vessels
- Glands
  - Mucin-secreting glands

Pancreas

- **Exocrine** (via ducts)
  - Digestive enzymes
- **Endocrine** (via bloodstream)
  - Glucagon
  - Insulin
  - Somatostatin

*Enzyme production is regulated by duodenal **secretin** (↑ bicarbonate secretion) and **CCK** (↑ proenzyme secretion).*

Exocrine Pancreas

- Function: Produces digestive enzyme precursors (proenzymes), which are activated by trypsin in the lumen of the small intestine. Trypsinogen is first activated to trypsin by enterokinase.
  - Trypsinogen
  - Pepsinogen
  - Amylase
  - Lipase
  - Deoxyribonuclease
  - Ribonuclease
- Components: **Pancreatic acini**
- Cell types: **Centroacinar cells**

*Pancreatic digestive enzymes are activated only after they reach the **small intestine**, where trypsinogen is converted to trypsin via enterokinase. **Trypsin** then converts the other inactive digestive enzymes.*

Endocrine Pancreas

- Function: Regulates blood glucose levels
- Components: **Islets of Langerhans**
- Cell types: See Table below

Major Cells of the Pancreatic Islets

Somatostatin is also released by the hypothalamus to inhibit pituitary secretion of GH.

Cell Type	Major Product	Function
Alpha	Glucagon	↑ **blood glucose levels** ↑ glycogenolysis, gluconeogenesis, and hepatic lipase
Beta	Insulin	↓ **blood glucose levels** ↑ cellular glucose uptake, utilization, and storage (as glycogen)
Delta	Somatostatin	Inhibits insulin and glucagon secretion

Components

▪ Kidneys
▪ Ureters
▪ Urinary bladder
▪ Urethra

Functions of Kidneys

▪ Removes metabolic waste
▪ Conserves body fluids
▪ Synthesizes erythropoietin
▪ Synthesizes renin
▪ Hydroxylates vitamin D

Pyramids are conical structures in the medulla composed of groups of medullary straight tubules, collecting ducts, and vasa recta. Usually 8–12 per kidney.

Components of Kidneys (Figure 2–11)

▪ **Capsule:** Tough, thin outer covering
▪ **Cortex:** Outer portion
  ▪ Renal (Malpighian) corpuscles
    ▪ **Glomerulus:** 10–20 capillary loops
    ▪ **Bowman's capsule:** Double-layered epithelial covering
  ▪ Proximal tubules
  ▪ Distal tubules
  ▪ Cortical collecting ducts
▪ **Medulla:** Inner portion
  ▪ Medullary collecting ducts
  ▪ Loop of Henle
  ▪ Vasa recta

Medullary rays are striations in the cortex (radiating from the medulla) composed of groups of cortical straight tubules and collecting ducts.

Juxtaglomerular Apparatus (JGA)

▪ **Macula densa:** Part of distal convoluted tubule
▪ **Juxtaglomerular cells:** Modified smooth muscle cells; secrete **renin**
▪ **Extraglomerular mesangial cells:** Phagocytic cells

JG cells produce renin, which regulates blood pressure.

Nephron

▪ Functions
  ▪ Filtration
  ▪ Absorption
  ▪ Secretion
  ▪ Excretion
▪ Components
  ▪ Glomerulus
  ▪ Bowman's capsule
  ▪ Proximal convoluted tubule
  ▪ Loop of Henle (descending, ascending, thick, thin)
  ▪ Distal convoluted tubule

The nephron is the functional unit of the kidney. There are millions per kidney.

TYPES OF NEPHRONS

Nephron	Location of Renal Corpuscles	Length of Loop of Henle
Cortical	Outer cortex	Short
Intermediate	Middle cortex	Medium
Juxtamedullary	Base of medullary pyramid	Long

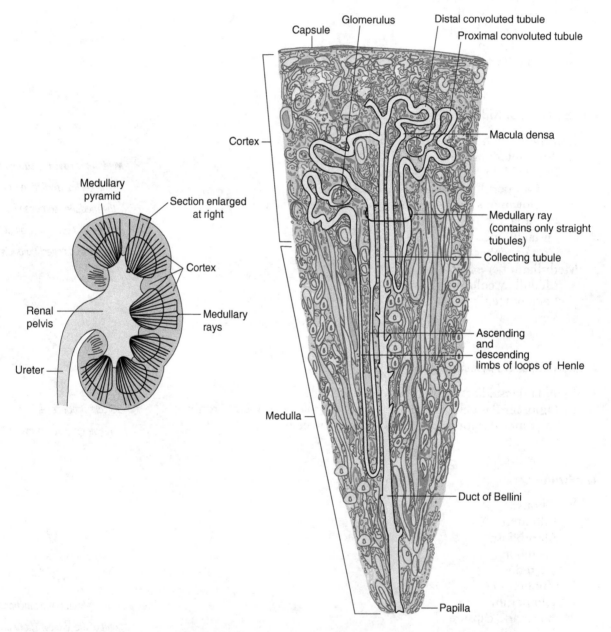

FIGURE 2–11. Schematic diagram of a kidney and nephron structure.

Reproduced, with permission, from Ross MH, Romrell LJ, Kaye GI. *Histology: A Text and Atlas.* 3rd ed. Philadelphia: Williams & Wilkins; 1995.

Urethra

- The male urethra is long (20 cm) and has three segments:
  - **Prostatic urethra:** Travels from the urinary bladder through the prostate gland. Widest and most dilatable.
  - **Membranous urethra:** Travels from the end of the prostate through the body wall to the penis. Shortest and least dilatable.
  - **Penile urethra:** Travels through the length of the penis within the corpus spongiosum. Longest and narrowest.
- The female urethra is short (3–5 cm), and extends from the urinary bladder to the vaginal vestibule.

▶ REPRODUCTIVE SYSTEM

Testis

- Produces **sperm** and steroids (**testosterone**).
- **Tunica albuginea:** Thick connective tissue capsule that covers the testis.
- Covered by a thick connective tissue capsule called the **tunica albuginea.**
- Composed of many lobules, each containing 1–4 **seminiferous tubules,** the site of **spermatogenesis.**
- **Epididymis:** Sits on the posterior aspect of the testis. Contains the ductus epididymis. Stores sperm. Epithelial cells have stereocilia, which increase surface area for nutrient absorption for sperm.
- **Seminal fluid:** Secretions from seminal vesicles and prostate.

Major Cellular Components of the Male Reproductive System

Cell	Location	Function
Leydig cell	Seminiferous tubules	Produces testosterone
Sertoli cell	Seminiferous tubules	Produces testicular fluid
Sperm cell	Produced in seminiferous tubules, but mature and are stored in the epididymis	Produces sperm

Intra- and Extra-Testicular Duct System

Seminiferous tubules (testis)
↓
Rete testis (testis)
↓
Efferent ductules (testis)
↓
Ductus epididymis (epididymis)
↓
Ductus (vas) deferens (spermatic cord)-joins seminal vesicle duct
↓
Ejaculatory duct (enters into urethra)

Spermatic cord:
- *Ductus (vas) deferens*
- *Testicular artery and veins*
- *Lymph vessels*
- *Autonomic nerves*

Prostate Gland

- Surrounds the proximal urethra
- Secretes acid phosphatase, fibrinolysin, and citric acid

Penis

- Composed of three major masses of tissue surrounded by a dense fibroelastic capsule (**tunica albuginea**):
    - **Corpora cavernosa:** Two *dorsal* sections of erectile tissue
    - **Corpus spongiosum:** One *ventral* section containing the urethra

Ovarian follicle development:

1. Primordial oocytes (surrounded by granulosa cells).

2. Multilayered theca interna secretes estrogen.

3. Surrounding stromal cells form theca externa.

4. Split in theca interna forms Graafian follicle.

Ovary

- Elliptical organs supported by broad ligament of uterus.
- Produces **ova** and steroids (**estrogen** and **progesterone**).
- Composed of two regions:
    - **Inner medulla:** Contains vasculature, nerves, and CT.
    - **Outer cortex:** Contains **ovarian follicles,** the site of **oogenesis.**

Oviducts (Fallopian Tubes)

- Extend bilaterally from the ovaries to the uterus.
- Divided into four sections (from ovary → uterus):
    - **Infundibulum:** Just adjacent to the ovary. Contains fingerlike extensions called **fimbriae.**
    - **Ampulla:** Longest section of the oviduct. Site of fertilization.
    - **Isthmus:** Just adjacent to the uterus.
    - **Uterine:** Opening into the uterus.

Uterus

- Site of embryonic and fetal development.
- Composed of three layers:
    - **Endometrium:** Mucosal layer shed during menstruation.
    - **Myometrium:** Thickest layer containing smooth muscle.
    - **Perimetrium:** External layer containing connective tissue.
- Contains uterine glands.
- The cervix is the lower section of the uterus, connecting it to the vagina. Its mucosa is *not* shed during menstruation.

Vagina

- Lined by nonkeratinized stratified squamous epithelium.
- Does *not* contain glands.

Although both skin and oral mucosa have stratified squamous epithelial surfaces and subepithelial connective tissues, there are some important differences in terminology and structures.

Mammary Glands

- Contain **tubuloalveolar glands** (produce milk), sebaceous glands (glands of Montgomery), and sweat glands.
- Milk is produced by both **merocrine** and **apocrine** secretion.
- Lactation is regulated by sex hormones produced during pregnancy, and is under the control of the pituitary and the hypothalamus.

▶ INTEGUMENT

Functions of Skin

- Protection: Against physical, chemical, and biological agents
- Sensory: Touch, pain, pressure, etc
- Homeostasis: Regulates body temperature and water loss

- Synthesis: Produces vitamin D from UV light
- Excretion: Via sweat glands

Layers of Skin

- **Epidermis:** Stratified squamous keratinized epithelium (from innermost → outermost).
  - **Stratum basale (germinativum):** Site of all epithelial mitotic activity (contains *melanocytes*, keratinocytes, and other specialized cells). Least cytodifferentiated. Cuboidal to low columnar in shape.
  - **Stratum spinosum:** Spinous (prickle cell) layer. Cells have peripheral cytoplasmic processes. *Langerhans cells* often extend into this layer.
  - **Stratum granulosum:** Cells appear flattened and may contain *keratohyalin granules*. Organelles are diminished.
  - **Stratum lucidum:** Clear cell layer found only in *thick skin* (palms, soles). Cells appear flattened with few (if any) organelles.
  - **Stratum corneum:** Keratinized cell layer. Cells appear flattened and pyknotic with few (if any) organelles.
  - **Basement membrane:** Links the epidermis and dermis via **hemidesmosomes**.
    - **Lamina lucida**
    - **Lamina densa (basal lamina)**
      - *Type IV collagen*
      - Proteoglycans
      - Laminin
      - Fibronectin
      - Anchoring fibrils (type VII collagen)
    - **Reticular lamina**
      - Reticular fibers (type III collagen)
- **Dermis:** Thicker portion of skin. Dense CT, vasculature, lymphatics, nerves, sweat glands, sebaceous glands, hair follicles.
  - **Papillary layer:** Thinner, cellular, less fibrous. Dermal papillae are the projections that interdigitate with the epidermal rete pegs (ridges), creating a variably tortuous epidermal-dermal interface. Contains **blood vessels** that supply overlying epidermis.
  - **Reticular layer:** Thicker, fibrous, less cellular.
- **Hypodermis:** Loose CT, vasculature, lymphatics, and **adipose tissue** (provides insulation, energy storage, and anchorage).

> ***Epidermal layers (from innermost to outermost):***
>
> **B**ad **S**printers **G**et **L**eg **C**ramps:
>
> **B**asale
> **S**pinosum
> **G**ranulosum
> **L**ucidum
> **C**orneum

SPECIALIZED EPIDERMAL CELLS

- Concentrated in the basal cell layer.
- **Melanocytes:** Produce melanin (pigment).
- **Keratinocytes:** Produce keratin (protection). Have well-developed tonofibrils and desmosomes.
- **Langerhans cells:** Antigen-presenting cells. Often extend into stratum spinosum.
- **Merkel cells:** Touch-sensory cells (touch).

NEURONAL ENDINGS OF SKIN

- **Free nerve endings:** Most abundant nerve endings. Detect touch, temperature, pain. Extend into stratum granulosum. Not encapsulated.
- **Pacinian corpuscles:** Pressure and vibration receptors.
- **Meissner's corpuscles:** Touch receptors.
- **Ruffini endings:** Mechanoreceptors.

Hair

- Regulate body temperature
- Composed of keratinized cells
- Produced by hair follicles:
  - Bulb
  - Internal root sheath
  - External root sheath
  - Arrector pili muscle

Types of Sweat Glands

Type	Function	Cells	Secretion	Location	Innervation
Eccrine	Regulates body temperature	Clear Dark Myoepithelial Duct	Sweat	Entire body except lips and parts of external genitalia	SNS (parasympathetic)
Apocrine	Produces pheromones	Myoepithelial Duct	Odorless serous secretion	Axilla, areola, nipple, circumanal region, external genitalia	SNS (sympathetic)

Sebaceous Glands

- Sebocytes: Secrete **sebum**, an oily substance that coats hair-covered skin.
- Outgrowths of external root sheaths of hair follicles.

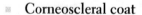

▶ EYE

Layers of Eye

See Figure 2–12.
From outermost → innermost:

- Corneoscleral coat
  - **Cornea:** Transparent portion (anterior 1/6) of eye.
  - **Limbus:** Transitional zone between cornea and sclera.
  - **Sclera:** "White" portion (posterior 5/6) of eye.
- Uvea
  - **Choroid:** Vascular layer. Dark brown color.
  - **Ciliary body:** Smooth muscle (lens accommodation). See Figure 2–13.
  - **Iris:** Smooth muscle (changes pupil diameter). Pigmented portion of eye.
    - **Pupil:** Central aperture of iris.
- Retina
  - **Pigment epithelium:** Melanin-containing cells.
  - **Neural retina:** Rods and cones.

CHAMBERS

- Anterior chamber: From cornea → iris
- Posterior chamber: From iris → lens
- Vitreous chamber: From lens → neural retina

Aqueous humor is the watery fluid within the anterior and posterior chambers.

Vitreous humor is the transparent watery gel within the vitreous chamber.

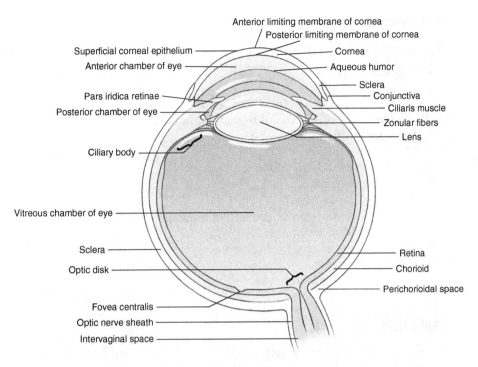

FIGURE 2–12. General structure of the eye.

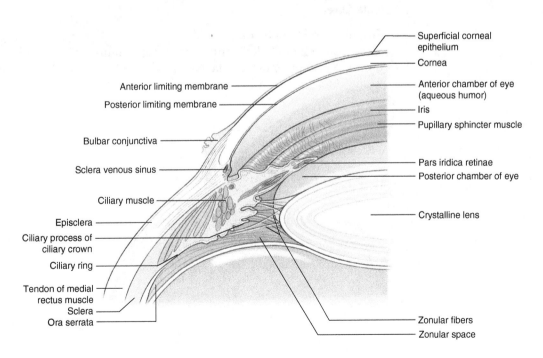

FIGURE 2–13. Ciliary zone.

Reproduced, with permission, from Riordan-Eva P, Hoyt WF. *Vaughan and Asbury's General Ophthalmology*, 17th ed. New York: McGraw-Hill, 2008.

Vitamin A is a source of retinal, an essential component of rods. Dietary deficiency of vitamin A results in the inability to see in dim light ("night blindness").

Ten Layers of Retina

From outermost → innermost:

1. Pigment epithelium
2. Photoreceptor cells
   - **Rods:** Sensitive to **light**; contain **rhodopsin**
   - **Cones:** Sensitive to **color**; contain **iodopsin**
3. External limiting membrane
4. Outer nuclear layer
   - Nuclei of rods and cones
5. Outer plexiform layer
6. Inner nuclear layer
   - Nuclei of horizontal, amacrine, bipolar, and Müller's cells
7. Inner plexiform layer
8. Ganglion cell layer
9. Optic nerve fibers
10. Internal limiting membrane

Optic Disc

- Collection of retinal ganglion cell nerve fibers (axons) leaving eye as **optic nerve**. The right and left optic nerves meet at the **optic chiasm**.
- Central artery and vein of the retina also exit here. The central artery (branch of ophthalmic artery) pierces the optic nerve and gains access to retina by emerging from center of optic disc and fans out.
- Small **blind spot** on the retina; 3 mm to nasal side of macula.
- Only part of retina without rods or cones.

Macula Lutea

- Just temporal to optic disc
- Responsible for detailed central vision (eg, reading)
- **Fovea:** Very center of macula. No blood vessels. Very high concentration of cones. Area of sharpest vision.

CHAPTER 3

Oral Histology

Oral Mucosa

LAYERS OF ORAL MUCOSA (SEE FIGURE 3–1)

From outermost → innermost:

- **Stratified squamous epithelium:** Keratinized or nonkeratinized.
  - **Stratum corneum:** Keratinized cell layer. Cells appear flattened and pyknotic with few (if any) organelles.
  - **Stratum granulosum:** Cells appear flattened and may contain *keratohyalin* granules. Organelles are diminished.
  - **Stratum spinosum:** Spinous (prickle cell) layer. Cells have peripheral cytoplasmic processes. Langerhans cells often extend into this layer.
  - **Stratum basale (germinativum):** Site of all epithelial mitotic activity. Least cytodifferentiated. Cuboidal to low columnar in shape.
- **Basement membrane:** Contains **type IV collagen** and **laminin.** Epithelial attachment to the basement membrane is mediated by *hemidesmosomes.*
- **Subepithelial connective tissue:** Contains collagen and elastic fibers, ground substance, blood vessels, nerves, and inflammatory cells.
  - **Lamina propria**
    - **Papillary layer:** Connective tissue **papillae** are the projections that interdigitate with the epithelial **rete pegs (ridges),** creating a variably tortuous epithelial–connective tissue interface.
    - **Reticular layer:** Constitutes the remainder of the lamina propria.
- **Submucosa.** Present in areas of high compression. Often indistinguishable with the lamina propria.

SPECIALIZED EPITHELIAL CELLS

- **Melanocytes:** Produce melanin.
- **Keratinocytes:** Produce keratin, not present in all oral mucosa.
- **Langerhans cells:** Antigen-presenting cells.
- **Merkel cells:** Touch-sensory cells.

TYPES OF ORAL MUCOSA

See Table 3–1.

- *All* oral mucosa contains **stratified squamous epithelium.**

Gingiva

See Figures 3–2 and 3–3.

- The fibrous, keratinized tissue that surrounds a tooth and is contiguous with the periodontal ligament and oral mucosa.
- Contains a stratified squamous **keratinized** epithelium with rete pegs.
- Extends from the **gingival margin** (the most coronal portion of the gingiva) to the **mucogingival junction (MGJ).** The MGJ separates the gingiva from the alveolar mucosa.
- Color ranges from pink to brown, depending on the amount of melanin expression, which is correlated with cutaneous pigmentation.

Oral mucosa layers (from outermost to innermost):
California Girls String Bikinis

- **C**orneum
- **G**ranulosum
- **S**pinosum
- **B**asale

Most specialized epithelial cells concentrate in the basal cell layer; however, ***Langerhans cells*** *may extend into the stratum spinosum.*

Chronic ***mouth breathing*** *often results in pronounced gingival erythema, especially in the anterior regions.*

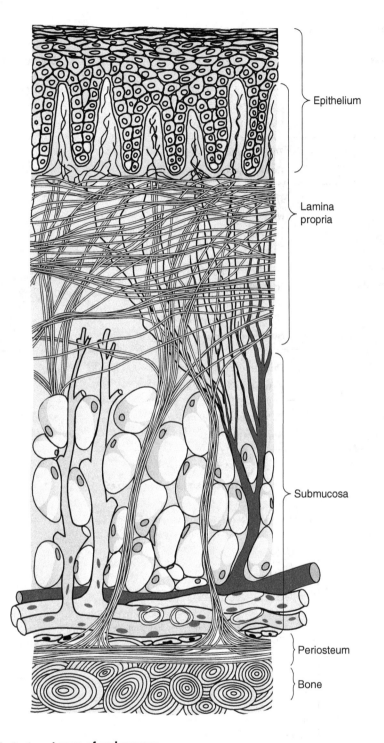

FIGURE 3-1. Layers of oral mucosa.

Reproduced, with permission, from Ten Cate AR. *Oral Histology: Development, Structure, and Function.* 4th ed. St Louis: Mosby; 1994.

ZONES OF GINGIVA

- **Attached gingiva:** Firmly bound to periosteum and cementum. About 40% of the adult population exhibits **stippling** of the attached gingiva, which is an orange-peel-like surface characteristic caused by the intersection of epithelial rete pegs.

The free gingival groove separates the attached and unattached (marginal) gingiva. The mucogingival junction separates the gingiva from the alveolar mucosa.

TABLE 3-1. The Three Major Types of Oral Epithelium

MUCOSA TYPE	LOCATION	EPITHELIUM	SUBMUCOSA
Masticatory	Gingiva	*Thick* stratified squamous **Keratinized** (75% para) May show stippling (40%)	Indistinct
	Hard palate	*Thick* stratified squamous **Keratinized** (mostly ortho)	Thin
Lining	Soft palate	*Thin* stratified squamous **Nonkeratinized** Taste buds	Thick
	Alveolar mucosa Floor of the mouth	*Thin* stratified squamous **Nonkeratinized**	Thick
	Buccal mucosa	*Thick* stratified squamous **Nonkeratinized**	Thin
	Lips	*Thin* stratified squamous **Keratinized** (ortho and para)	Thin
	Ventral tongue	*Thin* stratified squamous **Nonkeratinized**	Thin
Specialized	Dorsal tongue	*Thick* stratified squamous *Both* **keratinized** and **nonkeratinized** Taste buds	Indistinct

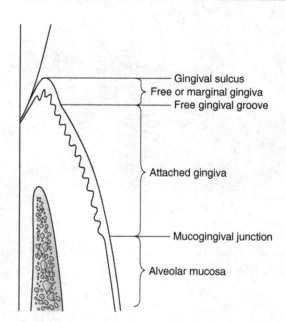

- Gingival sulcus
- Free or marginal gingiva
- Free gingival groove
- Attached gingiva
- Mucogingival junction
- Alveolar mucosa

Denture abrasion may cause the masticatory mucosa (gingiva and hard palate) to become more orthokeratinized.

FIGURE 3-2. Gingival anatomy.

Reproduced, with permission, from Carranza FA. *Clinical Periodontology*, 8th ed., page 60, copyright 1996 by Elsevier.

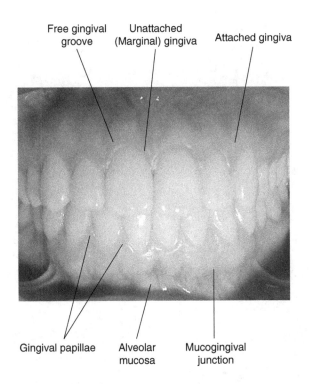

Free gingival groove · Unattached (Marginal) gingiva · Attached gingiva

Gingival papillae · Alveolar mucosa · Mucogingival junction

FIGURE 3–3. Healthy gingival anatomy.

Note the gingival stippling in the maxillary anterior region. Stippling occurs in about 40% of the adult population.

- **Free (unattached, marginal) gingiva:** Located coronal to the attached gingiva and is separated from the tooth surface by the **gingival sulcus.**
  - **Interdental papilla:** The triangular portion of the free gingiva located in the interproximal embrasures between teeth just apical to their contact areas.
  - **Gingival col:** The depression in the interdental gingiva connecting the buccal and lingual papilla immediately apical to the contact areas of adjacent teeth. Its epithelium is generally **nonkeratinized,** and its presence is based solely on the presence of an interdental contact.

Dentogingival Junction

- The attachment of the gingiva to the tooth.
- Consists of epithelial (**epithelial attachment**) and connective tissue (**connective tissue attachment**) components.
- Forms as the oral epithelium fuses with the reduced enamel epithelium (REE) during tooth eruption. As the tooth reaches its fully erupted position, cells of the junctional epithelium replace those of the REE.

DENTOGINGIVAL EPITHELIUM

- **Sulcular epithelium:** Stratified squamous **nonkeratinized** epithelium without rete pegs that extends from the gingival margin to the junctional epithelium. It lines the gingival sulcus (Figure 3–4).

*Biologic width is defined as the length of the dentogingival junction. In humans, the average width of epithelial attachment is 0.97 mm and 1.07 mm for the connective tissue attachment, creating a mean biologic width of **2.04 mm.***

In the presence of inflammation (eg, gingivitis), rete pegs will be present in the sulcular and junctional epithelia.

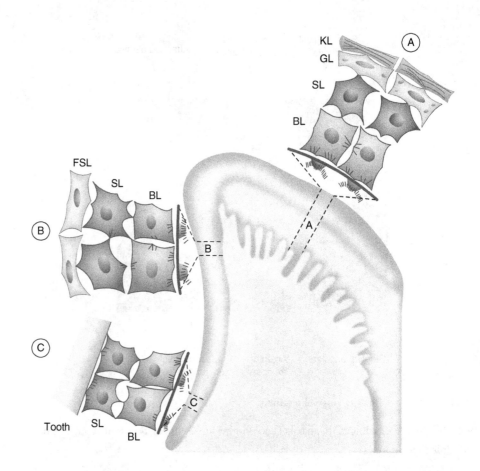

FIGURE 3-4. **Dentogingival epithelium. A: Gingival epithelium; B: Sulcular epithelium; C: Junctional epithelium. BL: Basal cell layer; SL: Spinous cell layer; FSL: Flattened spinous layer; GL: Granular cell layer containing keratohyaline granules; KL: Keratinized layer.**

Reproduced, with permission, from Rose LF, Mealey B, Genco R. *Periodontics: Medicine, Surgery, and Implants.* St Louis: Mosby; 2004.

The subepithelial connective tissue provides the cellular signaling that determines epithelial expression.

■ **Junctional epithelium:** Stratified to single-layer (at its apical extent) **nonkeratinized** epithelium without rete pegs that adheres to the tooth surface at the base of the sulcus. It provides the epithelial attachment to the tooth. Junctional epithelial cells have higher turnover rates and larger intercellular spaces than sulcular and gingival epithelia. It consists of two basal laminae:
   ■ **External basal lamina:** Attaches to underlying connective tissue as elsewhere in the body.
   ■ **Internal basal lamina:** Attaches to the cementum via *hemidesmosomes.* It is unlike other basal laminae in that it does not contain type IV collagen.

DENTOGINGIVAL CONNECTIVE TISSUE

■ **Type I collagen** makes up the bulk of the connective tissue.
■ Other major components include fibroblasts, leukocytes, mast cells, elastic fibers, proteoglycans, and glycoproteins.

GINGIVAL FIBER GROUPS

See Figure 3–5.

- Support the gingiva and aid in its attachment to alveolar bone and teeth.
- They are continuous with the PDL.
- Resist gingival displacement.
- Found at the gingival level.
- Do not confuse these with PDL fibers!
    - **Dentogingival fibers:** Fan laterally from cementum into the adjacent CT.
    - **Alveologingival fibers:** Fan coronally from the alveolar crest into the adjacent CT.
    - **Dentoperiosteal fibers:** Extend from cementum over the alveolar crest, and turn apically to insert into the periosteum of the buccal side of the alveolar bone.
    - **Circumferential fibers:** Surround the tooth in a circular fashion. Help prevent rotational forces. Located in lamina propria of marginal gingiva.

*The connective tissue adjacent to the sulcular and junctional epithelia generally contains an **increased inflammatory infiltrate** compared to that adjacent to the oral epithelium. PMNs and other leukocytes continually migrate between these epithelial cells into the sulcus, and account for a significant portion of **gingival crevicular fluid (GCF)** along with plasma proteins, epithelial cells, and bacteria.*

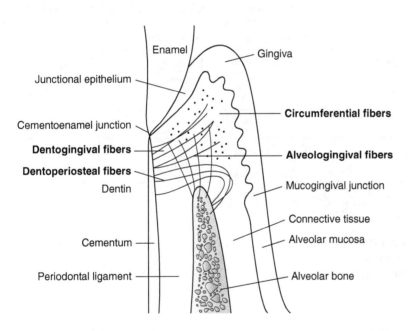

FIGURE 3–5.   The gingival fibers.

Comparison of the Major Tissues of Teeth and the Periodontium

	Enamel	Dentin	Cementum	Alveolar Bone	Pulp
Mineral composition	96%	70%	55%	50%	<5%
Organic composition	4%	30%	45%	50%	>95%
Embryologic origin	Ectoderm	Ectomesenchyme (neural crest)	Ectomesenchyme (neural crest)	Ectomesenchyme (neural crest)	Ectomesenchyme (neural crest)
Formative cell	Ameloblast	Odontoblast	Cementoblast	Osteoblast	Fibroblast Mesenchymal
Formative cells differentiated from	IEE	Dental papilla	Dental follicle	Dental follicle	Dental papilla
Tissue type	Epithelial	Connective	Connective	Connective	Connective
Viability	No	Repair	Repair	Remodeling	Yes
Incremental lines	Neonatal Retzius (daily)	Neonatal Owen von Ebner (daily)	Resting	Resting Reversal	None
Sensitivity	No	Yes	No	Yes	Yes (pain)
Nutritive supply	None	Pulp	PDL (diffusion)	Vessels (diffusion)	Vessels

Dentin

- An elastic, avascular, mineralized tissue that is harder than bone but softer than enamel
- Color is generally yellowish

ORIGIN

- Differentiated ectomesenchymal cells of the dental papilla

DENTINOGENESIS (SEE FIGURE 3–6)

- Organization
  - The odontoblasts become elongated and the organelles become polarized by ameloblastic induction.
- Mantle dentin formation
  - The dentin matrix formed by odontoblasts starts at the DEJ and progresses inward toward the eventual pulp. The dentin matrix first produced by the odontoblasts consists largely of type I collagen and ground substance, known as **predentin.**
  - As the odontoblasts retreat inward, they leave cytoplasmic extensions called **odontoblastic processes** (Tomes' fibers) at the DEJ. These

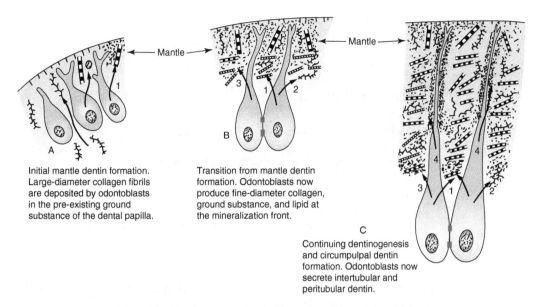

Initial mantle dentin formation. Large-diameter collagen fibrils are deposited by odontoblasts in the pre-existing ground substance of the dental papilla.

Transition from mantle dentin formation. Odontoblasts now produce fine-diameter collagen, ground substance, and lipid at the mineralization front.

Continuing dentinogenesis and circumpulpal dentin formation. Odontoblasts now secrete intertubular and peritubular dentin.

FIGURE 3–6. Dentinogenesis. A: Initial mantle dentin formation. Large-diameter collagen fibrils are deposited by odontoblasts in the pre-existing ground substance of the dental papilla. B: Transition from mantle dentin formation. Odontoblasts now produce fine-diameter collagen, ground substance, and lipid at the mineralization front. C: Continuing dentinogenesis and circumpulpal dentin formation. Odontoblasts now secrete intertubular and peritubular dentin.

Reproduced, with permission, from Ten Cate AR. *Oral Histology: Development, Structure, and Function.* 4th ed. St Louis: Mosby; 1994.

processes are housed in **dentinal tubules,** which form channels from the DEJ/DCJ to the pulp.

- The odontoblastic processes release **matrix vesicles** containing calcium, which crystallize and rupture. These crystals act as a nidus for the formation of more **hydroxyapatite** (HA) crystals in and around the organic dentin matrix.
- This initial 150 μm of dentin in known as **mantle dentin.**

- Circumpulpal dentin formation
  - Once mantle dentin is formed, odontoblasts (with well-developed rough ER and Golgi bodies) begin to secrete collagen fibrils perpendicularly to
  · the odontoblastic processes, as well as other organic substances such as lipids, phospholipids, and phosphoproteins.
  - Mineralization occurs by globular calcification by which globules of HA fuse to form a calcified mass. Occasionally, the globules fail to fuse, leaving hypomineralized **interglobular dentin** in between.
  - The odontoblastic processes shrink in width, providing a space for a hypermineralized **peritubular dentin** to form. If several adjacent dentinal tubules become occluded with this peritubular dentin, it takes on a glassy appearance and is called **sclerotic dentin.**
  - Most of the circumpulpal dentin produced is between the tubules, known as **intertubular dentin.**
  - **Dead tracts** are groups of necrotic odontoblastic processes within the dentinal tubules (often caused by trauma).
- Reparative dentin formation
  - **Reparative dentin** is formed only at specific sites of injury.
  - The types I and III collagens in its matrix are produced by differentiated odontoblast-like cells from the pulp. The tubular pattern is often distorted due to an increased rate of its formation.

$HA = Ca_{10}(PO_4)_6(OH)_2$

$FA = Ca_{10}(PO_4)_6F_2$

Coronal dentinal tubules follow an S-shape (primary curvature); radicular tubules are generally straight. There are more tubules concentrated near the pulp than the DEJ.

CLASSIFICATIONS OF DENTIN

- By time of formation
    - **Mantle:** The first 150 μm of dentin formed. Located closest to enamel (CEJ) and cementum (CDJ)
    - **Circumpulpal:** All dentin formed thereafter until tooth formation is complete
    - **Reparative:** Formed in response to trauma (eg, caries, restorations, attrition, erosion, abrasion, etc)
    - **Sclerotic:** Results from calcification of the dentinal tubules as one ages over time. Helps prevent pulpal irritation
- By root completion
    - **Primary:** Formed before root completion. Tubules are most regular.
    - **Secondary:** Formed after root completion, but not in response to trauma.
    - **Tertiary:** Formed in response to trauma (eg, caries, restorations, attrition, erosion, abrasion, etc). Tubules are least regular.
- By proximity to dentinal tubules
    - **Peritubular:** *Hyper*mineralized dentin formed within the perimeter of dentinal tubules as odontoblastic processes shrink.
    - **Intertubular:** *Hypo*mineralized dentin located between the dentinal tubules. Makes up the bulk of the dentin formed.
    - **Interglobular:** *Hypo*mineralized dentin located between improperly fused HA globules.
- By location
    - **Coronal**
        - May contain hypomineralized **interglobular dentin.**
        - May contain **dead tracts.**
    - **Radicular**
        - May contain hypomineralized **Tomes' granular layer.**

CROSS STRIATIONS AND INCREMENTAL LINES

- **Daily imbrication line of von Ebner:** Daily periodic bands.
- **Contour lines of Owen:** Wide rings produced by metabolic disturbances during odontogenesis that run perpendicular to dentinal tubules.
- **Neonatal line:** A more pronounced contour line of Owen formed during the physiologic trauma at birth.

Odontoblasts move at a rate of 4–8 μm/day.

EFFECTS OF AGING ON DENTIN

- ↑ sclerotic dentin (↓ dentinal tubule diameter due to continued deposition of peritubular dentin).
- ↑ reparative dentin formation.
- ↑ dead tracts.

CLINICAL IMPLICATIONS

- **Dentinal hypersensitivity:** Can occur for several reasons:
    - Myelinated nerve fibers have been found in dentinal tubules which can be directly stimulated.
    - Changes in dentinal tubule fluid pressures may affect pulpal nerve fibers directly or may cause damage to odontoblasts, releasing inflammatory mediators in the pulp.

DEFORMITIES OF DENTIN

- **Dentinogenesis imperfecta:** Generally *autosomal dominant* defects in dentin formation. Teeth exhibit an opalescent color and have bulb-shaped crowns. The dentin is abnormally soft (allowing enamel to easily chip) and pulp chambers are often obliterated.
    - **Type I:** Often occurs with osteogenesis imperfecta (**blue sclera** is a common finding).
    - **Type II:** Not associated with osteogenesis imperfecta.
    - **Type III:** Very rare form which exhibits multiple pulp exposures of the primary dentition.
- **Dentin dysplasia:** *Autosomal dominant* defects in dentin formation and pulp morphology. Tooth color is usually normal. Often called "**rootless teeth**" because root dentin is usually affected more often than coronal dentin. Roots are short, blunt, or absent.

Enamel

- The most calcified and brittle substance in the human body.
- Color ranges from yellowish to grayish-white.
- Semitranslucent.

ORIGIN

- Differentiated ectodermal cells of the inner enamel epithelium.

AMELOGENESIS

- Organization
    - The ameloblasts become elongated and the organelles become polarized *before* the same occurs to odontoblasts.
- Formation (see Figure 3–7)
    - The enamel matrix produced by ameloblasts starts virtually perpendicularly to the DEJ and progresses outward toward the eventual tooth surface. The oldest enamel is located at the DEJ underlying a cusp or cingulum.
    - Ameloblastic activity starts immediately *after* mantle dentin formation.
    - As ameloblasts retreat, **Tomes' processes** are formed around which enamel matrix proteins are secreted, most of which are almost instantly partially mineralized to form enamel matrix. This determines the structure and morphology of the tooth.
- Maturation
    - Final mineralization occurs with inorganic ion influx and removal of protein and water by cyclic ameloblastic activity, forming **hydroxyapatite (HA)** crystals.
    - As the HA crystals accumulate, they are tightly stacked in elongated units called **enamel rods (prisms)**. The rods are surrounded by a **rod sheath** and separated by an **inter-rod substance** that consists of HA crystals aligned in a different direction than the rods themselves.
    - Each keyhole-shaped enamel rod is formed by **four** ameloblasts (one for the head and three for the tail).
    - At cusp tips, the enamel rods appear twisted and intertwined in a formation known as **gnarled enamel**.

Amelogenin constitutes about 90% of the enamel matrix protein secreted. Other proteins include enamelin and tuftelin.

Most enamel rods extend the width of the enamel from the DEJ to the outer enamel surface.

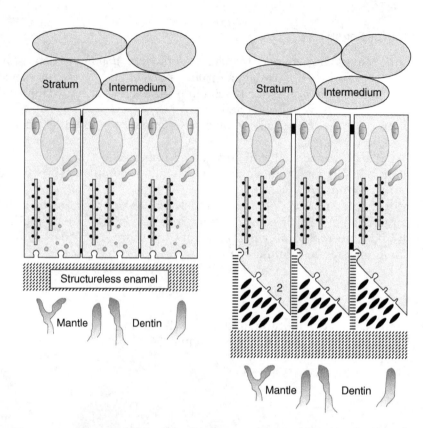

FIGURE 3-7. Enamel formation. Structureless enamel initially forms across the straight face of each ameoloblast. As the ameloblasts retreat from the DEJ, Tomes' processes are formed, and enamel matrix is secreted and mineralized at different orientations (1 and 2).

Reproduced, with permission, from Ten Cate AR. *Oral Histology: Development, Structure, and Function.* 4th ed. St Louis: Mosby; 1994.

■ **Protection**
  ■ When enamel maturation is complete, the outer enamel epithelium, stratum intermedium, and stellate reticulum collapse onto the ameloblastic layer, forming the **reduced enamel epithelium (Nasmyth's membrane)**. This is worn away soon after tooth eruption and quickly replaced by the **salivary pellicle.** Hemidesmosomes are also produced, which are critical in providing epithelial attachment to the tooth.

CROSS STRIATIONS AND INCREMENTAL LINES

■ **Daily imbrication lines:** Daily periodic bands.
■ **Striae of Retzius:** More pronounced weekly periodic bands.
  ■ Shallow depressions, called **perikymata,** are formed on the enamel surface where these lines reach the tooth surface. Perikymata disappear with age due to attrition of the raised areas between them.
■ **Neonatal line:** A more apparent stria of Retzius formed during the physiologic trauma at birth.
■ **Hunter–Schreger bands:** Alternating light and dark zones produced only as an *optical phenomenon* during light microscopy of longitudinal ground sections.

THE DENTINO–ENAMEL JUNCTION (DEJ)

■ **Enamel tufts:** *Hypo*calcified, fan-shaped enamel protein projecting a short distance into the enamel.

Enamel matrix is produced at a rate of 4 µm/day.

The DEJ is scalloped, which provides more surface area for enamel–dentin adhesion.

206

- **Enamel lamellae:** *Hypo*calcified enamel defects that can extend all the way to the enamel surface. They generally consist of enamel protein or oral debris.
- **Enamel spindles:** Trapped odontoblastic processes in the enamel.

EFFECTS OF AGING ON ENAMEL

- **Attrition:** Enamel wear by masticatory forces.
- **Discoloration:** Becomes darker as more dentin becomes visible.
- ↓ **permeability:** Enamel crystals have accepted more ions, especially fluoride.

CLINICAL IMPLICATIONS

- Since enamel is **translucent,** its color depends on its thickness. The more translucent the enamel, the more yellow it appears because the underlying dentin becomes more visible.
- **Tetracycline** antibiotics can be incorporated into mineralizing tissues by chelation to divalent cations. This leads to a **brownish-gray banding** within the enamel. Drugs from this family should not be given until about age 8 (about the time the second molar completes calcification).

DEFORMITIES OF ENAMEL

- **Amelogenesis imperfecta:** Autosomal dominant or recessive enamel defects of three basic types:
    - **Hypoplastic:** Enamel has abnormal thickness or pitting, but normal hardness. Defect in enamel *matrix formation.*
    - **Hypocalcified:** Enamel has normal thickness, but is soft and chalky. Defect in enamel *mineralization.*
    - **Hypomaturation:** Enamel has normal thickness, but abnormal hardness. Mild forms exhibit "snow-capped" incisal edges, while severe forms lose their translucency. Defect in enamel *maturation.*
- **Enamel hypoplasia:** Enamel is hard, but deficient in amount. Caused by defective or altered enamel *matrix formation.* Can be acquired or developmentally-induced.
    - **Fluorosis:** Enamel is *selectively permeable* to water and certain ions. This allows fluoride (in drinking water and topical applications) to concentrate in enamel apatite, forming fluorapatite, which is highly resistant to acid dissolution. Fluoride concentrations greater than 5 parts per million, however, affect ameloblastic enamel matrix secretion, leading to the appearance of **enamel mottling** and a **brownish pigmentation.**
    - **Nutritional deficiencies:** Deficiencies of vitamins A, C, and D and calcium often lead to enamel pitting.
    - **Infections:** Febrile diseases at the time of amelogenesis can halt enamel formation, leaving bands of malformed surface enamel.
- **Congenital syphilis:** Often causes incisors to look screwdriver-shaped (**Hutchinson incisors**) and molars to look globular (**mulberry molars**).

Pulp

- The soft connective tissue that supports the dentin and is contained inside the **pulp chamber** of the tooth.
- Communicates to the periodontal tissues via the **apical foramen** and **accessory canals.**

Fluoride:

- *Tasteless, odorless, colorless*
- *Excreted rapidly by kidneys*
- *Deposited in calcified tissues*
- *Passes slowly through placental barrier*

Hutchinson's triad *of congenital syphilis:*

- *Blindness (interstitial keratitis)*
- *Deafness (CN VIII injury)*
- *Dental anomalies (notched "Hutchinson" incisors, mulberry molars, peg-shaped laterals)*

Pulp capping is more successful in young teeth because of:

- *Large apical foramen*
- *Highly cellular / vascular, fewer fibers, more tissue fluid*
- *No collateral circulation*

*Virtually all of the nerve bundles of the pulp terminate as **free nerve endings** that are specific for **pain**, regardless of the type of stimulation.*

ORIGIN

- Ectomesenchymal cells of the dental papilla.

CLASSIFICATIONS OF PULP

- By location
  - Coronal: Found in the pulp horns.
  - Radicular: Found in pulp canals.

FUNCTIONS OF PULP

- Formative: Has mesenchymal cells that ultimately form dentin.
- Nutritive: Nourishes the avascular dentin.
- Sensory: Free nerve endings provide pain sensation.
- Protective: Produces reparative dentin as needed.

ZONES OF PULP (SEE FIGURE 3–8)

From outer → inner:

- **Odontoblastic zone:** A single layer of odontoblasts lining the pulp chamber.
- **Cell-free zone of Weil:** Devoid of cells (except during dentinogenesis). Contains the parietal plexus of nerves (Raschkow's plexus) and a plexus of blood vessels (including arteriovenous anastamoses).

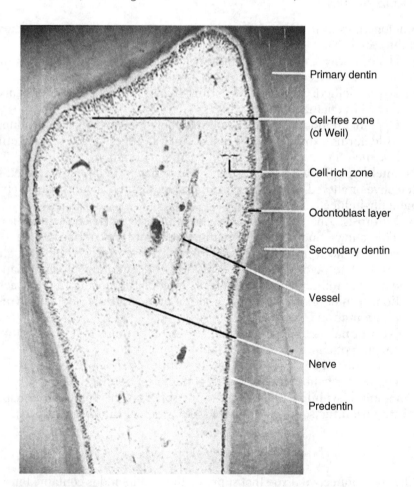

FIGURE 3-8. Zones of pulp.

Reproduced, with permission, from Ten Cate AR. *Oral Histology: Development, Structure, and Function.* 4th ed. St Louis: Mosby; 1994.

- **Cell-rich zone:** Contains **fibroblasts** and undifferentiated mesenchymal cells.
- **Pulp core:** Contains fibroblasts, macrophages, leukocytes, blood and lymph vessels, myelinated (mostly Aδ) and unmyelinated (C) sympathetic nerve fibers, collagen types I and III (55:45 ratio), and ground substance. There are no elastic fibers.

PULP CALCIFICATIONS

- **Denticles (pulp stones):** Concentric layers of mineralized tissue
  - **True:** Surround dentinal tubules or odontoblastic processes.
  - **False:** Surround dead cells or collagen fibers.
  - **Free:** Located freely (unattached) in the pulp chamber.
  - **Attached:** Attached to the pulp chamber wall.
  - **Interstitial:** Embedded in the pulp chamber wall.
- **Dystrophic calcifications:** Calcifications of collagen bundles or collagen fibers surrounding blood vessels and nerves.

EFFECTS OF AGING ON PULP

- ↑ collagen fibers and calcifications.
- ↓ pulp chamber volume (due to continued dentin deposition), apical foramen size, cellularity, vascularity, and sensitivity.

Cementum

- An avascular tissue about 10 μm thick that covers the radicular dentin.
- Composition most closely resembles bone.

ORIGIN

- Differentiated ectomesenchymal cells of the dental follicle.

FUNCTIONS OF CEMENTUM

- **Support:** Provides attachment for teeth (Sharpey's fibers).
- **Protection:** Helps prevent root resorption during tooth movement.
- **Formative:** Continual apical cementum deposition accounts for continual tooth eruption and movement.

CEMENTOGENESIS

- During root formation, ectomesenchymal cells of the dental follicle migrate through gaps in Hertwig's epithelial root sheath and orient themselves along radicular dentin. Here, they differentiate to **cementoblasts** and secrete **cementoid** (cementum matrix).
- As the cementoblasts retreat away from the dentin, the matrix is calcified and a new layer of cementum matrix is secreted. These layers form **resting lines,** which can be seen microscopically.
- Cementoblasts may be trapped in their own matrix. When this occurs, they are known as **cementocytes,** which reside in **lacunae.** They receive nutrients via **canaliculi** that extend to the periodontal ligament.
- Cementum is constantly produced at the apical portion of the root to account for the continual eruption of teeth. Deposition of excessive cementum is known as **hypercementosis.**

CLASSIFICATIONS OF CEMENTUM

- By formation
  - **Primary:** First formed cementum. Covers coronal cementum, is acellular, and consists of extrinsic collagen fibers.
  - **Secondary:** Overlies primary cementum. Covers apical cementum, may be either acellular or cellular, and consists of mixed collagen fibers.
- By cellularity
  - **Cellular:** Contains cementocytes, cementoblasts, and cementoclasts. Most commonly found in apical areas of cementum.
  - **Acellular:** Devoid of cells. Most commonly found in coronal areas of cementum.
- By collagen fibers
  - **Intrinic fibers:** Produced by cementoblasts. Arranged parallel to the tooth surface.
  - **Extrinsic fibers:** Produced by the PDL. Arranged perpendicular to the tooth surface. As they become trapped in the cementum, they are known as Sharpey's fibers.
  - **Mixed fibers:** Combination of intrinsic and extrinsic fibers.

APPROXIMATION WITH ENAMEL AT THE CEJ

See Figure 3–9.

EFFECTS OF AGING ON CEMENTUM

- ↑ cementum deposition.

CLINICAL IMPLICATIONS

- Cementum enables orthodontic tooth movement because it is more resistant to resorption than alveolar bone.

Alveolar Bone

- **Alveolar bone:** A general term to describe the bone in the maxilla and mandible which houses the teeth.
- **Interalveolar septum:** The bony projection separating two alveoli.
- **Interradicular septum:** Alveolar bone between the roots of multirooted teeth.

The only function of alveolar bone is to support teeth. During tooth development, it grows in all dimensions to accommodate the new dentition. When a tooth is lost, it continually resorbs until complete alveolar ridge atrophy occurs.

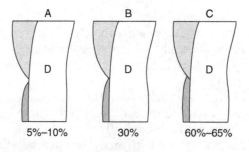

FIGURE 3–9. Cementum morphology at the CEJ.

A. Cementum does not reach enamel; B. Cementum meets enamel; C. Cementum overlaps enamel. Reproduced, with permission, from Carranza FA. *Clinical Periodontology*, 8th ed. page 61, copyright 1996 by Elsevier.

ORIGIN

- Differentiated ectomesenchymal cells of the dental follicle.

COMPONENTS OF ALVEOLAR BONE

- **Alveolar bone proper:** The thin layer of **cortical bone** that immediately surrounds the teeth and into which PDL fibers (Sharpey's fibers) are embedded. It is also called **bundle bone, lamina dura,** or **cribriform plate.**
- **Supporting alveolar bone:** The part of the alveolus that surrounds the alveolar bone proper. It consists of the following:
  - **Cortical bone (cortical plate):** Forms the buccal and lingual outer surfaces of the maxilla and mandible. It is generally thicker in the mandible and in posterior (molar) regions.
  - **Cancellous bone (spongy bone, trabecular bone):** Fills the area between the cortical plates. It makes up the majority of alveolar bone.

CLINICAL IMPLICATIONS

- The radiographic appearance of the **lamina dura** is determined as much by the x-ray beam angulation as it is by its integrity.
- The radiographic presence (or absence) of the crestal lamina dura has no correlation with periodontal attachment loss.

The new alveolar bone deposited during orthodontic treatment is intramembranous bone.

Periodontal Ligament (PDL)

See Figure 3–10.

- A soft connective tissue located between the tooth and alveolar bone.
- Approximately **0.2 mm wide** but varies with tooth function and age.

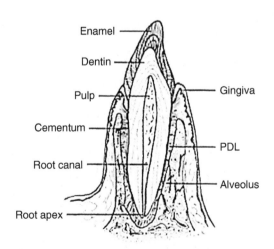

Enamel

Dentin

Pulp

Gingiva

Cementum

Root canal

PDL

Alveolus

Root apex

FIGURE 3–10. The tooth and its periodontium.

*The **periodontium** is the attachment apparatus of the tooth. It consists of:*

- *Cementum*
- *Alveolar bone proper*
- *PDL*

Reproduced, with permission, from Liebgott B. *The Anatomical Basis of Dentistry.* Toronto: BC Decker, 1986.

ORIGIN

- Differentiated ectomesenchymal cells of the dental follicle.

Orthodontic tooth movement is possible because the PDL actively responds to externally applied forces.

FUNCTIONS OF THE PDL

- **Support:** Provides attachment of the tooth to the alveolar bone.
- **Formative:** Contains cells responsible for formation of the periodontium.
- **Nutritive:** Contains a vascular network providing nutrients to its cells.
- **Sensory:** Contains afferent nerve fibers responsible for pain, pressure, and proprioception.
- **Remodeling:** Contains cells responsible for remodeling of the periodontium.

CONTENTS OF THE PDL

- Cells and cellular elements
    - **Fibroblasts:** Most common cell of the PDL.
    - Cementoblasts and cementoclasts.
    - Osteoblasts and osteoclasts.
    - Macrophages, mast cells, and eosinophils.
    - Undifferentiated mesenchymal cells.
    - **Ground substance:** Proteoglycans, glycosaminoglycans, glycoproteins, and water (70%).
    - **Epithelial rests of Malassez:** Remnants of HERS. Found closer to cementum than alveolar bone.
    - **Cementicles:** Calcified masses either attached or unattached to root surfaces.
- Fibers (See Figure 3–11.)
    - **Principal collagen fibers:** Composed mostly of type I collagen, but also type III collagen.
        - **Transseptal:** Extend interproximally over the alveolar crest from the cementum of one tooth to that of an adjacent tooth. Resist mesial-distal forces.

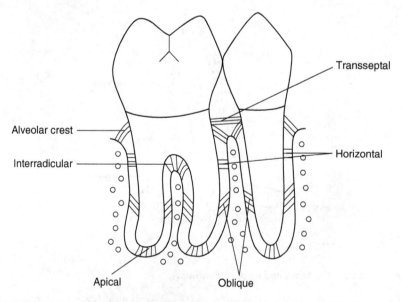

FIGURE 3-11. The principal PDL fibers.

- **Alveolar crest:** Extend obliquely from cementum just apical to the junctional epithelium to the alveolar crest. Resist vertical (intrusive/extrusive) forces.
- **Horizontal:** Extend at right angles from cementum to alveolar bone. Resist lateral (tipping) and rotational forces.
- **Oblique:** Extend obliquely from cementum to alveolar bone. They are the *most abundant* principal fibers. Main resistance to masticatory (intrusive and rotational) forces.
- **Apical:** Extend from cementum to alveolar bone at root apices. Resist vertical (extrusive) forces.
- **Interradicular:** Extend from radicular cementum to interradicular alveolar bone. Only present in multirooted teeth. Resist vertical (intrusive/extrusive) and lateral (tipping) forces.
- **Oxytalan fibers:** Elastic-like fibers that run parallel to the tooth surface and bend to attach to cementum. They are largely associated with blood vessels.
- Blood vessels (see Figure 3–12)
  - The vasculature of the PDL arises from the **maxillary artery**. Vessels can reach the PDL from various sources:
    - **Periosteal vessels:** Branches from the periosteum. This is the *primary source* of PDL vasculature.
    - **Apical vessels:** Branches of the dental vessels that supply the apical regions of the PDL.
    - **Transalveolar vessels:** Branches of transseptal vessels that perforate the alveolar bone proper.
    - **Anastomosing vessels** of the gingiva.
- Nerve fibers
  - Arise from branches of the **trigeminal nerve (CN V).**
    - Free nerve endings: Transmit pain. *Most abundant.*
    - Ruffini corpuscles: Provide mechanoreception.
    - Coiled endings.
    - Spindle endings.

Sharpey's fibers *are the portions of the principal fibers that insert into cementum or alveolar bone proper. They are thicker on the alveolar bone side.*

Blood vessels in the interdental papilla anastomose freely with periodontal and interalveolar vessels.

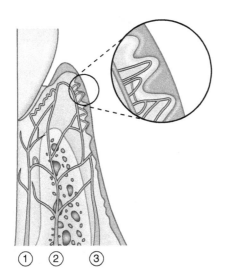

FIGURE 3–12. **Gingival vasculature. Arterial branches extend from the apical aspect of the periodontal tissues though the PDL (1), alveolar bone (2), and along the periosteum (3), forming anastamoses and capillary loops in the gingival connective tissue.**

- Lymphatics
  - All drain to the **submandibular lymph nodes**, *except* mandibular incisors which drain to the submental nodes.

EFFECTS OF AGING ON THE PDL

- ↓ PDL width.
- ↓ cellularity and fiber content.

CLINICAL IMPLICATIONS

- Teeth in **hypofunction** have a decreased PDL width with fibers arranged parallel to the root.
- Teeth in **hyperfunction** have an increased PDL width.

Developmental Biology

Odontogenesis

INITIATION

See Figure 4–1.

- Starts at week 6 in utero.
- Underlying ectomesenchymal cells induce the overlying ectoderm (oral epithelium) to proliferate, forming a localized thickening at the site of each tooth called the **dental lamina.**
- Defects in this stage result in anodontia or supernumerary teeth.

BUD STAGE

See Figure 4–1.

- Starts at week 8 in utero.
- Both ectodermal and ectomesenchymal cells **proliferate,** creating the round shape of each tooth bud.

CAP STAGE

See Figure 4–1.

- Starts at week 9 in utero.
- The **enamel organ** begins to form, which is composed of a single layer of cells at the convex region (**outer enamel epithelium, OEE**) and the concave region (**inner enamel epithelium, IEE**). Between the two epithelial layers is

It is the underlying ectomesenchyme that determines the type of tooth to be formed.

---

*The **tooth germ** is composed of:*

- Enamel organ
- Dental papilla
- Dental follicle

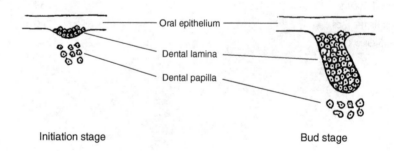

Oral epithelium
Dental lamina
Dental papilla

Initiation stage

Bud stage

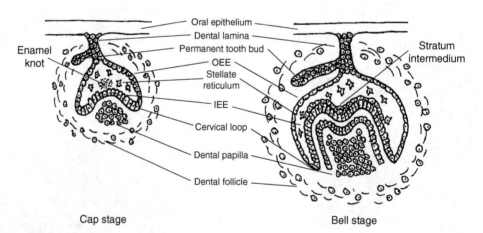

Enamel knot

Oral epithelium
Dental lamina
Permanent tooth bud
OEE
Stellate reticulum
IEE
Cervical loop
Dental papilla
Dental follicle

Stratum intermedium

Cap stage

Bell stage

FIGURE 4–1. **Odontogenesis.**

the loosely arranged **stellate reticulum.** Some cells of the stellate reticulum become densely packed near the IEE and are known as the **enamel knot.**

- The **dental papilla** is composed of condensed ectomesenchymal cells located within the concavity of the enamel organ.
- The **dental follicle (dental sac)** is the capsulelike encasing of mesenchyme surrounding the enamel organ.
- The **succedaneous dental lamina** begins to form adjacent to the primary enamel organ.
- Defects in this stage result in dens-in-dente, gemination, fusion, and tubercles.

BELL STAGE

See Figure 4–1.

- Starts at week 11 in utero.
- Morphodifferentiation and histodifferentiation of specific cells occurs.
- The **enamel organ** is now well-defined and composed of the following:
    - **OEE:** Outermost layer of the enamel organ.
    - **IEE:** Innermost layer of the enamel organ.
    - **Stratum intermedium:** Forms directly lateral to the IEE.
    - **Stellate reticulum:** Becomes more sparsely arranged due to increased proteoglycan synthesis.
- The enamel knot disappears.
- The cells of the IEE become tall and columnar (now called **preameloblasts**) *first.*
- The cells of the dental papilla closest to the IEE become tall and columnar (now called **preodontoblasts**) *after* the preameloblasts are formed.
- The dental lamina disintegrates. Its remnants are known as **epithelial rests of Serres.**
- Defects in this stage result in dentinogenesis imperfecta, amelogenesis imperfecta, and macrodontia / microdontia.

APPOSITIONAL STAGE

- Starts at week 14 in utero.
- The **reduced enamel epithelium (REE)** forms when the stellate reticulum collapses, merging the OEE with the IEE.
- Odontoblasts secrete dentin matrix *first.*
- Ameloblasts secrete enamel matrix *after* dentin is first formed.
- Root formation (see below) begins.
- The dental papilla forms pulp tissue.
- The dental follicle forms cementum, alveolar bone, and PDL.
- Defects in this stage result in enamel dysplasia, concrescence, and enamel pearls.

MINERALIZATION STAGE

- Starts at 4–6 months in utero.
- Starts at the **DEJ** (where odontoblasts and ameloblasts first secrete matrix).
- Takes about 2 years to complete.

ROOT FORMATION

See Figure 4–2.

Korff's fibers are the thick, coarse bundles of collagen fibers in the periphery of the pulp associated with dentin matrix formation.

The differentiation of the IEE cells to preameloblasts induces the differentiation of preodontoblasts from mesenchymal cells of the dental papilla.

Remember the chronological order of enamel and dentin formation. Root, pulp, and periodontium formation occurs after these events.

1. Differentiation of ameloblasts
2. Differentiation of odontoblasts
3. Deposition of dentin matrix
4. Deposition of enamel matrix

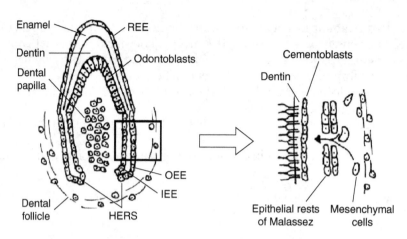

FIGURE 4-2. **Root formation.**

- Begins at the **cervical loop** (where the IEE and OEE join) *after* enamel is first formed.
- As the cervical loop elongates, **Hertwig's epithelial root sheath (HERS)** is formed, which shapes the root(s) and ultimately surrounds the majority of the dental papilla. Its most apical segment, the **epithelial diaphragm,** turns medially, ensuring that the root tapers as odontogenesis proceeds.
- As root formation continues, the tooth erupts, leaving the epithelial diaphragm always at the same location. This eventually forms the **apical foramen.**
- As radicular dentin is formed, HERS begins to disintegrate, leaving behind patches of epithelial cells called **epithelial rests of Malassez.** The collapse of HERS enables ectomesenchymal cells of the dental follicle to contact dentin and differentiate into the formative cells of the periodontium: cementoblasts (forming cementum), osteoblasts (forming alveolar bone proper), and fibroblasts (forming the PDL).

Remember these epithelial remnants:

- *Serres: From dental lamina*
- *Malassez: From HERS*

It is believed that the epithelial rests of Malassez are the source of the epithelium of odontogenic cysts.

ERUPTION

See Figure 4–3.

- As the tooth erupts into the oral cavity, the REE fuses with the oral epithelium, forming the **dentogingival junction (epithelial attachment).**

Nasmyth's membrane (the primary enamel cuticle) is the epithelial coating that covers newly erupted teeth.

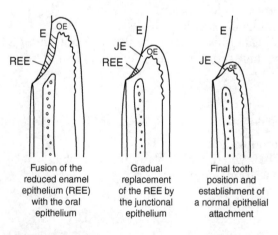

FIGURE 4-3. **Tooth eruption.**

- This later migrates apically along the tooth to its normal position in which the most apical cells of the JE are at the CEJ. A delay in this apical migration is known as **delayed (altered) passive eruption.**

Gametogenesis

- See Figure 4–4 for stages of meiosis in sperm and egg.
- See Figure 4–5 for sperm development.
- See Figure 4–6 for mature sperm.
- See Figure 4–7 for oocyte maturation.

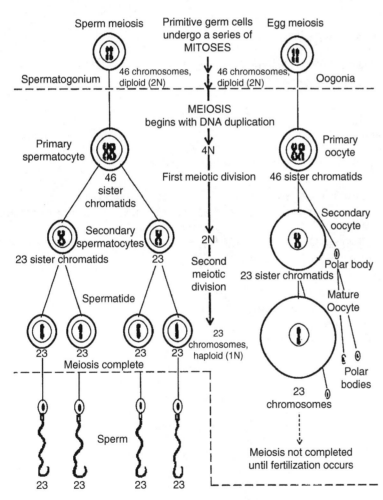

23, 46 = number of chromosomes; 1N, 2N, 4N = number of chromatid copies (N = 23)

FIGURE 4–4. **Stages of meiosis in sperm and egg.**

Reproduced, with permission, from Sweeney LJ. *Basic Concepts in Embryology.* New York: McGraw-Hill, 1998.

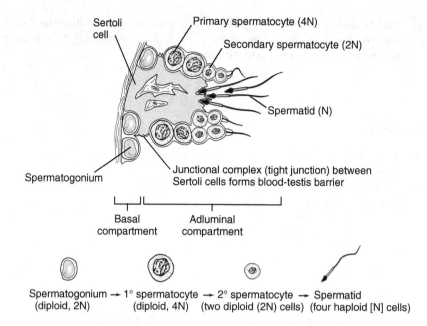

FIGURE 4-5. **Sperm development.**

Reproduced, with permission, from Bhushan V, Le T, Amin C. *First Aid for the USMLE Step-1*. New York: McGraw-Hill, 2003.

Fertilization usually occurs in the uterine tube. Implantation normally occurs in the uterus; if not, it is ectopic.

FERTILIZATION

- Capacitation and acrosomal reaction of sperm.
- Entry of spermatozoon.
    - Inhibition of polyspermy.
        - Acrosome reaction: Sperm releases enzymes to penetrate outer surface of egg.
        - Cortical (zona) reaction: Sperm alters zona pellucida, preventing other sperm from binding.
    - Meiosis II occurs in oocyte.
        - Barr body (second polar body).
    - Fusion of male and female pronuclei.
        - = Zygote.
        - Restores diploid (46).

Acrosome contains a packet of enzymes to penetrate and fertilize the egg-acrosome reaction.

Acrosome is derived from Golgi; the middle piece contains numerous mitochondria; the tail is flagellum (9 x 2 + 2).

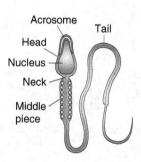

FIGURE 4-6. **Mature sperm.**

Reproduced, with permission, from Bhushan V, Le T, Amin C. *First Aid of the USMLE Step-1*. New York: McGraw-Hill, 2003.

Meiosis II occurs only if fertilization occurs.

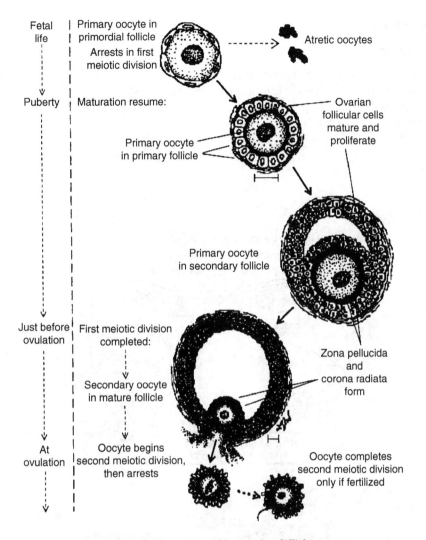

FIGURE 4-7. Maturation of the oocyte and its ovarian follicle.

Reproduced, with permission, from Sweeney LJ. *Basic Concepts in Embryology.* New York: McGraw-Hill, 1998.

Sperm become motile in the epididymis.

IMPLANTATION

See Figure 4–8.

- Occurs by the end of the first week.
- Trophoblast cells invade endometrial epithelium.
- Trophoblast produces hCG.
- See Figure 4–9 for cleavage stages.

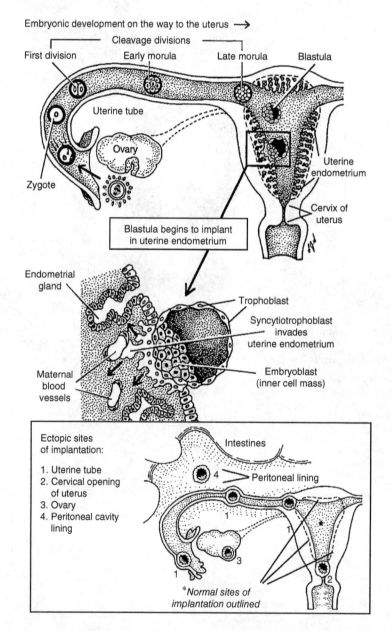

FIGURE 4–8. Development of the embryo and its travels during week 1.

Reproduced, with permission, from Sweeney LJ. *Basic Concepts in Embryology.* New York: McGraw-Hill, 1998.

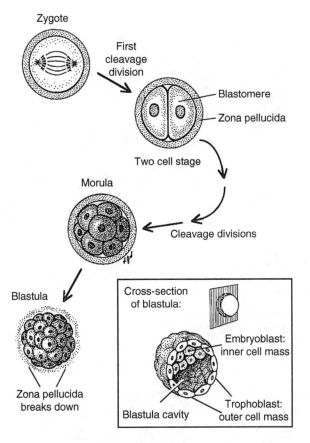

FIGURE 4–9. Cleavage stages: morula and blastula.

Reproduced, with permission, from Sweeney LJ. *Basic Concepts in Embryology.* New York: McGraw-Hill, 1998.

BILAMINAR DISC

- Occurs in the second week.
- Epiblast (primary ectoderm).
  - Amniotic cavity.
  - Ultimately gives rise to:
    - Ectoderm.
    - Mesoderm.
- Hypoblast (primary endoderm).
  - Lining of yolk sac.

See Figure 4–10 for placentation.
See Figure 4–11 for twinning.

Decidual reaction occurs during week 2. Pregnant endometrium enlarges, accumulates lipid and glycogen.

Allantois forms on day 16.

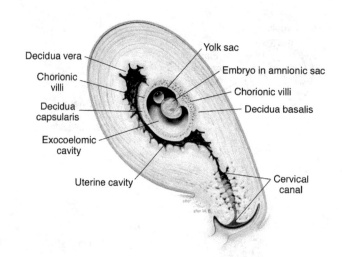

FIGURE 4–10. Placentation.

Reproduced, with permission, from Cunningham FG, et al (eds). *Williams Obstetrics*, 21st ed. New York: McGraw-Hill, 2001.

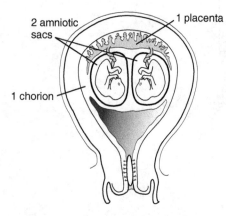

1 zygote splits evenly to develop 2 amniotic sacs with a single common chorion and placenta.

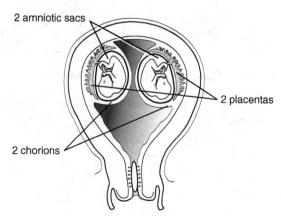

Dizygotes develop individual placentas, chorions, and amniotic sacs.

Monozygotes develop 2 placentas (separate/fused), chorions, and amniotic sacs.

FIGURE 4–11. Twinning.

Reproduced, with permission, from Bhushan V, Le T, Amin C. *First Aid for the USMLE Step-1*. New York: McGraw-Hill, 2003.

Primitive blood formation occurs in the allantois, yolk sac, liver, spleen, and bone.

FETAL CIRCULATION

See Figure 4–12.
- Oxygenated blood to heart via
  - Umbilical vein.
  - Inferior vena cava.
- Foramen ovale
  - Allows most of the oxygenated blood to bypass the pulmonary circuit.
  - Pumps out the aorta to the head.

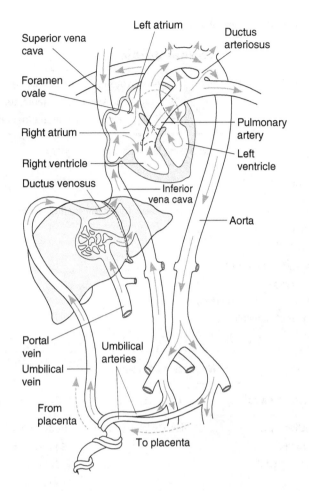

FIGURE 4–12. Fetal circulation.

Reproduced, with permission, from Hay WW, Hayward AR, Levin MJ, Sondheimer JM. (eds). *Current Pediatric Diagnosis & Treatment*, 16th ed. New York: McGraw-Hill, 2003.

After birth the foramen ovale closes to become the fossa ovalis, the ductus arteriosis closes to form the ligamentum arteriosum, and the umbilical vein closes to form the ligamentum teres hepatis.

- Deoxygenated blood returned via
  - Superior vena cava.
  - Mostly pumped through the pulmonary artery and ductus arteriosus to the:
    - Feet.
    - Umbilical arteries.

EMBRYOLOGIC BODY AXES

See Table 4–1 for germ layer derivatives.
See Figure 4–13 for anatomic orientation of the embryo.
See Figure 4–14 for germ layer derivatives.
See Figure 4–15 for stages of fetal life.

Foramen Ovale

- In fetal heart allows blood to flow from RA to LA.
- Bypass pulmonary circuit .
  - Because oxygenated blood comes from the mother/placenta.
- Closes with fibrous connective tissue to become fossa ovalis in the adult.

TABLE 4-1.   Germ Layer Derivatives

ECTODERM DERIVATIVES

Epithelium of skin (superficial epidermis layer)	All nervous tissue: formed by neuroectoderm: Brain and spinal cord (neural tube) All peripheral nerve tissue (neural crest)

ENDODERM DERIVATIVES

EPITHELIAL LININGS OF:

The gastrointestinal tract Organs that form as buds from the endoderm tube: Pharyngeal gland derivatives* Respiratory system Digestive organs (liver, pancreas) Terminal part of urogenital systems	Hypoblast endoderm: Gametes migrate to gonads

MESODERM DERIVATIVES

ALL CONNECTIVE TISSUES†	ALL MUSCLE TYPES:	EPITHELIAL LININGS OF:
General connective tissues Cartilage and bone Blood cells (red and white)	Cardiac, skeletal, smooth	Body cavities Some organs: Cardiovascular system Reproductive and urinary systems (most parts)

*Pharyngeal derivatives: palatine tonsils, thymus, thyroid, parathyroids.
†Some connective tissues in the head are derived from neural crest.

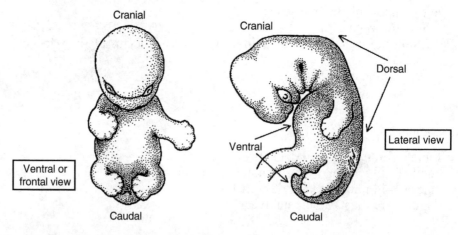

FIGURE 4-13.   Embryonic body axes.

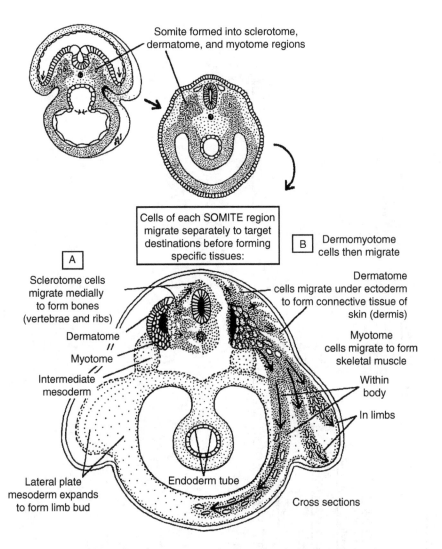

Somite formed into sclerotome, dermatome, and myotome regions

Cells of each SOMITE region migrate separately to target destinations before forming specific tissues:

A

B Dermomyotome cells then migrate

Sclerotome cells migrate medially to form bones (vertebrae and ribs)

Dermatome cells migrate under ectoderm to form connective tissue of skin (dermis)

Dermatome

Myotome cells migrate to form skeletal muscle

Myotome

Intermediate mesoderm

Within body

In limbs

Lateral plate mesoderm expands to form limb bud

Endoderm tube

Cross sections

FIGURE 4–14. **Dermatome, myotome, and sclerotome derivatives.**

Reproduced, with permission, from Sweeney LJ. *Basic Concepts in Embryology.* New York: McGraw-Hill, 1998.

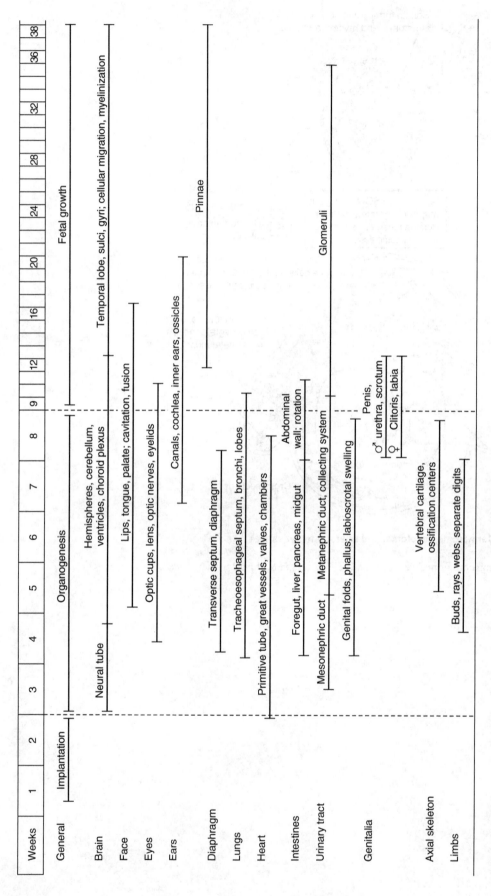

FIGURE 4–15. **Stages of fetal life.**

Reproduced, with permission, from Hay WW, Hayward AR, Levin MJ, Sondheimer JM. (eds). *Current Pediatric Diagnosis & Treatment*, 16th ed. New York: McGraw-Hill, 2003.

Embryology of the Central Nervous System

See Figure 4–16.

- Neural plate.
- Neural tube.
- Alar plate: Alar = sensory (posterior, dorsal).
- Basal plate: Basal = motor (anterior, ventral).
- See Figure 4–17 for formation of the nervous system.

Organogenesis occurs from week 3 to 8.

The neural plate invaginates to form neural groove with neural folds on each side on day 18 of embryonic life (two neural folds fuseforming the neural tube). Neuroectoderm (ectoderm of neural plate) gives rise to CNS (brain and spinal cord).

Week 4 of embryologic development:

- Neural tube is closed.
- Four pairs of branchial arches are visible externally.
- Characteristic C-shaped curvature of embryo is appreciated due to folding.
- Upper and lower limb buds appear.

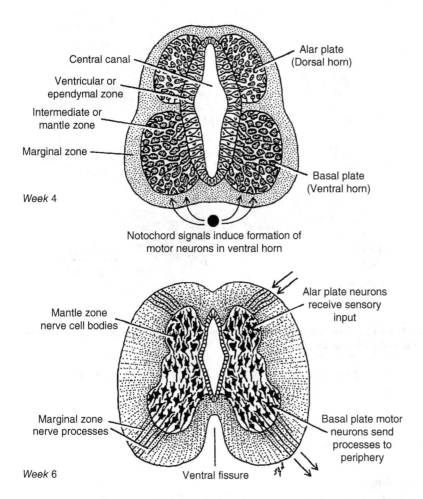

FIGURE 4–16. Development of regional specialization across the neural tube.

Reproduced, with permission, from Sweeney LJ. *Basic Concepts in Embryology.* New York: McGraw-Hill, 1998.

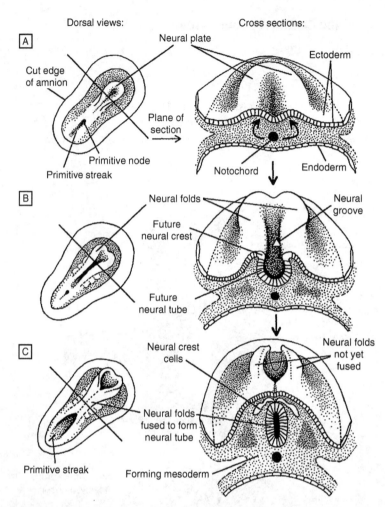

FIGURE 4–17. Neuroectoderm forms the neural tube and neural crest in late week 3 (A and B) and early week 4 (C).

Reproduced, with permission, from Sweeney LJ. *Basic Concepts in Embryology*. New York: McGraw-Hill, 1998.

EMBRYOLOGY OF THE BRAIN

Brain stem = midbrain + hindbrain

Brain stem = midbrain + pons + medulla.

Embyologic Division	Subset	Second Subset	Adult Derivative
Forebrain	Prosencephalon	Telencephalon	Cerebrum, basal ganglia
		Diencephalon	Thalamus Hypothalamus Epithalamus Subthalamus Posterior pituitary (neurohypophysis)
Midbrain	Mesencephalon		Midbrain
Hindbrain	Metencephalon		Pons
	Myelencephalon		Medulla oblongata

NEURAL TUBE CELLS

	Gives Rise To
Neural crest	Sensory ganglia (CNs V, VII, IX, X)
	Dorsal root ganglia (in peripheral nervous system)
	Schwann cells (peripheral)
	Melanocytes and odontoblasts
	Enterochromaffin cells
	Neurons in parasympathetic and sympathetic ganglia (adrenal medulla)
	Leptomeninges (pia and arachnoid)
	Parafollicular cells (C-cells) of parathyroid
Neuroepithelial	Neuroblasts → neurons
	Ependymal cells (lining ventricles, central canal)
	Glioblasts-astrocytes, oligodenrocytes (myelin in CNS)
Mesenchymal (mesoderm)	Microglia

Embryology of the Cardiac System

AORTIC ARCH DERIVATIVES

See Figure 4–18.

- Aortic arch arteries
- Form during week 4.
- Arise from distal truncus arteriosus (aortic sac).
- Associated with corresponding pharyngeal arch.
- Connect to the paired dorsal aortae.
  - Dorsal aortae fuse in week 5 to form:
    - Descending thoracic aorta.
    - Abdominal aorta.

See Figure 4–19 for cardiac development.
See Figure 4–20 for heart embryology.

The cardiovascular system is derived from mesoderm.

Atrial Septal Defect

- Results from incomplete fusion of septum primum and septum secundum.
- Often asymptomatic until middle age.
- Located near the foramen ovale.

Patent Foramen Ovale

- *Failure of complete fusion of foramen ovale.*
- Usually of no hemodynamic significance.

Aortic Arch	Adult Analogue
1	Maxillary artery
2	Hyoid artery
	Stapedial artery
3	Common carotid artery
	ICA (first part)
4	Aortic arch
	Right subclavian (proximal)
5	Involutes
6	Pulmonary arteries (proximal)
	Ductus arteriosus

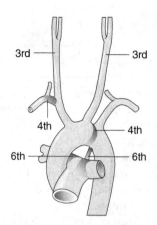

FIGURE 4–18. **Aortic arch derivatives.**

Reproduced, with permission, from Bhushan V, Le T, Amin C. *First Aid for the USMLE Step-1.*
New York: McGraw-Hill, 2003.

Embryology of the Gastrointestinal System

Segment	Artery	Innervation	Derivatives
Foregut	Celiac trunk	Vagus nerve (parasympathetic) Splanchnic nerve (sympathetic) Thoracic nerve	Esophagus Stomach Duodenum (1st part) Liver Gallbladder Pancreas
Midgut	SMA	Vagus nerve (parasympathetic) Splanchnic nerve (sympathetic)	Duodenum (2nd–4th parts) Jejunum Ileum Appendix Ascending and transverse colon
Hindgut	IMA	Pelvic splanchnic (S2–S4) nerve (parasympathetic) Lumbar splanchnic nerve (sympathetic)	Colon (distal to splenic flexure) Sigmoid Rectum

Ectodermal derivatives to GI tract:

- Oropharynx (mucosa, tongue, lips, parotid, enamel)
- Rectum (distal to pectinate line)
- Anus

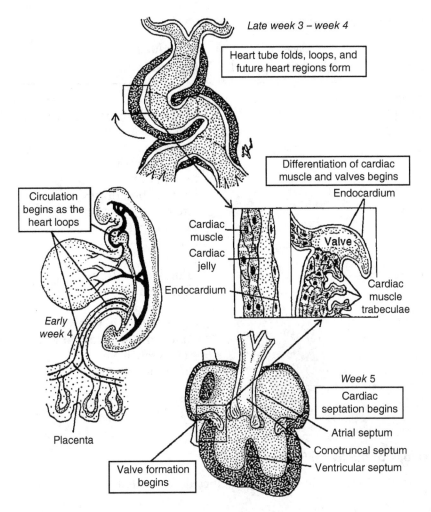

FIGURE 4–19. Overview of cardiac development.

Reproduced, with permission, from Sweeney LJ. *Basic Concepts in Embryology.* New York: McGraw-Hill, 1998.

Heart embryology

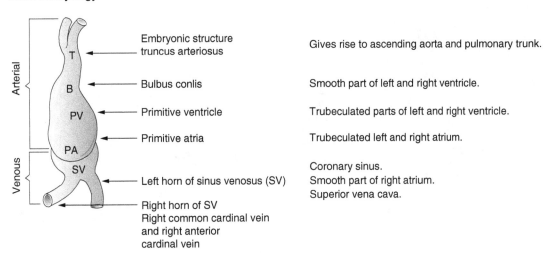

Embryonic structure truncus arteriosus	Gives rise to ascending aorta and pulmonary trunk.
Bulbus conlis	Smooth part of left and right ventricle.
Primitive ventricle	Trubeculated parts of left and right ventricle.
Primitive atria	Trubeculated left and right atrium.
Left horn of sinus venosus (SV)	Coronary sinus. Smooth part of right atrium. Superior vena cava.
Right horn of SV Right common cardinal vein and right anterior cardinal vein	

FIGURE 4–20. Heart embryology.

Reproduced, with permission, from Bhushan V, Le T, Amin C. *First Aid for the USMLE Step-1.* New York: McGraw-Hill, 2003.

233

Embryology of the Renal System

Structure	Week of Development	Structures Formed
Pronephros	4	Regresses
Mesonephros	4	Mesonephric duct (gives rise to): Ductus deferens Epididymis Ejaculatory duct Seminal vesicle Ureteric bud (forms): Ureter Renal pelvis Calyces Collecting tubules
Metanephros	5	Adult kidney (from): Ureteric bud Metanephric mass Kidney forms in pelvis but "ascends" to abdomen with fetal growth Ureters lengthen

Wolffian duct

(mesonephric duct).

Embryonic duct develops into

deferent duct, etc. in males;

obliterated in females.

Embryology of the Renal System

See Figure 4–21 for the three stages of kidney development.

- From intermediate mesoderm
  - Nephrogenic cord gives rise to:
    - Pronephros.
    - Mesonephros.
    - Metanephros.

See Figure 4–22 for embryology of the pancreas.

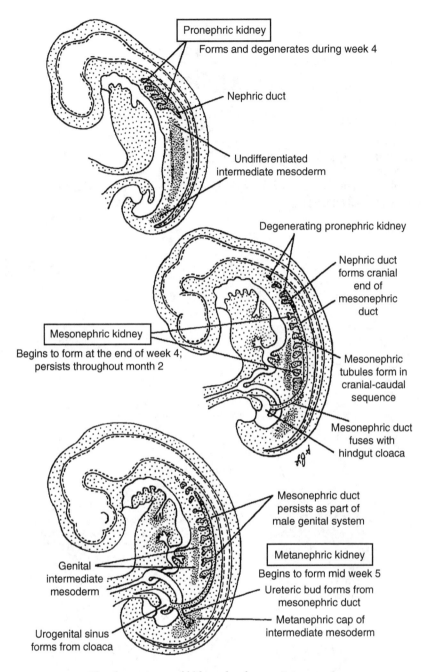

FIGURE 4-21. **The three stages of kidney development.**

Reproduced, with permission, from Sweeney LJ. *Basic Concepts in Embryology*. New York: McGraw-Hill, 1998.

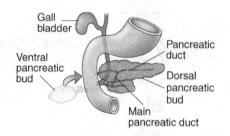

FIGURE 4–22. **Embryology of the pancreas.**

Reproduced, with permission, from Bhushan V, Le T, Amin C. *First Aid for the USMLE Step-1*. New York: McGraw-Hill, 2003.

► **EMBRYOLOGY OF THE FACE AND PHARYNGEAL ARCHES**

See Figure 4–23 for formation of the neurocranium and viscerocranium.

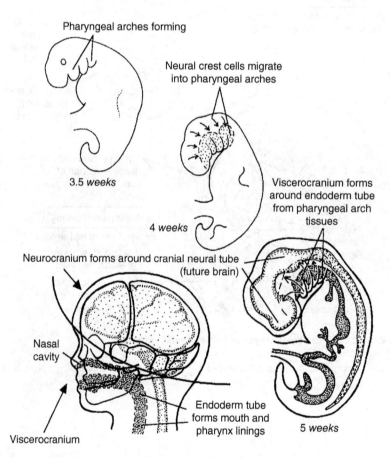

FIGURE 4–23. **Formation of neurocranial and viscerocranial regions of the head.**

Reproduced, with permission, from Sweeney LJ. *Basic Concepts in Embryology*. New York: McGraw-Hill, 1998.

Branchial Arches

- Rounded, mesodermal ridges (neural crest cells).
- Form from proliferative activity of neural crest cells.
- Each arch contains nerve, artery, muscle, and cartilaginous bar.
  - Nerves (CNs V, VII, IX, X) are **branchiomeric** because they originate from the branchial arches.
    - Not from somites.
    - Develop about week 4 of life.
  - At the end of week 4 the arches are well-defined and visible externally.
  - During week 4 the first branchial arch divides into:
    - Mandibular process.
    - Maxillary process.
    - Weeks 5–6, arches are smaller, not seen on surface.
    - Arches 1–3 play role in forming face and oral cavity.
  - Arch 1
    - Mandible
    - Maxilla (most)
  - Arches 2 and 3
    - Tongue

> *Third arch*
> - Hyoid bone
> - Tongue formation (root-posterior third)
> - Hypobranchial eminence

See Figure 4–24 for derivatives in the pharyngeal region.

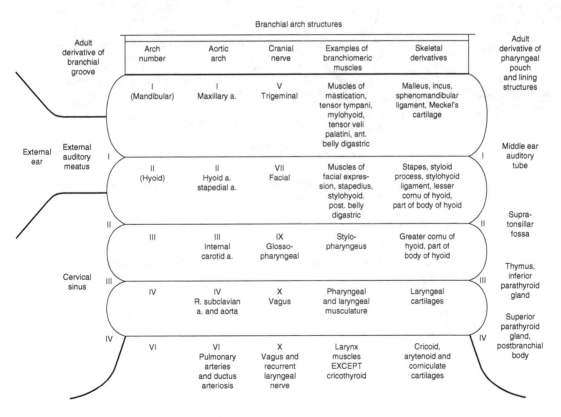

FIGURE 4-24. Derivatives in the pharyngeal region.

Reproduced, with permission, from Carlson BM. *Patten's Foundations of Embryology.* 5th ed. New York: McGraw-Hill, 1988.

First arch

- See Figure 4–25.
- Meckel's cartilage
  - Model for the mandible.
- Dissolutes with only minor contribution to ossification.
- Mandibular process (forms mandible).
- Maxillary process (forms maxilla, zygoma, squamous temporal).
- Tongue formation (anterior two-thirds).
  - Tuberculum impar (median tongue bud)
  - Lateral lingual swellings (2) (distal tongue buds)

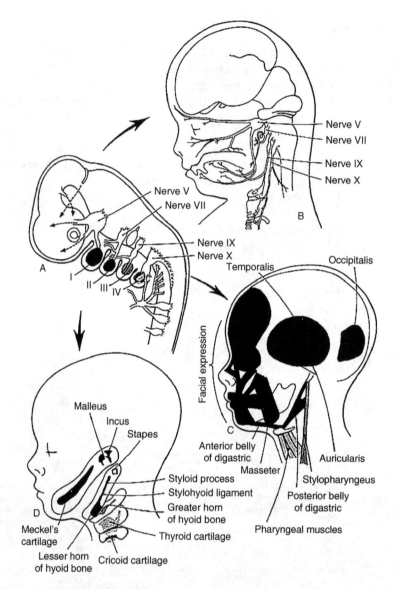

FIGURE 4–25. **Schematic diagram showing major derivatives of structures that constitute the branchial arches.**

(A) 5-week embryo; (B–D) 4- to 5-month fetuses. The gray tones of structures in C and D correspond to those of the branchial arches depicted in A.

Reproduced, with permission, from Carlson BM. *Patten's Foundations of Embryology*. 5th ed. New York: McGraw-Hill, 1988.

Pharyngeal Pouches

See Figure 4–26.

▪ Paired evaginations of pharyngeal endoderm that lines inner aspects of branchial arches

Pouch	Structures
1	Tympanic membrane
	Auditory tube
	Middle ear cavity
2	Lymphatic nodule
	Palatine tonsil
3	Inferior parathyroid gland
	Thymus
4	Superior parathyroid gland
	Ultimobranchial body
	▪ Gives rise to thyroid parafollicular/C-cells
	▪ Calcitonin
5	Rudimentary structure (becomes part of pouch 4)

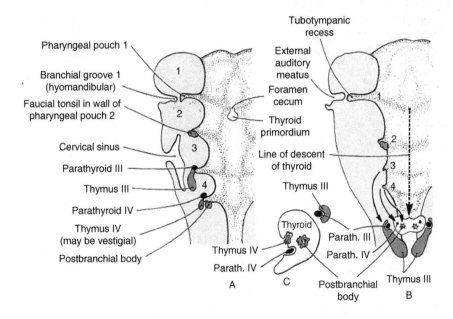

FIGURE 4-26. **Diagrams showing the origin of the pharyngeal derivatives.**

(A) The primary relationships of the several primordial to the pharyngeal pouches. (B) Course of migration of some of the primordial from their place of origin. (C) Definitive relations of parathyroids, postbranchial body, thymus, and thyroid as they appear in a transverse section of the right lobe of the thyroid taken above the level of the isthmus. Abbreviation: *Parath.*, parathyroid. Reproduced, with permission, from Carlson BM. *Patten's Foundations of Embryology.* 5th ed. New York: McGraw-Hill, 1988.

The mandible and maxilla, except the mandibular condyles, are formed by intramembranous ossification.

Most of the upper lip is formed by the maxillary processes.

The corner of the mouth is formed by the fusion of the maxillary and mandibular processes.

The vestibular lamina separates the lips and cheeks externally and jaw structures internally in the developing embryo.

The stomodeum is the primitive mouth; lined by ectoderm.

The plane passing through the right and left anterior pillars marks the separation between the oral cavity and oropharynx in the adult.

Nasal processes are proliferations of mesenchyme at the margins of the nasal placodes. The nasal placodes develop on the lower part of the frontonasal process, on each side.

Formation of the Face

MANDIBLE

- Two mandibular processes (branchial arch 1) merge.
- Medial ends merge at week 4.
- Mandibular processes → merge to form lower lip.

MAXILLA

- Two maxillary processes (branchial arch 1) merge.
  - Form upper cheek regions and most of upper lip.

FRONTAL NASAL PROCESSES

- Form with growth of forebrain.
- Develop into forehead and nose.
- Two medial nasal processes merge.
- Form philtrum of upper lip.

NASAL PLACODES

- Thickened areas of specialized ectoderm.
- Located on either side of the frontal nasal process.
- Give off elevations at their margins.
- Lateral nasal processes (2).
  - Form sides/alae of nose.
- Medial nasal processes (2).
  - Form bridge of nose.
  - Nostrils.
  - Upper lip philtrum.

Mouth and Oral Cavity

See Figure 4–27.

- Begins as a slight depression on the stomodeum.
- Located between branchial arch 1 and the forebrain.
- **Buccopharyngeal membrane** (oropharyngeal membrane)
  - Thin bilaminar membrane.
  - Composed of ectoderm externally and endoderm internally.
  - Separates the stomodeum from the primitive pharynx (until rupture).
  - Ruptures around week 3½ (~24 days).
  - Connecting the primitive mouth and primitive pharynx.

See Figure 4–28 for formation of the nasal cavities and the teeth.

FORMATION OF THE PALATE

See Figure 4–29.

Lateral cleft lip occurs because the maxillary and medial nasal processes fail to fuse. Cleft lip can be unilateral or bilateral.

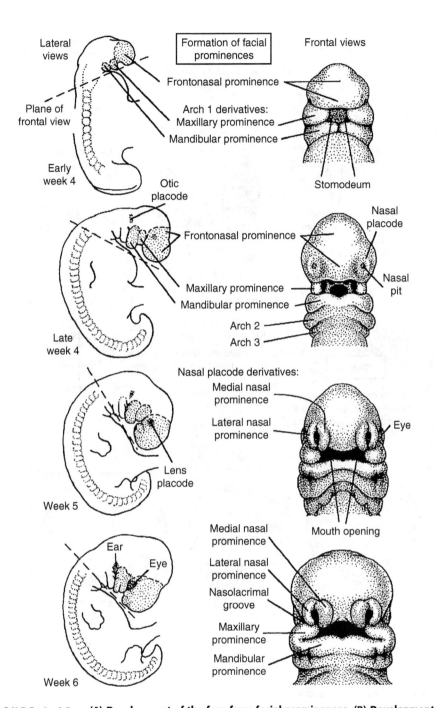

FIGURE 4–27. **(A) Development of the face from facial prominences. (B) Development of the mature face and formation of cleft lip defects.**

Reproduced, with permission, from Sweeney LJ. *Basic Concepts in Embryology.* New York: McGraw-Hill, 1998.

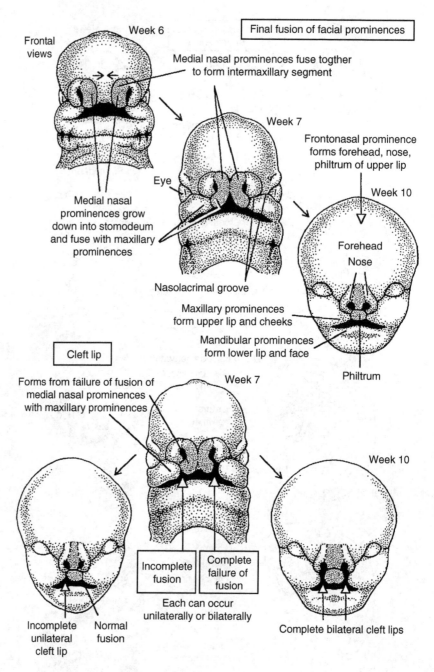

FIGURE 4–27. (Continued)

PRIMARY PALATE

- Forms from merging of the **two median nasal processes.**
- Becomes the premaxillary part of the maxilla.
    - Maxilla anterior to incisive foramen in adults.
    - Contains central and lateral incisors.

SECONDARY PALATE

- Forms from the two maxillary processes (lateral palatine processes).
- Forms hard and soft palates.
- Extends from incisive foramen posteriorly.

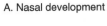

A. Nasal development

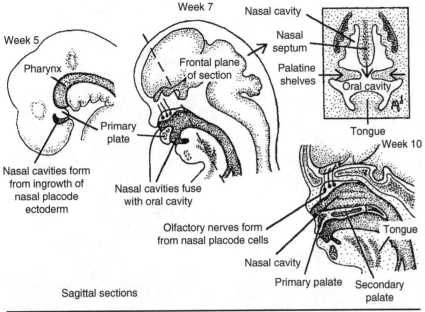

Sagittal sections

B. Tooth development

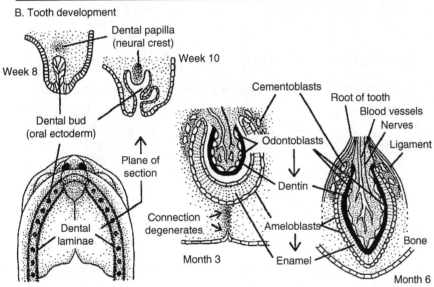

FIGURE 4–28. Formation of (A) the nasal cavities and (B) the teeth.

Reproduced, with permission, from Sweeney LJ. *Basic Concepts in Embryology.* New York: McGraw-Hill, 1998.

CLEFT PALATE

▪ Occurs with failure to fuse >1 of the following:
  ▪ Lateral palatine processes (palatal shelves).
  ▪ Nasal septum.
  ▪ Primary palate.

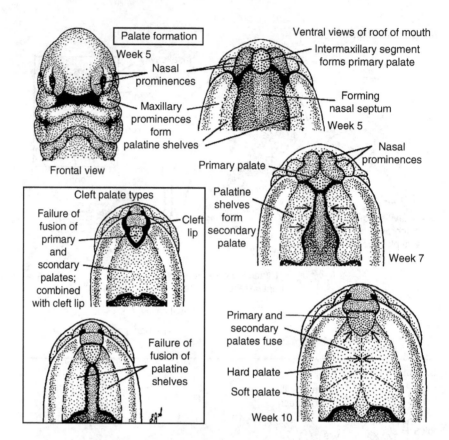

FIGURE 4-29. Normal formation of the mouth and palate and defects in palate formation.

Reproduced, with permission, from Sweeney LJ. *Basic Concepts in Embryology.* New York: McGraw-Hill, 1998.

Embryologically, the tongue is derived from the first four pharyngeal arches; and innervation comes from associated nerves of those arches (arch 1, V; arch 2 VII; arch 3 IX; arch 4, X).

Bifid tongue occurs because of lack of fusion of distal tongue buds (lateral swellings).

VARIATIONS OF CLEFT LIP AND PALATE

- May involve uvula only, or extend through hard and soft portions of palate.
- Cleft uvula only.
- Unilateral cleft of secondary palate.
- Bilateral cleft of secondary palate.
- Complete unilateral cleft.
  - Lip.
  - Alveolar process (of maxilla).
  - Primary palate.
- Complete bilateral cleft (except secondary palate).
  - Lip.
  - Alveolar process (of maxilla).
  - Anterior palate.
  - Secondary palate (unilateral).
- Complete bilateral cleft.
  - Lip.
  - Alveolar process.
  - Anterior (primary) palate.
  - Posterior (secondary) palate.

TONGUE DEVELOPMENT

See Figure 4–30.

- Begins in the first week with the formation of the tuberculum impar.
- Tuberculum impar.
  - Median, triangular elevation.
  - Appears on floor of pharynx, just in front of foramen cecum.

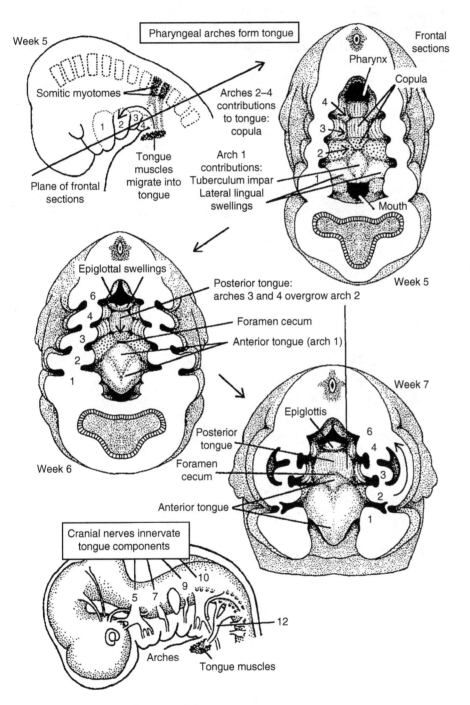

FIGURE 4–30. Development of the tongue.

Reproduced, with permission, from Sweeney LJ. *Basic Concepts in Embryology.* New York: McGraw-Hill, 1998.

Anterior Two-Thirds of Tongue

- Lateral lingual swellings (distal tongue buds [2]).
- Form on each side of the tuberculum impar.
- From the proliferation of mesenchyme (arches 1, 2, 3).
- Swellings fuse to form the anterior two-thirds of tongue.

Posterior Third of Tongue:

- Formed by two elevations.
  - Copula (arch 2).
  - Hypobranchial eminence (arch 3).

SECTION 2

Biochemistry-Physiology

CHAPTER 5

Physical-Chemical Principles

- **Covalent bonds:** *Strong* molecular interactions mediated by shared electrons.
- **Noncovalent bonds:** *Weak, reversible* molecular interactions.
  - **Ionic bonds:** Mediated by opposite electrostatic charges.
  - **Hydrogen bonds:** Mediated by a shared hydrogen atom.
  - **Van der Waals bonds:** A nonspecific attraction (occurs when any two atoms are 3–4 Å apart).

- Polar.
- Triangular.
- Highly cohesive.
- Excellent solvent for polar molecules.
- Weakens ionic and H-bonds.

Carbonic Anhydrase

Most CO_2 is transported in the blood as bicarbonate.

See Figure 5–1.

- Catalyzes the reaction between CO_2 and H_2O.
- Extremely *fast* enzyme.
- Located largely in **erythrocytes** and **kidneys.**
- A metalloenzyme: contains zinc.

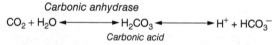

$$CO_2 + H_2O \xleftrightarrow{\text{Carbonic anhydrase}} H_2CO_3 \xleftrightarrow{} H^+ + HCO_3^-$$
Carbonic acid

FIGURE 5–1. **Carbonic anhydrase reaction.**

Enthalpy *is the heat content of a system.*
Entropy *is the degree of disorder of a system.*

- **First law:** The total energy of a *closed* system is conserved.
- **Second law:** The entropy of a *closed* system always increases.

- **Direct calorimetry:** Direct measurement of the amount of heat produced in a given system.
- **Indirect calorimetry:** Measurement of the amount of heat produced in terms of inhaled O_2 and exhaled CO_2.

Enzymes

- Highly specific catalysts for biochemical reactions.
- Classified according to their mechanism of action.

TABLE 5–1. Examples of Metallic Coenzymes of Various Enzymes

COENZYME	ENZYME
Copper	Cytochrome oxidase
Iron	Catalase
	Peroxidase
Magnesium	Hexokinase
	Glucose-6-phosphatase
	Pyruvate kinase
Nickel	Urease
Zinc	Carbonic anhydrase
	Alcohol dehydrogenase

Metals and *B-complex vitamins* serve as the majority of nonprotein coenzymes.

- Composed of *proteins* combined with nonprotein structures (either organic or inorganic) that aid in their function:
    - Coenzymes
    - Cofactors
    - Prosthetic groups

DEFINITIONS (TABLE 5–1)

- **Coenzyme:** Nonprotein portion of an enzyme.
- **Apoenzyme:** Protein portion of an enzyme. Catalytically inactive by itself.
- **Haloenzyme:** Complete, catalytically active enzyme.
    - Haloenzyme = Apoenzyme + Coenzyme
- **Isozymes:** Enzymes with subtle molecular differences that catalyze the same reaction.

CLASSIFICATION

- **Oxidoreductases:** Catalyze redox reactions.
- **Transferases:** Catalyze the transfer of functional groups.
- **Hydrolases:** Catalyze bond cleavage by hydrolysis.
- **Isomerases:** Catalyze a change in molecular structure.
- **Lyases:** Catalyze bond cleavage by elimination.
- **Ligases:** Catalyze the union of two molecules.

Enzyme Classification:
Over The **HILL**

Enzyme Mechanics

INDUCED-FIT MODEL

See Figure 5–2.

- Substrate-binding induces a conformational change in an enzyme.
- The energy produced by these changes enables the reactions to progress.

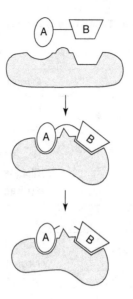

FIGURE 5–2. **The induced-fit model of enzyme biomechanics.**

Reproduced, with permission, from Murray RK. *Harper's Illustrated Biochemistry*, 26th ed. New York: McGraw-Hill, 2003.

Enzyme Kinetics

SUBSTRATE CONCENTRATION

See Figures 5–3 and 5–4.

K_m reflects the affinity of the enzyme for its substrate.

V_{max} is directly proportional to the substrate concentration.

K_m is indirectly proportional to enzyme affinity.

- Increasing substrate concentration increases reaction rate only until the enzyme-binding sites are saturated.
- Maximum reaction velocity (V_{max}) is achieved when any further increase in substrate concentration does not increase reaction rate.
- The Michaelis constant (K_m) is the substrate concentration when the initial reaction velocity (v_i) is *half* of the maximum reaction velocity (V_{max}).
- Illustrated mathematically by the **Michaelis–Menten equation.**

GIBBS FREE ENERGY CHANGE (ΔG)

$$\Delta G = \Delta G_P - \Delta G_S$$

ΔG provides no information about the reaction rate and is independent of the path of the reaction.

- Determines reaction *direction*.
- If $\Delta G_S > \Delta G_P$, then ΔG will be *negative* and the reaction will proceed spontaneously toward equilibrium.
- Equilibrium is attained when $\Delta G = 0$.

$$v_i = \frac{V_{max} \cdot [S]}{K_m + [S]}$$

FIGURE 5–3. **Michaelis–Menten equation.**

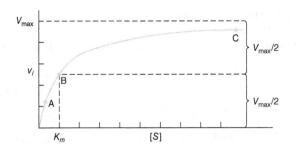

FIGURE 5-4. The effect of substrate concentration on reaction kinetics.

Reproduced, with permission, from Murray RK. *Harper's Illustrated Biochemistry*, 26th ed. New York: McGraw-Hill, 2003.

- Reactions are based on their ΔG (see Table 5–2).
  - Exergonic
  - Endergonic

REACTION DIRECTION

- Determined by the ΔG

REACTION EQUILIBRIUM

A. $A + B + Enz \longleftrightarrow C + D + Enz$

B. $K_{eq} = \dfrac{[C][D][Enz]}{[A][B][Enz]}$

- A: Any reaction with enzyme present.
- B: Equilibrium constant of the reaction.
- Enzymes have *no effect* on reaction equilibrium.

REACTION RATE

- Determined by the **activation energy.**
- Attaining activation energy requires an increase in reactant **kinetic energy.**
- Kinetic energy is largely influenced by *temperature* and *substrate concentration.*
- Enzymes *lower* the activation energy of a reaction, accelerating the rate.
- Influenced by five major factors. (See Table 5–3.)

Activation energy is the energy needed to initiate a reaction.

TABLE 5-2. Classification of Reactions Based on ΔG

REACTION TYPE	ΔG	ENERGY FLOW
Exergonic	Negative	Released
Endergonic	Positive	Required

TABLE 5-3. Factors Influencing Reaction Rate

CONTRIBUTING FACTOR	CHANGE IN FACTOR	CHARACTERISTICS
pH	Extreme changes can alter the charged state of the enzyme or substrate.	Enzymes function within an optimal pH range.
Temperature	An ↑ in temperature will ↑ the reaction rate.	Extreme ↑ in temperature can cause enzyme denaturation.
Enzyme concentration	An ↑ in enzyme concentration will ↑ the reaction rate.	
Inhibitor concentration	An ↑ in inhibitor concentration will ↓ the reaction rate.	
Substrate concentration	An ↑ in substrate concentration will ↑ reaction rate *only until* the enzyme-binding sites are saturated.	Enzymes have a limited number of active sites.

Kompetitive inhibition:
K_m increases; V_{max} does not change.
Non-Kompetitive inhibition:
K_m does Not change;
V_{max} decreases.

Enzyme Inhibition

COMPETITIVE INHIBITION

See Figure 5–5.

- Inhibitor and substrate compete for the **same binding site.**
- Inhibition can be reversed with increased substrate concentration.
- *No effect* on V_{max}.
- K_m is *increased.*

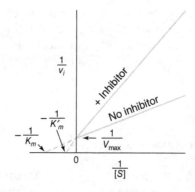

FIGURE 5-5. Competitive inhibition.

Reproduced, with permission, from Murray RK. *Harper's Illustrated Biochemistry*, 26th ed. New York: McGraw-Hill, 2003.

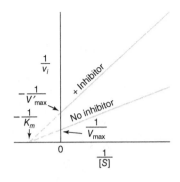

FIGURE 5-6. Noncompetitive inhibition.

Reproduced, with permission, from Murray RK. *Harper's Illustrated Biochemistry*, 26th ed. New York: McGraw-Hill, 2003.

NONCOMPETITIVE INHIBITION

See Figure 5–6.

- Inhibitor and substrate bind simultaneously.
- The **two binding sites** do not overlap.
- Inhibition cannot be reversed with increased substrate concentration.
- V_{max} is *decreased*.
- *No effect* on K_m.

*A noncompetitive inhibitor is an **allosteric inhibitor.***

UNCOMPETITIVE INHIBITION

- Inhibitor binds *only after* the substrate is bound first.
- The **two binding sites** do not overlap.
- V_{max} is *decreased*.
- K_m is *decreased*.

IRREVERSIBLE INHIBITION

- Inhibitor irreversibly alters the molecular structure of an enzyme, prohibiting its continued activity.

Aspirin irreversibly inhibits cyclooxygenase by acetylating serine.

Enzyme Regulation

COVALENT MODIFICATION

- Reversible or irreversible enzymatic modification alters enzyme conformation, thus affecting its activity.
  - Phosphorylation (kinases)
  - Dephosphorylation (phosphatases)
  - Methylation (methyltransferases)

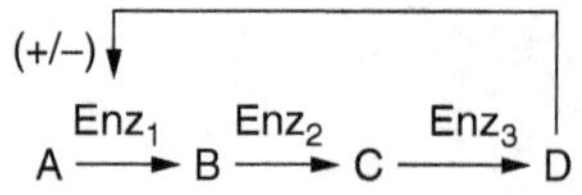

$$(+/-) \downarrow \quad \text{Enz}_1 \quad \text{Enz}_2 \quad \text{Enz}_3$$
$$A \xrightarrow{} B \xrightarrow{} C \xrightarrow{} D$$

FIGURE 5–7. **Feedback regulation.**

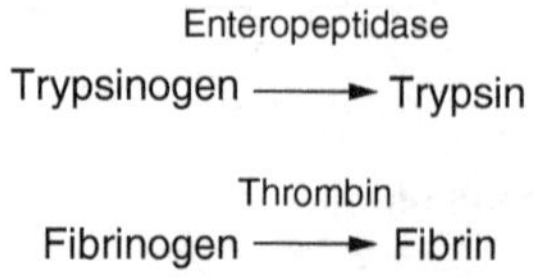

Enteropeptidase
$$\text{Trypsinogen} \xrightarrow{} \text{Trypsin}$$

Thrombin
$$\text{Fibrinogen} \xrightarrow{} \text{Fibrin}$$

FIGURE 5–8. **Examples of protease activity.**

ALLOSTERIC REGULATION

▪ **Allosteric enzyme:** A regulatory enzyme that has both an **active site** (for the substrate) and an **allosteric site** (for the effector).
▪ If the effector is present, it binds to the allosteric site causing a conformational change to the active site, which then changes (increases or decreases) the enzymatic activity.
▪ If no effector is present, the enzyme can still act on substrate normally (via the active site) to produce product.
▪ A form of **feedback regulation** in which an enzyme of a metabolic pathway is controlled by the end product of that same pathway. (See Figure 5–7.)
▪ Often catalyzes a committed step early in a metabolic pathway.
▪ Simple Michaelis–Menten kinetics are *not* followed.

PROTEASE ACTIVITY

See Figure 5–8.

▪ **Proenzyme (zymogen):** Catalytically inactive enzyme precursor.
▪ Proteases cleave the protein fragment (propeptide) of the zymogen, activating the enzyme.

Zymogens are enzymatically inactive precursors of proteolytic enzymes.

CHAPTER 6

Biological Compounds

Carbohydrate Structure

GLUCOSE

- The most fundamental carbohydrate; required for carbohydrate metabolism, storage, and cellular structure.
- If carbohydrates are not absorbed by dietary intake, they are generally converted to glucose in the *liver*.

CARBOHYDRATE CLASSIFICATION

- **Monosaccharides:** The simplest carbohydrates.
  - Further classified by:
    - Number of carbon atoms: Trioses, tetroses, pentoses, hexoses, heptoses.
    - Functional group: Aldoses (aldehyde) or ketoses (ketone) (Figures 6–1 and 6–2).
      - **Reducing sugars:** Contain aldehyde groups that are *oxidized* to carboxylic acids. For example: glucose, fructose, galactose, maltose, lactose.
    - Isomerism:
      - D-form: Hydroxyl group on right. Most common form.
      - L-form: Hydroxyl group on left.
- **Disaccharides:** Glycosidic condensation of two monosaccharides.
  - Maltose → glucose + glucose; via maltase.
  - Sucrose → glucose + fructose; via sucrase.
  - Lactose → glucose + galactose; via lactase.
- **Oligosaccharides:** Glycosidic condensation of 2–10 monosaccharides.
- **Polysaccharides:** Glycosidic condensation of >10 monosaccharides.
  - Mostly used as storage molecules or cellular structural components.
  - Can be linear or branched.

Sucrose is a non-reducing sugar.

Only monosaccharides can be absorbed in the small intestine. Disaccharides are hydrolyzed first by brush border enzymes.

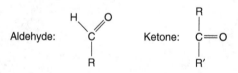

FIGURE 6–1. Functional Groups.

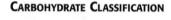

FIGURE 6–2. (A). Important aldoses.

The structures of important ketoses:

Dihydroxyacetone

$$CH_2OH$$
$$|$$
$$C=O$$
$$|$$
$$CH_2OH$$

D-Xylulose

$$CH_2OH$$
$$|$$
$$C=O$$
$$|$$
$$HO-C-H$$
$$|$$
$$H-C-OH$$
$$|$$
$$CH_2OH$$

D-Ribulose

$$CH_2OH$$
$$|$$
$$C=O$$
$$|$$
$$H-C-OH$$
$$|$$
$$H-C-OH$$
$$|$$
$$CH_2OH$$

D-Fructose

$$CH_2OH$$
$$|$$
$$C=O$$
$$|$$
$$HO-C-H$$
$$|$$
$$H-C-OH$$
$$|$$
$$H-C-OH$$
$$|$$
$$CH_2OH$$

D-Sedoheptulose

$$CH_2OH$$
$$|$$
$$C=O$$
$$|$$
$$HO-C-H$$
$$|$$
$$H-C-OH$$
$$|$$
$$H-C-OH$$
$$|$$
$$H-C-OH$$
$$|$$
$$CH_2OH$$

FIGURE 6–2. (Continued) (B). Important ketoses.

Reproduced, with permission, from Murray RK. *Harper's Illustrated Biochemistry*, 26th ed. McGraw-Hill, 2003.

Storage of Polysaccharides

STARCH

- A homopolymer of glucose linked by α–1, 4 glycosidic bonds.
- The major glucose storage molecule in *plants*.
- Contains unbranched helical *amylose* (15–20%) and branched (α–1, 6) *amylopectin* (80–85%).
- **Amylases:** The key enzymes in starch catabolism. (See Table below.)
- **Dextrins:** D-glucose polymer intermediates in starch hydrolysis. "Limit dextrins" are the fragments that remain following hydrolysis.

Isomaltase cleaves α-1, 6 branch points.

Major Amylases Important for Starch Hydrolysis

Amylase	Cleaves	Hydrolysis Products
α-Amylase	α-1,4 linkages (internal)	Maltose + dextrins
β-Amylase	α-1,4 linkages (from nonreducing ends)	Maltose
γ-Amylase (glucamylase)	α-1,4 linkages α-1,6 linkages	Glucose

α-**Amylase** is secreted by both the pancreas and the parotid gland.

GLYCOGEN

- A homopolymer of glucose linked by α-1, 4 glycosidic bonds.
- The major glucose storage molecule in *animals*.
- Contains numerous branch points via α-1, 6 glycosidic linkages.

Glycogen is stored in the liver.

Major Enzymes Important for Glycogenolysis

Enzyme	Function
Glycogen phosphorylase	Cleaves α-1,4 linkages
Glucantransferase	Exposes α-1,6 branch points
Amylo-α-1,6 glucosidase	Cleaves α-1,6 linkages

Glycogen Storage Diseases

Disease	Enzyme Deficiency	Glycogen Accumulates in	Clinical Features	Inheritance
von Gierke disease (type I glycogenosis)	Glucose-6-phosphatase	Liver Kidney	Hepatomegaly Renomegaly Stunted growth 50% mortality	Autosomal recessive
Pompe disease (type II glycogenosis)	Lysosomal glucosidase Muscle hypotonia	Lysosomes Heart Skeletal muscle	Hepatomegaly Cardiomegaly	Autosomal recessive
McArdle syndrome (type V glycogenosis)	Muscle glycogen phosphorylase	Skeletal muscle	Muscle cramping Myoglobinuria	Autosomal recessive

INULIN

▪ A homopolymer of *fructose*.
▪ Highly water soluble.
▪ Used to determine glomerular filtration rate (GFR).

Structural Polysaccharides

GLYCOSAMINOGLYCANS (GAGs)

See Table 6–1.

Bacterial cell walls contain a heteropolysaccharide consisting of alternating N-acetylglucosamine + N-acetylmuramic acid residues.

▪ Heteropolymer chains containing *repeating disaccharide units* of an **amino sugar** (N-acetylglucosamine, N-acetylgalactosamine) and a **uronic acid** (glucaronic acid, iduronic acid).
▪ The major structural polysaccharides of extracellular matrix (ECM), connective tissue (CT), and outer cell membrane surfaces.
▪ Because they contain sulfate and carboxyl groups, GAGs are *highly negatively charged* and *easily attract water,* enabling them to cushion their surrounding structures.
▪ Accumulation of various GAGs (due to enzyme deficiencies) results in several syndromic diseases.

Mucopolysaccharide Storage Diseases

Disease	Enzyme Deficiency	Accumulation of	Clinical Features	Inheritance
Hurler's syndrome	α-L-iduronidase	Heparan sulfate Dermatan sulfate	Developmental retardation Corneal clouding Gargoylism	Autosomal recessive
Hunter's syndrome	L-iduronate sulfatase	Heparan sulfate Dermatan sulfate	Mild Hurler syndrome No corneal clouding	X-linked recessive

TABLE 6–1. Major Glycosaminoglycans

GAG	PROMINENT LOCATION	COMPONENTS
Chondroitin sulfate • *Most abundant* GAG	Cartilage Bone Tendon Ligament Heart valves	N-acetylgalactosamine + D-glucuronic acid
Hyaluronic acid • *Most unique* GAG • Shock absorbing • Does not form a proteoglycan • Does not contain sulfur	ECM Synovial fluid Vitreous humor	N-acetylglucosamine + D-glucuronic acid
Heparan sulfate	Basement membranes	N-acetylglucosamine + L-glucuronic acid (or L-iduronic acid)
Heparin • Highly sulfated • Anticoagulant	Mast cell granules	N-acetylglucosamine + L-glucuronic acid (or L-iduronic acid)
Dermatan sulfate	Skin Blood vessels Heart valves	N-acetylgalactosamine + L-iduronic acid
Keratan sulfate	Cornea Cartilage Bone	N-acetylglucosamine + galactose

Hyaluronidase splits hyaluronic acid:

- *Promotes depolymerization of ECM*
- *Lowers HA viscosity and increases CT permeability*

PROTEOGLYCANS (PGs)

- Complex carbohydrates that have a central protein molecule to which many GAGs are attached in a radial (brush-like) pattern. (See Figure 6–3.)
- 95% polysaccharide; 5% protein.
- Linkage of GAGs to the central protein involves a trisaccharide: 2 galactose + 1 xylose.
- Central protein is rich in *serine* and *threonine*.
- Located mostly in the ECM.

CELLULOSE

- A homopolymer of β-D-glucopyranose linked by β-1, 4 bonds.
- Major component of **plants.**
- Cannot be digested by humans.

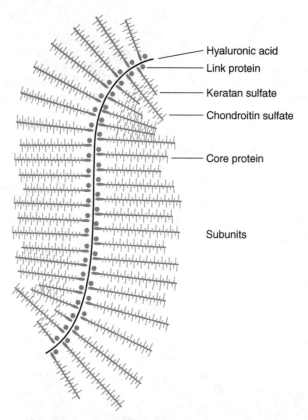

FIGURE 6–3. **Schematic representation of the proteoglycan aggrecan.**

Cariogenic bacteria synthesize glucans (dextrans) and fructans (levans) from their metabolism of dietary sucrose, which aid in their adherence to teeth.

CHITIN

▣ A homopolymer of N-acetyl-D-glucosamine linked by β-1, 4 glycosidic bonds.
▣ Major component of insect and crustacean **exoskeletons.**

Bacterial Polysaccharides

DEXTRAN

▣ A homopolymer of **glucose** formed by the hydrolysis of sucrose via glucosyl transferase (dextran sucrase).
▣ Produced by *Streptococcus mutans.*

$$\text{Sucrose} \xrightarrow[\textit{Glucosyl transferase}]{} \text{Fructose + Glucan (Dextran)}$$

LEVAN

▣ A homopolymer of **fructose** formed by the hydrolysis of sucrose via levan sucrase.
▣ Increases adhesion of bacteria to tooth surfaces.
▣ Stored intracellularly as reserve nutrients for bacteria.

Complex Carbohydrates

GLYCOPROTEINS

- Proteins with covalently linked oligosaccharide (glycan) chains.
- Function: Structural components, transport molecules, enzymes, receptors, and hormones.
- Examples: Collagens, proteoglycans, immunoglobulins, selectins, fibronectin, laminin, thyroid-stimulating hormone (TSH), and alkaline phosphatase.

GLYCOLIPIDS

- Sphingolipids with attached carbohydrates.
- Derived from ceramide.
- Commonly found on outer cell membrane surfaces, especially in brain and other nervous tissues.
- Examples: Gangliosides, galactosylceramide, and glucosylceramide.

Saliva

- A *hypotonic* fluid with an average pH ranging from 6 to 7.
- Salivary duct cells reabsorb Na^+/Cl^- in exchange for K^+/HCO_3^-.
- Contains mostly water, electrolytes, and organic factors.
- Elevated caries risk when salivary flow <0.7 mL/min.

Major Components of Saliva

Function	Major Salivary Component	Purpose
Antimicrobial	Secretory IgA	Opsonization
	Lysozyme	Hydrolyzes peptidoglycan
	Lactoperoxidase	Catalyzes H_2O_2 oxidation of bacterial substrates
Buffering	Bicarbonate	Maintains pH
Cleansing	Water	Washes away debris
Digesting	α-Amylase	Hydrolyzes starch
Lubricating	Mucins	Coats food for swallowing
Dental integrity	Calcium, phosphate	Enamel mineralization
	Glycoproteins	Pellicle formation

SALIVARY SECRETIONS

- **Serous** (watery) → contain α-amylase.
- **Mucous** (viscous) → contain mucins.

Salivary Glands and Their Primary Secretions

Salivary Gland	Primary Secretion
Parotid	Serous
Submandibular	Mixed
Sublingual	Mucous
Minor (except von Ebner)	Mucous

von Ebner's salivary glands are serous. Located in circumvallate papillae of tongue.

Parasympathetic action has greatest effect on salivary control.

SALIVARY CONTROL

- Controlled by the autonomic nervous system.
- **Parasympathetic** action → *serous* secretions.
- **Sympathetic** action → *mucous* secretions.

▶ **PROTEINS**

- Consist of chains of amino acids (*polypeptides*), which are arranged in specific three-dimensional conformations.

Amino Acids

See Tables 6–2 through 6–4.

Basic amino acid structure.

- Building blocks of polypeptides.
- Basic structure consists of a central α-carbon atom surrounded by four groups: a hydrogen atom, carboxyl group, amino group, and an R-group specific to each amino acid.
- All amino acids found in proteins are stereoisomers in the *L-configuration*.

PEPTIDE BONDS

- Amino acids are *covalently* linked by peptide bonds at their amino (N-terminus) and carboxyl (C-terminus) groups.
- Generally short, polar, and allow the α-carbon to rotate freely about its axis (Proline has a restricted a-carbon rotation due to its 3° amine).
- Generally a *trans* (not *cis*) bond.
- Very stable; generally require proteolytic enzymes to break them.
- Do not ionize at physiologic pH.

D-amino acids are found in some antibiotics and bacterial cell walls.

***Glycine** is the only amino acid that has two of the same group (hydrogen atoms) bonded to the α-carbon.*

TABLE 6–2.   Classification of Amino Acids by R-Group

R-GROUP	AMINO ACIDS
Aliphatic	Alanine, glycine, isoleucine, leucine, valine
Hydroxylic	Serine, threonine, tyrosine
Acidic	Asparagine, aspartate, glutamate, glutamine
Basic	Arginine, histidine, lysine
Aromatic	Histidine, phenylalanine, tryptophan, tyrosine
Thiol	Cysteine, methionine
Imino	Proline

TABLE 6-3. Classification of Amino Acids by Dietary Necessity

DIETARY NECESSITY	CHARACTERISTIC	AMINO ACIDS
Essential (9)	Must be obtained from dietary intake Dietary lack can result in negative nitrogen balance	Phenylalanine Valine Threonine Tryptophan Isoleucine Methionine Histidine Lysine Leucine
Nonessential (11)	All synthesized from **glucose** in TCA cycle (from α-ketoacids, α-amino acids, transaminases, vitamin B$_6$), *except* tyrosine, which is derived from phenylalanine	Arginine Aspartate Asparagine Alanine Cysteine Glycine Glutamate Glutamine Proline Serine Tyrosine

Essential amino acids:
PriVaTe TIM HaLL

DISULFIDE BONDS

- Strong, covalent bonds between thiol (–SH) group of two cysteine residues that stabilizes structure of proteins and prevent denaturation.
- Abundant in insulin and Ig.

CLASSIFICATION

- By R-group. (See Table 6–2.)
- By dietary necessity. (See Table 6–3.)
- By metabolic end product. (See Table 6–4.)

TABLE 6-4. Classification of Amino Acids by Metabolic End Product

METABOLIC CATEGORY	AMINO ACIDS
Ketogenic Yields *acetyl-CoA*	Leucine, lysine
Glucogenic Yields *pyruvate*	Arginine, aspartate, asparagine, alanine, cysteine, histidine, methionine, glycine, glutamate, glutamine, proline, serine, threonine, valine
Both	Isoleucine, phenylalanine, tryptophan, tyrosine

Epinephrine and norepinephrine are produced by the adrenal medulla. They cause potent vasoconstriction and bronchodilation.

Serotonin is released largely by gastric mucosa and platelets, causing vasoconstriction. It is a potent neurotransmitter in the CNS.

Histamine is released largely by basophils and mast cells, causing vasodilation and bronchoconstriction.

H1 *receptors mediate type I hypersensitivity.*
H2 *receptors mediate gastric acid and pepsin secretion.*

Nitric oxide is released largely by vascular endothelium, causing vasodilation.

Heme is a major component of hemoglobin and myoglobin.

Protein structures are determined by ***x-ray diffraction*** *analysis.*

AMINO ACID DERIVATIVES

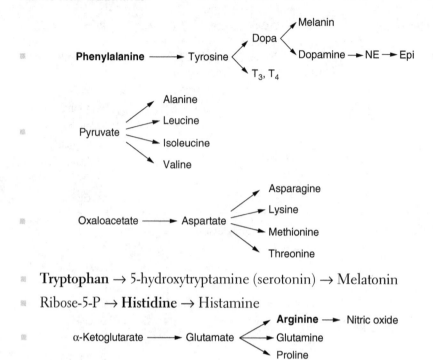

- Tryptophan → 5-hydroxytryptamine (serotonin) → Melatonin
- Ribose-5-P → **Histidine** → Histamine

DEFECTS OF AMINO ACID METABOLISM

Disease	Affected AA	Deficiency	Effects
Phenylketonuria (PKU)	Phenylalanine	Phenylalanine hydroxylase	Developmental retardation, ↓ skin/ hair pigmentation Need to take tyrosine supplements
Albinism	Tyrosine	Tyrosinase	Lack of melanin pigmentation
Alkaptonuria	Tyrosine	Homogentisic acid oxidase	Excessive urinary excretion of homogentisic acid (causing **black urine**), pigmented sclera
Cystinuria	Cysteine	Renal reabsorption of cysteine	Excessive urinary excretion of cysteine, kidney stones

Protein Structure

- **Primary structure:** The specific sequence of amino acids in a polypeptide chain. Each amino acid in the polypeptide chain is called a **residue**.
- **Secondary structure:** The folding of portions of a polypeptide chain.
    - *α*-**Helix:** Coiled configuration.
    - *β*-**Pleated sheet:** Zigzag or pleated configuration.
    - *β*-**Turn:** Reverse turns that link two sides of a *β*-pleated sheet.

Amino acid
sequence   – Gly – X – Y – Gly – X – Y – Gly – X – Y –

2° structure

Triple helix

FIGURE 6–4. **Collagen structure.**

Reproduced, with permission, from Murray RK. *Harper's Illustrated Biochemistry*, 26th ed. McGraw-Hill, 2003.

- **Tertiary structure:** The overall three-dimensional conformation of a polypeptide. Each portion of the polypeptide that can perform a biochemical or physical function is called a **domain.**
- **Quarternary structure:** The spatial arrangement of two or more polypeptide chains. Each polypeptide is known as a **subunit.** Associated via noncovalent interactions.

Physiologically Relevant Proteins

COLLAGEN

See Figure 6–4 for collagen structure and Figure 6–5 for collagen synthesis.

- 1/3 of body's protein.
- Consists of three polypeptide α-chains wound around one another to form a **triple helix.**
- Produced by many cells: *fibroblasts,* epithelial cells, odontoblasts, osteoblasts, and chondrocytes.
- It is the organic matrix in dentin and cementum.

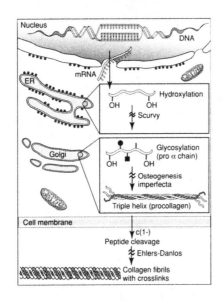

*Vitamin C is required for the hydroxylation of **proline** and **lysine** during collagen synthesis.*

FIGURE 6–5. **Collagen synthesis.**

Reproduced, with permission, from Bhushan V. *First Aid for the USMLE Step 1.* McGraw-Hill, 2006:85.

- 35% glycine; 21% proline; 11% alanine.
- Fibers have high tensile strength.

COLLAGEN SYNTHESIS

The amount of hydroxyproline and hydroxylysine provide a good estimate of collagen content since they are not found in many other proteins.

- Intracellular events
    - rER: Synthesis of α-chains with **glycine-x-y** sequence.
    - rER: Hydroxylation of proline and lysine residues, forming **hydroxyproline** and **hydroxylysine**. Requires vitamin C.
    - Golgi: Glycosylation of α-chains, forming **procollagen**, a triple helix containing N- and C-terminal propeptides.
- Extracellular events
    - Endopeptidases cleave the N- and C-terminal propeptides of procollagen, forming **tropocollagen**.
    - Cross-linking of tropocollagen molecules, forming collagen fibrils. Requires oxidation of lysine via lysine oxidase (contains copper).

Types of Collagen

Tropocollagen is the longest known protein. Found in all collagen and reticular fibers, except in the thymus.

Type	Location
I	Skin, bone, tendon, sclera, dentin, cementum, gingiva, PDL
II	Cartilage, vitreous humor
III	Embryonic CT, organ CT, blood vessels, pulp, PDL
IV	Basement membrane
V	Widely distributed CT, dentin, gingiva, PDL
VII	Anchoring fibrils of basement membrane

ELASTIN

*Elastin does **not** contain **hydroxylysine**, which makes it much more elastic than collagen.*

- Fibers are extremely elastic, "rubber-like."
- Found in skin, ligaments, arterial walls.
- Synthesis can occur simultaneously with collagen.
- Synthesized similarly to collagen:
    - Amino acid sequence of the proelastin polypeptide chain is typically **glycine-x-y**. Other residues include proline, lysine, alanine, and hydroxyproline (to a lesser extent).
    - Endopeptidases cleave the N- and C-terminal propeptides of proelastin, forming **tropoelastin**.
    - Cross-linking of tropoelastin molecules via *desmosine*, forming elastin fibers. Requires oxidation of lysine via lysine oxidase (contains copper).

PLASMA PROTEINS

- Synthesized in the **liver** (*except* gamma globulins).
- Act as buffers to stabilize pH.

Major Plasma Proteins

Plasma Protein	Plasma Content	Examples	Function
Albumin	60%	Albumin	Maintains plasma osmotic pressure Transports various molecules (calcium, copper, free fatty acids, bilirubin, steroid hormones, drugs)
Fibrinogen (Factor I)	4%	Fibrinogen	Hemostasis
α-Globulins	10%	Lipoproteins (HDL) Prothrombin Erythropoietin Angiotensinogen α_2-Macroglobulin	Transports cholesterol esters Hemostasis Erythrocyte synthesis Regulates blood pressure Protease inhibition
β-Globulins	10%	Lipoproteins (LDL) Transferrin	Transports cholesterol Transports copper and iron
γ-Globulins	15%	Immunoglobulins	Antibodies
Complement proteins	<1%	C3, C5, etc	Bacterial cell lysis Inflammation

IMMUNOGLOBULINS

See also Chapter 21, "Immunology and Immunopathology."

HEMOGLOBIN

See Tables 6–5 and 6–6 and Figure 6–6.

■ Transports O_2 in erythrocytes.

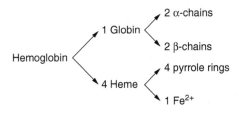

■ Each heme reversibly binds one molecule of O_2 when the iron is in a reduced ferrous (Fe^{2+}) state.
■ Heme binds carbon monoxide (CO) with a greater affinity than O_2.
■ Hb binds ~15% of the CO_2 carried in venous blood (the majority is carried by bicarbonate).
■ Mutations of α and β subunits result in numerous hemoglobin types.

Methemoglobinemia *is a condition in which Fe^{2+} (ferrous) is oxidized to Fe^{3+} (ferric), which cannot bind oxygen. Methemoglobin is formed due to decreased activity of methemoglobin reductase–a side effect of drugs (eg, sulfonamides) or a hereditary phenotype of increased hemoglobin M.*

TABLE 6–5.   The Major Types of Hemoglobin

Hb Type	Characteristic	Cause of Abnormality
Hb A	Normal Hb	N/A
Hb F	Fetal Hb	N/A
Hb C	Chronic anemia	Lysine replaces glutamate
Hb H	α-Thalassemia	Defect of α chain genes (composed of four β chains)
Hb M	Methemoglobinemia	Tyrosine replaces histidine
Hb S	Sickle-cell anemia	Valine replaces glutamate

TABLE 6–6.   Comparison of Hemoglobin and Myglobin

Globin	Location	Hemes (no.)	O$_2$ Usage	O$_2$ Affinity
Hemoglobin	Erythrocyte	4	Transport	+
Myoglobin	Muscle	1	Storage	+++

Heme *is a cyclic structure composed of four pyrrole rings with a central **iron** atom.*

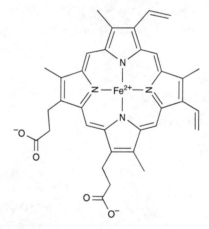

FIGURE 6–6.   Heme.

Reproduced, with permission, from Murray RK. *Harper's Illustrated Biochemistry*, 26th ed. New York: McGraw-Hill, 2003.

MYOGLOBIN

- Stores O$_2$ in muscle.
- Similar structure to hemoglobin.
- Contains only *one* heme: can only associate with one O$_2$ molecule.
- Has much higher affinity for O$_2$ than hemoglobin.

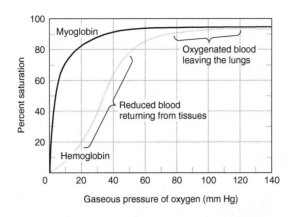

Shift to right (Bohr effect):

↑ CO_2, acid, 2,3-DPG, altitude, temp., metabolic need; ↓ O_2 affinity, pH.

Shift to left:

↓ CO_2, acid, 2,3-DPG, temp., metabolic need; ↑ O_2 affinity, pH.

Oxygen-binding curves of hemoglobin and myoglobin.

Reproduced, with permission, from Murray RK. *Harper's Illustrated Biochemistry*, 26th ed. McGraw-Hill, 2003, as modified, with permission, from Scriver CR, et al. (ed.) *The Molecular and Metabolic Basis of Inherited Disease*, 7th ed. New York: McGraw-Hill, 1995.

▶ LIPIDS

STRUCTURE

- Highly *hydrophobic* molecules.
- Soluble in *nonpolar* solvents such as chloroform, ether, and other organic solvents.
- Functions:
    - Cellular structure
    - Metabolism
    - Transportation
    - Storage

FATTY ACIDS

- Basic building blocks of most lipids.
- All are aliphatic (non-aromatic) carboxylic acids.
- Most are esters, although some exist as unesterified free fatty acids.
- The carbon chain can be *saturated* or *unsaturated*.
- Have an *even* number of carbon atoms with a terminal carboxyl group.
- Most are nonessential (can be synthesized).
- Only a few are essential (found in vegetable oils and animal fats):
    - **Linolenic acid:** ω-3 fatty acid
    - **Linoleic acid:** ω-6 fatty acid
    - **Oleic acid:** ω-9 fatty acid
    - **Arachidonic acids**

$$C_\omega H_3 — (CH_2)_n — C_\beta H_2 — C_\alpha H_2 — C \overset{O}{\underset{OH}{}}$$

Basic fatty acid structure.

CLASSIFICATION

- By number of double bonds.
  - **Saturated:** No double bonds.
  - **Monounsaturated:** One double bond, usually in "cis" configuarion.
  - **Polyunsaturated:** Multiple double bonds.

LIPID TYPES

- Triacylglycerols
- Phospholipids
- Steroids
- Eicosanoids

*Triglycerides are **not** found in cell membranes.*

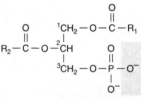

Basic triglyceride structure.

TRIACYLGLYCEROLS (TRIGLYCERIDES)

- Consists of three fatty acids acylated to a glycerol molecule.
- Important source of energy.
- Stored in *adipose tissue*.
- Transported in the plasma by *lipoproteins*.
- Increased TGs linked to atherosclerosis, heart disease, and stroke.

PHOSPHOLIPIDS

- Consists of two fatty acids acylated to two carbons of a glycerol molecule and a phosphate group esterified to the third carbon.
- Hydrophilic head (phosphate group); hydrophobic tail (fatty acids).
- Derive from *phosphatate*.
- Major constituents of cell and mitochondrial membranes.
- Precursors for second messengers and metabolic intermediates.
- Increased TGs linked to atherosclerosis, heart disease, and stroke.

Basic phospholipid structure.

Accumulation of sphingomyelins causes Niemann-Pick disease.

Three Major Types of Phospholipids

Phospholipid	Function	Major Constituent
Lecithins (phosphatidycholines)	Water-soluble emulsifiers Plasma membrane constituent	Choline
Cephalins (phosphatidylethanolamines)	Nerve tissue components	Ethanolamine
Sphingomyelins	Plasma membrane constituent Nerve tissue constituent	Ceramide Choline

CHOLINE

- $N^+(CH_3)_3\text{-}CH_2\text{-}CH_2\text{-}OH$
- An essential nutrient.
- Found mostly in phospholipids.
- Found as *lecithin* in plasma cell membrane.
- Precursor of *betaine*, an osmolyte used by kidney to control water balance.
- Component of *sphingomyelin*, which forms myelin sheath. Insulates nerve fibers and aids in rapid conduction on nerve impulses.
- Source of methyl group required for *lipoprotein* formation in liver.
- Necessary for *acetylcholine* formation.
- Active component of *lung surfactant*.

Choline deficiency causes abnormal fat metabolism and can lead to fatty liver disease and hepatic cirrhosis.

STEROIDS

- **Cholesterol** is the most basic steroid.
- Major constituent of cell membranes and lipoproteins.
- Commonly present as a cholesterol ester.
- Conversion of HMG-CoA → mevalonate via HMG-CoA reductase is the *rate-limiting step*.
- Precursor molecule for other steroids:
  - Bile salts
  - Sex hormones
  - Adrenocortical hormones
  - Vitamin D

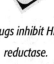

Statin drugs inhibit HMG-CoA reductase.

EICOSANOIDS

- 20-carbon long polyunsaturated fatty acids.
- Derivatives of **arachidonic acid.**
- **Phospholipase A₂ (PLA₂)** releases arachidonic acid from plasma membrane phospholipids upon hormone or cytokine stimulation or cellular damage.

Corticosteroids inhibit phospholipase A₂ (PLA₂).

Eicosanoids

Eicosanoid	Formative Pathway	Examples	Function
Prostanoids	Cyclooxygenase (COX)	Prostaglandins	Vasodilation Inflammatory Pain Gastric protection
		Prostacyclins	Vasodilation ↓ platelet aggregation
		Thromboxanes	Vasoconstriction ↑ platelet aggregation
Leukotrienes	5-Lipoxygenase (5-LOX)	Various leukotrienes	Bronchoconstriction Inflammatory
Lipoxins	15-Lipoxygenase (15-LOX)	Various lipoxins	Anti-inflammatory

Aspirin and nonsteroidal anti-inflammatory drugs (NSAIDs) inhibit cyclooxygenase (COX).

Prostaglandins:
- *Modulate hormones*
- *Act locally*
- *Metabolized rapidly*

Eicosanoid formation pathways.

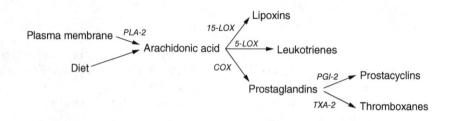

Lipid Transport

LIPOPROTEINS

LDL is the major carrier of cholesterol in the blood. It is taken up by cell-mediated endocytosis.

- Transport lipids in blood plasma.
- Composed of a nonpolar lipid core surrounded by a single layer of amphipathic phospholipids and cholesterol (see Figure 6–7).
- Characterized by the protein moiety embedded in their outer layer (**apoprotein**).
- Contain triglycerides (16%), phospholipids (30%), cholesterol (14%), cholesterol esters (36%), and free fatty acids (4%).
- *Choline* is essential for the secretion of lipoproteins from hepatocytes, especially very low density lipoproteins (VLDL).

HDL is produced de novo in the liver.

__Familial hypercholesterolemia__ is caused by an autosomal dominant defect of the low-density lipoprotein (LDL) receptor, leading to increased plasma LDL cholesterol and atherosclerosis.

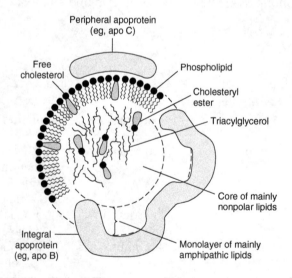

FIGURE 6–7. **Lipoprotein structure.**

Reproduced, with permission, from Murray RK. *Harper's Illustrated Biochemistry*, 26th ed. McGraw-Hill, 2003.

The Major Lipoproteins

Lipoprotein	Density	Protein (%)	Major Lipid Content	Carries Lipid From	Carries Lipid To
Chylomicron	+	1	Dietary TG	Small intestine	Extrahepatic tissues
Chylomicron remnants	++	7	Cholesterol	Chylomicrons of extrahepatic tissues	Liver
VLDL	++	10	Endogenous TG	Liver	Extrahepatic tissues
IDL (VLDL remnants)	+++	11	TG, Cholesterol	VLDL of extrahepatic tissues	Liver
LDL	+++	20	Cholesterol	Liver	Extrahepatic tissues
HDL	++++	30–55	Cholesterol	Extrahepatic tissues	Liver

BILE SALTS

- Aid in lipid absorption (emulsification and solubilization).
    - Absorption via **micelles** (water-soluble complexes).
    - Decrease surface tension of particles to break them into smaller sizes.
- Formed from cholesterol in the liver.
- Almost exclusively absorbed in the *ileum* and returned to the liver via the **enterohepatic (portal) circulation.**
- Those that are not reabsorbed are excreted.
- Surplus bile salts are stored in the **gall bladder.**
- Two major bile salts enter bile as *glycine* or *taurine* conjugates (occurs in peroxisomes):
    - **Glycocholic acid:** Glycine + cholic acid.
    - **Taurocholic acid:** Taurine + cholic acid.

Lipid Storage

- Most lipid triglycerides are stored in **adipose tissue.**

LIPID (LYSOSOMAL) STORAGE DISEASES

See Table 6–7.

- Inherited disorders of the **reticuloendothelial system.**
- Caused by incomplete lysosomal breakdown of sphingolipids and mucopolysaccharides within phagocytes, leading to their accumulation.
- Most are common to Ashkenazi Jewish ancestry.

TABLE 6–7. Lipid Storage Diseases

DISEASE	DEFICIENT ENZYME	ACCUMULATED LIPID	CLINICAL FEATURES	INHERITANCE
Gaucher's disease	β-Glucocerebrosidase	Glucocerebrosides	Splenomegaly Hepatomegaly Anemia Skin pigmentation (brown) *Most common*	Autosomal recessive
Niemann-Pick disease	Sphingomyelinase	Sphingomyelin	Splenomegaly Hepatomegaly Cherry red spot on macula *Rapidly fatal*	Autosomal recessive
Tay-Sachs disease	Hexosaminidase A	Gangliosides	CNS degeneration Developmental retardation Cherry red spot on macula *Rapidly fatal*	Autosomal recessive
Fabry's disease	α-Galactosidase	Ceramide trihexoside	Peripheral neuropathy Skin lesions (angiokeratomas) Renal failure Cardiovascular	X-linked recessive
Krabbe's disease	Galactocerbrosidase	Galactocerebroside	Peripheral neuropathy Optic atrophy Developmental retardation	Autosomal recessive

CHAPTER 7

Metabolism

See Figure 7–1 for summary of metabolic pathways.

KEY INTERMEDIATES

See Figure 7–2.

- Glucose-6-phosphate
- Pyruvate
- Acetyl-CoA

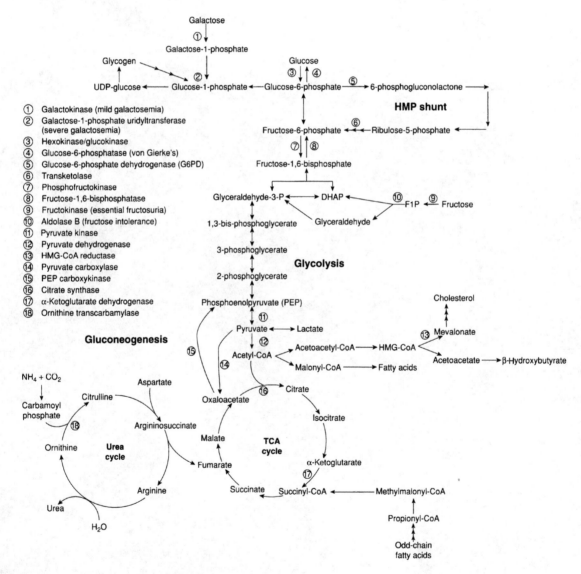

① Galactokinase (mild galactosemia)
② Galactose-1-phosphate uridyltransferase (severe galactosemia)
③ Hexokinase/glucokinase
④ Glucose-6-phosphatase (von Gierke's)
⑤ Glucose-6-phosphate dehydrogenase (G6PD)
⑥ Transketolase
⑦ Phosphofructokinase
⑧ Fructose-1,6-bisphosphatase
⑨ Fructokinase (essential fructosuria)
⑩ Aldolase B (fructose intolerance)
⑪ Pyruvate kinase
⑫ Pyruvate dehydrogenase
⑬ HMG-CoA reductase
⑭ Pyruvate carboxylase
⑮ PEP carboxykinase
⑯ Citrate synthase
⑰ α-Ketoglutarate dehydrogenase
⑱ Ornithine transcarbamylase

FIGURE 7–1. Summary of metabolic pathways.

Reproduced, with permission, from Bhushan V, et al. *First Aid for the USMLE Step 1.* New York: McGraw-Hill, 2006.

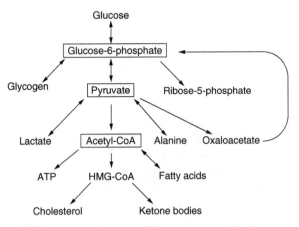

FIGURE 7-2. Common metabolic intermediates.

Rate-Limiting Steps (Table 7–1)

TABLE 7-1. **Rate-Limiting Enzymes of Major Metabolic Pathways**

METABOLIC PATHWAY	ENZYME
Glycolysis	Phosphofructokinase (PFK)
Gluconeogenesis	Fructose bisphosphatase-2
TCA cycle	Isocitrate dehydrogenase
Glycogen synthesis	Glycogen synthase
Glycogenolysis	Glycogen phosphorylase
HMP shunt	Glucose-6-phosphate dehydrogenase (G6PD)
Urea cycle	Carbamoyl phosphate synthetase
Fatty acid synthesis	Acetyl-CoA carboxylase (ACC)
Fatty acid oxidation	Carnitine acyltransferase
Ketogenesis	HMG-CoA synthase
Cholesterol synthesis	HMG-CoA reductase

▶ ATP PRODUCTION

See Table 7–2.

- **Substrate-level phosphorylation:** $ADP + P_i \rightarrow ATP$.
- **Oxidative phosphorylation:** Major source of ATP (*aerobic*).

TABLE 7-2. Net ATP Production per Molecule of Glucose

PROCESS	LOCATION	PHOSPHORYLATION	NET ATP PER GLUCOSE
Embden-Meyerhof pathway	Cytosol	Substrate level	2
Entner-Doudoroff pathway	Cytosol	Substrate level	1
TCA cycle	Mitochondrial matrix	Substrate level	2 (as GTP)
ETC	Inner mitochondrial membrane	Oxidative	32 (G3P shuttle) 34 (malate-aspartate shuttle)

Photophosphorylation occurs in plants as a result of photosynthesis. Also involves an ETC.

► CARBOHYDRATE METABOLISM

▪ Determines the fate of *glucose.*
▪ **ATP production per molecule of glucose.** The table below assumes that the NADH produced in glycolysis is carried into mitochondria via the malate–aspartate shuttle. If the glycerol-3-phosphate (G3P) shuttle is used, the net ATP production would be 36.

ATP Production per Molecule of Glucose

Metabolic Pathway	ATP Produced
Glycolysis (cytosol)	
2 ATP consumed (by hexokinase and PFK)	−2
4 ATP formed	+4
2 NADH formed	
Pryuvate → Acetyl-CoA (mitochondrial matrix)	
2 NADH formed	
TCA Cycle (mitochondrial matrix)	
2 GTP formed	+2
6 NADH formed	
2 FADH$_2$ formed	
ETC (inner mitochondrial membrane)	
10 NADH oxidized	+30
2 FADH$_2$ oxidized	+4
	+38

Each NADH yields ~3 ATP.
Each FADH$_2$ yields ~2 ATP.

GLYCOLYSIS

▪ Also called the Embden–Meyerhof Pathway. (See Figures 7–3.)
▪ Occurs in the *cytosol,* in the absence of O$_2$.
▪ Converts glucose (as glucose-6-phosphate) → two molecules of pyruvate.
▪ Conversion of fructose-6-phosphate → fructose-1, 6-biphosphate via **phosphofructokinase (PFK)** is the *rate-limiting step.*

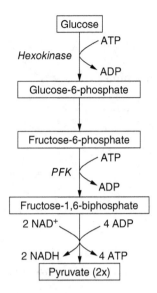

FIGURE 7-3. **Major reactions of glycolysis.**

Fluoride inhibits *enolase,* the enzyme that converts 2-phosphoglycerate → phosphoenolpyruvate.

- Stoichiometry of glycolysis:

Glucose + 2 P_i + 2 ADP + 2 NAD^+ → 2 Pyruvate + 2 ATP + 2 NADH + 2 H^+ + 2 H_2O

METABOLIC FATES OF PYRUVATE

Because erythrocytes do not have mitochondria, glycolysis always ends in lactate. The lactic acid is converted back to glucose via the Cori cycle. (see Fig 7–5).

Type of Reaction	Enzyme	Product	Function
Oxidation	Pyruvate dehydrogenase	Acetyl-CoA	ATP production Fatty acid synthesis
Reduction	Lactate dehydrogenase	Lactate	Anaerobic glycolysis
Carboxylation	Pyruvate carboxylase	Oxaloacetate	Gluconeogenesis Replenishes TCA cycle
Transamination	Alanine aminotransferase	Alanine	Amino acid synthesis

- ATP-requiring reactions:
  - Hexokinase/Glucokinase: glucose → glucose-6-phosphate
  - PFK: fructose-6-phosphate → fructose-1,6-bisphosphate
- ATP-producing reactions:
  - Phosphoglycerate kinase: 1,3-bisphosphoglycerate → 3-phosphoglycerate
  - Pyruvate kinase: phosphoenolpyruvate → pyruvate

PYRUVATE DEHYDROGENASE

- Pyruvate + NAD$^+$ → Acetyl-CoA + CO$_2$ + NADH
- Requires five cofactors:
    - Pyrophosphate (B$_1$, thiamine)
    - FAD (B$_2$, riboflavin)
    - NAD (B$_3$, niacin)
    - CoA (B$_5$, pantothenate)
    - Lipoic acid

THE LACTIC ACID CYCLE

- Also called the Cori cycle (See Figure 7–4.)
- Occurs in the *liver*
- Prevents lactic acidosis
- Converts lactate → glucose, which is then reoxidized via glycolysis
- Provides quick ATP production during *anaerobic* glycolysis in muscle and erythrocytes
- Results in net loss of 4 ATP per cycle

THE CITRIC ACID CYCLE

- Also called the Krebs cycle and the tricarboxylic acid cycle. (See Figures 7–5.)
- Occurs in the *mitochondrial matrix.*
- Completes the metabolism of glucose.
- Oxidizes acetyl-CoA.
- Reduces NAD$^+$ and FAD → NADH and FADH$_2$, which are reoxidized in the ETC to produce ATP.
- Tightly regulated by both *ATP* and *NAD$^+$*.
- Stoichiometry of TCA cycle:

Acetyl-CoA + 3 NAD$^+$ + FAD + P$_i$ + GDP + 2 H$_2$O → 2 CO$_2$ + 3 NADH + FADH$_2$ + GTP + 2 H$^+$ + CoA

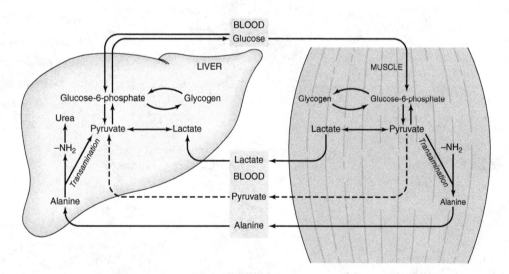

FIGURE 7–4. The Cori cycle.

Reproduced, with permission, from Murray RK. *Harper's Illustrated Biochemistry*, 26th ed. New York: McGraw-Hill, 2003.

THE ELECTRON TRANSPORT CHAIN

- Also called the respiratory chain (See Figure 7–5.)
- Occurs in the *inner mitochondrial membrane*.
- Produces ATP via **oxidative phosphorylation** of ADP.
- Reoxidizes NADH and $FADH_2$ back $\rightarrow$ NAD^+ and FAD as electrons flow through a series of *four* cytochrome complexes of increasing redox potential (along a proton gradient).
- **Cytochromes** contain a central iron atom (similar to hemoglobin), which can exist in an oxidized ferric (Fe^{3+}) state or a reduced ferrous (Fe^{2+}) state.
- Cytochromes receive electrons from the reduced form of coenzyme Q (ubiquinone).
- Cytochromes carry electrons as flavins, iron-sulfur groups, hemes, and copper ions.

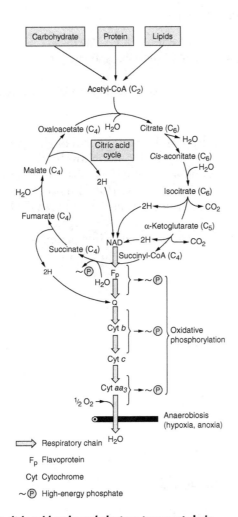

FIGURE 7–5. **The citric acid cycle and electron transport chain.**

Reproduced, with permission, from Murray RK. *Harper's Illustrated Biochemistry*, 26th ed. New York: McGraw-Hill, 2003.

CYTOCHROME COMPLEXES OF THE ETC

Coenzyme Q is also known as **ubiquinone.**

Cytochrome Complex	Enzyme	Electron Transfer
Complex I	NADH-Q reductase	NADH → ubiquinone
Complex II ▪ Does not pump protons	Succinate-Q reductase	$FADH_2$ → ubiquinone
Complex III	Cytochrome reductase	Ubiquinone → cyt c
Complex IV ▪ Requires copper	**Cytochrome oxidase**	$Cyt\ c + H^+ + O_2 \to H_2O$ ▪ O_2 is the final e^- receptor

THE PENTOSE PHOSPHATE PATHWAY

- Also called the hexose monophosphate shunt.
- Stoichiometry of the pentose phosphate pathway (PPP):

$$\text{Glucose-6-phosphate} + 2\ NADP^+ + H_2O \to \text{Ribose-5-phosphate} + 2\ NADPH + 2\ H^+ + CO_2$$

No ATP is produced from the PPP.

The NADPH produced from the PPP helps to rid erythrocytes of free radicals and H_2O_2. **G6PD deficiency** *causes hemolytic anemia due to a ↓ in NADPH production, and subsequent ↑ of oxidizing agents in RBCs.*

- Occurs in the *cytosol.*
- An alternative to glycolysis in the metabolism of glucose.
- Coverts glucose-6-phosphate → ribose-5-phosphate.
- Conversion of glucose-6-phosphate → 6-phosphogluconolactone via **glucose-6-phosphate dehydrogenase (G6PD)** is the *rate-limiting step.*
- Produces **ribose** (for nucleotide synthesis) and **NADPH** (for fatty acid and steroid synthesis).
- Not all cells use the PPP (most active in liver, adipose tissue, adrenal cortex, thyroid, mammary gland, testis, and erythrocytes).

GLUCONEOGENESIS

- Stoichiometry of gluconeogenesis:

$$\text{Pyruvate} + 2\ ATP + GTP + NADH + 2\ H_2O \to \text{Glucose-6-phosphate} + 2\ ADP + GDP + 3\ P_i + NAD^+ + H^+$$

- Occurs mostly in the *liver* and kidneys
- *Not* a direct reversal of the glycolysis
- Converts *amino acids* → glucose or glycogen in states of carbohydrate need
- Clears *lactic acid* (from anaerobic glycolysis) and *glycerol* (from fatty acid metabolism)
- Under strict hormonal regulation

GLYCOGEN SYNTHESIS AND CATABOLISM

- Enzymatic regulation of glycogen metabolism:

Glycogen is a branched polymer of glucose residues.

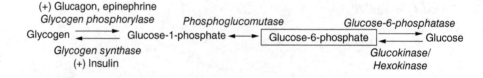

- **Glycogen synthase:** Key regulatory enzyme in its synthesis. Uses UDP-glucose and the nonreducing end of glycogen as its substrate.
    - **Glycogenin:** Primer for glycogen synthase by catalyzing the addition of glucose to itself.
- **Glycogen phosphorylase:** Key regulatory enzyme in its catabolism.
- Under strict hormonal regulation.

Glucagon and epinephrine stimulate glycogenolysis and gluconeogenesis, whereas insulin triggers glycogen formation and cellular glucose uptake.

▶ LIPID METABOLISM

FATTY ACID SYNTHESIS

See Figure 7–6.

- Occurs in the *cytosol* of mostly hepatocytes.
- The *irreversible* conversion of acetyl-CoA → **malonyl-CoA** via acetyl-CoA carboxylase is the *rate-limiting step*.
- Conversion of acetyl-CoA → **malonyl-CoA** is the *rate-limiting step*.
- **Citrate–malate shuttle** transports acetyl groups from mitochondria to the cytosol.

Coenzyme A (CoA) is a pantothenic acid (B5)-containing coenzyme involved in both fatty acid synthesis and catabolism.

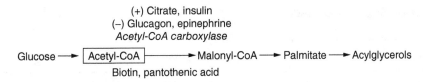

FIGURE 7–6. **Overview of fatty acid synthesis.**

TRIGLYCERIDE LIPOLYSIS

See Figure 7–7.

- Occurs in *adipocytes*.
- The glycerol is phosphorylated and ultimately oxidized in glycolysis.
- The free fatty acids are transported to the *liver* for β-oxidation.
- **Triacyglycerol lipase** is under strict hormone regulation.

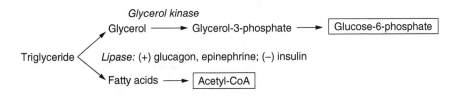

FIGURE 7–7. **Overview of triglyceride lipolysis.**

β-OXIDATION

See Figure 7–8.

- Occurs in the *mitochondrial matrix* of **hepatocytes.**
- Converts acyl-CoA → **acetyl-CoA.**
- Fatty acids are carried into the mitochondrial matrix by a **carnitine**-mediated enzyme system.

In humans, fatty acids cannot be converted to glucose.

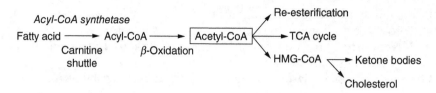

FIGURE 7-8. Overview of β-oxidation.

*Of the three ketone bodies, **acetone** is not used for energy production. Its accumulation can cause breath with a fruity odor.*

- Under certain metabolic states (starvation, diabetes mellitus), much of the acetyl-CoA is converted to **ketone bodies:**
  - Acetoacetate: synthesized by cleavage of HMG-CoA
  - β-Hydroxybutyrate
  - Acetone
- Ketone bodies are a source of fuel in extrahepatic tissues such as skeletal and cardiac muscle.
- **Ketosis** is the accumulation of ketone bodies leading to ketoacidosis and diabetic coma.

METABOLIC FATES OF ACETYL-CoA

Fate	Pathway
ATP production	Via TCA cycle and the ETC
Cholesterol synthesis	Via HMG-CoA reductase
Ketone body synthesis	Via HMG-CoA lyase
Fatty acid synthesis	Via malonyl-CoA

▶ PROTEIN METABOLISM

- Both dietary and structural proteins are degraded daily to their amino acid constituents by various proteases and peptidases. (See Figure 7–9.)

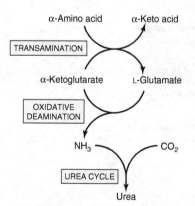

FIGURE 7-9. Key reactions and intermediates in the formation of urea.

Reproduced, with permission, from Murray RK. *Harper's Illustrated Biochemistry*, 26th ed. New York: McGraw-Hill, 2003.

TRANSAMINATION

▪ Amino acids are used to synthesize other *amino acids* (and proteins) or *metabolic intermediates* (pyruvate, acetyl-CoA, oxaloacetate, succinyl CoA, and α-ketoacids).

▪ **Aminotransferases (transaminases)** cleave the α-amino nitrogen of most amino acids, leaving hydrocarbon skeletons, which are degraded to the various glucogenic and ketogenic intermediates.

▪ Requires either *pyridoxal phosphate or pyridoxamine phosphate*, forms of pyridoxine (**vitamin B$_6$**), as a coenzyme.

▪ The transamination of pyruvate to alanine yields either α-ketoglutarate or oxaloacetate.

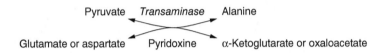

▪ See Figure 7–10 for key metabolic intermediates formed from the carbon skeletons of amino acids.

Only lysine, serine, and threonine are not transaminated.

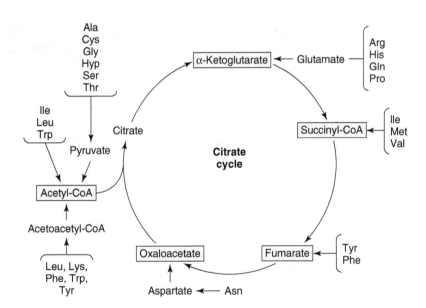

FIGURE 7–10. Key metabolic intermediates formed from the carbon skeletons of amino acids.

Reproduced, with permission, from Murray RK. *Harper's Illustrated Biochemistry*, 26th ed. New York: McGraw-Hill, 2003.

BIOCHEMISTRY-PHYSIOLOGY

Transaminase	Also Known As	Location	↑ Levels May Suggest
Aspartate aminotransferase (AST)	Serum glutamate-oxaloacetate transaminase (SGOT)	Liver Cardiac muscle Skeletal muscle Kidneys Brain RBCs	Acute hepatitis Myocardial infarction Acute renal disease Acute hemolytic anemia
Alanine aminotransferase (ALT)	Serum glutamate-pyruvate transaminase (SGPT)	Mostly liver	Acute hepatitis

METABOLISM

OXIDATIVE DEAMINATION

Glutamate is the only amino acid that undergoes rapid oxidative deamination.

- An alternative to transamination in the metabolism of amino acids.
- Results in the formation of **α-ketoacids** (for energy) and **ammonia** (for urea formation).
- Oxidative deamination of glutamate:

Glutamate dehydrogenase

L-Glutamate + NAD(P)$^+$ + H$_2$O $\longleftrightarrow$ α-Ketoglutarate + NAD(P)H + NH$_4^+$ + H$^+$

- The reaction is reversible but favors the formation of glutamate.
- Occurs mostly in the liver and kidneys.
- In humans, the vast majority of oxidative deamination derives from **glutamate**; the major enzyme responsible is **glutamate dehydrogenase.**
- Other amino acids that can undergo oxidative deamination are asparagine, histidine, serine, and threonine (Table 7–3).

TABLE 7–3. **Enzymes Involved in Oxidative Deamination**

ENZYME	DEAMINATES	PRODUCES
Glutamate dehydrogenase	Glutamate	α-Ketoglutarate + NH$_4^+$
Histidinase	Histidine	Urocanic acid + NH$_4^+$
Serine dehydratase	Serine	Pyruvate + NH$_4^+$
Asparaginase	Asparagine	Aspartic acid + NH$_4^+$

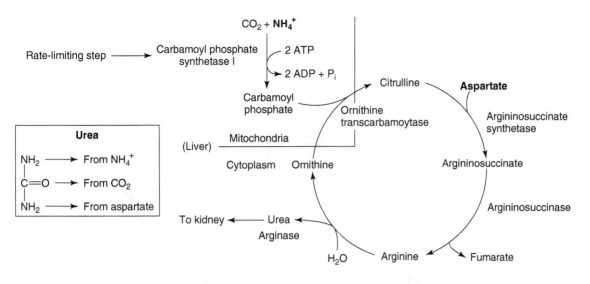

CO$_2$ + NH$_4^+$

Rate-limiting step ⟶ Carbamoyl phosphate synthetase I

2 ATP

2 ADP + P$_i$

Carbamoyl phosphate

Ornithine transcarbamoytase

Citrulline

Aspartate

Argininosuccinate synthetase

(Liver) Mitochondria

Cytoplasm   Omithine

Argininosuccinate

Argininosuccinase

To kidney ⟵ Urea ⟵

Arginase

Fumarate

H$_2$O   Arginine

Urea

NH$_2$ ⟶ From NH$_4^+$

C═O ⟶ From CO$_2$

NH$_2$ ⟶ From aspartate

FIGURE 7–11. **Key metabolic intermediates formed from the carbon skeletons of amino acids.**

Reproduced, with permission, from Le T, Bhushan V, Vasan N. *First Aid for the USMLE Step 1 2011.* 21st ed. New York: McGraw-Hill, 2011.

THE UREA CYCLE

- Occurs in the *cytosol* and *mitochondrial matrix* of **hepatocytes.**
- Eliminates the **ammonia** (NH$_4^+$) produced by oxidative deamination in the form of urea (Figure 7–11).
- Stoichiometry of the urea cycle:

CO$_2$ + NH$_4^+$ + 3 ATP + Aspartate + 2 H$_2$O → Urea + 2 ADP + 2 P$_i$ + AMP + PP$_i$ + Fumarate

- The excess nitrogen is converted to **urea** and excreted by the kidneys.
- Complete block of the cycle leads to extensive ammonia accumulation. For example, liver cirrhosis (eg, from alcoholism) results in ↓ carbamoyl phosphate synthase. It is *fatal* since there is no alternative pathway.

*The urea cycle requires **3 ATP**.*

The amount of nonprotein nitrogen in the blood is primarily due to urea.

▶ BACTERIAL METABOLISM

ENTNER–DOUDOROFF PATHWAY

- An alternative method of **glycolysis** to the Embden-Meyerhof or pentose phosphate pathways.
- Used most commonly by *aerobic* bacteria.
- Converts glucose → pyruvate + glyceraldehyde-3-phosphate.
- Produces 1 ATP per glucose via substrate-level phosphorylation.

Molecular Biology

*A **nucleoside** is a nucleotide (sugar + base) without esterified phosphate groups.*

▶ **NUCLEOTIDES**

- Building blocks of DNA and RNA.
- Functions:
    - Protein synthesis
    - Nucleic acid synthesis
    - Signal transduction pathways
- Composed of three basic compounds:
    - **Nitrogenous base**
        - Purine
        - Pyrimidine
    - **Pentose sugar**
        - Deoxyribose
        - Ribose
    - **Phosphate group(s)**

▶ **BASE PAIRING**

See Figure 8–1 for base pairing in DNA.

Purines:

Pure Ag (silver)
Purines are **A**denine and **G**uanine.

Pyrimidines:

CUT the **PY** (pie)
Cytosine, **U**racil, **T**hymine are the **Py**rimidines.

Organization

- Purines pair with pyrimidines.
- Held together via **hydrogen bonds**.
    - Adenine—Thymine/Uracil (**two** H-bonds).
    - Guanine—Cytosine (**three** H-bonds).

The strongest bonds (three hydrogen bonds) are between **C**ytosine and **G**uanine, like **C**razy **G**lue.

Adenine and Thymine/Uracil are held by two hydrogen bonds.

FIGURE 8–1. Base pairing in DNA.

Reproduced, with permission, from Murray, RK. *Harper's Illustrated Biochemistry*, 26th ed. New York: McGraw-Hill, 2003.

Comparison of Purines and Pyrimidines

Nucleotide	DNA Bases	RNA Bases	Metabolic Defects	Catabolize to	Catabolic Defects
Purines	Adenine (A) Guanine (G)	Adenine (A) Guanine (G)	Antifolate drugs Anticancer drugs	Uric acid	Gout Hyperuricemia G-6-P deficiency
Pyrimidines	Thymine (T) Cytosine (C)	Uracil (U) Cytosine (C)	UV light Methotrexate Other anticancer drugs	β-Alanine β-Amino- isobutyrate	Rare (highly water soluble)

Biosynthesis

- Nucleotide synthesis.

$$\text{Ribose-5-phosphate} \xrightarrow{\text{ATP}} \text{5-phosphoribosyl-1-pyrophosphate} \rightarrow \text{Purines}$$
$$\textbf{(PRPP)}$$
$$\downarrow$$
$$\text{Orotic acid} \rightarrow \text{Orotate monophosphate} \rightarrow \text{Pyrimidines}$$

- Uric acid synthesis.

$$\text{Purines} \rightarrow \text{Xanthine} \rightarrow \text{Uric acid}$$
$$\textit{Xanthine oxidase}$$

Tetrahydrofolic acid (TFA):

- *Used by several enzymes in purine/pyrimidine synthesis.*
- *Target for antimetabolites (eg, methotrexate).*

The catabolism of nucleotides results in no ATP production.

▶ **NUCLEIC ACIDS**

- Extremely *polar* and *hydrophilic*.
- The "backbone" consists of pentose sugars linked by **phosphodiester bonds** at the third and fifth carbon atoms.
- The two polynucleotide chains are considered **antiparallel** and **complementary** (one chain runs in the 5′ → 3′ direction; the other runs in the 3′ → 5′ direction).

*DNA and RNA are differentiated in the laboratory by the **Feulgen reaction**, which is specific for deoxyribose.*

Comparison of DNA and RNA

Nucleic Acid	Strands	Sugar	Bases
DNA	Double	Deoxyribose	A-T, G-C
RNA	Single	Ribose	A-U, G-C

The melting temperature of the double helix is a function of base composition: a higher G-C content increases the melting temperature and stability.

DNA

See Figure 8–2 for the backbone structure of a single DNA strand.

RNA

See Figure 8–3 for the backbone structure of a single RNA strand.

Three Major Types of RNA

RNA	Site of Synthesis	Function	Note
Ribosomal (rRNA)	Nucleolus	Major component of ribosomes	*Most prevalent* RNA
Transfer (tRNA)	Nucleus	Carries amino acids from cytosol to ribosomes	Contains an **anticodon** (complementary to mRNA codons)
Messenger (mRNA)	Nucleus	Carries genetic code from DNA to ribosomes	*Least prevalent* RNA. Contains **codons** (complementary to DNA template and tRNA anticodon)

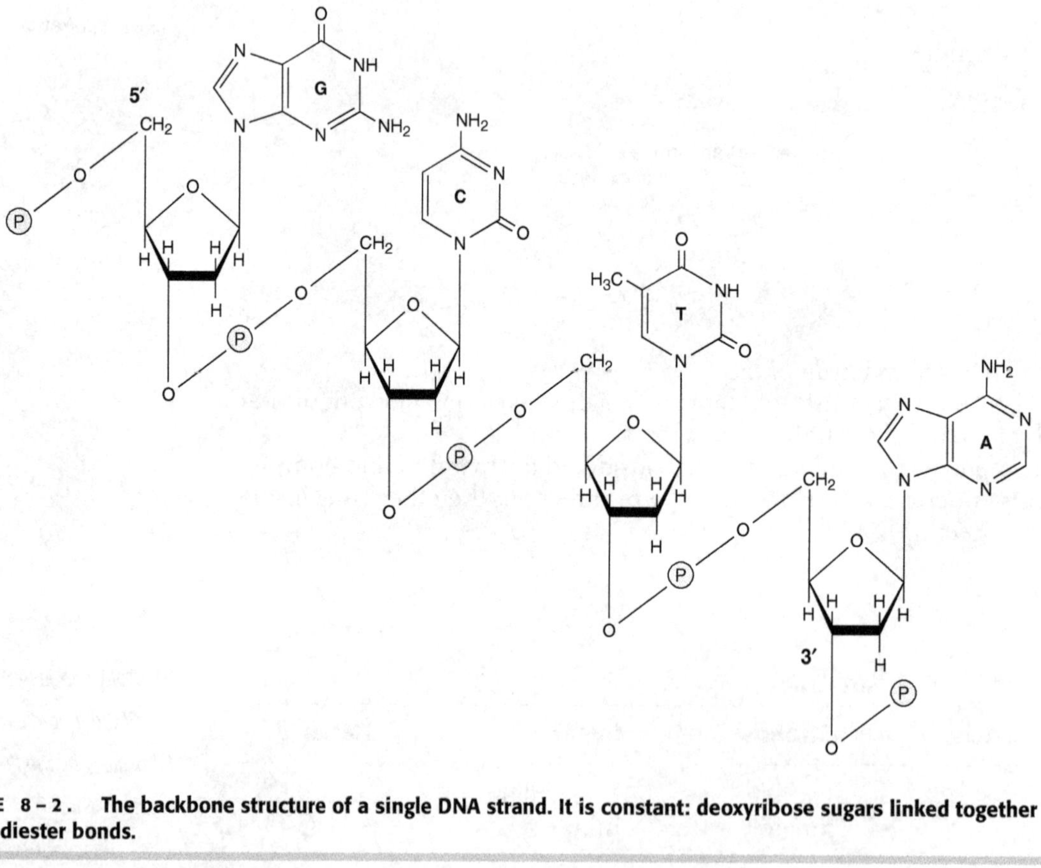

FIGURE 8-2. **The backbone structure of a single DNA strand. It is constant: deoxyribose sugars linked together via phosphodiester bonds.**

Reproduced, with permission, from Murray RK. *Harper's Illustrated Biochemistry*, 26th ed. New York: McGraw-Hill, 2003.

FIGURE 8–3. The backbone structure of a single RNA strand. It is constant: ribose sugars linked together via phosphodiester bonds.

Reproduced, with permission, from Murray RK. *Harper's Illustrated Biochemistry*, 26th ed. New York: McGraw-Hill, 2003.

▶ DNA ORGANIZATION

Nucleosomes

See Figures 8–4 and 8–5.

- Consists of DNA wrapped around a **histone** octomer.
- Held by *ionic bonds*.

*Histones are composed largely of **arginine** and **lysine**, which are positively charged due to their free amino group. They bond tightly to the negatively charged phosphate groups of DNA.*

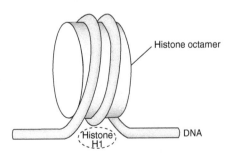

FIGURE 8–4. Nucleosome structure.

Reproduced, with permission, from Murray RK. *Harper's Illustrated Biochemistry*, 26th ed. New York: McGraw-Hill, 2003.

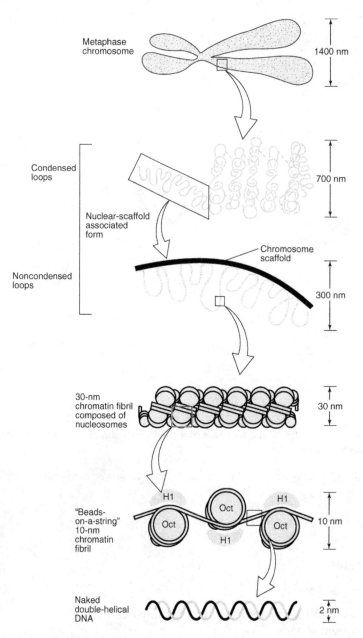

FIGURE 8–5. DNA organization.

Reproduced, with permission, from Murray RK. *Harper's Illustrated Biochemistry*, 26th ed.
New York: McGraw-Hill, 2003.

*Chromatin looks like beads
of nucleosomes on a string
of DNA.*

Chromatin

▪ Consists of nucleosomes, enzymes, gene regulatory proteins (transcription
factors), and small amounts of RNA.

▶ **DNA SYNTHESIS**

See Figure 8–6.

▪ **Helicase:** Unwinds the DNA molecule.
▪ **Topoisomerase:** Secures the replication fork, where the two DNA strands
are separated into leading and lagging strands.

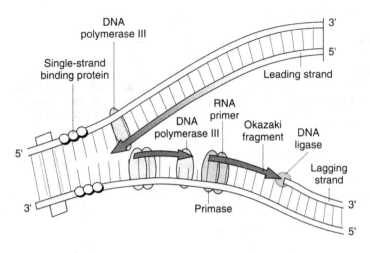

FIGURE 8–6. **DNA synthesis.**

Reproduced, with permission, from Bhushan V et al. *First Aid for the USMLE Step 1:* 2006.
New York: McGraw-Hill, 2006.

- **DNA polymerase:** Forms new complementary strands in the **5′ → 3′** direction.
  - **Leading strand:** Runs in the 3′ → 5′ direction. Synthesized continuously.
  - **Lagging strand:** Runs in the 5′ → 3′ direction. Synthesized in segments (**Okazaki fragments**).
- **DNA ligase:** Joins Okazaki fragments.
- **Exonuclease:** Removes the nuclueotide primer.
- **DNA gyrase:** Reforms the supercoiled structure once the replication fork has passed.

▶ **TRANSCRIPTION AND TRANSLATION**

See Figure 8–7.

RNA Synthesis (Transcription)

- DNA is used as a template to form RNA.
- Occurs in the *nucleus.*
- DNA is unwound and the replication fork is exposed.
- **RNA polymerase** binds to a promoter site on the DNA strand.
- Synthesis occurs in the **5′ → 3′** direction.
- Posttranscriptional modifications:
  - Addition of a **5′ cap** and a **3′ poly(A) tail.**
  - RNA splicing:
    - Removal of **introns** (noncoding segments).
    - Subsequent joining of **exons** (coding segments).

Protein Synthesis (Translation)

- An mRNA template is used to determine the specific amino acid sequence for polypeptide synthesis.
- Occurs in the *cytoplasm* (in ribosomes).
- A *small* ribosomal subunit binds to mRNA.

70s ribosomes (50s + 30s) are found in prokaryotic cells.

80s ribosomes (60s + 40s) are found in eukaryotic cells.

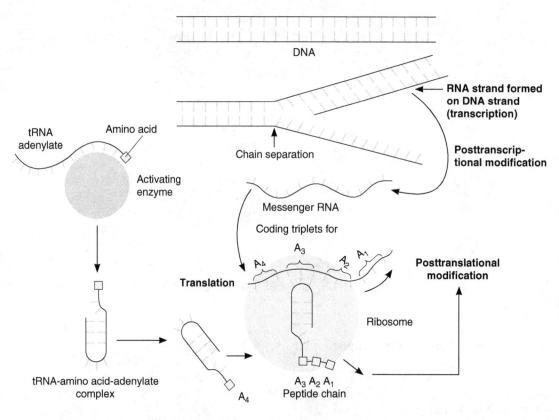

FIGURE 8-7. Transcription and translation.

Reproduced, with permission, from Ganong WF. *Review of Medical Physiology*, 21st ed. New York: McGraw-Hill, 2003.

- **Aminoacyl-tRNA synthetase:** Adds each amino acid to tRNA.
- The complementary *anticodon* of tRNA (carrying the first amino acid) binds to the mRNA start codon.
- A *large* ribosomal subunit attaches, forming a complete ribosome.
- Synthesis occurs in the $5' \rightarrow 3'$ direction until a stop codon is reached.

Important Codons

Codon	Amino Acid	Function
AUG	Methionine (Met)	Initiation
UAA, UAG, UGA	None (Nonsense)	Termination

▶ **MUTATIONS**

- Caused by mutagenic chemicals, radiation, UV light, and some viruses.
- Due to failure of DNA repair mechanisms.

Point Mutations

- Substitution of one base with another.
  - **Missense mutation:** Results in a codon that causes an altered amino acid sequence (eg, valine replaces glutamate causing sickle cell anemia).
  - **Nonsense mutation:** Results in a *stop codon* that causes polypeptide chain termination.
  - **Transverse mutation:** A purine is replaced with a pyrimidine, or vice versa (the purine–pyrimidine orientation is changed).
  - **Transition mutation:** A purine is replaced with another purine, or a pyrimidine is replaced with another pyrimidine (the purine–pyrimidine orientation is not changed).

Frameshift Mutations

- Deletion or insertion of one or two base pairs, changing the reading frame of the DNA template and the amino acid sequence.

Repeat Mutations

- Amplification of the sequence of three nucleotides.

▶ CLINICAL CONSIDERATIONS

Reverse Transcriptase

- Forms a complementary strand of DNA from the original RNA.
- HIV contains only a single-stranded RNA molecule and its own reverse transcriptase.

Recombinant DNA Technology

- **Restriction endonucleases:** Cleave DNA at various points to allow addition of various vectors, plasmids, cosmids, or bacteriophages.
- **DNA ligases:** Join DNA fragments.
- **DNA polymerase:** Adds nucleotides.
- **Exonucleases:** Remove nucleotides.

Polymerase Chain Reaction (PCR)

- Amplifies a target sequence of DNA.
- Extremely sensitive, selective, and fast.
- Used extensively in forensic medicine.
- Laboratory sequence:
  1. Denaturation of the DNA sample into two strands
  2. Anneal primers to each strand
  3. Copy each strand by a *heat-stable DNA polymerase*
  4. Repeat cycle resulting in exponential amplification of sample

Wobble effect: Degeneracy resides in the last nucleotide of the triplet. Thus, several codon-anticodon pairings may result in the same amino acid based solely upon the 3rd nucleotide.

UV light produces pyrimidine dimers in DNA, which interfere with replication and transcription. These lesions are typically removed by exonuclease.

AZT inhibits reverse transcriptase function.

The first organism used for DNA cloning was E. coli.

Blotting Techniques

▪ Identify specific DNA/RNA/protein fragments within a given tissue sample

Blot Technique	Identifies	Probe
Southern	DNA	cDNA
Northern	RNA	cDNA
Western	Protein	Antibody
Southwestern	Protein-DNA	cDNA

CHAPTER 9

Membranes

- Function as barriers, separating the contents of cells and organelles.
- **Asymmetric** sheetlike structures consisting of an outer and an inner surface.
  - Outer: More carbohydrates (glycoproteins, glycolipids) and glycosphingolipids.
  - Inner: More phospholipids.
- **Selectively permeable,** enabling only small, **nonpolar** molecules (O_2, CO_2, etc) and **water** to easily pass.
- Contain lipids, proteins, and carbohydrates in varying ratios.
- Lipids and integral proteins generally interact *noncovalently*, allowing molecules to move freely within the membrane.

Fluidity of plasma membrane:

- *Increases with higher temperature*
- *Decreases with lower temperature.*

Phospholipids constitute the majority of membrane lipids.

▶ FLUID MOSAIC MODEL

See Figure 9–1 for the fluid mosaic model of plasma membrane structure.

▶ MEMBRANE COMPONENTS

Lipids

- Form an **amphipathic lipid bilayer** suspended in water with *hydrophilic head groups* (on the outer and inner surfaces) and *hydrophobic tail groups* (on the inside of the bilayer).
- Types of plasma membrane lipids:
  - **Phospholipids**
    - Phosphoglycerides
      - Phosphatidylcholine (lecithin)
      - Phosphatidylethanolamine (cephalin)

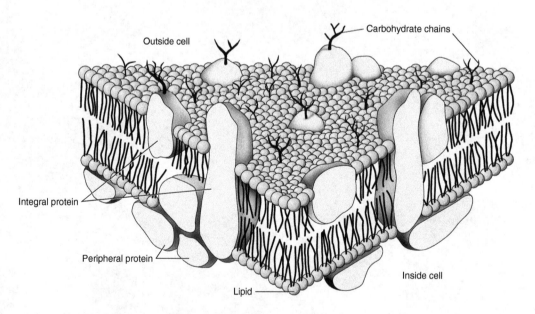

FIGURE 9–1.   The fluid mosaic model of plasma membrane structure.

Reproduced, with permission, from Murray RK. *Harper's Illustrated Biochemistry*, 26th ed. New York: McGraw-Hill, 2003.

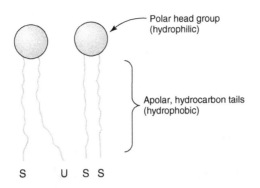

FIGURE 9-2. Membrane phospholipids. S: Saturated; U: Unsaturated.

Reproduced, with permission, from Murray RK. *Harper's Illustrated Biochemistry*, 26th ed. New York: McGraw-Hill, 2003.

Formation of lipid bilayer arises via two opposing forces:

- *Attractive: between hydrocarbon chains (via van der Waals forces).*
- *Repulsive: between polar head groups.*

- Phosphatidylglycerol (cardiolipin)
- Phosphatidylserine
- Phosphatidyinositol
- Sphingomyelin
- **Glycosphingolipids**
  - Galactoceramide
  - Glucosylceramide
  - Gangliosides
- **Cholesterol** and other steroids
- See Figure 9–2 for membrane phospholipids.

Proteins

- Function as receptors, transport channels, enzymes, antigens, and other structural components.
- Two types of plasma membrane protein:
  - **Integral:** Amphipathic proteins that are embedded within either one or both (traverse the entire membrane) portions of the lipid bilayer.
  - **Peripheral:** Proteins that weakly bind to hydrophilic head groups on the inner or outer membrane surfaces.

Carbohydrates

- Attach to proteins and lipids *only* on the *external surface* of cell membranes.

▶ MOVEMENT THROUGH MEMBRANES

Membrane Transport

See Figure 9–3 for the types of movement of substances through membranes.

Transport Proteins

- **Uniport:** Transport of a single molecule in both directions.
- **Coupled:** Transport of one molecule depends on the presence of another (different) molecule.
  - **Symport:** Transports molecules in the *same* direction.
  - **Antiport:** Transports molecules in *opposite* directions.

*Both active transport and facilitative diffusion are characterized by **competitive inhibition**.*

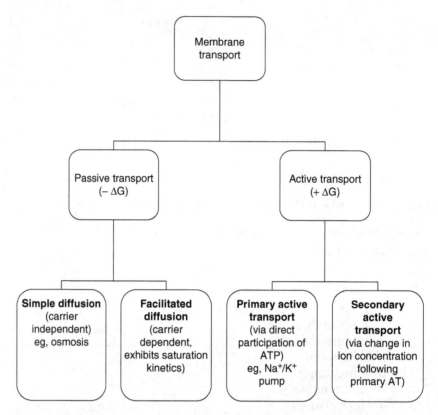

FIGURE 9–3. **Outline of the types of movement of substances through membranes.**

Glucose Transporters

- Facilitative *bidirectional* transporters of glucose.
    - GLUT-1: Erythrocytes, brain
    - GLUT-2: Liver, pancreas
    - GLUT-3: Neurons
    - GLUT-4: Muscle, adipose tissue
    - GLUT-5: Intestines, testes

CHAPTER 10

Neurophysiology

▶ CENTRAL NERVOUS SYSTEM

CNS = brain + spinal cord

▶ PERIPHERAL NERVOUS SYSTEM

- All nerves outside the brain and spinal cord:
  - Cranial nerves.
  - Spinal nerves.
  - Nerve plexuses.
  - Associated spinal and autonomic ganglia.

▶ AUTONOMIC NERVOUS SYSTEM

- ANS = nervous system involved in controlling involuntary functions.
  - Sympathetic.
  - Parasympathetic.

Brain

See embryology of the nervous system, Chapter 4—forebrain, midbrain, hindbrain.

CEREBRAL CORTEX

TWO CEREBRAL HEMISPHERES

- Right and left.
- Connected by corpus callosum.
  - Thick white matter tract; nerve fibers.

FOUR LOBES PER HEMISPHERE

- Frontal lobes.
  - Control skilled motor behavior (precentral gyrus).
- Parietal lobes.
  - Interpret somatosensory input (postcentral gyrus).
- Occipital lobes.
  - Interpret visual input.
- Temporal lobes.
  - Interpret auditory input.

Beyond the primary function of each lobe, much of the cerebral cortex works together for associative and higher order functions (including ideation, language, and thought).

Diencephalon

Thalamus + hypothalamus

THALAMUS

- Ovoid mass of gray matter.
- Ascending input (all sensory stimuli **except** olfactory) is relayed through the thalamus to the cerebral cortex.
- Descending output (from cortex) can also pass through/synapse within thalamus.

Hypothalamus

- Collection of nerve cells (nuclei).
- Lies subcortical (at base of cerebrum).
- Controls homeostatic processes.
  - Often associated with autonomic nervous system.
- Regulates:
  - Body temperature
  - Appetite
  - Water balance (thirst)
  - Sexual activity
  - Sleep
  - Emotions
  - Pituitary secretions: Releasing hormones to the pituitary gland (endocrine system)
  - Autonomic functions: GI and cardiac activity, etc

Heat Regulation

- Controlled by the posterior hypothalamus.
  - Both heat generation and heat loss.
- Goal is to keep human body temperature constant.
  - Heat gained = heat loss.

SHIVERING

- Potent mechanism for heat production.
- When body core temperature drops the shivering reflex is triggered,
  - Causes fibrillation of muscle for heat production.

HEAT LOSS

- When environmental temperature < body temperature,
  - Want to produce more heat.
- When exercise or warm environment,
  - Want to give off excess heat:
    - Vasodilation of skin vessels.
    - ↑ sympathetic outflow to sweat glands.

Heat Transfer

Heat Transfer	Conduction	Convection	Evaporation

Emission of heat in the form of infrared rays.
 	
Body is continually exchanging heat by radiation with objects in the environment.[b]
	Flow of heat energy from warmer to cooler environment (down gradient).
	
	Usually, transfer of thermal energy with direct contact between two objects.
		Movement of heat by currents in the medium, eg, wind.
		
		Air molecules exchange heat with body surface and continue to breeze past (replaced by other molecules).
			Conversion of a liquid into vapor. Heat is lost when water evaporates from body surfaces.[a]
			
			Two-way evaporation occurs on body surfaces:
			▪ Insensible water loss
			  ▪ Respiratory
			  ▪ Skin
			▪ Sweating
			▪ Active fluid secretion by sweat glands

[a]For sweat to produce cooling effects, it must evaporate. It is a more effective means of cooling in low humidity environments than high humidity environments because of the gradient.

[b]The body surface temperature is higher than the surface temperature of most objects in the environment.

Limbic System

▪ Primitive brain area.
▪ Located deep in the temporal lobe.
▪ Communicates with the cerebral cortex.
▪ Initiates basic drives:
  ▪ Hunger
  ▪ Aggression
  ▪ Emotional feelings
  ▪ Sexual arousal
▪ Consists of:
  ▪ **Hippocampus**
    ▪ Functions in learning and memory.
  ▪ **Amygdala**
    ▪ Center of emotions.
    ▪ Communicates with autonomic system (fight or flight).
    ▪ Oxytocin and ADH receptors.

▶ MOTOR CONTROL AND COORDINATION

Basal Ganglia

▪ Located deep to cerebral cortex.
▪ Controls complex patterns of voluntary motor behavior (inhibitory).
▪ Includes:
  ▪ Caudate nucleus.
  ▪ Putamen.
  ▪ Globus pallidus.
  ▪ Substantia nigra.
  ▪ Subthalamic nucleus.

Motor pathway:

Motor cortex (precentral gyrus)

↓

Upper motor neuron

↓

Internal capsule

↓

Corticospinal tract

↓

*(Cerebral peduncles –
midbrain)*

↓

*(Pyramids – medulla – fibers
cross)*

↓

Ventral horn (spinal cord)

↓

Lower motor neuron

↓

Muscle

Cerebellum

- Lies posteroinferior to cerebrum, superoposterior to brain stem.
- Morphologically divided:
    - Two lateral hemispheres.
    - Middle portion (Vermis).
- Functions (excitatory):
    - Maintains muscle tone.
    - Coordinates muscle movement.
    - Controls balance.

Note: The basal ganglia and cerebellum modify movement on a minute-to-minute basis. The output of the cerebellum is excitatory, whereas that of the basal ganglia is inhibitory.

These two systems work together to achieve smooth, coordinated movement. Movement disorders result from aberration to each of these systems, eg, Parkinson's (loss of DA neurons in basal ganglia), Huntington's (loss of neurons in basal ganglia, triple repeat disease), dysmetria, ataxia (see pathology).

▶ BRAIN STEM

Lies immediately inferior to cerebrum, just anterior to cerebellum.

Midbrain (Mesencephalon)

- Connects dorsally with the cerebellum.
- Large voluntary motor nerve tracts pass through.
- Location of:
    - CN III, IV nuclei (connect with VI via MLF).
    - Substantia nigra. (See also "Parkinson's Disease" in Neuropathology)

Pons

- Between the midbrain and medulla.
- Connects to the cerebellum posteriorly.
- Location of:
    - CN V, VI, VII, VIII nuclei.

Medulla Oblongata

- Most inferior segment of vertebrate brain.
- Continues with the spinal cord below.
- Joins the spinal cord at foramen magnum.
- Contains:
    - Important regulatory centers:
        - Area postrema—vomiting.
        - Swallowing.
        - Cardiac.
        - Vasomotor.
        - Respiratory.
    - CN IX, X, XI, XII nuclei.

PNS is composed of:

- **Afferent neurons:** From sensory receptors to CNS.
- **Efferent neurons:** From CNS to muscles, organs, and glands (and their associated ganglia and plexuses).

Subdivisions of the Peripheral Nervous System

Somatic Nervous System	Autonomic Nervous System

12 pairs of cranial nerves.
31 pairs of spinal nerves.
Both sensory and motor neurons.
Innervates skeletal muscle (voluntary).
Motor:
No synapse in peripheral ganglion.
  ▪ Uses 1 efferent neuron from the CNS to end-organ (LMN).
Sensory:
Synapse within dorsal root ganglion (peripheral) prior to CNS.
Modalities:
  ▪ Touch.
  ▪ Movement (position sense).
  ▪ Temperature.
  ▪ Pain.
	2 subdivisions:
	  ▪ Sympathetic.
	  ▪ Parasympathetic.
	Action is largely involuntary.
	Controls:
	Glands (exocrine and endocrine).
	Cardiac muscle.
	Smooth muscle.
	Visceral organs.
	Not skeletal muscle.
	Motor:
	Synapses within autonomic ganglion.
	  ▪ Uses 2 efferent neurons from CNS to effector.

Refer to the illustrations in the "Neuroanatomy" section.

BASIC ANATOMIC PATHWAY

Preganglionic neuron (within CNS).

↓

Ganglion (cell bodies of postganglionic neurons; outside of the CNS).

↓

Postganglionic neuron (outside of the CNS).

↓

Effector organ.

Autonomic Ganglia

- Collections of cell bodies of the postganglionic neurons (unmyelinated).
- **Sympathetic:** Sympathetic chain ganglia (near spinal cord) (paravertebral):
  - Short preganglionic neuron.
  - Long postganglionic neuron.
- **Parasympathetic:** Ganglia at, within organ (eg, celiac ganglion):
  - Long preganglionic neuron.
  - Short postganglionic neuron.

Remember: Both parasympathetic and sympathetic preganglionic neurons are cholinergic (release Ach). However, parasympathetic postganglionic neurons are cholinergic (muscarinic receptors); sympathetic postganglionic neurons are largely adrenergic (release norepinephrine, which binds to sympathetic receptors). The exception is in sweat glands and blood vessels in skeletal muscle. Here the postganglionic sympathetic neurons are cholinergic (release Ach at muscarinic receptors).

Remember: Prevertebral ganglia have longer preganglionics.

BIOCHEMISTRY-PHYSIOLOGY

NEUROPHYSIOLOGY

Parasympathetic Nervous System

- Craniosacral: Composed of:
  - CN nuclei (ie, III-ciliary, VII- submandibular and pterygopalatine, IX-otic).
  - S2–S4 (pelvic splanchnic).
- Major nerve is the vagus nerve (CN X): Originates in medulla.
- **Preganglionic neuron (myelinated)**
  - Cholinergic (releases Ach).
  - Binds nicotinic cholinergic receptors on postganglionic neurons (ganglia within effector).
- **Postganglionic neuron (unmyelinated)**
  - Cholinergic (releases Ach).
  - Binds muscarinic cholinergic receptors in the tissue.

Postganglionic Receptors

	Nicotinic		Muscarinic
	N1 (N_N) stimulated by: nicotine blocked by: hexamethonium	N2 (N_M) stimulated by: muscurin blocked by: atropine	M
Principal location	Autonomic ganglia <ul><li>Both symp and parasymp preganglionics release Ach on N_N</li></ul>	Motor endplate (NMJ)	Effector organs (including sweat glands under sympathetic control)
Effect(s)	Excitatory <ul><li>Nerve transmission</li><li>Postganglionics are activated</li></ul>	Excitatory <ul><li>Muscle contraction</li></ul>	Excitatory or inhibitory blood vessels in skeletal muscle

Sympathetic Tone Only:
adrenal medulla
sweat glands
pilorector muscles
blood vessels

NOTES

- All preganglionic autonomic neurons (both sympathetic and parasympathetic) and all postganglionic parasympathetic neurons are cholinergic (use Ach as NT).
- Cholinergic effects of preganglionic autonomic systems (at ganglia of sympathetic and parasympathetic systems) are excitatory.
- Cholinergic effects of postganglionic parasympathetic fibers are either excitatory or inhibitory, depending on the end-organ (eg, parasympathetic fibers innervating heart ↓ HR).

Paravertebral ganglia→
sympathetic chain versus
Prevertebral ganglia →
celiac, SMA, IMA, inferior
hypogastric

Sympathetic Nervous System

- Thoracolumbar.
  - Composed of spinal segments T1–L3.
- Exerts widespread effect because of high ratio of postganglionic to preganglionic fibers.
  - Each sympathetic preganglionic neuron branches extensively and synapses with numerous postganglionic neurons.

- **Preganglionic neuron (myelinated)**
    - Cholinergic (releases Ach).
    - Binds nicotinic cholinergic receptors on postganglionic neurons (ganglia within effector).
    - Each preganglionic parasympathetic neuron synapses with many postganglionic parasympathetic neurons.
- **Postganglionic neuron (unmyelinated)**
    - Adrenergic (releases NE).
    - Binds adrenergic receptors in the tissue **except** sweat glands and skeletal muscle blood vessels.

ADRENERGIC RECEPTORS

- Membrane receptor proteins.
- G-protein-coupled receptors.
- Located on autonomic effector organs.
- Bound by catecholamine ligands (epinephrine, norepinephrine).
- Norepinephrine (NE) stimulates mainly alpha receptors.
- Epinephrine stimulates both alpha and beta equally.

Three cervical sympathetic ganglia supply the head and neck (superior, middle, and inferior). These are paravertebral ganglia. Other ganglia of the SNS include the celiac ganglion, superior mesenteric ganglion, and inferior mesenteric ganglion.

Alpha- and Beta-Adrenergic Receptors

	Alpha-1 (α-1)	Alpha-2 (α-2)	Beta-1 (β-1)	Beta-2 (β-2)
Principal location	Vascular smooth muscle: Skin Mucosa GI	Presynaptic nerve terminals—decrease synaptic transmission Platelets—platelet aggregation Fat cells—inhibit lipolysis GI tract wall	Heart	Skeletal muscle Bronchial smooth muscle
Effect(s)	Vasoconstriction	Inhibition (relaxation or dilation)	↑ Heart rate ↑ Contractility	Vasodilation Bronchodilation

Monoamine oxidase (MAO) is an enzyme that catalyzes oxidative deamination of monoamines (including NE, serotonin, and epinephrine). The deamination process ↑ breakdown (metabolism) of excess NTs that accumulate at postsynaptic terminals.

Gray ramus communicans—carry unmyelinated post-ganglionic sympathetic nerves to peripheral organs.

Summary of Autonomic Effects

	Sympathetic	Parasympathetic
	Adrenergic	Cholinergic
Pupils	Mydriasis (dilate)	Miosis (constrict)
Salivation	Thick (mucous)	Watery (ready to eat)
Bronchi	Bronchodilation	Bronchoconstriction
Heart rate	↑	↓
Adrenal medulla	Causes epi and NE release	No effect

White ramus communicans—all sympathetic preganglionic neurons enter the paravertebral chain via white ramus.

- See also the "Neuroanatomy" section.
- Spinal cord is part of the CNS.
- White matter tracts:
  - Composed of myelinated nerve fibers bundles.
  - Surround gray matter horns.
- Form ascending and descending tracts.
- Axons of a tract have the same origin, termination, and function.
- Tracts are often named for origin and termination (eg, spinothalamic tract).
- Tracts are sensory or motor (see the following chart).

Sensory (Ascending)	Motor (Descending)
Spinothalamic	Corticospinal (pyramidal)
▫ Pain	Extrapyramidal
▫ Temperature	
Dorsal column, medial lemniscus	
▫ Touch	
▫ Pressure	
▫ Vibration	
▫ Proprioception (position)	

Tracts can be:

- **Ipsilateral:** Axons run on same side as cell bodies.
- **Contralateral:** Axons run on opposite side (have crossed over).

Spinal cord anatomy:
- Dorsal horn
  - Sensory.
  - Receives fibers from the dorsal root ganglia.
- Ventral (anterior) root
  - Motor.

SENSORY PATHWAY

Receptor
↓
Peripheral nerve (sensory fibers)
↓
Dorsal root ganglion (synapse) (primary neuron)
↓
Spinal cord
↓
Spinal tracts (spinothalamic or dorsal column, medial lemniscus)
↓
Brain stem nuclei (gracile/ cuneate nucleus in medulla; secondary neuron)
↓
Thalamus (tertiary neuron; VPL)
↓
Decussates after synapse
↓
Cortex (postcentral gyrus of parietal lobe)

BIOCHEMISTRY-PHYSIOLOGY

NEUROPHYSIOLOGY

RECEPTORS

- Receive information from internal or external environment.
- Send nerve impulses to CNS.
- Two broad types: According to location of stimuli.
- **Exteroreceptors:** Receive external stimuli (from body surface):
  - Touch.
  - Pressure.
  - Pain.
  - Temperature.
  - Light.
  - Sound.
- **Interoreceptors** (visceroreceptors): Receive input from internal environment of body:
  - Pressure.
  - Pain.
  - Chemical changes.

PROPRIORECEPTORS

- Type of interoceptor.
- Relays information concerning position of body parts (in space).
- Separate from visual input.
  - *Kinesthetic sense*
- Located in muscles, tendons, joints.
- Communicate with the vestibular apparatus.

> *There are many types of joint receptors:*
> - Nonencapsulated
>   - Free nerve endings: Pain.
> - Encapsulated
>   - Pacinian: Vibration, pressure.
>   - Ruffini: Stretch.
> - Neuromuscular spindles
>   - Stretch.
> - Neurotendons
>   - Tension.

Nonencapsulated versus Encapsulated Receptors

Nonencapsulated Receptors	Encapsulated Receptors (corpuscles)
Free nerve endings Pain primarily, touch, pressure, tickle, hot/cold. Terminal ends have no myelin. In epithelial cells, skin, cornea, alimentary tract, connective tissue, haversian system of bone, dental pulp.	**Meissner's corpuscles—rapidly adapting** Mechanoreceptors, allow 2-point discrimination. In dermal papilla of skin. Ovoid stack of Schwann cells.
Merkel's disc—slow adapting Tactile (touch, pressure) (fine detailed surface patterns). In hairless skin—fingertips, pressure. Found in basal layer.	**Pacinian corpuscles (rapidly adapting)** Vibration, pressure. In dermis, subcutaneous tissue, ligaments, joints. Concentric lamellae of flattened cells.
Hair follicle receptors Mechanoreception—bending hair stimulates, touch. Fiber winds around hair.	**Ruffini's corpuscles (slow adapting)** Stretch, continuous pressure states In dermis of hairy skin. Large unmyelinated nerve fibers ending within bundles of collagen fibers.

Receptors Classified by Stimulus Type

	Mechanoreceptor	Thermoreceptor	Nociceptor	Chemoreceptor	Photoreceptor
Stimulus	Pressure or stretch	Temperature	Pain	Chemicals (inhaled, ingested, or in blood)	Light
Examples	Pacinian corpuscles Muscle spindles (Golgi tendon organs) Meissner's corpuscles Hair cells	Free nerve endings	Free nerve endings	Taste receptors Smell receptors Osmoreceptors Carotid body O_2 receptors	Retina ▪ Rods ▪ Cones

Hair cells transduce senses of hearing and balance.

Osmoreceptors and carotid body O_2 receptors monitor pH and gas levels.

▶ SOMATOSENSORY PATHWAYS

Sensory Tracts (Ascending)

See Figure 10–1 for somatosensory pathways.

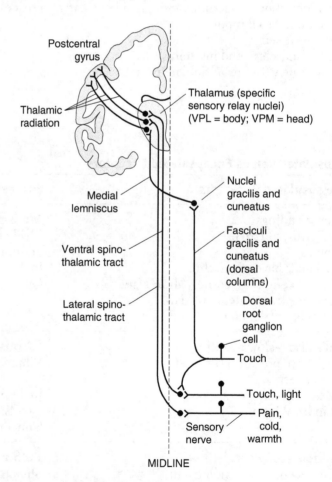

FIGURE 10–1. Somatosensory pathways.

Reproduced, with permission, from Ganong WF. *Review of Medical Physiology*, 22nd ed. New York: McGraw-Hill, 2005.

SPINOTHALAMIC TRACT (ANTEROLATERAL SYSTEM)

- **Lateral spinothalamic tract:** Transmits pain and temperature.
- **Anterior spinothalamic tract:** Transmits light touch.

PATHWAY

Sensory nerve
↓
Dorsal horn of spinal cord gray matter (travel in Lissauers tract and then synapse on secondary neurons)
↓
Cross to opposite side of cord via anterior white commisure (decussate at level enters cord) via Lissaure's tract; secondary neuron
↓
Ascend contralateral spinal cord (through anterior and lateral white matter columns/tracts)
↓
Thalamus (tertiary neuron, in VPL)
↓
Somatosensory cortex (parietal lobe)

DORSAL COLUMN, MEDIAL LEMNISCUS SYSTEM

- Conveys touch, pressure, and vibration.

PATHWAY

Sensory nerve
↓
Dorsal horn of spinal cord gray matter
↓
Ascend ipsilateral spinal cord
↓
Posterior columns: Fasciculus gracilis (fibers from lower extremities) and Fasciculus cuneatis (fibers from upper extremities)
↓
Synapse in medulla (nucleus gracilis and cuneatis)
↓
Internal arcuate fibers decussate and ascend contralateral brain stem in medial lemniscus
↓
Thalamus
↓
Somatosensory cortex

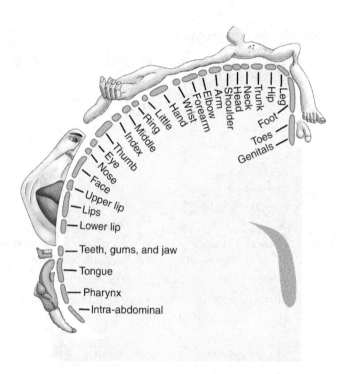

FIGURE 10-2. **Somatosensory cortex.**

Reproduced, with permission, from Ganong WF. *Review of Medical Physiology*, 22nd ed.
New York: McGraw-Hill, 2005.

SOMATOSENSORY CORTEX (POSTCENTRAL GYRUS)

See Figures 10–2 and 10–3 for somatosensory cortex.

- Representation is homunculus (representation of body proportional to sense).

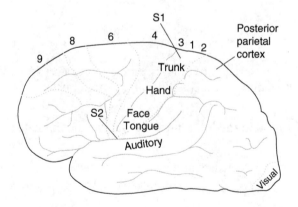

FIGURE 10-3. **Somatosensory cortex.**

Reproduced, with permission, from Ganong WF. *Review of Medical Physiology,* 22nd ed.
New York: McGraw-Hill, 2005.

Descending Motor Tracts (Efferent or Descending Pathways)

▪ The upper motor neuron tracts sending signals from the brain muscles.

MOTOR PATHWAY

Motor area of brain (precentral gyrus of frontal lobe)
↓
Upper motor neurons (= descending motor tracts, eg, corticospinal tract)
↓
Lower motor neurons
↓
Skeletal muscle

Upper Motor Neurons

▪ Originate in white matter of brain.
▪ Form two major systems:
  ▪ Corticospinal tract (pyramidal system).
  ▪ Extrapyramidal system.

Corticospinal Tract (Pyramidal System)

See Figure 10–4 for corticospinal tract (pyramidal system).

▪ Two components:
  ▪ **Lateral** (70–90%).
  ▪ **Anterior/ventral** (10–30%).
▪ Travel via primary motor cortex through internal capsule to medulla.
  ▪ **Decussate in medulla (pyramids).**
  ▪ Continue down opposite side of spinal cord →
    anterior horn → lower motor neurons → muscles.
  ▪ Right brain controls left somatic muscles.
▪ Control fine, skilled movements of skeletal muscle.

Extrapyramidal System

▪ Collection of smaller tracts:
  ▪ **Rubrospinal** (red nucleus in midbrain—voluntary movements).
  ▪ Important for somatic muscle control, posture
  ▪ **Reticulospinal**—important for somatic motor control and autonomic function control (reticular nuclei, pons, and medulla) (reticular formation (diffuse brain stem nuclei); coordinate locomotion, mediate autonomic).
  ▪ **Olivospinal** (inferior olive—motor learning).
  ▪ **Vestibulospinal** (vestibular nuclei—control limb extensors, head and neck (gaze)) mediates vestibular end organ and cerebellum upon extensive muscle tone and balance.
  ▪ **Tectospinal** (superior colliculus—coordinate neck, head, and eye movements).
▪ Travel from premotor area of frontal lobe (and other areas) to pons.
  ▪ **Decussate in pons.**
  ▪ Continue down opposite side of spinal cord →
    anterior horn → lower motor neurons → muscles.
  ▪ Right brain controls left lower motor neuron.
▪ Controls gross motor movement, posture, and balance.

This tract is called pyramidal system because fibers of the corticospinal tract form the pyramids in the medulla.

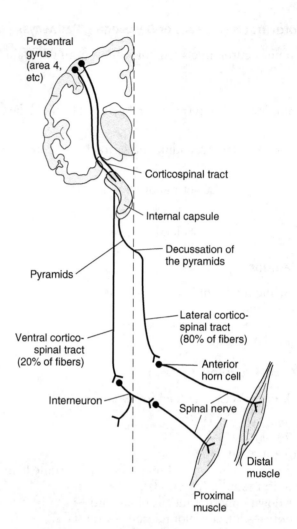

FIGURE 10-4. **Corticospinal tract (pyramidal system).**

Reproduced, with permission, from Ganong WF. *Review of Medical Physiology,* 22nd ed. New York: McGraw-Hill, 2005.

Lesion on one side causes:

- Ipsilateral motor loss (corticospinal).
- Ipsilateral touch/sensory loss.
- Contralateral pain and temperature loss (spinothalamic).
- Example: If you hemitransect the right side of the spinal cord, you lose right-sided (ipsilateral) motor control (corticospinal) and left-sided (contralateral) pain and temperature sense (spinothalamic).

Resting Membrane Potential (All Cells!)

- Charge differential or voltage set up across the resting nerve membrane.
  - Due to separation of charged particles (ions and proteins) between extracellular and intracellular fluids.

- *Polarized membrane*
  - More positive ions (cations) outside (extracellular).
  - More negative ions (anions) inside (intracellular).
- Charge separation occurs because:
  - **K⁺ leak** (resting K⁺ conductance)
    - + charges leave cell down electrochemical gradient.
    - *Most important determinant of RMP.*
  - **Na⁺/K⁺ pump**
    - Using ATP, establishes the Na⁺ and K⁺ gradient; creates gradient to allow K⁺ leak to occur.
    - Pump is electrogenic: 2 K⁺ in for every 3 Na⁺ pumped out = net loss of + charges from the cell.
- RMP: ranges between –40 and –85 mV.
  - RMP in humans (most cells) is ~ –70 mV (close to K), skeletal muscle –90 mV, cardiac muscle –90 mV
    - Threshold for depolarization: ~ –50 mV

Visceral smooth muscle and cardiac pacemaker cells lack a stable RMP.

Action Potential

- Initiated by depolarizing stimulus (depolarization).
- RMP becomes more positive (less negative).
  - Ion channels open.
  - Positive ions move from outside to in.
  - As positive ions go intracellularly, RMP becomes positive.
- Na⁺ (sodium)
  - Na⁺ entry initially causes more Na⁺ channels to open.
  - Membrane potential approaches that of sodium equilibrium potential.
  - Once threshold reached, the action potential (AP) will fire.
  - Threshold = 20 mV+.
- All or none phenomenon.
  - If don't reach threshold, don't get AP.
  - AP is same with supra threshold and threshold stimuli.

$E_{Na} = 67$ mV
$E_K = -90$ mV
$E_{Cl} = -80$ mV
$E_{Ca} = 123$ mV

REFRACTORY PERIOD

- Period of time after an AP that the membrane cannot again be stimulated, ie, another AP cannot be initiated.

ABSOLUTE REFRACTORY PERIOD

- No stimulus, no matter how large, will stimulate an AP (corresponds to close of voltage-sensitive Na⁺ channel).

RELATIVE REFRACTORY PERIOD

- A larger than usual stimulus will stimulate an AP, ie, the threshold is increased (due to increased permeability to K⁺ channel).

Repolarization (Figure 10–5)

- Membrane potential returns to normal following an AP.
- ↓ **Na⁺ permeability** (rapid).
- Block Na⁺ entry.
- ↑ **K⁺ permeability** (in to out)(slower).
- K⁺ leaks out of the cell.

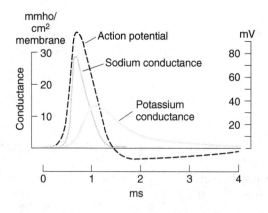

FIGURE 10-5. Repolarization.

Reproduced, with permission, from Ganong WF. *Review of Medical Physiology,* 22nd ed.
New York: McGraw-Hill, 2005:59. As modified from Hodgkin AL. Ionic movements and
electrical activity in giant nerve fibers. *Pro R Soc Lond Ser* B 1958;143:1.

Hyperpolarization

- During repolarization there is an overshoot in the more negative direction.
- Membrane potential briefly becomes more negative than RMP before returning to RMP.
- This is because of ↑ **K⁺ conductance.**
  - K⁺ channels stay open.
  - K⁺ efflux is greater than in resting.

Note: Hyperpolarization is responsible for the relative refractory period (cell remains hypoexcitable). Influx of Cl⁻ will also hyperpolarize and make AP more difficult to generate.

Remember:
Excitable cells

- Neurons
- Muscle cells
- Cardiac pacemaker

► LOCAL ANESTHETICS

- Block sodium channels (↓ Na⁺ permeability).
  - Bind to inactivation gates of fast, voltage-gated Na⁺ channels,
    - keeping them closed and
    - prolonging absolute refractory period.
- ↓ Membrane excitability → cannot generate AP → no nerve impulse conduction.
- Reversible.
- K, Cl, Ca conductances are *unchanged.*

Local Anesthetics

- Affect small myelinated fibers first (size rule).

  Unmyelinated C-fibers (slow, dull, long lasting) (smallest)

  ↓

  Small myelinated nerve fibers (pain, temp)

  ↓

  Larger A-fibers (touch proprioception, Golgi tendon)

Excitatory

- Depolarize (more positive) the postsynaptic membrane potential.
  - Brings it closer to threshold.
  - ↑ probability of AP in postsynaptic neuron.
- Creates an excitatory postsynaptic potential (EPSP).
- Glutamate is the major excitatory neurotransmitter.

EPSPs can combine, using summation (2 forms) to reach threshold and initiate an AP.

Inhibitory

- Hyperpolarize (more negative) the postsynaptic membrane potential.
  - Moves it away from threshold.
  - ↓ probability of AP in postsynaptic neuron.
- Creates an inhibitory postsynaptic potential (IPSP).
- Result of ↑ membrane permeability to either Cl^- or K^+.
- Examples of inhibitory NTs:
  - Glycine.
  - GABA.
    - Both bind receptors and open Cl^- channels (↑ Cl^- permeability).

The inhibitory or excitatory effects of NTs depend on their binding characteristics to receptors.

Spatial Summation

- Two excitatory inputs arrive at a postsynaptic neuron simultaneously.
  - Converging circuit.
  - Arrival of impulses from *multiple* presynaptic fibers at same time.

Temporal Summation

- Two excitatory inputs arrive at a postsynaptic neuron in rapid succession.
  - ↑ frequency of nerve impulses from a *single* presynaptic fiber.

- Nerve impulse = action potential spreads along plasma membrane.

Saltatory Conduction

- Occurs in myelinated fibers (remember: Schwann cells (periphery) and oligodendrocytes (CNS)).
- ↑ velocity of nerve transmission along myelinated fibers.
- Conserves energy because:
  - Only the Ranvier node depolarizes.
    - Less energy for Na^+/K^+ ATPase to reestablish resting ion gradients.
    - Na^+/K^+ pumps reestablish concentration gradient only at Ranvier nodes.
  - Allow repolarization to occur with less transfer of ions.
- Electrochemical basis behind saltatory conduction is ↓ **membrane capacitance** (increase distance between charges; less charges necessary).

Neurotransmitter Review:

MAO—catalyze oxidative deamination of NE, serotonin, epi
ACh—voluntary movement, skeletal muscles/movement of viscera
NE—wakefulness, arousal
DA—voluntary movement and motivation, pleasure, addiction, love
Serotonin—memory, emotion, sleep/wake, temperature
Glycine—spinal reflexes and motor behavior
Histamine—sleep/wake, inflammation

BIOCHEMISTRY-PHYSIOLOGY

NEUROPHYSIOLOGY

MYELIN

- Prevents movement of Na^+ and K^+ through the membrane.
  - Na^+, K^+ conductance only at Ranvier nodes.
- ↓ membrane capacitance.
- ↑ membrane resistance.

Saltatory conduction is a faster way to conduct an impulse down the axon (up to 100 m/sec).

NODES OF RANVIER

- Exposed nerve membrane where depolarization occurs.
  - Continue fueling spread of AP during nerve transmission.
- Located every 0.2–2 mm along the myelin sheath.
- APs could not be produced if the myelin sheath were continuous.
- APs travel down axon and "jump" from node to node.

CONTINUOUS CONDUCTION

- Occurs in unmyelinated fibers.
- Nerve transmission (AP) travels along entire membrane surface.
- Relatively slow conduction (1.0 m/sec).

Conduction velocity depends on:
- *Diameter of nerve fiber.*
  - *↑ diameter → ↑ resistance to flow → ↑ velocity.*
- *Presence of myelin sheath.*

Problems with Nerve Conduction

WALLERIAN DEGENERATION

- Axon is cut.
- The axon remnant distal to the cut (away from the cell body) degenerates because axonal transport is interrupted.
- Regeneration of axons possible if endoneurial sheath is intact (neurolemma).
  - Occurs at a rate of 2–4 mm/day.
  - If cell body is irreversibly injured, the entire neuron degenerates.

Neurilemma: Thin membrane spirally wrapping the myelin layers of fibers, especially peripheral nerves and axons of unmyelinated nerve fibers. All axons of the PNS have it.

NEUROPRAXIA

- Transient block (bruise).
- Incomplete paralysis or loss of sensation.
- Rapid recovery.

Fibers of CNS (brain and spinal column) are not enclosed by neurilemma–regenerated severed axons are rare.

AXONOTMESIS

- Axon damaged, but connective sheath remains intact.
- Wallerian degeneration occurs distally but then regeneration can occur.

NEUROTMESIS

- Complete transaction of nerve trunk.
- Results in:
- Motor
  - Flaccid paralysis.
  - Atrophy of end-organ.

In CNS, neurons are myelinated by oligodendrocytes and lack a neurilemma.

- Sensory
  - Total loss of cutaneous sensation.

▶ SYNAPSE

Functional connection, anatomical junction between

- Nerve axon (presynaptic axon) and
- Target cell
  - Nerve (postsynaptic neuron)
  - Muscle (NMJ)
  - Gland

Synapse controls direction of nerve impulse

PRESYNAPTIC NEURONS

- Transmit information toward a synapse.

SYNAPTIC CLEFT

- Space between presynaptic terminal and postsynaptic cell.

POSTSYNAPTIC NEURONS

- Transmit away from a synapse (dendrite → axon).

NERVE IMPULSES

- Travel in only one direction because synapses are polarized.

Neuronal Excitability

- Nerves are excited (APs generated) electrically or chemically.
  - Ligand-gated (NT binding) (most common).
  - Voltage-gated channels.
  - Mechanically gated (stretching).

Types of Synapse

- Chemical synapse (most common).
  - Ligand-gated: Use NTs.
- Electrical synapse.

Depolarization of the presynaptic cell initiates a response in the postsynaptic cell either by release of NTs (most common) or by direct passage of electrical current.

Site of interneuronal communication can involve one axon to one dendrite, one axon to many dendrites, or many axons to one dendrite.

CHEMICAL SYNAPSE

- Most common type.
- Consists of:
  - Presynaptic membrane.
    - Synaptic vesicles within this terminal contain a NT.
  - Synaptic cleft.
    - Space between the presynaptic and postsynaptic membranes.
  - Postsynaptic membrane.
    - Membrane of postsynaptic neuron that contains specific receptors for the NT.

SYNAPTIC TRANSMISSION

- Release of NTs.
- NTs are stored in synaptic vesicles within the presynaptic axon terminal.
- AP depolarizes the presynaptic membrane, causing:
  - Voltage-gated Ca^{2+} channels opened (on the presynaptic membrane).
    - ↑ Ca^{2+} influx.
  - Ca^{2+} causes the synaptic vesicles to fuse with membrane.
  - NTs are released by exocytosis into synaptic cleft.
  - NTs diffuse across cleft.
  - Bind to specific receptors on postsynaptic cell.
- The time required for this process to occur is called synaptic delay.

CHEMICAL NEUROTRANSMITTERS

- Mediate most connections.
- Small molecule NTs (contained within vesicles):
  - Glutamate, GABA, glycine, ACh, 5HT, NE, Epi, etc.
- Neuropeptides (large dense vesicles):
  - Somatostatin, endorphins, enkephalins, opioids, etc.

ELECTRICAL SYNAPSE

- Gap junctions; minority.
- Cytoplasm of adjacent cells is connected by gap junctions.
- Allows passage of local electrical currents (ions and small molecules) (from APs in presynaptic neuron) to pass directly to postsynaptic neuron.
  - Rare in the CNS.
  - Common in cardiac and smooth muscle.
  - Ensure a group of neurons act together; Synchronize groups of neurons.
  - Important in embryonic development (morphogenic gradients).

▶ NEUROMUSCULAR JUNCTION (NMJ)

Synapse between lower motor neuron (efferent nerve) and muscle.

- Presynaptic terminal (lower motor neuron axon)
  - Releases ACh.
- Postsynaptic membrane (skeletal muscle membrane).
  - Displays nicotinic receptor (N_M).

- Threshold is –65 mV → all or nothing!
  - ~35 ACh required.

SEQUENCE

ACh binds N_M

↓

Na^+ channels open on the motor end-plate (ligand-gated ion channel)

↓

Muscle fiber depolarized (Na^+ influx)

↓

Voltage-gated Na^+ channels on the sarcolemma open

↓

AP stimulated in skeletal muscle fiber

↓

AP travels down the transverse tubules (dihydropyridine receptors (voltage-gated Ca^{2+} channel))

↓

Ca^{2+} release from the sarcoplasmic reticulum (ryanodine receptor in SR (mechanically activated))

↓

Muscle contraction (Ca^{2+} binds troponin, troponin moves off actin, myosin can bind, etc)

> AP in LMN → Ca^{2+} voltage-gated channel opens → Ca^{2+} in → ACh vesicles fuse and released into synaptic cleft → ACh binds to Nm.

In the NMJ, AChE is located on the muscle end-plate.

If AChEs are inhibited, get prolongation of end-plate potential (EPP).

Acetylcholine Metabolism

- Synthesized in the presynaptic terminal of the motor neuron from which it is released.
  - Acetyl CoA + choline – (choline acetyltransferase)→ ACh (acetylcholine).
- Stored in synaptic vesicles.
- Released into synaptic cleft (generates effect).
- Breakdown:
  - ACh – (acetylcholinesterase [AChE])→ acetate + choline.

> Two enzymes involved in ACh metabolism:
>
> - Choline acetyltransferase: ACh generation.
> - Acetylcholinesterase (AChE): ACh breakdown.

▶ SPECIAL SENSES

Vision

General eye anatomy (Chapter 2).

EYEBALL

- Grossly divided into two segments:
- **Anterior segment**
  - Consists of two chambers (anterior and posterior).
  - Filled with aqueous humor (watery fluid).
- **Posterior segment**
  - Filled with vitreous humor (thick, gelatinous material).

STRUCTURAL COMPONENTS

- Sclera
  - Tough, white outer layer.
  - Maintains size and form of the eyeball.
- Cornea
  - Transparent dome on the anterior eye surface.
  - Protective function.
  - Helps focus light on retina at back of eye.
- Choroid
  - Lining of the inner aspect of the eyeball beneath the retina; very vascular.

COMPONENTS THAT CONTROL LIGHT ENTERING THE EYE AND FOCUS LIGHT ON THE RETINA

- Pupil
  - Circular opening (black area) in the middle of the iris.
  - Light enters the eye to reach retina through this opening.
  - Lens is located behind this aperture.
  - Size of the pupil is controlled by muscles in the iris.
- Iris
  - Circular colored area of the eye (amount of pigment in the iris determines the color of the eye).
  - **Miosis**: Constriction of pupil:
    - Sphincter pupillae (iris sphincter) closes iris.
    - Response to:
      - Increased light.
      - Drugs (eg, narcotics).
      - Pathologic conditions.
      - Parasympathetic stimulation.
  - **Mydriasis**: Dilation of the pupil (term often used for prolonged papillary dilation):
    - Dilator pupillae (iris dilator) opens iris.
    - Response to:
      - Decreased light.
      - Sympathetic stimulation (fight or flight).
      - Drug.
      - Disease.

- Lens
  - Directly behind the iris and pupillary opening.
  - Focuses light on the retina.
  - Controlled by ciliary muscle (within the ciliary body).
- Ciliary body
- Functions:
  - Accommodation.
    - Ciliary muscle alters the lens refractory power (to focus light on the retina).
  - Produces aqueous humor.
  - Holds lens in place.

- Retina
  - Innermost layer of the eye on the posterior surface.
  - Receives visual stimuli.
  - Communicates via CN II with the brain (visual cortex).
  - Photoreceptors (visual receptors) of retina (on deepest surface to incoming light).

- **Rods (higher sensitivity, lower acuity)**
  - Contain rhodopsin (photopigment).
  - Perceive different degrees of brightness: Responsible for night vision (dark adaptation).
  - Relative lack of color discrimination.
  - Located mostly at the periphery of the retina.
- **Cones (higher acuity (fovea); color)**
  - Each contains one of three photopigments.
  - Each being sensitive to a particular wavelength of light.
  - Three types: Red, green, blue.
    - Primarily responsible for color vision.
  - Principal photoreceptors during daylight or in brightly lit areas.
    - Located in the center of the retina, especially in the fovea.
- **Photopigments**
  - Four photopigments:
    - Rhodopsin (rods).
    - Red, green, and blue (cones).
  - Each photopigment contains:
    - Opsin (protein) bound to
    - Retinal (a chromophore molecule).
    - Together they compose rhodopsin.
  - The difference among the opsin molecules allows a photopigment to have specificity for a particular type or color of light.

Rods are more abundant, have higher sensitivity, and lower acuity compared with cones.

Retinal (a vitamin A aldehyde) is constant among all photopigments and is produced from vitamin A.

VISUAL PATHWAY

See Figure 10–6.

Light
↓
(passes through cornea, lens, aqueous humor, vitreous humor, and onto retina)
↓
Retina (rods & cones)
↓
Bipolar neurons
↓
Ganglion cells
↓
Optic disc
↓
Optic nerve (exits through optic foramen)
↓
Optic chiasm (temporal visual fields decussation; crossing of images on nasal side of each retina)
↓
Lateral geniculate (of thalamus)
↓
Optic radiations
↓
Visual cortex (area 17) and visual association cortex (18, 19)

Oxidation of vitamin A (retinol) leads to retinal.

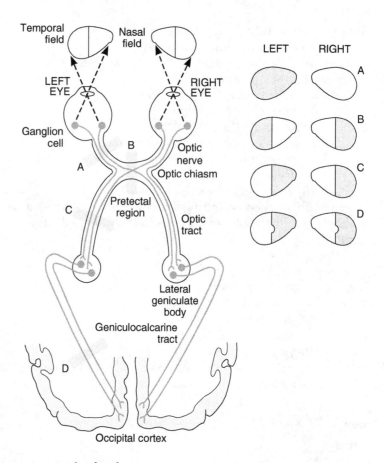

FIGURE 10-6.   Visual pathway.

Reproduced, with permission, from Ganong WF. *Review of Medical Physiology*, 22nd ed. New York: McGraw-Hill, 2005.

General visual pathway:

Light enters eye → retina →

optic nerve (CN II) → visual

cortex (occipital lobe). Up is

down and right is left in

occipital cortex.

LESIONS ALONG THE VISUAL PATHWAY

- Left anopsia (A)
- Bitemporal hemianopsia (B)
- Right homonomous hemianopsia (C)
- Right hemianopsia with macular sparing (D)

Disturbances of Vision

	Myopia (Nearsightedness)	Hyperopia (Farsightedness)	Astigmatism	Presbyopia
Problem	Eyeball too long. Focal point of far objects is focused in front of the retina. Near objects are focused correctly.	Eyeball too short. Focal point of near objects is focused behind the retina. Distant objects are focused correctly.	Curvature of lens is not uniform.	Loss of lens elasticity with advancing age. Eye cannot focus sharply on nearby objects.
Treatment	Concave lenses.	Convex lenses.	Cylindric lenses.	Often with bifocals.

Anatomy of the Ear

EXTERNAL EAR

- Auricle (Pinna)
  - Directs sound waves.
- External auditory canal (meatus)
  - Contains hair and cerumen (wax).
  - Serves as resonator and conduit.

MIDDLE EAR

- Tympanic cavity.
- Air-filled cavity in temporal bone.
  - Auditory tube: Equalizes pressure.
  - Ossicles (malleus, incus, stapes): Transmit sounds from tympanic membrane to oval window → to inner ear → converting them to higher pressure sounds that are able to travel through fluid.

INNER EAR

See Figure 10–7.

- Formed by bony labyrinth and membranous labyrinth
- Vestibule (saccule and utricle)
  - Associated with sense of balance and linear acceleration (static position)
- Semicircular canals
  - Concerned with equilibrium and angular momentum.
- Cochlea (two membranes: vestibular and basilar)
  - Responsible for hearing.
  - Spiral organ (organ of Corti).
    - Receptors (hair cells) for hearing.
    - Basic functional unit of hearing.
    - Transforms fluid vibrations from sound waves (mechanical energy) into a nerve impulse (electrical energy).

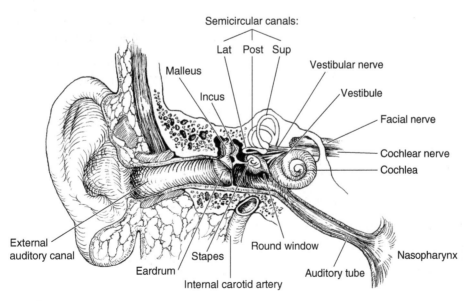

FIGURE 10–7. Inner ear.

Reproduced, with permission, from Ganong WF. *Review of Medical Physiology,* 22nd ed. New York: McGraw-Hill, 2005.

Pitch = Frequency.

Loudness = Amplitude.

Unlike other sensory systems, hearing has bilateral central representation (ie, sound from one ear reaches auditory cortex in both hemispheres).

Superior olivary nuclei are important in sound localization. Parallel nuclei involved in vision: inferior olivary, superior colliculus, and lateral geniculate.

Presbycusis = hearing loss that gradually occurs because of changes in the inner or middle ear in individuals as they grow older.

Sound amplification:

- Lever action of ossicles
- Concentration of sound waves from tympanic membrane to oval window

Organ of Corti lies on basilar membrane and is bathed in endolymph.

Organ of Corti is the basic functional unit of hearing– transforms the sound waves (mechanical energy) into fluid vibrations into a nerve impuse (electrical energy).

Hearing

- Ability to detect sound.
- Human hearing range = 20–20,000 Hz.

CHARACTERISTICS OF A SOUND WAVE

- **Pitch**
  - Related to the frequency of the sound wave.
  - ↑ frequency = ↑ pitch.
    - Frequency is measures in hertz (Hz) or cycles per second.
- **Loudness** (amplitude)
  - Related to the intensity and the amplitude of the wave.
  - ↑ amplitude = ↑ intensity = ↑ loudness.
    - Intensity is measured in decibels (dB).
- **Timbre** (quality)
  - Related to the presence of additional sound-wave frequencies superimposed on the principal frequency.

HEARING PATHWAY

Sound vibration (external ear (pinna to canal))
↓
Tympanic membrane (middle ear)
↓
Ossicles (malleus → incus → stapes)
↓
Oval window
↓
Waves in perilymph (bony labyrinth)
↓
Endolymph (membranous labyrinth)
↓
Bending of hairs (stereocilia)
↓
Hair cell depolarization within tectorial membrane or organ of Corti in cochlea (between basilar and vestibular membanes)
↓
Short axons to spiral ganglion (located within bony modiolus)
↓
Long axons form the cochlear nerve
↓
Synapse w/cochlear nuclei (dorsal and ventral)
↓
Superior olivary nucleus (ipsi- and contralaterally)
↓
Lateral lemniscus
↓
Inferior colliculus
↓
Medial geniculate of thalamus
↓
Transverse temporal gyrus (Heschl's gyrus)

▶ TASTE

- Direct detection of chemical composition via contact with chemoreceptor cells.
- Food broken down; taste-producing molecules bind with protein from Ebner's glands.
  - These bound molecules stimulate taste bud receptors.
  - von Ebner's glands secrete lingual lipase.

Review of salivary glands:
Parotid–serous
Sublingual–mucus
Submandibular–mixed
Minor–mucus
**except von Ebner's glands which are serous and also begin lipid hydrolysis, essential component of taste

▶ TASTE BUDS

- Made of gustatory receptor cells that synapse with sensory nerve fibers.
- Located:
  - Within the fungiform and vallate papillae of the tongue:
    - **Fungiform papillae**
      - Rounded.
      - Located mostly at the tongue tip of the tongue (which is innervated by VII).
      - Contain ~5 taste buds.
    - **Vallate papillae (circumvallate)**
      - In "V" arrangement on the back of the tongue (which is innervated by IX). Contain ~100 taste buds.
      - Associated with von Ebner's glands (as are foliate papillae).
  - On the mucosa of the epiglottis, palate, and pharynx.

Filiform papillae *on dorsum of the tongue do **not** usually contain taste buds. They are the most numerous papillae.*

There are five basic tastes:

- *Sweet*
- *Sour*
- *Bitter*
- *Salt*
- *Umami (MSG (monosodium glutamate))*

Each taste is sensed on all parts of the tongue, by each type of taste bud.

TASTE PATHWAY (ALL IPSILATERAL)

Taste bud, receptor cell
↓
CN VII, IX, X
↓
Nucleus of the solitary tract (within medulla)
↓
Ipsilateral VPM of thalamus
↓
Insular cortex (to facial area of post-central gyrus). (Note: insular cortex is where parietal infolds next to temporal.)

*Both foliate and fungiform papillae are **not** keratinized. Filiform and circumvallate **are** keratinized.*

TASTE DISTURBANCES

See Figure 10–8.

- **Ageusia:** Complete loss of taste.
- **Dysgeusia:** Disturbed sense of taste.

Review:
Filliform papillae–V-shaped cones w/o taste buds, most numerous, mechanical, characterized by increased keratin.
Foliate papillae–extreme posterior/lateral tongue, in front of vallate papillae.

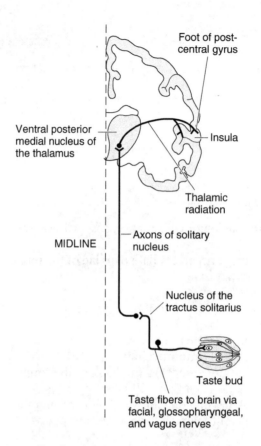

FIGURE 10–8. Taste disturbances.

Reproduced, with permission, from Ganong WF. *Review of Medical Physiology,* 22nd ed. New York: McGraw-Hill, 2005.

▶ SMELL

- Detection of inhaled odors.
- Chemoreceptor cells associated with the olfactory nerve (CN I). Note that the neuron is a chemoreceptor not separate like taste.

Smell Pathway

See Figure 10–9.

Odorant particles (dissolve in mucous from Bowman's glands)
↓
Bipolar olfactory cells (within nasal mucosa)
↓
Olfactory nerve (passes through cribriform plate)
↓
Olfactory bulb on cribiform plate (synapses with mitral and tufted cells)
↓
Olfactory tract (outgrowth of brain)
↓
Primary olfactory cortex and amygdala

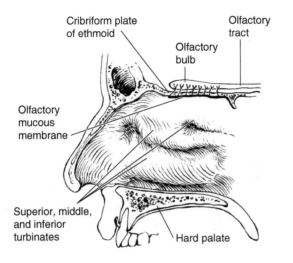

FIGURE 10-9. Smell pathway.

Reproduced, with permission, from Waxman, SG. *Clinical Neuroanatomy,* 25th ed. New York: McGraw-Hill, 2003.

DISTURBANCES OF SMELL

- **Anosmia:** Absence of smell.
  - Disease of olfactory mucous membranes (common cold, allergic rhinitis).
  - Kallman syndrome (hypogonadism, GnRH deficiency).
- **Hyposmia:** Diminished smell.
- **Dysosmia:** Distorted smell.

Kallman syndrome—hypogonadism caused by deficiency of GnRH created by hypothalamus, association with asnosmia.

Muscle Physiology

- The largest tissue type in the human body.
- Converts chemical energy to mechanical energy.
- Three types:
  - Skeletal
  - Cardiac
  - Smooth

Major Cellular Components

- **Sarcolemma:** The plasma membrane of muscle cells.
- **Sarcoplasm:** The cytoplasm of muscle cells.
- **Sarcoplasmic reticulum (SR):** A network of channels extending throughout the sarcoplasm that stores Ca^{2+}.
- **Myofilaments:** Mediate muscle contraction. Located in the sarcoplasm.
  - **Thin filaments:** ~6–8 nm in diameter.
    - **Actin:** Globular (G) actin is arranged in double helical chains called fibrous (F) actin.
    - **Troponin:** Attached to each tropomyosin molecule.
    - **Tropomyosin:** Blocks actin-binding sites during rest.
  - **Thick filaments:** ~15 nm in diameter.
    - **Myosin**
      - **Light meromyosin (LMM):** Makes up the rod-like backbone of myosin filaments.
      - **Heavy meromyosin (HMM):** Forms the shorter cross-bridges which bind to actin during contraction.

Comparison of Skeletal, Cardiac, and Smooth Muscle

Characteristic	Skeletal	Cardiac	Smooth
Striations	Yes	Yes	No
Nucleation	Multinucleated	Single	Single
Nucleus location	Peripheral	Central	Central
Innervation	Motor	Autonomic	Autonomic
Movement	Voluntary	Involuntary	Involuntary
Contraction by	A.P.	Intrinsic	A.P./hormones
Syncytium	No	Yes	Yes
Ca^{2+} source	SR	SR/extracellular	SR/extracellular
T-tubules	Yes	Yes	No
Regulation	Actin	Actin	Myosin
Troponin	Yes	Yes	No

Innervation

- Afferent nerves: Sensory receptor → CNS.
- Efferent nerves: CNS → muscle cell.

Histology

See Figure 11–1.

- Cells are long and **multinucleated.**
- Nuclei are generally elongated and peripherally located.
- The major structural unit is the **myofibril:**
  - **Thick filaments** (contain myosin).
  - **Thin filaments** (contain actin, troponin, and tropomyosin).
  - Myosin cross-bridges link the two filaments.
- The **sarcomere** is the functional (contractile) unit of the myofibril. Defined as the area between two Z lines.
- **Cross-striations** are apparent due to alternating light and dark banding of the myofibrils.
  - **A band**: Dark band contains myosin. Never changes length.
  - **H band**: Light band that bisects the A band. Shortens during contraction.
  - **I band**: Light band containing actin. Shortens during contraction.
  - **Z line**: Dark band that bisects the I band. Anchor for actin.
  - **M line**: Dark band that bisects the H band. Anchor for myosin.

Satellite cells are responsible for skeletal muscle regeneration.

Two t-tubules lie within a single sarcomere.

As thin and thick filaments overlap, the H and I bands are shortened, thereby contracting each sarcomere.

The d**A**rk band is the **A** band.
The l**I**ght band is the **I** band.

HAZI *(hazy)*:

The **H** band bisects the **A** band.
The **Z** line bisects the **I** band.

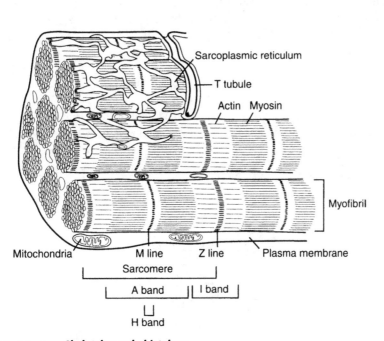

FIGURE 11–1. Skeletal muscle histology.

Reproduced, with permission, from Bhushan V, et al. *First Aid for the USMLE Step 1: 2006.* New York: McGraw Hill, 2006.

*Weight lifting causes muscle **hypertrophy**, increasing skeletal muscle cell size, not number. Contrarily, muscle disuse causes a decrease in muscle size.*

*Each **motor unit** consists of the following:*

- *α-Motor neuron*
- *Synaptic cleft*
- *Associated muscle fibers*

*Occurs via **actin-linked** regulation.*

Connective Tissue

- Contains a rich supply of blood vessels and nerves required for nerve conduction.
- Divided into three layers:
  - **Epimysium:** Surrounds the entire muscle.
  - **Perimysium:** Surrounds muscle bundles (fascicles).
  - **Endomysium:** Surrounds each muscle fiber.

Motor Innervation

- One α-**motor neuron** innervates several skeletal muscle fibers (axon is highly branched).
- When a motor neuron transmits an action potential, ALL of the fibers it innervates contract simultaneously.
- All motor neurons are arranged in various positions within the **ventral horn** of the spinal cord.
- **Fractionation:** Not necessary to activate all motor units in a muscle.
- **Size principle:** Motor units are recruited in order of size of motor unit. With greater muscle force, larger motor units are recruited.

Contraction

- When an action potential reaches the neuromuscular junction, **acetylcholine** is released from vesicles within the axon terminus and binds to postsynaptic nicotinic receptors on the sarcolemma. This, in turn, increases the membrane permeability of Na^+ and K^+ and depolarizes the muscle cell.
- See Figure 11–2.

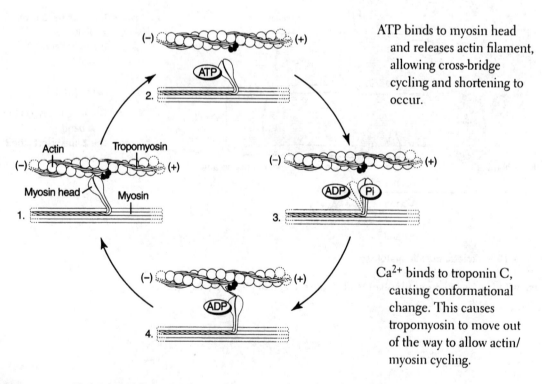

ATP binds to myosin head and releases actin filament, allowing cross-bridge cycling and shortening to occur.

Ca^{2+} binds to troponin C, causing conformational change. This causes tropomyosin to move out of the way to allow actin/ myosin cycling.

FIGURE 11-2. Skeletal muscle contraction.

Reproduced, with permission, from Bhushan V, et al. *First Aid for the USMLE Step 1*: 2006. New York: McGraw-Hill, 2006.

- The action potential travels along the sarcolemma and through a system of **t-tubules,** which extend from the outer surface of the muscle fiber to the SR of two adjacent sarcomeres.
- Ca^{2+} released from the terminal cisternae of each SR bind to **troponin C,** which is attached to the **tropomyosin** molecule of thin filaments. This causes a conformational change in the shape of tropomyosin, allowing the actin filament to interact with the myosin cross-bridge.
- An **ATP** molecule bound to myosin is hydrolyzed to ADP + P_i. When the ADP + P_i is released from myosin, the actin filament is pulled closer toward the center of the sarcomere, shortening its length (**power stroke**).
- As long as Ca^{2+} and ATP are available, this cycle continues, further contracting the muscle. If more muscle force is needed, more motor units are activated.
- During relaxation, Ca^{2+} is taken up by the SR, causing the release of actin from the myosin cross-bridges. Tropomyosin returns to its normal configuration, blocking this interaction.

Contraction (Twitch) Speed

- Oxidative capacity of muscle fibers is related to
  - Number of capillaries
  - Myoglobin content
  - Number of mitochondria

Comparison of Skeletal Muscle by Twitch Speed

Characteristic	Slow (Type I)	Fast (Type II)
Function	Postural/endurance	Rapid/powerful movement
Rate of fatigue	Low	High
Contraction speed	Slow	Fast
Fiber diameter	Small	Large
Color	Red	White
Myoglobin content	High	Low
Mitochondria content	High	Low
Capillary content	High	Low
ATP source	Oxidative phosphorylation	Anaerobic glycolysis of stored glycogen
ATPase activity	Low	High
Glycogen content	Low	High
SR content	Low	High

Fiber Types

- **Extrafusal fibers**
  - Make up the majority of skeletal muscle.
  - Innervated by α-**motor neurons.**
- **Intrafusal fibers**
  - Located within the bulk of the muscle.
  - Encapsulated.
  - Innervated by γ-**motor neurons**.
  - Includes muscle spindle and Golgi tendon organs.

*Both extrafusal and intrafusal fibers run **parallel** with each other and attach to tendons at either end of the muscle.*

Sensory Innervation

- Encapsulated intrafusal nerve fibers.
- Stretch receptors.
- Fine-tunes muscle tone.
- Run parallel with extrafusal muscle fibers.

Receptor	Location	Efferent Terminals	Afferent Terminals	Sensory Function	Characteristic
Muscle spindle - Nuclear bag fibers	Muscle belly	γ-motor	Ia	Detect *dynamic* Δ in muscle **length**	Activate α-motor neurons
- Nuclear chain fibers			Ia, II	Detect *static* Δ in muscle **length**	
Golgi tendon organ	Muscle tendon	None	Ib	Detect Δ in muscle **tension**	Inhibit α-motor neurons

Type Ia fibers (annulospiral endings): Largest and fastest. Rapid adaptation to change in muscle length.

Type II fibers (flower-spray endings): Non-adaptive.

The stretch reflex maintains muscle tone.

Spinal Reflexes

- Reflex arcs:
  1. Receptor
  2. Sensory (afferent) neuron
  3. Integration center (CNS)
  4. Interneuron
  5. Motor (efferent) neuron
  6. Effector

Reflex Type	Receptor	Sensitivity	Action	Example
Stretch (myotactic)	Muscle spindle	Δ in length	Contraction	Knee-jerk reflex
Tendon (inverse myotatic)	Golgi tendon organ	Δ in tension	Relaxation	Pick up something too heavy and drop it
Flexor-withdrawal (nociceptive)	Nociceptor	Δ in temperature	Flexion	Touch something hot and withdraw hand, causing pain

Histology

- Cells have a similar contractile structure (myofilaments) and **striated** (actin, myosin) appearance as skeletal muscle cells.
- Fibers are firmly linked by *desmosomes*.
- Nuclei are centrally located.
- More mitochondria between myofibrils.
- Richer in myoglobin.
- Cells have many **branches**, which communicate to adjacent cardiac muscle cells via *gap junctions*.
- **Intercalated discs** coordinate the action of cardiac muscle cells.
- Cells do *not* undergo mitosis: Injury results in fibrosis with loss of function at that site.

Innervation

- Mediated by its own **intrinsic contractile activity.**
- There are **no motor units.**
- The **autonomic nervous system** (both sympathetic and parasympathetic fibers) controls the *rate* and *strength* of myocardial depolarization.

Muscle Contraction

- Ca^{2+} enters the myocytes via specific **calcium channels**, which are regulated by **cAMP protein kinases.**
- The influx of Ca^{2+} enables the release of more Ca^{2+} from the SR, initiating troponin-C binding and eventual muscle contraction.
- Relaxation occurs when Ca^{2+} exits the myocytes through a regulated **Ca^{2+}-Na^+ exchange system.**

Cardiac muscle behaves as a ***functional syncytium.***

An increase in cardiac demand causes a ***compensatory hypertrophy,*** *increasing cardiac cell* ***size,*** *not number.*

The sinuatrial (SA) node is known as the pacemaker of the heart.

Occurs via ***actin-linked regulation,*** *but relies more on* ***extracellular*** Ca^{2+} *than skeletal muscle because its SR is less extensive.*

The plateau in the cardiac muscle action potential is due to the influx of Ca^{2+}.

Histology

- Commonly found in tubular organs such as blood vessels, the GI tract, and the respiratory tract, but also in ciliary bodies of the eye and hair follicles.
- Cells are small in diameter but very long.
- Nuclei are single and centrally located.
- Myofibrils are **not striated.**
- **No t-tubules** are present.
- SR system is poorly developed.

Innervation

- Mediated by the **autonomic nervous system** (both sympathetic and parasympathetic).
- However, there is a considerable synaptic distance from the nerve terminal to the sarcolemma because the autonomic axons terminate in the surrounding connective tissue.

Smooth muscle behaves as a ***functional syncytium.***

Smooth muscle contraction can also be stimulated by ***hormones*** *such as epinephrine and oxytocin.*

BIOCHEMISTRY–PHYSIOLOGY

MUSCLE PHYSIOLOGY

- Because not all smooth muscle cells are directly innervated, they rely on cell-cell *gap junctions* to propagate the action potential.
  - **Single unit**: Numerous gap junctions between adjacent cells. Fibers contract spontaneously without nerve impulses. Examples: GI, uterus, ureters, arterioles.
  - **Multi-unit**: Cells lack gap junctions. Fibers are directly innervated. Examples: Iris, vas deferens, arteries.

Muscle Contraction

See Figure 11–3.

*Occurs via **myosin-linked regulation**; thin filaments **lack troponin,** so they are always ready to interact with myosin.*

- Ca^{2+} (from the SR or extracellular sources) enters the smooth muscle cell cytoplasm and binds to **calmodulin**.
- Calmodulin activates **myosin light-chain kinase**, which transfers a P$_i$ from an ATP molecule to the myosin light-chain.
- The phosphorylation of myosin enables it to interact with actin in the same manner as skeletal and cardiac muscle.
- Relaxation occurs when Ca^{2+} is taken up by the SR or plasma membrane and the myosin light-chain kinase becomes inactivated.
- Contraction is slow and prolonged. Each contraction cycle requires one ATP.

Maintains contraction for extended periods of time because the cross-bridges detach very slowly, allowing them to stay attached longer.

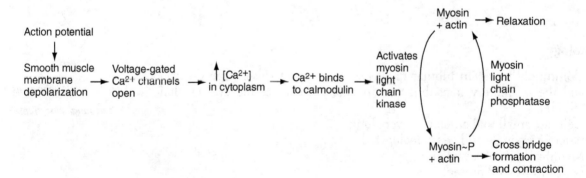

FIGURE 11–3. Smooth muscle contraction.

CHAPTER 12

Circulatory and Cardiac Physiology

Blood Flow

- $F = P/R$ (flow = pressure/resistance). $I = V/R$.
- $Q = \Delta P/R$.
- Q = flow.
- Flow is proportional to pressure difference at two ends of vessel.
- Flows from high pressure to low pressure.
- Inversely proportional to resistance along the vessel.
- Greatest in
  - Large straight vessels.
  - Low turbulence.
  - Low viscosity.
  - Low resistance.

PERFUSION PRESSURE

- Pressure at the arterial end minus pressure at venous end.

Resistance

- Poiseuille's law ($F = P\pi r^4/8nL$) describes the flow rate of liquid through a tube.
- The resistance to flow is determined by the equation ($R = 8nL/\pi r^4$).
  - n = viscosity.
    - Hematocrit (HCT)
      - Affect is greater in larger vessels than smaller.
      - Overall vascular resistance is not affected unless severe (eg, polycythemia).
    - Decrease in deformation of cells.
    - Plasma concentration (eg, increase in protein, multiple myeloma).
  - L = length of tube.
  - r = radius.
    - Type and size of vessel.
    - Regulation of tone (sympathetic nervous system, medications, local factors).
    - Pathologic narrowing of vessel.
- $R\pi 1/r^4$.
- If radius (r) increases by 2, the resistance (R) drops 16 ×. ** most powerful relationship with resistance.

The RADIUS has the most powerful relationship with resistance.

Remember:
artery → arteriole →
capillary → venule →
vein

SERIES RESISTANCE

- $R_{total} = R_1 + R_2 + R_3 + R_4 \ldots$

PARALLEL RESISTANCE

- Recruitment of capillaries serves to lower the resistance and therefore increases the flow.
  $1/R_{total} = 1/R_1 + 1/R_2 + 1/R_3 + 1/R_4 \ldots$

Resistance and conductance are inversely related.

*Resistance to flow of blood offered by the entire systemic circulation is called **total peripheral resistance (TPR)**.*

Capillaries have the largest cross-sectional area and the lowest blood flow velocity

Inverse relationship between area and velocity of blood flow.

$$V = Q/A$$

where Q = flow and A = cross-sectional area

When the vena cava is somewhat collapsed, as it often is, it has a lower cross-sectional area and a higher velocity of blood flow when compared to the aorta.

Properties of Flow

See Figure 12–1.

- **Laminar flow** (streamline)
- Low Reynolds number
  - In straight vessels.
  - Layer closest to vessel surface does not move.
  - Layer in center moves at maximum velocity.
  - Laminar flow occurs up to a certain critical velocity.
    - Turbulent flow occurs above critical velocity.

- **Turbulent flow**
- High Reynolds number
  - Occurs above critical velocity.
  - Reynolds number.
  - Represents probability for turbulent flow.
  - Related to:
    - Velocity.
    - Diameter of vessel.
    - Blood viscosity.
  - Examples of turbulence:
    - Constricted, atherosclerotic vessel.
    - Ascending aorta.
    - Anemia.

Velocity of Blood Flow

- Fastest to slowest:
  - Vena cavae.
  - Aorta.
  - Large veins.
  - Small arteries.
  - Arterioles.
  - Capillaries.

See Figure 12–2 for systemic blood flow and changes in pressure and velocity.

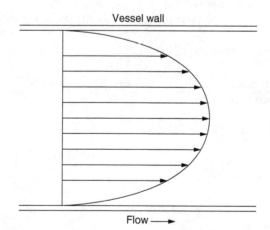

FIGURE 12–1. Properties of flow.

Reproduced, with permission, from Ganong WF. *Review of Medical Physiology*, 22nd ed. New York: McGraw-Hill, 2005.

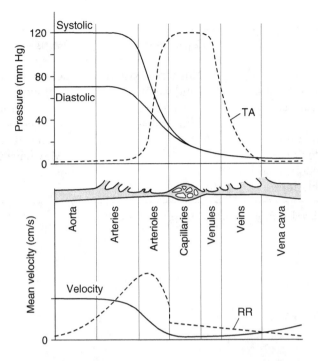

FIGURE 12-2. Systemic blood flow—changes in pressure and velocity.

Reproduced, with permission, from Ganong WF. *Review of Medical Physiology*, 22nd ed. New York: McGraw-Hill, 2005.

LAPLACE'S LAW

- Wall stress = Pr/t.
  - P = pressure.
  - r = radius.
  - t = wall thickness.
- **In vessels:** A thin-walled, distended vessel, under large amounts of pressure has more wall tension/stress and is at greater risk for rupture.
- **In the heart:** A dilated, thin-walled myocardium, under increasing pressure and volume has higher wall tension (and the myocardial oxygen demand is elevated).
  - P within the ventricle depends on afterload (eg, TPR, aortic stenosis).
  - r within the ventricle depends on preload (amount of venous return).
  - t thickness of the ventricle: Increased thickness decreases wall stress to a point, then
  - Oxygen demand increases because of greater muscle mass.
  - Oxygen supply decreases by narrowing coronary vessels.

Blood Vessel Types and Characteristics

Arteries*	Arterioles	Capillaries	Veins
Oxygenated blood carried under high pressure from heart to body. Muscular walls. High pressure. Low compliance.	Regulate blood flow into capillaries. *Primary resistance vessels.* Tissue metabolites, humoral factors affect vasoconstriction and vasodilation.	Nutrient, oxygen, and waste exchange. Thin walls.	Carry deoxygenated blood back to heart. Large lumens. High compliance (volume reservoirs). May have valves.

*Pulmonary and umbilical arteries carry deoxygenated blood. Pulmonary vein carries oxygenated blood.

Oxygen Exchange

CAPILLARIES

At rest most capillaries are closed. In active tissue they dilate and perfuse. In inflammation capillary leakiness is mediated by substance P, bradykinin, etc.

- Greatest total area.
- Large surface area.
- Slowest velocity of an individual blood cell.
  - Allows time for oxygen, nutrient exchange/diffusion.

ARTERIOLES

- Account for:
  - Largest drop in BP (~50% drop from arteries to arterioles).
  - Highest proportion of peripheral vascular resistance.
- Pressure decreases as blood moves through systemic circulation.
  - This pressure gradient is required for blood flow.

▶ BLOOD VOLUME

Venules are small veins that collect blood from capillaries (coalesce into larger veins).

Most is held within the **systemic venous circulation:**

- >60% in systemic veins.
- >10% in systemic arteries.
- <10% in arterioles and capillaries.
- 9% in pulmonary vessels.
- 7% in heart.

▶ CAPACITANCE

- Ability to hold blood volume.
- Act as a reservoir.

- Veins.
    - Capacitance vessels.
    - Dilate to accommodate blood volume.
    - Hold 50–60% of blood volume.

In hypovolemia, veins/venules constrict.

- Sympathetic mediated.
- Compensatory.
    - No clinical manifestations with 15–20% blood loss.
    - Helps maintain mean systemic filling pressure in the face of blood loss.
    - Preload is maintained with venous constriction.

Arterial constriction system has much less effect on mean systemic filling pressure.

- Arterial system contains relatively small amount of blood.
- Arterial constriction increases afterload.

Capillaries do not constrict because they lack smooth muscle in their walls.

Comparison of Pulmonary and Systemic Circulations

	Pulmonary Circulation[a]	Systemic Circulation[b]
BP	↓	↑
Resistance	↓	↑
Compliance	↑ (store blood without changing BP).	↓
Circuit[c]	Right heart → pulmonary artery → lungs → pulmonary vein → left heart (oxygenated).	Left heart → aorta → systemic arteries/arterioles/capillaries → venules/veins → SVC, IVC → right heart (deoxygenated).

[a]Pulmonary arteries supply only the lung gas exchange areas (alveoli).
[b]Systemic circulation supplies the body with oxygenated blood. Note that the bronchial arteries are part of the systemic circulation that supplies the lung tissue and bronchi for cellular metabolism (*not* gas exchange).
[c]Volume of blood flow is 5 L/min in both circuits (systemic and pulmonary).

▶ TOTAL PERIPHERAL RESISTANCE

- TPR (peripheral vascular resistance).
- Vascular resistance of the systemic circulation.
- Mean arterial pressure minus central venous pressure divided by the cardiac output (MAP – CVP)/CO.
- Increases with sympathetic activation; arteriolar constriction.

Because MAP = CO × TPR, the sympathetic/adrenergic system ↑ MAP by both:

- *↑ CO (via ↑ HR and SV).*
- *↑ TPR (by vasoconstriction, α_1).*

	↑TPR	↓TPR

Example	Cold
	Vasoconstriction
	  ▪ α_1 (sympathetic nervous system)
		Exercise
		Vasodilation
		  ▪ Especially in skeletal muscle
		    ▪ β_2 (sympathetic nervous system)
		  ▪ Local metabolites
		    ▪ Lactate
		    ▪ K^+
		    ▪ Adenosine

Sympathetic activation ↓ venous compliance and ↑ venous return (returns more blood to heart). This ↑ CO, via the Starling mechanism, and more blood is pumped back into arterial circulation.

Factor	Regulates
TPR	Blood flow from systemic circulation into venous circulation.
CO	Blood flow from veins back into arterial system.
Compliance	Amount of blood in systemic veins.

▶ BLOOD PRESSURE

Hypertension: Wall:lumen ratio ↑, arteriolar and capillary density ↓. See pathology for further discussion of pathogenesis.

- BP = CO × TPR.
- Systolic pressure/diastolic pressure (120/80).
- **Pulse pressure** = SBP − DBP.
  - Normal is (120 − 80) = 40.
  - Increases with age because of stiffened arteries (atherosclerosis, arteriosclerosis).
- **Mean arterial pressure (MAP)** = ~DBP + pulse pressure/3.
  - MAP = CO × TPR.
  - Vascular compliance − increase in volume/increase in pressure.
  - Average pressure throughout the course of the cycle.
  - MAP is slightly less than halfway between SBP and DBP because diastole is longer than systole.

Pulse Pressure

Narrow	Wide

Decreased arterial compliance (stiff, less distensible wall)
  ▪ HTN/atherosclerosis
  ▪ Aortic stenosis
  ▪ Cardiac tamponade
  ▪ Heart failure
Decreased SV (less blood ejected with each beat)
	AV malformations
	Aortic regurgitation
	Anemia
	Atherosclerosis
	Fever

Cardiac Output

- Cardiac output (CO) = amount of blood pumped per minute.
- $CO = HR \times SV$.
- Stroke volume (SV).
    - Amount of blood ejected with each beat.
    - $SV = {\sim}EDV - ESV$.
    - Average SV is 70–80 mL.
- HR
    - Bradycardia = <60 bpm.
    - Tachycardia = >100 bpm.
- Average resting CO is ~5.6 L/min for men (10–20% less for women).
- Varies depending on body activity, age, body size, and condition of heart.
- $CO = O_2$ consumption/$([O_2]$ pulmonary vein $- [O_2]$ pulmonary artery).

EJECTION FRACTION

- Proportion of end diastolic blood pumped out during diastole.

- $EF = EDV - ESV/EDV$ (or SV/EDV).

FRANK–STARLING MECHANISM

- Most important determinant of CO is venous return. (See Figure 12–3.)

$\uparrow$ venous return (EDV): $\uparrow$ ventricular filling in diastole: $\uparrow$ preload

$\downarrow$

$\uparrow$ cross bridges between actin and myosin

$\downarrow$

$\uparrow$ contraction force of cardiac muscle

$\downarrow$

$\uparrow$ CO

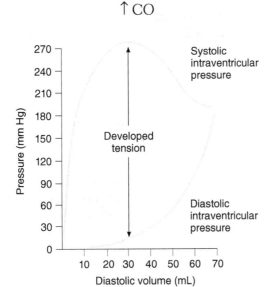

FIGURE 12–3. **Frank–Starling mechanism.**

Reproduced, with permission, from Ganong WF. *Review of Medical Physiology*, 22nd ed. New York: McGraw-Hill, 2005.

- The fibrous pericardium prevents the heart from overdistending during diastole, keeping it working at an effective point on Starling's curve. With compensatory cardiac enlargement (occurring slowly) the pericardium also expands, becoming more lax. In this case the ventricle can overfill (fall off Starling's curve).
- Conversely, a pericardium that is too stiff (or a pericardial space filled with fluid) results in underfilling or incomplete filling of the ventricle, leading to diastolic dysfunction and reduced stroke volumes.

Determinants of Cardiac Function

Myocardial Oxygen Supply	Myocardial Oxygen Demand
Arterial O$_2$ content Coronary blood flow ▪ Coronary perfusion pressure ▪ Patency	HR Contractility Wall stress (LaPlace's Law)

Imbalance between myocardial oxygen supply and demand causes ischemia (angina) and myocardial infarction (MI).

Heart Rate and Contractility

▪ Increase with sympathetic activation and certain drugs.
▪ However, remember that sympathetic activation also ↑TPR.
▪ Remember, CO = HR × SV.

Phospholamban (PLN):

▪ Normally inhibits SERCA (sarcoplasmic reticulum calcium pump)
▪ When phosphorylated by PKA, inhibition is relieved, ↑ contractility

	Heart Rate	Contractility
Effect	Chronotrope A chronotrope ↑ HR by increasing rate of SA node depolarization ↑HR will ↑CO until very high rate – when filling time is ↓	Inotrope Sympathetic or drug-mediated stimulation causes ↑ intracellular Ca^{2+}, which ↑ contraction force ↑ force of contraction ↑ SV (and therefore CO)

▪ **LaPlace's Law** = Wall stress = Pr/t
 ▪ P = pressure → **afterload**.
 ▪ r = radius → **preload**.
 ▪ t = thickness.

	Preload	Afterload
Definition	Filling of the ventricles (EDV)	Force against which the heart contracts
Determinants	Venous return* Radius of the ventricle (chamber size and expansion)	TPR (sympathetic activation, atherosclerosis) BP Aortic outflow tract (eg, narrowed in aortic stenosis—fixed increase in afterload)

*Frank–Starling mechanism says that venous return (preload) has a greater effect on CO than does TPR (afterload). The best way to ↑ CO is to ↑ preload (↑ venous return).

Venous Return

See Figure 12–4.

- ▦ **Skeletal muscle contraction**
    - ▦ Contraction pushes blood in veins back to heart.
    - ▦ Rhythmic contraction of leg muscles + presence of valves increase/allow venous return.
    - ▦ Counteracts force of gravity (that tends to pool blood in feet).
- ▦ **Compliance**
    - ▦ Intrathoracic pressure
        - ▦ ↑ intrathoracic pressure: ↑ venous compliance : ↓ venous return.
        - ▦ ↓ intrathoracic pressure : ↓ venous compliance : ↑ venous return.
    - ▦ Sympathetic nervous system
        - ▦ ↑ sympathetic tone: ↓ venous compliance (some constriction): ↑ venous return.

At very high heart rates (eg, >150–200) CO actually falls. ↑↑↑HR → ↓diastolic filling → ↓SV → ↓CO. So even though ↑HR (which ordinarily ↑CO), the ↓SV is to such a great extent that CO actually ↓ (so will BP↓).

Coarctation of the aorta increases afterload. There is a difference when measuring BP between arms and legs (or left and right arms, pre- versus post-ductus). This type of differential BP may also be present in older patients with atherosclerosis or dissection.

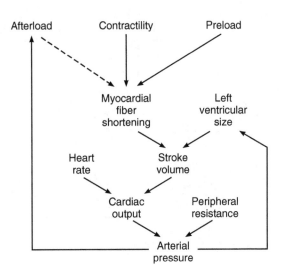

FIGURE 12–4. **Venous return.**

Reproduced, with permission, from Ganong WF. *Review of Medical Physiology*, 22nd ed. New York: McGraw-Hill, 2005.

Cardiac Cycle

	Diastole (Filling Phase)[a]	Isovolumetric Contraction	Systole (Ejection Phase)	Isovolumetric Relaxation
AV valves	Open.	Closed.	Closed.	Closed.
Pulmonic, aortic valves [b]	Closed.	Closed.	Open.	Closed.
Heart sound		S1 ("lub")[c] Sound of the AV valves (mitral and tricuspid) closing. This sound begins systole (ventricular contraction).		S2 ("dub") Sound of the semilunar valves (aortic and pulmonic) closing. This sound begins diastole (ventricle filling).[d]
	Blood enters ventricles through the open AV valves: ■ 70–80% passive. ■ 20–30% b/c atrial "kick" (contraction). Diastole is the long phase of the cycle.		Blood is ejected out the open aortic and pulmonic valves.	

[a] The coronary arteries are perfused during diastole.
[b] The aortic valve closes before the pulmonic, causing a splitting of S2 (this is accentuated on inspiration).
[c] S1 is louder and longer than S2.
[d] The pericardium helps regulate ventricular filling. (See the earlier section on the "Frank–Starling Mechanism.")

Splitting:
↑blood to R heart because of intrathoracic pressure. At same time ↓ blood to L heart because retained in lung vasculature. Pulmonary valve closes after aortic.

Pressure–Volume Loop

See Figure 12–5.
See Figure 12–6 for the cardiac cycle.

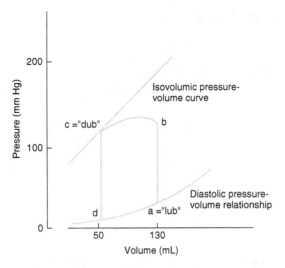

FIGURE 12-5. Pressure-volume loop.

Reproduced, with permission, from Ganong WF. *Review of Medical Physiology*, 22nd ed. New York: McGraw-Hill, 2005.

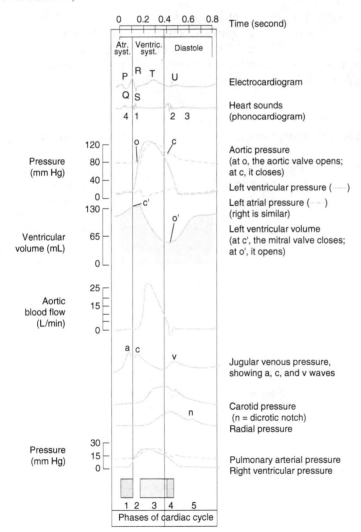

Letter "a" is from atrial "kick".

FIGURE 12-6. Cardiac cycle.

Reproduced, with permission, from Ganong WF. *Review of Medical Physiology*, 22nd ed. New York: McGraw-Hill, 2005.

Heart Murmurs with Valvular Disease

Diastolic	Systolic
Aortic insufficiency	Aortic stenosis
Mitral stenosis	Mitral regurgitation

Electrical Conduction of the Heart

See Figure 12–7.
- **Automaticity**
  - The spontaneous phase 4 depolarization that generates Aps.
  - These electrical signals conduct to atrial tissue, causing it to contract.
  - SA node → AV node → ventricular bundles (His/Purkinje) → ventricular myocytes → *ventricular contraction*.
- **Refractory period**
  - Long refractory period of heart allows relaxation (diastolic filling) and prevents the heart from going into reentry (arrhythmia).
  - Takes 0.22 seconds for AP to spread through the heart.
  - Ventricular muscle's refractory period is 0.25–0.30 second.
  - Atrial muscle's refractory period is 0.15 second.

As opposed to cardiac muscle, skeletal muscle has a short refractory period.

- This allows successive stimulation, a short time after initial contraction.
- Tetany serves to increase strength of contraction.

Absolute Refractory Period	Relative Refractory Period
During this, another AP cannot be elicited, regardless of magnitude of stimulus. Determined by Na$^+$ channel inactivation/gate closure.	Immediately follows the absolute refractory period. Continues until the membrane potential returns to resting level. During this, it is possible to generate another AP but need larger stimulus. Prevents reentry of ventricles.

Cardiac Conductive Tissues

Nodal/Pacemaker Tissue	Cardiac Myocytes
Phases 0–4. Phase 0 dependent on Ca^{2+}.	Gap junctions relay electrical signals, causing contraction. Phases 0–4. Phase 0 dependent on Na$^+$.

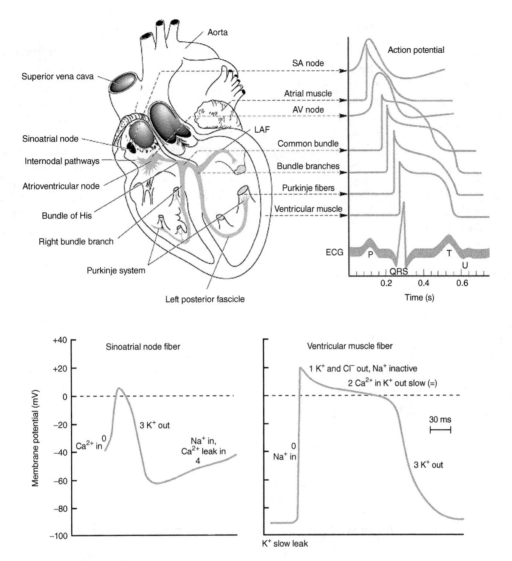

FIGURE 12–7. Electrical conduction of the heart.

Reproduced, with permission, from Ganong WF. *Review of Medical Physiology*, 22nd ed. New York: McGraw-Hill, 2005.

Nodal/Pacemaker Conduction System

SA Node	Internodal Pathways	AV Node	His-Purkinje System
Located in posterior wall of RA near opening of SVC. Pacemaker of the heart (starts the depolarization). Depolarizes at intrinsic rate that drives depolarization of rest of heart. Transmits signals faster than AV. Atria contract before ventricles, preventing fast, arrythmogenic beats from reaching the ventricle.	Transmits depolarization wave from the SA node to the LA and AV node.[a]	Located in the lower right interatrial septum. The impulse is delayed in AV node (~0.13 s) (slow conduction rate). Atria to contract before ventricles.	Fiber network arising in AV node. Purkinje fibers originate from R and L bundle branches.[b] Extend to papillary muscles and lateral walls of ventricles. Depolarization wave travels extremely fast through bundle branches and Purkinje fibers. Total elapsed time is 0.03 sec.

[a] Aside from AV node, the atria and ventricles are electrically isolated.
[b] His-Purkinje fibers fan across subendocardial surface of ventricles from endocardium outward through the myocardium. As cardiac impulse spreads, these fibers cause ventricles to depolarize and contract.

▶ ELECTROCARDIOGRAM (ECG)

- Records the flow of electrical impulses through the heart.

See Figure 12–8 for ECG waves.

- To read ECG:
  - Remember that a single lead corresponds to an anatomic territory.
  - Look at multiple leads together for voltage abnormalities and axis deviations.
  - Look at a single lead for arrhythmias.

ECG Leads

Standard Bipolar	Standard Unipolar	Chest leads
I—right arm (−), left arm (+)	AVR—right arm (+)	V1, V2, V3, V4, V5, V6 represent 6 places along chest wall.
II—right arm (−) and left leg (+)	AVL—left arm (+)	
III—left arm (−) and left leg (+)	AVF—left leg (+)	

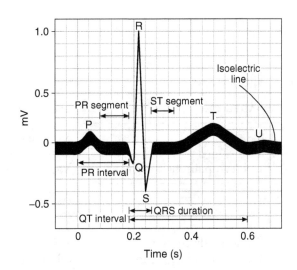

FIGURE 12-8. Waves of the ECG.

Reproduced, with permission, from Ganong WF. *Review of Medical Physiology*, 22nd ed. New York: McGraw-Hill, 2005.

QT = time between ventricular depolarization and repolarization

ECG of Partial Heart Block: PR prolonged with extra P before QRS

ECG Waves

P	PR Interval	QRS	ST Segment	T[a,b,c]
Atrial depolarization	Length between depolarization of atria and depolarization of ventricles (~0.16 s).	Ventricular depolarization. During phase 0, atrial repolarization occurs within QRS. Highest Na$^+$ influx; maximum ventricular Na$^+$ channel conductance. Shape of QRS complex is dictated by spread of the AP throughout the ventricular muscle.	Length corresponds to AP duration in ventricular muscle. Entire ventricle is depolarized. During phase 2, prolonged calcium conductance through slow channels.	Ventricular repolarization.
Prior to atrial contraction	Varies w/ HR (↑HR : ↓ PR).	Prior to contraction.	Isoelectric.	

[a] U wave is occasionally found in ECGs. This is caused by repolarization of papillary muscle, or it can be seen with hypokalemia.
[b] QT interval is the period between ventricular depolarization and repolarization (~0.35 s).
[c] The isoelectric point between T and P waves (ventricle is at resting membrane potential) occurs during ventricular diastole (when ventricle is filling with blood) and is shortened at high HRs.

Autonomic Control of the Heart

	Sympathetic	Parasympathetic
Control center	Medulla	Medulla
Nerve	T1–4 (sympathetic chain)	Vagus nerve (CN X)
NT	NE	ACh
HR	↑ ↑ SA nodal discharge ↑ Rate of depolarization through heart ↑ Intracellular Ca^{2+} ↑ Ventricular contraction force	↓ ↓ SA nodal discharge ↓ Rate of depolarization through heart

The right vagus nerve supplies the SA node; the left vagus nerve innervates the AV node.

Bainbridge Reflex

- Stretch of atria (with ↑ blood volume) causes ↑ HR and, therefore, ↑ CO.
- Mediated by stretch receptors in atria.
- Receptor cells are sensitive to pressure and stretch.
  - Mediated by vagal (CN X) afferents to the medulla.
    - Efferent loop is slowing of vagal output.
- Pumps more blood out of pulmonary system to the systemic system.
  - This helps prevent pulmonary edema.

Receptors

Receptor type	Baroreceptor	Chemoreceptor
Effect exerted	HR, BP	Respiration > vasomotor

Baroreceptors

- Modulate intravascular pressure and HR over a short time period.
- Activated by ↑ BP.
- Causes ↓ HR, vasodilation, ↓ BP.

BARORECEPTOR REFLEX (VALSALVA)

- ↑ BP/↑ stretch of baroreceptors → ↑ parasympathetic afferent output (CN IX, X) → medulla → ↑ vagal efferent tone (CN X) (↓ sympathetic tone) → ↓ HR, ↓ BP (vasodilation, venodilation) → ↓ CO.
- Antagonist to Bainbridge reflex.

Carotid Sinus[a]	Aortic Arch Baroreceptor[a]
Spindle-shaped dilation of receptors at the common carotid artery bifurcation (superior border of thyroid cartilage). Afferent = CN IX.	Receptors in the aortic arch. Afferent = CN X.

[a]These receptors are located in the adventitia of the vessels. They are extensively branched, knobby, coiled, and intertwined ends of myelinated nerve fibers (resemble Golgi tendon organs).

Stretch receptors in the atria and pulmonary circulations are stimulated by expansion of blood volume; they do not directly respond to changes in systemic arterial BP.

CAROTID SINUS SYNDROME

- Excessive stimulation of both carotid sinuses (eg, convulsive seizures) can lead to momentary loss of consciousness because of vagal discharge, venodilation, vasodilation.

RESPONSE TO SUDDEN STANDING

- $\downarrow$ BP in brain, upper body sensed by baroreceptors →
- $\downarrow$ parasympathetic firing (CN IX, X); (sympathetic discharge → $\uparrow$HR, $\uparrow$ conduction velocity, $\uparrow$ cardiac contractility, $\uparrow$ peripheral resistance $\uparrow$ vasoconstriction), $\downarrow$ renal blood flow $\uparrow\alpha_1$ vasocontriction of afferent artery; β_1 on JGA → $\uparrow$renin → $\uparrow$ angiotensin-II → aldosterone → $\uparrow$ blood back to heart ($\uparrow$preload because venoconstriction of large veins) → $\uparrow$ CO → return/maintain BP.

HEMORRHAGE OR HYPOVOLEMIA

COMPENSATIONS:

- Baroreceptor reflex ($\uparrow$ sympathetic, $\downarrow$ parasympathetic tone).
  - $\uparrow$ epinephrine from adrenal medulla.
  - $\downarrow$ vagal output from medulla ($\downarrow$ carotid sinus, $\downarrow$ aortic baroreceptor firing).
- RAAS (Renin-Angiotensin-Aldosterone system). See renal also.
  - AT-II, aldosterone and increase in TPR
    - AT-II: On efferent arteriole to preserve GFR.
    - Aldosterone: On cortical collecting duct, increase Na^+ reabsorption, K^+ excretion, H^+ secretion by intercalated cells.
- ADH
  - Capillary fluid shift
    - Increases water reabsorption in CCD.

Bainbridge reflex stimulated by stretch of atria versus Hering Breuer reflex which

- Prevents overinflation of lungs
- Pulmonary stretch receptors of smooth muscle in airways respond to excessive stretching
- Action potentials through vagus afferents to medulla and pons
- Inspiration inhibited and expiration occurs

Chemoreceptors

- Detect changes in blood oxygen, carbon dioxide, and hydrogen ion concentrations.
- Modulate respiratory center in brain (regulate respiratory activity).

Carotid Body	Aortic Body
Afferent CN IX	Afferent CN X

CHEMORECEPTOR PATHWAY

- See also Chapter 13, "Respiratory Physiology."
- $\uparrow CO_2$, $\uparrow H^+$, and/or $\downarrow O_2$ → stimulates chemoreceptors (carotid, aortic bodies) → $\uparrow$ parasympathetic afferent output (CN IX, X) → medulla (respiratory center) → $\uparrow$ ventilation (to breathe down CO_2) → ($\uparrow$ BP, $\uparrow$ HR secondary to simultaneous secretion of catecholamines from the adrenal medulla).
  - Increase in sensitivity to CO_2 and pH when <60 mm Hg.

Hormonal Regulation Systems

See Chapter 14, "Renal, Fluid, Acid–Base Physiology."

Exercise

- Mechanisms to meet $\uparrow$ demand to muscles during exercise ($\uparrow$ supply).
- $\uparrow$ CO because $\uparrow$ HR and $\uparrow$ SV.
- Sympathetic nervous system.
  - β_2 adrenergic receptors in muscle/pulmonary tree
    - Vasodilate
    - $\uparrow$ Blood flow to muscles
  - β_1 receptors in heart
    - $\uparrow$ HR
    - $\uparrow$ Contraction force (inotropic) (phospholumbar "releasing brake" on SERCA pump)
    - $\uparrow$ CO
  - α_1 in other parts of body
    - Vasoconstriction
    - $\uparrow$ Arterial pressure
- Enhanced venous return ($\uparrow$ preload).
  - $\downarrow$ Venous compliance
  - Pumping effect of the skeletal muscle
  - Vasoconstriction
- Local metabolites (released as $O_2 \downarrow 0$).
  - Adenosine, CO_2, lactic acid
    - Vasodilate: $\downarrow$ vascular resistance, $\uparrow$ blood flow

AUTOREGULATION OF BLOOD FLOW

- As blood flow $\uparrow$ to muscles during exercise, the adenosine is washed out.
- $\downarrow$ adenosine → arterioles and small arteries vasoconstrict → keeping blood flow at a normal rate (in face of $\uparrow$ arterial pressure).

Note: During exercise $\uparrow$ CO is slightly > $\downarrow$ TPR, so MAP $\uparrow$.

During exercise initially $\uparrow$ SV, then later $\uparrow$ HR (which is important, >50% of maximal work capacity is reached).

SVR $\downarrow$ during exercise (vasodilation, β_2, local metabolites). Blood flow to skeletal muscle can increase 20-fold during strenuous exercise.

► HEMATOCRIT (Hct)

- Percentage of RBCs in blood sample.
- Normal:
  - Male: 44–46.
  - Female: 40–42.
- Venous Hct is typically higher than arterial Hct because of "chloride shift."
  - More RBC mass in comparison to plasma. CO_2 from tissues gets converted by carbonic anhydrase → HCO_3 in RBC increases osmotic pressure → water rushes in → RBC greater volume

- See also Chapter 6, "Biological Compounds" and Chapter 13, "Respiratory Physiology," for discussion of hemoglobin (Hb).
- Normal:
  - Male: 15–16 g/dL.
  - Female: 13–14 g/dL.
- Severe anemia:
  - <7.5 g/dL.
  - $Hct = Hb \times 3$.

▶ ANEMIA

- ↓ Hct.
- ↓ RBC and/or ↓ Hb concentration.

Consequences of Anemia

- ↓ oxygen transport in blood.
- Fatigue, respiratory compensation, cardiac compensation.
- Hypoxia in the tissues.
  - Causes small arteries and arterioles to dilate (so ↑ blood return to the heart [preload]).
- Hypoxia in the pulmonary circulation results in vasoconstriction of those vessels (opposite to effect on other body tissues).

Compensations with Anemia

Cardiac Compensation	Respiratory Compensation
↑ CO	Bohr effect
Chemoreceptors sense ↓O_2	O_2–Hb curve shifts to the right ($\rightarrow$)
↑SV (↑ pulse pressure)	Unloads more O_2 to the tissues
↑HR (try to deliver more O_2 to tissues)	↑2, 3-DPG
↓Hct → ↓blood viscosity	↑CO_2
↓ resistance to flow → ↓ PVR	↑RBC H^+
↑ blood returns to the heart (↑ preload) (helps to increase SV)	

Types of Anemia and Associated Cell Size

↓ Production	↑ Destruction
Fe deficiency (microcytic)	Blood loss (normocytic)
Folate deficiency (megaloblastic) or macrocytic	Hemolysis (normocytic)
B_{12} deficiency (megaloblastic) or macrocytic	Hemoglobinopathies (microcytic)

Carbon Monoxide Poisoning

- CO competes with oxygen for Hb-binding sites and changes allosterics; CO has greater affinity (250×)
- Normal Hb level
- O_2 content ↓
  - Cherry red cheeks

Cyanosis

- Deoxygenated hemoglobin in tissues gives the skin/mucous membranes a blue tint.
- Does **not** occur in severe anemia because you need >5 g of deoxygenated Hb per 100 mL of blood to appreciate.

- Glycoprotein hormone produced in kidneys
- ↑ RBC production by bone marrow
- Acts at the hemocytoblast (pluripotent stem cell)
- ↓ Erythropoiesis → **anemia**
- ↑ Erythropoiesis → **polycythemia**
    - ↑ Blood viscosity, sluggish blood flow, ie, polycythemia vera (JAK2 mutation downstream of Epo Receptor)

Negative Feedback

- ↓ O_2 tension (anoxia/hypoxia) → ↑erythropoietin (HIF)
- ↑ O_2 → ↓ erythropoietin

Virchow's Triad

- Endothelial injury
- Stasis
- Hypercoaguability

Tissue factor (tissue thromboplastin) is part of the extrinsic pathway (it is not present in blood).

Hemostasis

- Three parts:
    - Vasoconstriction
    - Platelet aggregation/plug (primary)—platelets bind wWF on damaged endothelium
    - Coagulation (secondary)—crosslinking with fibrin meshwork

Coagulation

See Figure 12–9.

- Intrinsic and extrinsic pathways
  - Prothrombin is cleaved to thrombin.
    - Converted by prothrombin activator (Factor V_a).
  - Fibrinogen cleaved to fibrin.
    - Converted by thrombin.
  - Fibrin forms the clot and cross-links with the platelets.

Both intrinsic and extrinsic pathways are activated when blood vessels are damaged.

In cirrhosis, proteins, including prothrombin and fibrinogen, are deficient.

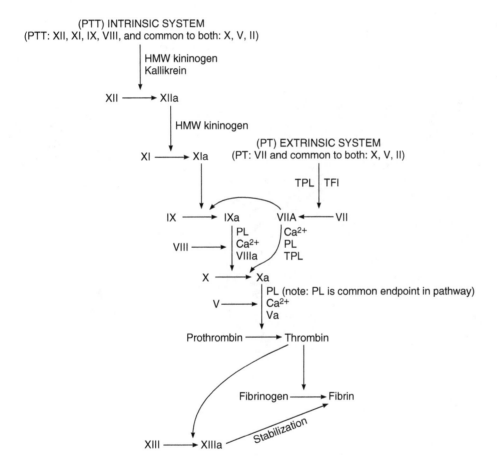

FIGURE 12–9. Intrinsic and extrinsic pathways of coagulation.

Reproduced, with permission, from Ganong WF. *Review of Medical Physiology*, 22nd ed. New York: McGraw-Hill, 2005.

Respiratory Physiology

See Figure 13–1.

- Total lung volume (TLV) = IRV + TV + ERV + RV.
- Vital capacity (VC) = TLV − RV.

Lung Volumes

Inspiratory reserve volume (IRV)	Air inspired with maximal inspiratory effort (after inspiring at TV).	**Inspiratory capacity (IC)**	Maximum air inspired up to TLC (limited by elastic recoil of lung) (TV + IRV).
Tidal volume (TV)	Air inspired or expired with a normal breath.		
Expiratory reserve volume (ERV)	Air pushed out after passive expiration (FRC − RV).	**Functional residual capacity (FRC)**	Air left in lungs after a normal passive expiration (ERV + RV).
Residual volume (RV)	Air remaining in lungs after maximal exhalation; cannot be measured by spirometry.		

RV is increased in older individuals and in chronic obstructive pulmonary disease (COPD) or asthma because of air trapping.

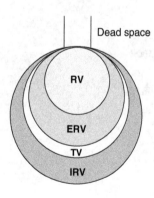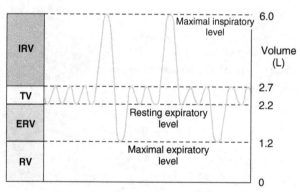

IRV = Inspiratory reserve volume TV = Tidal volume
ERV = Expiratory reserve volume RV = Residual volume

FIGURE 13–1. Lung volumes.

Reproduced, with permission, from Ganong WF. *Review of Medical Physiology*, 22nd ed. New York: McGraw-Hill, 2005.

Inspiration

- Active process
  - Requires muscular effort.
    - Mostly diaphragm at rest.
    - Intercostals used on exertion (accessory muscles).
- Inspiratory effort causes:
  - ↓ intrapleural pressure.
  - ↓ alveolar pressure.
  - Pressure gradient from mouth to alveoli.
  - Gas flow down pressure gradient.

Expiration

- Passive process (usually).
  - Due to lung recoil.
- Relaxation of inspiratory muscles causes:
  - ↑ intrapleural pressure (intrapleural pressure becomes less negative).
  - ↑ alveolar pressure.
  - Pressure gradient from alveoli to mouth.
  - Gas flow down pressure gradient.

FUNCTIONAL RESIDUAL CAPACITY

- FRC = At rest.
- Balance between inspiratory and expiratory forces.
  - Collapsing forces = Expanding forces.
- Muscle contraction is needed to ↑ or ↓ lung volume from FRC.

Collapsing Forces	Expanding Forces
Favors ↓ lung volume.	Favors ↑ lung volume.
・Elastic connective tissue of the lungs	・Elastic connective tissue of chest wall
↑ Surface tension helps *counteract* collapse.	
・Surfactant coating the alveoli	

ALVEOLAR PRESSURE

- Atmospheric pressure in resting position.
- 760 mm Hg (at FRC). $P_{alv} = 0$ mm Hg

INTRAPLEURAL PRESSURE

- Pressure within pleural cavity between outer surface lung and inner surface chest cavity.
- 756 mm Hg (at FRC) (< atomospheric pressure). $P_{pl} = -34$ mm Hg

Accessory muscles of inspiration:

- Scalene
- SCM
- Trapezium
- External intercostals

Accessory muscles of expiration:

- Intercostals (internal)
- Abdominal

VC = greatest amount of air that one can exchange in a forced respiration (inhalation + expiration).

ALVEOLAR VENTILATION

- (V_A) = RR × (TV – dead space air volume).
- Amount of gas that reaches the functional respiratory units (ie, alveoli) per minute.
- Amount of atmospheric air that can undergo gas exchange.
- Good gauge for breathing effectiveness.

RESPIRATORY RATE

- Breaths per minute.

TIDAL VOLUME

- TV = amount of air brought into/out of lungs with a normal breath.
- 500 mL.
  - 350 mL used for alveolar ventilation.
  - 150 mL dead space (fixed due to conducting airways).

DEAD SPACE

- V_D = Volume of air not participating in gas exchange.
- Anatomic dead space.
  - Typically 150 mL.
  - Volume of nonventilated gas in airways.
  - No gas exchange occurs within the nasal passages, pharynx, trachea, bronchi.
- Physiologic dead space.
  - Due to alveoli that are ventilated but not perfused.
  - Usually insignificant, unless there is disease.

MINUTE VENTILATION

- TV × RR = V_T.

ZONES OF THE LUNG

Conducting zone
(no gas exchange)
	Trachea
	Main bronchi 2 – left, 3 – right
	  lobar, segmental
	Bronchioles
	  (first place w/o cartilage)
	Terminal bronchioles

Respiratory zone (gas exchange occurs)	Respiratory bronchioles Alveoli

- Conducting zone airways contain mucous-secreting cells:
  - Goblet cells
  - Mucous cells
  - The epithelium is pseudostratified ciliated columnar.

- Respiratory zone, alveolar wall has:
  - Type I epithelial cells
  - Type II epithelial cells ↓ pneumocytes
    - Produce surfactant
  - See also Chapter 2

▶ GAS EXCHANGE IN THE LUNGS

- O_2 uptake, CO_2 elimination by the blood
  - O_2 diffusion (alveolus → blood)
  - CO_2 diffusion (alveolus ← blood)
- Depends on:
  - **Partial pressure gradient**
    - Pressure difference between two sides of the membrane.
    - Diffusion occurs from high to low pressure (down the gradient).
      - $P_ACO_2 > PaO_2$ (alveolar > pulmonary arterial); O_2 diffuses from alveoli → blood.
      - P_aCO_2 blood > P_ACO_2 in alveolus; CO_2 diffuses from blood → alveoli.
  - **Gas solubility**
    - Number of molecules dissolved in the liquid ↑ partial pressure of gas ↑.
    - Solubility is an intrinsic property of the gas.
    - Solubility ↑ as partial pressure ↑ (Henry's law). CO_2 more soluble than O_2.
  - **Thickness of membrane** (alveolus)
    - Rate of diffusion is inversely proportional to the diffusion distance.
      - ↑ diffusion as ↓ alveolar thickness.
  - **Alveolar surface area**
    - Rate of diffusion is directly proportional to surface area.
      - ↓ surface area (eg, emphysema), ↓ diffusion, ↓ gas exchange.

More CO_2 (HCO_3) in venous RBC →↑osmotic pressure →↑ water content →↑ volume of RBC, increased HC+??

▶ HEMOGLOBIN

- See also Biological Compounds, Chapter 6.
- Carries O_2 from lungs to tissues.
- Carries CO_2 from tissues to lungs.
- Normally:
  - 98% saturated with O_2 in lungs (arterial).
  - 75% saturated in tissues (venous).
    - $PaO_2 = 40$ mm Hg
  - 300 million Hb molecules in each erythrocyte.
    - Synthesis begins in erythroblasts.

O_2-Hb Dissociation Curve

See Figure 13–2.

The PO_2 determines the affinity of Hb for O_2 binding by causing a conformational change of Hb. Each O_2 binding increases the affinity for O_2 stepwise.

30 mm Hg → 50%

60 mm Hg → 90%

90 mm Hg → 99%

CO has 240 times the affinity for Hb as O_2 does. It, therefore, interferes with unloading of O_2 from Hb.

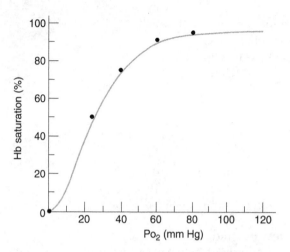

FIGURE 13-2. **Oxygen-hemoglobin dissociation curve for human blood at 37°C with a PO$_2$ of 40 mm Hg, a pH of 7.40, and a normal 2,3-DPG red cell concentration.**

Reproduced, with permission, from Doherty GM. *Current Surgical Diagnosis & Treatment*, 12th ed. New York: McGraw-Hill, 2006: 203.

2, 3-DPG is a product of glycolysis via the Ebden–Myerhoff pathway (see biochemistry section).

Shift	Left Shift	Right Shift
Effect	Favors O$_2$ uptake (eg, at lungs)	Favors O$_2$ release (to tissues)
Causes	↑ pH ↓ 2, 3-DPG ↓ temperature CO When PO$_2$ is low, Hb has a greater affinity for O$_2$ binding at the lungs (For a given PO$_2$, Hb is more saturated)	↓ pH ↑ PCO$_2$ ↑ 2, 3-DPG ↑ temperature When PO$_2$ is high, Hb does not bind O$_2$ as readily. O$_2$ is released to the tissues. Exercising muscle: Temperature ↑, pH goes ↓ (lactic acid ↑), 2, 3-DPG ↑

Example: O$_2$-Hb curve shifts to the right (→) in anemia. This helps unload O$_2$ to the tissues. It occurs because there is ↑ 2, 3-DPG, ↑ CO$_2$, and ↑ RBC H$^+$'s (↓ pH).

Bohr Effect

Curve shifts right (→) in an acidic environment (↓ pH) to help unload O$_2$ to the tissues.

- Hb has decreased affinity for O$_2$ when pH ↓.
- H$^+$'s ↑ as pH ↓.
- The H$^+$'s bond more actively to deoxygenated Hb than to oxyhemoglobin.
- As CO$_2$ ↑, pH ↓, curve shifts to the right (→).

Haldane Effect

- Oxygen tension affects the affinity of Hb for CO$_2$.
- High oxygen tension—lungs:
  - Hb ↑ O$_2$ binding; ↓ affinity for CO$_2$.
    - CO$_2$ released in the lungs (as ↑ O$_2$–Hb).

374

- Low oxygen tension—tissues:
  - Hb $\downarrow$ O$_2$ binding; $\uparrow$ affinity for CO$_2$ (binds H$^+$, forms carbamino compounds).
  - CO$_2$ uptake in the tissues (as $\downarrow$ O$_2$–Hb).

Amount of O$_2$ in Blood

- Dissolved O$_2$ + O$_2$ bound to Hb.

Dissolved O$_2$	O$_2$–Hb

Partial pressure of O$_2$ in blood (PO$_2$).
 Small fraction of the total O$_2$ carried in the blood.
     • 0.003 mL/dL blood/mm Hg PO$_2$.
	Hb + O$_2$ $\leftrightarrow$ HbO$_2$
	 Hb4(O$_2$)4
	 Hb-O$_2$ depends on:
	     • PO$_2$.
	 O$_2$ content (pulmonary function, anemia).
	 Hb concentration.
	     • Hb affinity for O$_2$.
	 %Hb bound with O$_2$ = O$_2$ saturation.

OXYGEN CONTENT

- Total amount of oxygen carried in blood (PO$_2$ + O$_2$–Hb).
- Determined mostly by the amount of hemoglobin and its saturation.
- Amount of hemoglobin is affected by anemia (production, loss, or destruction).
- The more hemoglobin in blood, the more O$_2$ that can be carried.

OXYGEN SATURATION

- The amount of Hb saturated with O$_2$.
- Corresponds to O$_2$–Hb curve.
- Determined by:
  - PO$_2$ (important; see table corresponding SaO$_2$: PO$_2$).
  - O$_2$ affinity of Hb altered by:
    - Changes in Hb molecule.
      - Intrinsic (hemoglobinopathies).
      - Extrinsic (eg, changes in pH, PCO$_2$, temperature, etc.).
      - Competition for Hb binding (eg, CO poisoning).

NORMAL VALUES

- Oxygen content (per 1 g Hb) = 1.34 mL of O$_2$.
- Hemoglobin concentration = ~15 g/dL.
  - Women: 12–16 g/dL.
    - Women have $\downarrow$ Hb concentrations than men
  - Men: 14–18 g/dL.
  - Infants: 14–20 g/dL.
- Oxygen concentration = ~20 g-mL/dL (or 15 g/dL × 1.34 mL)—just 20.1 mL.

Venous blood carries more CO$_2$ than arterial blood, and CO$_2$ uptake is facilitated in the tissues and CO$_2$ release is facilitated in the lungs.

AV fistula: Venous PCO$_2$ is lower than normal (because it bypassed the tissues); likewise venous PO$_2$ is higher (some O$_2$ is not dropped off at the tissues).

Blood Hb concentration does not affect O$_2$ saturation of Hb or PaO$_2$ (both PaO$_2$ and SaO$_2$ are independent of the Hb concentration).

With anemia, $\uparrow$ CO as compensation to maintain adequate oxygenation to the tissues.

OXYGEN-CARRYING CAPACITY OF BLOOD

Depends on:

- Oxygenation (from lungs).
    - FiO_2.
    - PaO_2 (gradient).
    - Effective gas exchange (no dead space or shunt).
- Hb concentration.
- Hb avidity for oxygen.
    - CO.
    - Left shift of curve.
- Perfusion.
    - Cardiac function.
    - Patency of vessels.
    - Adequacy of forward flow.

Carbon Dioxide

See Figure 13–3.

- Carbon dioxide (CO_2) is carried in blood as:
    - **Bicarbonate in serum** (most).
    - Bicarbonate in RBC.
    - Carbaminohemoglobin.
        - CO_2^+ NH_2 group of Heme (**not** Fe^{2+} of Heme like O_2 or CO).
    - Dissolved in blood (PCO_2).

Carbonic anhydrase is not present in the serum. Bicarbonate can be produced in serum by nonenzymatic means, but the process is slow.

CHLORIDE SHIFT

- Bicarbonate carried in serum is generated within the RBC.
- It is transported to the serum in exchange for Cl^-.
- Cycle:
    - CO_2 in blood diffuses passively into RBC.
    - Carbonic anhydrase (within RBC) combines intracellular CO_2 with H_2O to form bicarbonate and H^+.
    - Bicarbonate passes across the RBC membrane into serum in exchange for Cl^-.

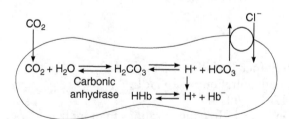

FIGURE 13-3. Carbon dioxide (CO_2) as carried in the blood.

Reproduced, with permission, from Ganong WF. *Review of Medical Physiology*, 22nd ed. New York: McGraw-Hill, 2005.

Causes of Hypoxemia

↓ FiO$_2$	Hypoventilation	V/Q Mismatch	Shunt	Diffusion Limitation (↓ DLCO)
↓ fraction of inspired O$_2$ (usually 21%). ▫ High altitude ▫ Incorrect ventilator settings	↓ respiratory drive (central) ▫ Narcotics ▫ Medullary injury ↓ ability for chest excursion (peripheral) ▫ Polio ▫ Chest trauma (rib fracture) ▫ Diaphragmatic injury ▫ Phrenic nerve paralysis	Unequal ventilation and perfusion Segment of lung is ventilated but not perfused (= dead space) Asthma ▫ COPD ▫ Interstitial lung disease ▫ Alveolar disease ▫ Pulmonary vascular disease	Segment of lung is perfused but not aerated. Intraalveolar filling ▫ Atelectasis ▫ Pneumonia ▫ Pulmonary edema ▫ Intracardiac shunt ▫ Vascular shunt	↓ surface area of blood gas barrier. ▫ Pneumonectomy ▫ Emphysema Thick blood–gas barrier ▫ Diffuse interstitial fibrosis ▫ Sarcoidosis ▫ Asbestosis ▫ ARDS ↓ Hb to carry oxygen ▫ Anemia ▫ PE

Hypoxemia

- ▫ Low oxygen level in blood (PO$_2$ <80).
- ▫ Causes of hypoxemia:
  - ▫ ↓ FiO$_2$
  - ▫ Hypoventilation
  - ▫ V/Q mismatch
  - ▫ Shunt
  - ▫ Diffusion limitation

Hypoxemia in COPD is secondary to both hypoventilation (↑ PCO) and V/Q mismatch (A-a gradient).

HYPOXIC VASOCONSTRICTION

- ▫ Mechanism to minimize V/Q mismatch.
- ▫ Example:
  - ▫ Shunt (air cannot get into alveolus).
    - ▫ Peanut occluding bronchiole (child).
    - ▫ Atelectasis.
  - ▫ Blood perfuses past the alveolus.
  - ▫ No/minimal gas exchange occurs.
  - ▫ Response is vasoconstriction of the pulmonary vasculature in that region.
    - ▫ ↓ amount of blood going to nonventilated segment of lung.
  - ▫ If this vasoconstriction secondary to hypoxia exists for long enough,
    - ▫ Get permanent secondary changes to the pulmonary vasculature.
    - ▫ Pulmonary hypertension.
    - ▫ Only place in body to constrict, not dilate.

Extreme hypercarbia (CO_2 ↑↑) depresses the CNS (including respiratory center) whereby respiratory compensation does not occur. Result is CO_2 narcosis.

Hypercarbia

- ↑ CO_2 in blood.
- Occurs because of either or both of the following:
  - ↑ CO_2 production.
  - ↓ V_A (alveolar ventilation)—hypoventilation.
- Compensation: hyperventilation.
- Headache.
- Confusion.
- Coma.

Hyperventilation

- ↑ rate and depth of breathing exceeding requirement for O_2 delivery and CO_2 removal
- Stimulated by:
  - **↓ PO_2 in normal circumstances** (non-COPD).
  - Chemoreceptor stimulation (↑CO_2, ↑H^+, ↓PO_2).
  - Effect on brain—emotional situations, anxiety.
- Results in:
  - ↓ CO_2: hypocapnia (hypocarbia).
  - Respiratory alkalosis (pH ↑).
  - ↑cerebrovascular resistance.
  - ↓ cerebral blood flow.
  - ↑PO_2 (and arterial oxygen concentration).

Effect of CO_2 on Cerebral Circulation

↑ PCO_2	↓ PCO_2
Vasodilation → ↑ cerebral blood flow.	Vasoconstriction → ↓ cerebral blood flow.

In shock, hyperventilation is caused by chemoreceptor stimulation (secondary to ↓ PO_2 (hypoxia) and ↑ H^+ (acidosis)) because of local stagnation of blood flow.

SYMPTOMS OF HYPERVENTILATION

- Related to ↓ cerebral blood flow.
- Example: anxiety → ↑ventilation → ↓ CO_2 → ↓ cerebral blood flow → neurologic symptoms:
  - Faintness/dizziness.
  - Blurred vision.
  - Also experience sensation of:
    - Suffocation.
    - Chest tightness.
- Terminate hyperventilation attack must:
  - ↑ PCO_2.
    - Breathing in and out of a plastic bag.
    - Inhale 5% CO_2 mixture.

Respiratory Drive

- Based on arterial PCO_2, specifically H^+.
- The H^+ (derived from CO_2) that acts at central chemoreceptors (medulla).

PATHWAY

- As $\uparrow PCO_2 \rightarrow CO_2$ diffuses from cerebral blood vessels into CSF → carbonic acid (H_2CO_3) is formed → dissociates into bicarbonate (HCO_3^-) and protons ($H+s$) → these protons ($H+s$) stimulate the central chemoreceptors → $\uparrow$ventilation.
  - CO_2 can diffuse from the blood vessels into CSF across the BBB because it is nonpolar.

$\uparrow$*RESPIRATORY DRIVE*

- Central chemoreceptors (medulla)
  - $\uparrow PCO_2$ (as its byproduct, H^+, in CSF or brain interstitial fluid sensed in medulla).
- Peripheral chemoreceptors (carotid or aortic bodies)
  - $\uparrow H^+$ (in blood or brain interstitial fluid).
  - $\downarrow PO_2$ (in blood)(<60 mm Hg).

FUNCTION OF RESPIRATORY REGULATION

- Keep alveolar PCO_2 stable (prevent hypercarbia or hypocarbia).
- Buffer acid–base changes.
- Prevent hypoxemia ($\uparrow PO_2$ when it falls).

$\uparrow PCO_2$ ($\uparrow H^+$ sensed in medulla) → $\uparrow$ respiration (blow off more CO_2) → $\downarrow PCO_2$ → $\downarrow$ respiration.

$\downarrow$ inspired O_2 has no effect on respiratory drive unless O_2 is <60 mm Hg; then it stimulates carotid and aortic chemoreceptors, resulting in $\uparrow$ respiration.

Respiratory Chemoreceptors

Receptors	Central Medullary chemoreceptors	Peripheral Carotid and aortic bodies (see Figure 13–4).
Affected by	$\uparrow H^+$ CSF, brain interstitial fluid. Major regulators of ventilation. **Not** respond to PO_2. **Not** respond to arterial PCO_2; it is PCO_2 that diffuses across into CSF then is converted to H^+.	$\uparrow PCO_2$. $\uparrow H^+$. $\downarrow PO_2$ (<60 mm Hg). Less important than central chemoreceptors (medulla). However, they respond more quickly and regulate abrupt changes in PCO_2.

	Carotid Body	**Aortic Body**
Afferent	CN IX	CN X
Efferent	Phrenic, intercostals nerves	Phrenic, intercostals nerves

Distinguish carotid and aortic bodies from carotid sinus and aortic baroreceptors (the latter two control changes in blood pressure and HR). CN IX (glossopharyngeal) provides afferent innervation for both carotid body and carotid sinus; CN X (vagus) is afferent for both aortic body and aortic baroreceptors.

Body = chemoreceptors
Sinus = baroreceptors

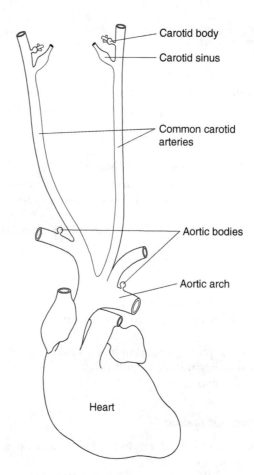

FIGURE 13–4.   Carotid and aortic bodies.

Reproduced, with permission, from Ganong WF. *Review of Medical Physiology*, 22nd ed. New York: McGraw-Hill, 2005.

Acid–Base Balance and Respiratory Changes

- See chart in Chapter 14.
- Primary respiratory processes: respiratory acidosis and alkalosis → metabolic compensation.
- Primary metabolic processes: metabolic acidosis and alkalosis → respiratory compensation.

Primary Metabolic Process	Respiratory Compensation	Mechanism
Metabolic acidosis. ▪ Diabetic ketoacidosis. ▪ Kussmaul breathing (deep, labored).	↑ respiration (hyperventilate). ▪ Blow off CO_2. ▪ ↓ alveolar CO_2. *Respiratory alkalosis.*	↑ H^+ stimulates central and peripheral chemoreceptors.

Metabolic alkalosis.
 ▪ ↓ HCL.
    ▪ Vomiting.
    NG suctioning.
	↓ respiration (hypoventilate).
	 ▪ ↑ alveolar CO_2.
	 ▪ ↑ H^+.
	 Respiratory acidosis.
	    ▪ pCO_2 elevated, not enough blown off.
		↓ H^+ ↓ stimulation to the central and peripheral chemoreceptors.

Hering–Breuer Reflex (Reflex to Prevent Overinflation)

- Inflate lungs → expiration.
- Deflate lungs → inspiration.
- Mediated by myelinated slow responding receptors (stretch receptors).
- Vagus nerve (afferent).

Pulmonary Chemoreflex

- Lung hyperinflation causes:
  - First apnea.
  - Then:
    - Rapid breathing (tachypnea).
    - Bradycardia.
    - Hypotension.
  - Mediated by:
    - J (juxtacapillary) (vagus nerve) receptors—in alveolar insterstitium.
      - C fiber endings (unmyelinated) close to pulmonary vessels ↓ O_2, hyperinflation, chemical administration.

The pulmonary chemoreflex is analogous to the Bezold–Jarisch reflex in the heart.

Pulmonary capillaries (endothelial cells and alveolar capillary bed) contain ACE (angiotensin-converting enzyme). ACE converts angiontensin-I to angiotensin-II (RAAS system).

	Stretch Receptors	J Receptors	Irritant Receptors
Located	Airway smooth muscle	Alveolar walls	Between airway epithelial cells
Stimulated by	Lung distention	Engorgement of capillary or alveolar walls with fluid pulmonary edema, pneumonia (eg, CHF)	Noxious substances (eg, dust, pollen) Histamine
Causes	Expiration (prevents overinflation; Hering–Breuer reflex)	Rapid shallow breathing Pulmonary chemoreflex	Coughing, bronchoconstriction

Respiratory Conditions

Condition	Description
Dyspnea	Difficulty breathing; unpleasant sensation.
Apnea	Cessation of breathing, usually transient (central versus peripheral).
Hyperapnea	Abnormally deep and rapid breathing.
Hypercapnia	$\uparrow CO_2$ in arterial blood, secondary to underbreathing ($\downarrow$ ventilation).
Hypocapnia	$\downarrow CO_2$ in arterial blood, secondary to overbreathing ($\uparrow$ ventilation).
Respiratory arrest	Cessation of breathing.
Hyperventilation	$\uparrow$ alveolar ventilation (greater than metabolic requirements); leads to $\downarrow PCO_2$ (with $\downarrow$ cerebral perfusion, fainting/syncope).
Hypoventilation	$\downarrow$ alveolar ventilation (less than needed for metabolic requirements); leads to $\uparrow PCO_2$.

Kussmaul breathing is rapid deep labored breathing in people with acidosis, in particular diabetic ketoacidosis.

High Altitude

- $\downarrow FiO_2$
- Results in:
  - Alveolar hypoxia ($\downarrow P_AO_2$).
  - Arterial hypoxemia ($\downarrow PaO_2$).
  - Secondary to $\downarrow$ barometric pressure.
- Compensation:
  - Pulmonary vasoconstriction (because of alveolar hypoxia).
  - $\uparrow$ erythropoietin ($\uparrow$ Hct, $\uparrow O_2$-carrying capacity).
  - $\uparrow$ mitochondrial density.
  - $\uparrow$ 2, 3-DPG (shifting O_2–Hb curve to the right, release O_2 to tissues).
  - $\uparrow$ respiratory rate (because of arterial hypoxia, secondary to $\downarrow$ barometric pressure; sensed by *peripheral chemoreceptors*; feeding back to medulla to $\uparrow$ respiratory rate).
  - Respiratory alkalosis (secondary to $\uparrow$ RR).
  - $\uparrow$ renal bicarbonate excretion, $\downarrow$ in H^+ excretion (compensation for respiratory alkalosis).

Renal, Fluid, and Acid–Base Physiology

Total Body Water

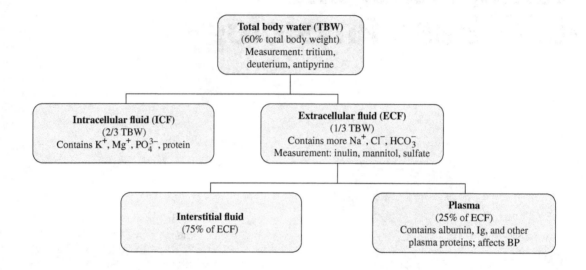

*Skin epidermis is nourished by
way of diffusion of interstitial
fluid (tissue fluid) from
capillary beds in the dermis;
this fluid bathes the cells.*

Intra- and Extracellular Fluids

	Extracellular Fluid	Intracellular Fluid
$[Na^+]$	142	10
$[K^+]$	4	140
%Body weight	15–20	35–40
Components (%BW)	Blood plasma (4–5)	NA
	Interstitial fluid (11–15)	
	Transcellular fluid	
	▪ CSF	
	▪ Intraocular	
	▪ Synovial	
	▪ Pericardial	
	▪ Pleural	
	▪ Peritoneal	

Starling Forces

- Forces that move fluid
  - Hydrostatic pressure
  - Oncotic pressure
- Fluid equilibrates between the intravascular and interstitial spaces.
- Fluid in the interstitial space
  - Is taken up by cells (becomes intracellular fluid)
  - Returns to the capillaries or
  - Returns to circulation via lymphatics.

Balance of Fluids

Hydrostatic Pressure	Oncotic Pressure (Colloid Osmotic Pressure)
"push"	"pull"
Force created by the column of fluid (water force promoting movement from one space to the other)	Force exerted by proteins, large molecules (that do not themselves readily diffuse)
"Water pushes toward the other space"	"Pulls water toward the protein"

- These forces force water from the intravascular space to interstitium or vice versa. Both hydrostatic and oncotic pressure exist for the intravascular space and the interstitium.
  - A combination of these forces dictates the movement of fluid.
  - **Fluid movement** = $k[(P_c + \pi_i) - (P_i + \pi_c)]$.
    - k = capillary perfusion coefficient.
    - P_c = capillary hydrostatic pressure.
    - π_i = interstitial oncotic pressure.
    - π_c = capillary oncotic pressure.
    - P_i = interstitial hydrostatic pressure.
- Promote fluid from capillaries to interstitium: $P_c + \pi_i$.
- Promote fluid from interstitium to capillaries: $P_i + \pi_c$.
- See Figure 14–1 for fluid capillary exchange.

See discussion of plasma proteins in Chapter 6, Biological Compounds.

Osmosis

See Figure 14–2.

- **Osmosis:** *Simple diffusion* of **water** caused by a concentration gradient.
- **Osmotic pressure:** The pressure developed as a result of net osmosis into a solution; depends on the *number* of solute particles present.
- **Osmolarity:** Osmotic pressure expressed in osmols/kg of *solution*.
- **Osmolality:** Osmotic pressure expressed in osmols/kg of *water*.

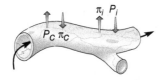

FIGURE 14–1. Fluid capillary exchange.

Reproduced, with permission, from Bhushan V, et al. *First Aid for the USMLE Step 1:* 2006. New York: McGraw-Hill, 2006.

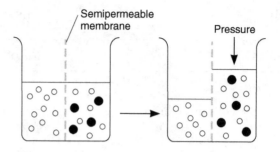

FIGURE 14-2. Osmosis.

Reproduced, with permission, from Ganong WF. *Review of Medical Physiology,* 22nd ed. New York: McGraw-Hill, 2005.

> *Nephrotic syndrome is defined by > 3.5 g protein in urine per day.*

▶ EDEMA

▪ Excess fluid in the interstitial space

Cause	↑ P_c	↓ π_c	↑ π_i	↓ P_i
Examples	CHF Cirrhosis	Nephrotic syndrome Protein-losing enteropathy Cirrhosis Malnutrition	Lymphatic blockage ▪ Elephantiasis ▪ Lymph node resection	

OTHER CAUSES OF EDEMA

▪ Increased capillary permeability (burns, sepsis, anaphylaxis/angioedema, ARDS).
▪ Inappropriate renal sodium and water retention.

Volume Expansion and Contraction

EXTRACELLULAR FLUID (ECF) EXPANSION

▪ Excess fluid in the intervascular or interstitial spaces.
▪ Evidence in physical examination.
  ▪ Rales
  ▪ Edema
  ▪ Hypertension
  ▪ Bulging fontanelle

> *SIADH: Syndrome of Inappropriate ADH Secretion. Excessive release of ADH from posterior pituitary or another source and usually caused by cancer.*

INTRACELLULAR FLUID (ICF) EXPANSION

▪ Excess fluid intracellularly.
▪ Gauged by serum Na^+.
  ▪ Low serum Na^+ = intracellular expansion.
  ▪ If chronic, formation of intracellular osmolytes prevents drastic influx of H_2O and cell burst.

Expansion (Overall Gain)	Examples	ECF Volume	ICF Volume	ECF Osmolarity	Hct	[Na⁺]	[Albumin]	UNa⁺ (Urinary Sodium Concentration)
(Hypo-) H_2O > Na^+	SIADH	↑	↑	↓	↓	↓	↓	↑
(Iso-) H_2O = Na^+	Isotonic NS	↑	–	–	↓	–	↓	↑
(Hyper-) H_2O < Na^+	Hypertonic NS	↑	↓	↑	↓	↑	↓	↑

Contraction (Overall Loss)	Examples	ECF Volume	ICF Volume	ECF Osmolarity	Hct	[Na⁺]	[Albumin]	UNa⁺
(Hyper-) loss H_2O > Na^+	Sweating, fever, DI	↓	↓	↑	↑	↑	↑	↓
(Iso-) H_2O = Na^+	Diarrhea	↓	–	–	↑	–	↑	↓
(Hypo-) H_2O < Na^+	Adrenal insufficiency	↓	↑	↓	↑	↓	↑	↓

Solutions

Solution	Characteristics	Effect on Cells	Example
Hypertonic	Solute > solvent	Shrink	>0.9% NaCl
Isotonic	Solute = solvent	No change	0.9% NaCl
Hypotonic	Solute < solvent	Swell	<0.9% NaCl

Isotonic solutions separated by a semipermeable membrane do not cause net movement of water or solutes. The osmotic potential is the same on either side of the membrane.

► ACID–BASE PHYSIOLOGY

Process	pH	HCO_3/PaCO₂	Compensation	pH	HCO_3/PaCO₂
Metabolic acidosis	↓	HCO_3^- ↓	Respiratory *(hyperventilate)*	↑	$PaCO_2$ ↓
Metabolic alkalosis	↑	HCO_3^- ↑	Respiratory *(hypoventilate)*	↓	$PaCO_2$ ↑
Respiratory acidosis	↓	$PaCO_2$ ↑	Metabolic *(conserve HCO_3)*	↑	HCO_3^- ↑
Respiratory alkalosis	↑	$PaCO_2$ ↓	Metabolic *(excrete HCO_3)*	↓	HCO_3^- ↓

Henderson–Hasselbalch Equation

- $pH = pKa + \log [A^-]/[HA]$.
- $pH = pK$ when an acid is half neutralized.

Isoelectric Point

- pH where the number of positive charges equals the number of negative charges.
- Solute has no electric charge at this pH.
  - Does not move an electric field (pI for that solute).
- Allows separation of proteins or amino acids based on charge.

Glycine has a net negative charge at any pH above its isoelectric point, so it moves toward the positive electrode (anode). At any pH below its isoelectric point (pI), glycine exhibits a net positive charge and moves toward the negative electrode (cathode).

Zwitterions (Dipolar Ions)

- Physiologic pH: Amino acids have both
  - Negatively charged carboxyl group ($-COO^-$) and
  - Positively charged amino group ($-NH_3^+$)

Buffer

- System to minimize pH changes
- Consists of
  - Weak acid (proton donor)
  - Conjugate base (a salt)(proton acceptor)
- Releases H^+ ions when the pH rises.
- Accepts H^+ when the pH drops.

In the oral cavity, the carbonic acid system helps neutralize dietary and bacteria-generated acids.

BUFFER SYSTEMS

- Sodium bicarbonate: carbonic acid buffer.
  - The major buffer in extracellular fluid, blood.
  - Breaks down to CO_2 and H_2O with respiratory elimination.
- Blood pH is ~ 7.4.
  - Range 7.35–7.45.
  - Usually >7.4: slightly alkaline/basic.
- Primary determinant is the bicarbonate and CO_2 ratio.
  - $pH = pKa + \log [HCO_3^-]/0.03 \times pCO_2$.
  - $pH = 6.1 + \log[HCO_3^-]/(0.03 \times pCO_2)$.
    - 6.1 is the pKa of the bicarb-CO_2 buffer system.

Control of Acid–Base Balance

- **Renal**
  - In tubules: H_2CO_3 (carbonic anhydrase) $\rightarrow$ H_2O + CO_2 $\rightarrow$ H^+ + HCO_3^-.
    - H^+ secreted, then excreted.
    - HCO_3^- reabsorbed.
    - NH_4 (ammonium) phosphates are excreted to compensate for acidity.
- **Buffers**
  - Bicarbonate
  - Hemoglobin
  - Albumin
- **Respiratory**
  - Blow off CO_2 (elevated CO_2 stimulates respiration).

- Regulates water and solute balance.
- Removes nitrogenous wastes (as urea) from blood.
  - Urea is a byproduct of protein breakdown.
    - Urea cycle in liver.

The urea cycle in the liver is important for disposal of ammonia.

Kidney Function

Filtration	Hormonal
Water and solute balance Excretion of wastes	Erythropoietin (stimulates RBCs) Renin (stimulates angiotensin, aldosterone system)

Urine

Characteristics	Contents
Clear, yellow Slightly acidic pH Specific gravity 1.005–1.030	Na^+ Cl^- K^+ Ca^{2+} Mg^{2+} Sulfates Phosphates HCO_3^- Uric acid Ammonia Creatinine Urobilinogen

Kidneys ordinarily excrete 1–2 L per day in urine.

180 L of glomerular filtrate are produced each day (99% reabsorbed).

Ammonia

- Waste product
- Sources:
  - Amino acids
    - Liver
    - Kidneys
    - Amines
    - Purines and pyrimidines

Nephron

See Chapter 2, Histology.

- Functional and structural unit of the kidney
  - Glomerulus
  - Bowman's capsule/space

- Tubules
  - Proximal convoluted
  - Loop of Henle
  - Distal convoluted
- Collecting duct
- Renal pelvis
- Ureter

Glomerulus is a tuft of capillaries (endothelial cells) that interface with Bowman's capsule (epithelial cells). Filtration occurs at this interface.

Renal Blood Supply

See Figure 14–3.

- Renal arteries branch from the aorta.
- Left renal artery is longer than the right.
  - Renal artery
  - Interlobar arteries
  - Arcuate arteries
  - Interlobular arteries
  - Afferent arteriole
  - Glomerulus
  - Efferent arteriole

Majority of glomerular filtrate occur at the proximal convoluted tubule (just distal to Bowman's space).

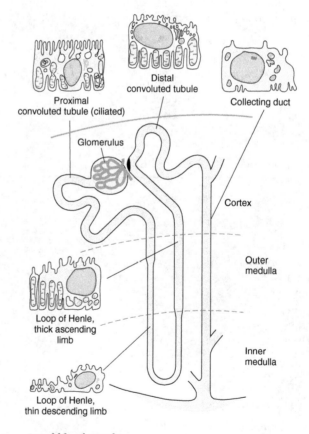

FIGURE 14–3. Renal blood supply.

Reproduced, with permission, from Ganong WF. *Review of Medical Physiology,* 22nd ed. New York: McGraw-Hill, 2005.

Filtration

See Figure 14–4.

- Renal blood flow delivered to glomerulus.
- Filtrate passes:
    - Endothelial cell barrier (glomerulus).
    - Epithelial cell barrier (Bowman's capsule).
- Filtrate enters Bowman's space, the first part of the tubule.

Reabsorption occurs by active transport, facilitated diffusion, and solvent drag. It can be paracellular or transcellular.

Reabsorption	Secretion	Excretion
Tubule back to circulation.	From tubular cell or circulation into tubular fluid.	Tubular fluid (and solute) that ends up as urine.

Substance	Reabsorption	Comments
H_2O	Proximal tubule Loop of Henle (descending) Distal tubule, collecting duct	Ascending loop is impermeable to H_2O ADH
Na^+	Proximal tubule (70%) Loop of Henle Distal tubule Collecting duct	Cl and H_2O follow passively Na/K/2Cl, impermeable to H_2O Na/K/2Cl cotransport Aldosterone Na^+ channel
Glucose	Proximal tubule	

Furosemide is a loop diuretic and thiazides work on the distal convoluted tubule.

Function of Nephron Segments

Segment	Reabsorption	Secretion
Proximal convoluted tubule.	H_2O, Na^+, K^+, Cl^-, HCO_3^-, amino acids, glucose, proteins	H^+, ammonia
Descending loop of Henle.	H_2O (impermeable to Na^+)	
Ascending loop of Henle.	Na^+, K^+, Cl^- (impermeable to H_2O)	
Distal convoluted tubule.	Na^+, Cl^- Ca^{2+} (regulated by **PTH**)	
Collecting duct.	H_2O (regulated by **ADH**) Na^+ (regulated by **aldosterone**)	K^+, H^+, ammonia, drugs

Reabsorption of NaCl (and impermeability to water) by the thick ascending loop is the basis of the countercurrent multiplier system.

Collecting duct drains multiple (> 1) nephron.

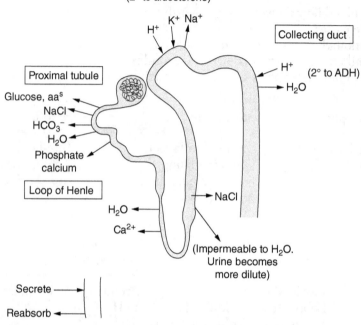

FIGURE 14–4. Filtration.

In the absence of ADH aquaporins are not expressed on the collecting duct membrane, therefore water reabsorption at the medullary collecting duct is much less pronounced and dilute urine is excreted.

If the vasa recta coursed straight through medulla, then water would move from the blood in the capillary into the interstitium (and interstitial solute would move into the capillary). This would dissipate the countercurrent gradient and decrease the concentrating ability.

▶ COUNTERCURRENT MECHANISM

- Countercurrent multiplier.
- Creation of a gradient to allow for concentrated urine.
- Occurs in:
  - Loop of Henle.
  - Collecting tubules (cortical and medullary).
  - Because these are anatomically located in both the medulla and cortex.
  - Mechanism:
  - Ascending loop:
    - **Active Na reabsorption (pumping)**
    - **Impermeability to water**
- This preferential egress of Na but not water creates:
- Dilute tubular fluid.
- Hyperosmotic interstitium.
- Urine is dilute at cortical collecting duct (water > Na).
- Urine concentrates as it descends medullary collecting duct.
- Because of the gradient created by hyperosmotic medulla
- Gradient ("pulls" water from the tubule).
- In presence of ADH
  - Aquaporins promote egress of water along this gradient.

Countercurrent Exchange

- Allows the hyperosmotic medullary gradient to be maintained.
- Hairpin (or loop) configuration of vasa recta capillaries.
- Minimizes removal of excess medullary interstitial solute.
- Maintains gradient so that urine can be concentrated.

EFFECTIVE RENAL PLASMA FLOW (ERPF)

- Volume of plasma flowing through the peritubular capillaries.
- Determined by calculation of paraaminohippuric acid (PAH).
  - PAH is completely secreted into the proximal tubule and excreted into the urine.
  - Therefore the volume of plasma cleared of PAH is ~ = ERPF.
- PAH is both filtered and secreted and used to estimate renal plasma flow.

$ERPF = U_{PAH} \times V/P_{PAH} = C_{PAH}$

RENAL BLOOD FLOW

Response to decreased renal blood flow.
- Decreased renal blood flow (eg, renal artery stenosis).
- Decrease in glomerular hydrostatic pressure (initially).
- Decrease in GFR.
  - Decreases NaCl delivery to the macula densa (Cl⁻ more important).
  - Causes JG cells to secrete renin.
  - AT-II is formed (aldosterone released).
  - AT-II constricts efferent arteriole.
  - Increases glomerular hydrostatic pressure.
  - GFR back to normal.

> **AT II functions:**
> - Constricts efferent arterioles, ↑GFR
> - Systemic vasoconstriction
> - Retention of Na/H$_2$O via proximal tubule Na$^+$/H$^+$ transporter
> - Aldosterone

GLOMERULAR FILTRATION RATE

- GFR = rate of filtrate formation at the glomerulus.
- Surrogate of renal function
- Determined by:
  - Hydrostatic pressures (Bowman's space and glomerulus).
  - Oncotic (colloid) pressures (Bowman's space and glomerulus).
  - Capillary filtration coefficient.
- Calculate using Cr or inulin clearance.
  - Freely filtered.
  - Not reabsorbed.
  - Minimally secreted into the urine.

GFR Increased ↑	GFR Decreased ↓

Increased renal perfusion (blood flow)
  Eg, dopamine, fenoldopam
  Afferent arteriole vasodilation
    Increases glomerular capillary hydrostatic pressure.
 	
Efferent arteriole vasoconstriction
    Increases glomerular capillary hydrostatic pressure.
    However, excessive constriction here will decrease RBF and GFR.
Decreased plasma oncotic pressure
    Eg, decrease plasma proteins
	Decreased renal perfusion
	    Eg, renal artery stenosis, low BP
	Afferent arteriole vasoconstriction
	Efferent arteriole vasodilation
	    Eg, ACE-I
	Increased hydrostatic pressure in Bowman's space
	    Eg, blocked ureter, outflow obstruction

> ACE-i used for renal failure to ↓ glomerular pressure.

$GFR = U_{Inulin} \times V/P_{Inulin} =$

$C_{Pinulin}$

Filtration fraction

$(FF) = GFR/RPF$

$(RPF = renal\ plasma\ flow)$

- Rate of substance is cleared from plasma.
- Clearance = (urine concentration × urine flow rate)/plasma concentration.
  - Use Cr or inulin clearance to estimate GFR.
  - Cr and inulin are freely filtered by the glomerulus.
  - Not secreted or reabsorbed.
  - Filtration rate and excretion rate are equal in steady state.

Excretion rate = GFR – reabsorption + secretion.

*Inulin clearance = rate insulin
cleared from plasma/unit
time = $U_{Inulin} \times V/P_{Inulin}$ =
$C_{PInulin}$ = GFR.
Note: Inulin is a starch.*

Net reabsorption:
*Solute clearance is less than
that of inulin.*
Net secretion:
*Solute clearance is greater
than that of inulin.*

*When GFR decreases by 50%,
Cr clearance is decreased by
about 50%. Cr excretion is
decreased and plasma Cr
level is increased.*

*Cr clearance is used to assess
renal function in the clinical
setting.*

Hormones and the Kidney

	Released from	Release Stimulated by	Site of Action	Effect
ADH	Posterior pituitary	Thirst	Distal tubule collecting duct	↑ H_2O resorption ↓ serum Na
		↑ Na^+ ($\uparrow$ osmolarity) ↓ extracellular fluid.	Aquaporins	↑ blood volume
Renin	Juxtaglomerular apparatus	↓ renal BP (or PaO_2) ↓ GFR ↓ Cl^- delivery to macula densa Sympathetic stimulation B1 receptors	Cleaves AT (made in liver) into AT-I ACE (in pulmonary capillaries) AT-I* → AT-II	AT-II Vasoconstrictor ↑ PVR efferent arteriole vasoconstrictor ↑ GFR Na^+, H_2O retention stimulates release of aldosterone
Aldosterone	Adrenal cortex (zona glomerulosa).	Renin via AT-II ↑ K^+	Collecting duct, ENaC channels	NaCl, H_2O reabsorption K^+ excretion HCO_3 reabsorption

*AT-I and AT-II = angiotensin I and II

See Figure 14–5.

- See the following chart for hormonal response to volume changes under normal circumstances.

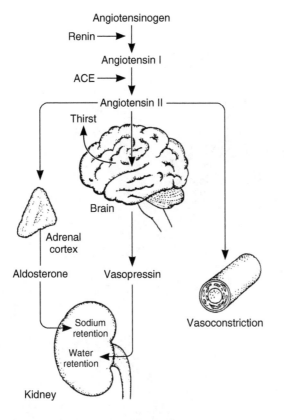

FIGURE 14-5. Hormonal response to volume changes.

Reproduced, with permission, from Ganong WF. *Review of Medical Physiology,* 22nd ed. New York: McGraw-Hill, 2005.

Volume Expansion	Volume Contraction
↓ ADH	↑ ADH
↓ renin-aldosterone	↑ renin-aldosterone
↑ ANP, BNP (natriuretic peptides) ↑renal Na⁺ excretion	↓ ANP, BNP (natriuretic peptides) − ↓ renal Na⁺ excretion
↑ baroreceptor response (↓ HR, ↓ BP)	↓ baroreceptor response (↑ HR, ↑ BP)

CHAPTER 15

Gastrointestinal Physiology

▪ Functions to digest and absorb nutritive substances, vitamins, nutrient, and fluids.

Nervous Control

▪ **Extrinsic**
  ▪ Mostly vagus (CN X, parasympathetic).
▪ **Intrinsic**
  ▪ **Enteric nervous system**
    ▪ **Myenteric plexus** (Auerbach's plexus): Between outer longitudinal and middle circular muscle layers.
    ▪ **Submucous plexus** (Meissner's plexus): Between the middle circular layer and the mucosa.

Hormonal Control

Hormone	Stimulus	Action
Gastrin[a]	Peptides, amino acids in gastric lumen; stomach distention.	Stimulates HCl secretion and gastric motility.
Cholecystokinin[b]	Fats, fatty acids, amino acids in duodenum.	↑ pancreatic digestive enzyme secretion. ↑ gallbladder contraction (bile secretion).
Secretin[b]	↓ pH in duodenum. HCL into duodenum.	↑ HCO_3 from pancreas (neutralizes H^+ in duodenum). ↓ gastric motility. ↓ gastric acid secretion.
GIP[b,c]	Fats and glucose in duodenum.	↓ gastric motility. ↓ gastric acid secretion. ↑ insulin release (β cells) in setting of ↑ BGL.
Somatostatin[d]	↑ acid and vagal tone.	↓ HCl and pepsinogen secretion, ↓ pancreatic and gallbladder secretion, ↓ insulin and glucagon secretion.
Ghrelin[e]	↑ before meals.	↑ GH, ATCH, cortisol, PRL.

[a]Gastrin is produced/secreted from G cells (enteroendocrine) in the stomach in response to a meal.
[b]Cholecystokinin, secretin, and GIP are all produced/secreted from duodenum. (CCK by I cells, secretin by S cells, GIP by K cells).
[c]GIP = gastric inhibitory peptide.
[d]Somatostatin released by D cells of pancreas, GI.
[e]Ghrelin relased by P/D cells of stomach.

Enterogastric reflex

▪ Duodenum distends with chyme.
▪ Pyloric pump inhibited.
▪ ↓ gastric motility and emptying.

ENTERO GASTRONE

▪ Includes:
  ▪ **Secretin**
  ▪ **Cholecystokinin**
  ▪ **Gastric inhibitory peptide (GIP)**

- All are released by small intestine in response to chime entering the duodenum:
  - Acidity (HCL)
  - Fats (FFAs)
  - Amino acids
- These hormones then enter the bloodstream.
  - Target organ is stomach.
    - ↓ gastric motility (↓ pyloric pump).
    - ↓ gastric emptying.

► GASTRIC SECRETIONS

- Gastric glands make 2–3 L secretions per day.
- pH of gastric secretion is 1.0–3.5.
- Secretions include:
  - **Mucous**
    - Adheres to stomach wall.
    - Lubricates the walls.
    - Protects the gastric mucosa from acidic secretions.
      - Mucous is alkaline.
  - **HCL**
    - Assists in digestion.
    - ↑ by Ach, gastrin, and histamine.
      - Secreted by parietal cells.
  - **Pepsinogen**
    - Converted to pepsin (when in contact with HCl).
    - Pepsin is a proteolytic enzyme.
      - Released by chief cells.
  - **Intrinsic factor**
    - Binds vitamin B_{12} to allow for its absorption in terminal ileum.
      - Released by parietal cells.
  - **Gastrin**
    - Hormone, bloodstream to parietal (oxyntic) cells in gastric glands.
    - Stimulates HCl secretion.

Peptic ulcers can result from:
- ↑ HCl (acid oversecretion).
- ↓ mucous (↓ ability of mucosal barrier to protect against acid).
- Also contribution by *H. pylori*.

Gastric Secretions by Region

Stomach Region	Gland(s)	Secretion(s)
Cardiac	Cardiac glands	Mucous
Fundus (and body)*	Gastric or fundic glands	
	Mucous neck cells	Mucous
	Parietal (oxyntic) cells	HCl and IF
	Chief cells	Pepsinogen
	Enteroendocrine cells	Gastrin
Pylorus	Pyloric glands	Mucous

*In the fundus there are 3 to 7 glands in the base of each gastric pit.

Stages of Gastric Secretion

- **Cephalic phase**
  - Smell, sight, taste, thought of food triggers reflexes to stimulate gastric secretion (parasympathetic activation).
- **Gastric phase**
  - Begins when food enters the stomach.
  - Stomach wall distends and ↑ pH triggers gastrin release.
  - Accounts for ~70% of gastric secretion.
- **Intestinal phase**
  - Begins when acidic, high-osmolarity food enters the intestine.
  - Gastric secretion is inhibited via
    - Enterogastric reflex.
    - Hormonal mechanisms (eg, secretin).

Chyme

- Semiliquid contents of the stomach.
  - Consist of partially digested foods and gastric secretions.
  - Passes through pyloric valve into duodenum.
- Volume and composition of chyme affect gastric motility and gastric emptying.
- Chyme is broken down by digestive enzymes in the small intestine.

Remember: CCK, secretin, and GIP are all produced in duodenum.

Gastric Emptying

Increased by	Decreased by
Eating	CCK
Gastric distention	Secretin
Gastrin	GIP
Vagal input (parasympathetic)	Duodenal distention (enterogastric reflex)

▶ **GI CONTRACTIONS**

Three major types.

1. Peristalsis

- Coordinated contractions with relaxation ahead.
- Propels chyme forward (from proximal to distal).
- Controlled by the enteric nervous system.
  - Local reflexes (stimulated by distention).

Contractions in the GI tract are influenced by mechanical, neural, and hormonal inputs. Myenteric (intrinsic) and parasympathetic (extrinsic) stimulation both increase contractile force.

2. Segmentation (Mixing)

- Most common in the small intestine.
- Rhythmic contractions in a piece of gut.
- Chops chyme and mixes it with digestive enzyme juices.
- Ensures chyme comes into maximum contact with the gut wall.
  - ↑ surface area for digestion and absorption.
- Stimulated by distention.
- Occurs at rate of 11–12 cycles per minute in duodenum.

- Progressively slower rate as you progress further down distally in the gut.
  - About 6–7 cycles per minute in terminal ileum.

3. Tonic Contractions

- Long duration—minutes to hours.
- Examples are sphincters located along GI tract.

Digestion and Absorption

| Component | Digestion | | Absorption |
	Enzyme[a]	Location	

Carbohydrates	Amylase (saliva)[b]
	Amylase (pancreas)
	Disaccharidases
	  Sucrase
	  Lactase
	  Maltase
		Upper GI
		  (mouth, stomach)
		Duodenum,
		  small intestine
		Small intestine
		  Brush border
			Na^+ cotransport
			  Glucose
			  Galactose
			Facilitated diffusion
			  Fructose

Proteins	Pepsin Trypsin Chymotrypsin Carboxypeptidase Peptidases	Stomach Pancreas Small intestine Brush border	Na^+ cotransport or Facilitated diffusion

Fats	Lingual lipase
	
	Pancreatic lipase
		Upper GI (mouth,
		  stomach)
		Small intestine
			Diffusion into
			  enterocyte
			Exocytosis into
			  lymph

[a]No human enzymes can hydrolyze cellulose.
[b]Ptyalin (a-amylase) is secreted by parotid glands. It hydrolyzes starch (into the disaccharide maltose).

DISACCHARIDE ABSORPTION

- Disaccharides and small glucose polymers are hydrolyzed at brush border by disaccharidases:
  - Lactase
  - Sucrase
  - Maltase
  - α-dextrinase
- Hydrolization forms:
  - Monosaccharides
  - Glucose
  - Galactose
- Disaccharides are absorbed by Na^+ cotransport (secondary active transporters are driven by the sodium gradient).
- Fructose absorption is mediated by facilitated diffusion.

> **Duodenum:** Fe^{2+}
> Jejunum- folate (celiac)
> Ileum- B12

PROTEIN ABSORPTION

- Proteins are broken down by peptidases on brush border.
- Protein breakdown gives rise to
  - Dipeptides
  - Amino acids
- Absorption immediately follows breakdown
  - Via secondary active transporters using sodium or hydrogen gradients.

TRIGLYCERIDES DIGESTION AND ABSORPTION

Triglycerides need to be broken into monoglyceride and free fatty acids.

- Triglycerides make up majority of dietary lipid.
- Digestion starts with lingual lipase.

Bile salts (amphipathic)
↓
Emulsify triglycerides (in duodenum)
↓
Pancreatic lipase, which breaks down emulsified triglycerides into:
↓
Monoglyceride + free fatty acids (FFAs)
↓
Monoglycerides + FFAs stay associated with bile salts as:
↓
Micelles (smaller fat droplets)
↓
Contact brush border and are absorbed into enterocyte by simple diffusion
↓
Endoplasmic reticulum were reconstituted as triglycerides
↓
Packaged as chylomicrons (triglycerides + cholesterol, lipoproteins, and other lipids)
↓
Chylomicrons into lymphatics by exocytosis.

Exocrine Pancreas

- Pancreatic secretion stimulated by:
  - Ach
  - Cholecystokinin
  - Secretin
- Enzymatic secretions from pancreatic acinar cells.
  - Protein breakdown:
    - Trypsin
    - Chymotrypsin
    - Carboxypepsidase
  - Carbohydrate breakdown:
    - Amylase
  - Fat breakdown:
    - Lipase
    - Cholesterol esterase
    - Phospholipase
- Enzymes are secreted in inactive form.
  - Activated in small intestine (contact acidic chyme).
- Pancreatic ductal cells secrete fluid high in bicarbonate.
  - pH of pancreatic secretions is 8.0 to 8.3.

Bile

- Produced by the liver.
- Stored in the gallbladder.
- pH ~7.8.
- Helps with lipid digestion and absorption.
    - Emulsification
    - Release (gallbladder contraction) stimulated by:
    - Cholecystokinin (hormone produced by wall of upper intestine).

pHs of Secretions

Secretion[a]	pH
Gastric	1.0–3.5
Pancreatic	8.0–8.3
Bile	7.8
Intestinal	7.5–8.0

[a]Intestinal secretions are mainly mucous. They are secreted by goblet cells and enterocytes.

▶ **LIVER**

Liver Functions

- Stores minerals and vitamins.
- Stores iron (Fe) as ferritin.
- Synthesizes cholesterol.
- Conjugates steroids.
- Metabolizes carbohydrates:
    - Regulates blood glucose level:
        - Glucose metabolism.
        - Glucose/carbohydrate storage.
        - Gluconeogenesis.
- Metabolizes lipids:
    - Synthesizes lipoproteins.
    - Regulates lipid metabolism.
- Metabolizes protein:
    - Deaminates AAs → urea (urea cycle).
    - Synthesizes AAs.
    - Synthesizes plasma proteins (eg, fibrinogen, prothrombin, clotting proteins).
- Detoxifies; reduces or eliminates toxic elements (eg, alcohol detoxification).
- Destroys damaged red blood cells.
- Phagocytosis of foreign antigens.
- Serves as bile reservoir.
    - Secretes bile.

Cholesterol Synthesis

- See also Chapter 7.
- Cholesterol is important for:
    - Bile salts (formed from cholesterol in liver)

Cholesterol synthesis in the liver is regulated by negative feedback. Statin allosterically inhibits HMG CoA reductase (↓ cholesterol formation from acetyl CoA).

Nonprotein nitrogen in the blood is made up primarily of urea.

- Steroid hormones
- Vitamin D

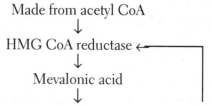

Made from acetyl CoA
↓
HMG CoA reductase ←
↓
Mevalonic acid
↓
Cholesterol (negative feedback to HMG CoA reductase)

Urea Cycle

- See also Chapter 7.
- Urea is the fate of most of the ammonia channeled to the liver.
- Deamination of amino acids results in ammonia (NH_3).
- Ammonia is toxic, fatal if it accumulates.
- Urea cycle converts NH_3 into urea:
  - $2 NH_3 + CO_2 \rightarrow$ urea (3 ATP are required).
  - Hydrolysis of arginine gives rise to urea.
- Ornithine regulates turn of the cycle (see biochemistry).
- Urea then passes to bloodstream to kidneys and is excreted in urine.

Glucose Metabolism

- See also Chapter 7.
- Glucose is required by all tissues, especially brain and RBCs.
- Liver maintains blood glucose level:
  - Liver releases glucose during exercise and between meals.
  - Released glucose is from one of two sources:
    - Glycogenolysis (breakdown of stored glycogen).
    - Gluconeogenesis (formation of new glucose).

Glucose

Glucose transporter review:

- glut1 - erythrocytes
- glut2 - renal, small intestine, liver, pancreatic B cell
- glut 3 - expressed in neuron, placenta
- glut 4 - insulin regulated, adipose, striated muscle tissue

- Glucose is the major fuel source derived from carbohydrate ingestion.
- The presence of glucose in urine occurs only when a person has exceeded the renal threshold (K_M) for glucose (eg, uncontrolled DM).
- During fasting liver glycogen ↓ because glycogenolysis occurs (to deliver glucose to the bloodstream).
- Skeletal muscle lacks glucose-6-phosphatase, so cannot deliver glucose to the bloodstream.
- The brain has no significant stores of glycogen and is completely dependent on blood glucose. The brain oxidizes nearly 140 g/day of glucose to CO_2 and H_2O, making ATP.

GLUCONEOGENESIS

- Synthesis of glucose from noncarbohydrate compounds.
- Mostly occurs in liver.
- ~10% occurs in kidneys.
- During prolonged starvation, the kidneys become major glucose-producing organs.

GLYCOGENESIS

- Glucose uptake to liver (via GLUT proteins).
- Glucokinase
  - Enzyme present only in the liver (expressed significantly only after a meal).
  - Converts glucose to glucose-6-phosphate, using ATP to catalyze the phosphorylation.

Other tissues use hexokinase to do the same thing as glucokinase.

Protein Metabolism

- Deamination of amino acids.
  - Convert to carbohydrates or fats for energy source.
- Amino acid synthesis.
  - Nonessential amino acids can be synthesized in the liver.

See the section on plasma constituents. Liver plasma protein synthesis accounts for 90% of plasma proteins.

Jaundice

- Yellowish discoloration of skin, sclera, and tissues.
- Secondary to hyperbilirubinemia (high levels of bile pigment bilirubin in the blood).
- Jaundice is common manifestation of liver disease.
- Occurs at any age and in either sex.

Under the tongue is the first location to spot jaundice.

Causes of Jaundice

Prehepatic (Hemolytic)	Hepatic (Hepatocyte Damage)	Posthepatic (Obstructive)
Hemolytic anemia	Hepatitis	Choledocholithiasis (presence of gallstones in common bile duct)
Malaria	Alcoholic liver disease Primary biliary cirrhosis	Pancreatic head cancer

BILIRUBIN

- Derived from broken-down hemoglobin.
- Carried to liver and is conjugated (converted into diglucuronide derivative) (conjugated with glucuronic acid by glucuronyltransferase).
- Excreted into the intestine as a component of bile.
- Normal plasma bilirubin concentration = 0.5 mg/100 mL.
- In jaundice, can rise to 40 mg/100 mL.

EtOH METABOLISM

$$\text{EtOH} \xrightarrow[\text{Alcohol dehydrogenase}]{\text{NAD}^+ \rightarrow \text{NADH}} \text{Acetaldehyde} \xrightarrow[\text{Acetaldehyde dehydrogenase}]{\text{NAD}^+ \rightarrow \text{NADH}} \text{Acetate}$$

- ↑ NADH production with alcoholism → ↑ gluconeogenesis and FA synthesis → steatosis

CHAPTER 16

Nutrition

Synthesized by intestinal
bacteria:
- Vitamin K
- B_2
- B_{12}
- Biotin
- Folic acid

- Essential organic compounds required for growth and metabolism.
- Most act as **coenzymes**.

Fat-Soluble Vitamins

See Table 16–1.
Synthesis of biologically active vitamin D:

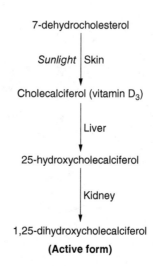

7-dehydrocholesterol

Sunlight | Skin

↓

Cholecalciferol (vitamin D_3)

Liver

↓

25-hydroxycholecalciferol

Kidney

↓

1,25-dihydroxycholecalciferol
(Active form)

*Excess fat-soluble vitamins
accumulate in body fat.
Excess water-soluble vitamins
are eliminated in urine.*

TABLE 16–1. The Fat-Soluble Vitamins

VITAMIN	FUNCTION	DEFICIENCY	OTHER FACTS
Vitamin A (Retinol)	Epithelial development, differentiation, and maintenance Growth and remodeling of bone	Night blindness Xerophthalmia (ocular tissue keratinization) Dry skin *Enamel* irregularities	Constituent of the visual pigments **rhodopsin** (rods) and **iodopsin** (cones)
Vitamin D (Calciferol)	Growth and mineralization of bone and teeth Ca^{2+} and $(PO_4)^{3-}$ metabolism	**Rickets** (children) **Osteomalacia** (adults)	*Most toxic* of fat-soluble vitamins
Vitamin E (Tocopherol)	**Antioxidant** (prevents free radical formation)	Neurologic dysfunction (premature infants)	*Least toxic* of fat-soluble vitamins
Vitamin K (Phylloquinone) (Menaquinones) (Menadione)	Activation of **prothrombin** and vitamin K–dependent clotting factors **(II, VII, IX, X)** Synthesis of γ-carboxyglutamate (chelates Ca^{2+})	Diminished blood clotting ↑ PT and INR (extrinsic clotting pathway)	Warfarin (Coumadin) blocks hepatic synthesis of vitamin K–dependent clotting factors Synthesized by intestinal bacteria

Water-Soluble Vitamins

See Table 16–2.

TABLE 16-2. The Water-Soluble Vitamins

VITAMIN	FUNCTION	DEFICIENCY	OTHER FACTS
Vitamin B_1 (thiamine)	Metabolism of carbohydrates and amino acids Decarboxylation of α-ketoacids	**Beriberi:** Peripheral nerve damage **Wernicke–Korsakoff syndrome:** CNS damage	Deficiency associated with alcoholism and malnutrition
Vitamin B_2 (riboflavin)	Component of **FAD** and **FMN** Antioxidant	**Cheilosis** Dermatitis Photosensitivity Glossitis	Synthesized by intestinal bacteria
Vitamin B_3 (niacin)	Component of **NAD** and **NADP**	**Pellagra:** 3 D's 　▨　Dementia 　▨　Dermatitis 　▨　Diarrhea	Formed from **tryptophan**
Vitamin B_5 (pantothenic acid)	Component of **coenzyme A** Fatty acid synthesis	Dermatitis Fatigue Sleep impairment Diarrhea	
Vitamin B_6 (pyridoxine)	Precursor of **pyridoxal phosphate** (a coenzyme in transamination reactions)	Fatigue Depression, mood swings Impaired growth Convulsions	Formed from **pyridine** Deficiency associated with oral contraceptive use
Vitamin B_{12} (cobalamin)	Formation of **methionine** Converts **methylmalonyl CoA → succinyl CoA** *Intrinsic factor* (IF) required for GI absorption	**Pernicious anemia:** 　▨　Megaloblastic anemia + demyelinating neurologic disorder 　▨　Caused by ↓ IF Glossitis Malabsorption associated with Crohn's disease	Not found in plant foods (only animal sources) Synthesized by intestinal bacteria Excreted solely in feces Contains cobalt
Folic acid (B_9)	Synthesis of **purines** (adenosine and guanine) and **thymidine** (required for DNA formation)	**Megaloblastic anemia** Glossitis	*Most common vitamin deficiency in U.S.* Inhibited by antimetabolites (eg, methotrexate) Essential for neural tube formation Synthesized by intestinal bacteria Stored in liver

(Continued)

TABLE 16–2. **The Water-Soluble Vitamins (Continued)**

VITAMIN	FUNCTION	DEFICIENCY	OTHER FACTS
Biotin (B$_7$) (vitamin H)	Protein and amino acid synthesis Converts **acetyl CoA → malonyl CoA** in fatty acid synthesis	Fatigue Depression Muscle pain Hair loss Dermatitis	Inactivated by **avidin** (a protein in egg whites) Synthesized by intestinal bacteria
Vitamin C (ascorbic acid)	Coenzyme for the hydroxylation of **proline** and **lysine** (in collagen synthesis) Antioxidant	**Scurvy:** Delayed wound healing, poor bone matrix formation, ↑ permeability of oral mucosa, capillary fragility	Deficiency associated with gingival disease and *dentin* irregularities

▶ MINERALS

- Essential inorganic elements required for structural and metabolic function.
- Functions of minerals:
  - Maintenance of acid–base balance
  - Coenzymes/catalysts for biochemical reactions
  - Components of essential body compounds
  - Transmission of nerve impulses
  - Regulation of muscle contractions
  - Maintenance of water balance
  - Growth of oral and other body tissues

Major Minerals

See Table 16–3 for the major minerals.

- Greater than 0.005% of body weight.

TABLE 16–3. The Major Minerals

ELEMENT	FUNCTION
Calcium	**Bone** and **tooth** formation Muscle contraction Nerve function Blood clotting
Chlorine	Membrane function (major *negative* ion in *extracellular fluid*) Water balance Digestion
Magnesium	Protein synthesis
Phosphorous	**Bone** and **tooth** formation Component of ATP Acid–base balance
Potassium	Membrane function (major *positive* ion in *intracellular fluid*) Acid–base balance Nerve function Water balance
Sodium	Membrane function (major *positive* ion in *extracellular fluid*) Acid–base balance Nerve function Water balance
Sulfur	**Cartilage** and **tendon** formation

*A deficiency in **calcium** results in osteopenia and osteoporosis. Their diagnosis is based on bone density scans.*

Calcium and iron are the minerals most lacking in the average American diet.

Minor Minerals

See Table 16–4 for the minor minerals.

- Less than 0.005% of body weight.

Transferrin *transports copper and iron in blood plasma.*

Fluoride toxicity causes:
- *Enamel mottling & discoloration*
- *↑ bone density*
- *Calcification*

Fe^{2+} *(ferrous): absorbed form via proximal duodenum.*
Fe^{3+} *(ferric): stored form bound to ferritin and hemosiderin.*

TABLE 16–4. **The Minor Minerals**

ELEMENT	FUNCTION	DEFICIENCY
Chromium	Glucose metabolism	
Cobalt	Constituent of **vitamin B₁₂** (cobalamin)	Pernicious anemia
Copper	**Iron** metabolism Maturation of collagen and elastin (cofactor for **lysyl oxidase**) Component of cytochrome oxidase	Microcytic anemia
Fluoride	Converts hydroxyapatite → fluorapatite (reduces solubility of enamel) Excreted by the kidney Passes the placental barrier Deposited in other calcified tissues	↑ caries risk
Iodine	Constituent of **thyroid hormones** Energy metabolism	**Cretinism** (children) **Myxedema** (adults)
Iron	Constituent of **hemoglobin** and **myoglobin** Constituent of **cytochromes** and cytochrome oxidase Stored as **ferritin** and **hemosiderin** intracellularly	Microcytic anemia
Manganese	Cofactor of several enzymes	
Molybdenum	Constituent of some enzymes	
Selenium	Fat metabolism Skeletal muscle function	Cardiomyopathy
Zinc	**Collagen** metabolism (constituent of MMPs) Taste/smell acuity Stabilizes cell membranes Cell-mediated immunity Component of carbonic anhydrase DNA synthesis	Delayed wound healing Hypogonadism

CHAPTER 17

Endocrine Physiology

Steroid Hormones

- Hormone response elements that bind to intracellular receptors to affect gene transcription
- Derivatives of cholesterol
  - *Cyclopentanoperhydrophenanthrene* core
- Sex hormones
  - Estradiol
  - Progesterone
  - Testosterone
- Adrenal hormones
  - Cortisol
  - Aldosterone
- **Not** water soluble
- Action:
  - Bind to intracellular receptors.
  - Form hormone response elements (HREs), complexes that activate or inactivate genes.

Amine Hormones

- Derived from amino acids
- Tyrosine
  - Thyroid hormones
    - Thyroxine (T_4)
    - Triiodothyronine (T_3)
  - Catecholamines
    - Norepinephrine
    - Epinephrine
    - Dopamine
- Tryptophan
  - Melatonin

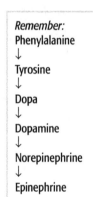

Remember:
Phenylalanine
↓
Tyrosine
↓
Dopa
↓
Dopamine
↓
Norepinephrine
↓
Epinephrine

Peptide Hormones

- Made in precursor form (pre-hormone).
- Transported in blood unbound.
- Secreted in secretory vesicles.
- Action:
  - Bind to plasma membrane receptor.
  - Generate second messenger.
- Peptide hormones include:
  - Anterior pituitary hormones: growth hormone (GH), thyroid-stimulating hormone (TSH), follicle-stimulating hormone (FSH), luteinizing hormone (LH), prolactin
  - Posterior pituitary hormones: antidiuretic hormone (ADH), oxytocin
  - Pancreatic hormones: insulin and glucagons
  - Parathyroid hormone (PTH)

Small Peptides	Larger Peptides	Glycoproteins
TRH	Insulin*	LH
GnRH	GH	FSH
Somatostatin	PTH	TSH
	hCG	

*Insulin works by ↑ tyrosine kinase activity of cytoplasmic portions of transmembrane receptors.

▶ HORMONE MECHANISMS

- A certain hormone affects its target cells (not necessarily all body cells).
- **Target cells** have hormone-specific receptors:
    - Intracellular receptor (steroid hormones)
    - Plasma membrane receptor (amine and peptide hormones)

Second Messenger

- Signals received at cell surface (extracellular receptor) are relayed to targets in the cytoplasm or nucleus by second messengers.
- Three major classes:
    - Cyclic nucleotides (cAMP, cGMP).
    - IP3 and DAG.
    - Ca²⁺ ions.

Protein kinases are involved in cAMP, cGMP, and IP3 pathways.

SECOND MESSENGERS USED BY COMMON HORMONES

cAMP	cGMP	IP3, DAG
Epinephrine*	ANP	ADH
Glucagon	NO	TSH
ACTH		Angiotensin
PTH		
TSH		
FSH		
LH		

*When glucagon, epinephrine, and PTH activate cAMP → ↑ glycolysis, ↑ gluconeogenesis.

AC is a protein enzyme located on the inner surface of the plasma membrane.

cAMP is metabolized by phosphodiesterase. So, phosphodiesterase shuts off the response of the second messenger.

cAMP MECHANISM

See Figure 17–1.

- Hormone/factor binds extracellular receptor (G protein–coupled receptor).
- G protein activated.
- Adenylate cyclase (AC) activated.
- ATP – (AC) → cAMP.
- ↑ cAMP.
    - Activates protein kinase A.
    - Stimulates gene transcription.
        - CREB (cAMP response element-binding protein).

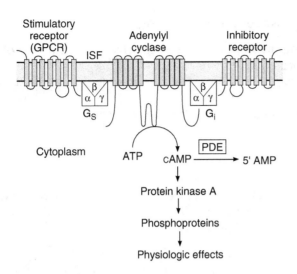

FIGURE 17–1. cAMP mechanism.

Reproduced, with permission, from Ganong WF. *Review of Medical Physiology,* 22nd ed. New York: McGraw-Hill, 2005.

GPCR (G protein–coupled receptor): When activated exchanges GDP for GTP on G alpha subunit. G alpha has ability to hydrolyze GTP with its inherent enzyme activity.

▶ PITUITARY AND HYPOTHALAMUS

Hypothalamus

▨ Part of forebrain involved in homeostasis control.
▨ Controls anterior and posterior pituitary.

HYPOTHALAMIC CONTROL OF THE ANTERIOR PITUITARY

▨ Hypothalamic releasing and inhibitory factors control secretion of anterior pituitary hormones.
▨ These factors are:
  ▨ Secreted within the hypothalamus then,
  ▨ Transported to anterior pituitary via small blood vessels (portal system).
    ▨ Hypothalamic–hypophyseal portal system.

	Hypothalamic Hormone	Anterior Pituitary Hormone
Releasing	Gonadotropin-releasing hormone (GnRH)	↑ FSH, ↑ LH
	Thyrotropin-releasing hormone (TRH)	↑ TSH
	Corticotropin-releasing hormone (CRH)	↑ ACTH
	Growth hormone–releasing hormone	↑ GH
Inhibitory	Dopamine (DA) somatostatin	↓ prolactin ↓ GH

Hypothalamic Control of the Posterior Pituitary

- Posterior pituitary hormones are synthesized in cell bodies of neurosecretory cells (located in hypothalamus).
- Axons project to and deliver hormones to pars nervosa of posterior pituitary.
- Brain neural inputs influence their release.

Hypothalamic Neurosecretory Cells	Hormones Produced
Supraoptic (ADH) and paraventricular (oxytocin) nuclei	ADH Oxytocin

Pituitary Gland

See Figure 17–2.

- Formed from:
    - Diencephalon (posterior pituitary).
    - Rathke's pouch (anterior pituitary).
        - In week 5 of development, Rathke's pouch and diencephalon come in contact.

Hypothalamic–Pituitary Endocrine Organ Axis

See Figures 17–3 and 17–4.

- **Hypothalamus:** Releasing factors
- **Pituitary:** Trophic hormones
- **Endocrine organ:** Hormones
    - Hormones exert metabolic affect.
    - Hormones give feedback on the system.

GH is the only anterior pituitary hormone that does not act directly on a target gland.

Neither ADH nor oxytocin is produced in the posterior pituitary (made in hypothalamus).

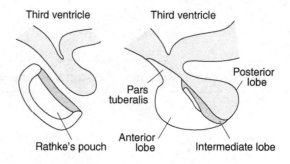

FIGURE 17-2. Pituitary gland.

Reproduced, with permission, from Ganong WF. *Review of Medical Physiology*, 22nd ed. New York: McGraw-Hill, 2005.

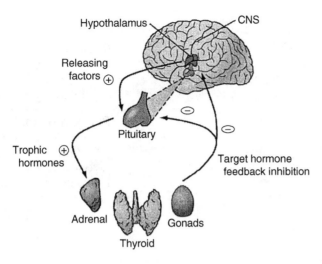

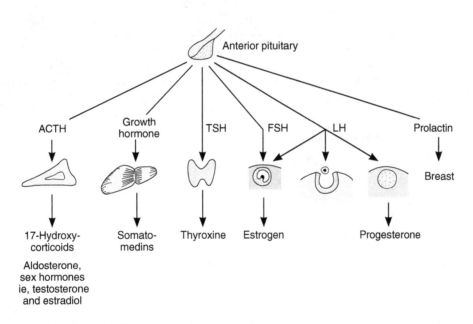

BIOCHEMISTRY–PHYSIOLOGY

ENDOCRINE PHYSIOLOGY

419

Posterior Pituitary Hormones

Hormone	ADH	Oxytocin
Produced	Hypothalamus (mainly, supraoptic nuclei)	Hypothalamus (supraoptic and paraventricular nuclei)
Stored	Posterior pituitary	Posterior pituitary
↑ release	↑ plasma Na^+ ↑ plasma osmolarity ↓ blood volume ↓ BP Nicotine Sweating SIADH	Suckling Cervical dilation Estrogen (↑ uterine oxytocin receptors)
↓ release	Ethanol Caffeine Drinking (↑ H_2O) Diabetes insipidus (DI)	Stress—catecholamines
Action	H_2O reabsorption of water from collecting duct: ↑ aquaporin expression Produce small volume of concentrated urine Conserve intravascular H_2O Helps control BP	Milk letdown* (ejection of milk with breast feeding) Uterine contraction with birthing Maternal behavior

Body fluid volume stays close to normal in DI provided the patient drinks enough water (↑ thirst) to make up for the ↑ passage of water in the urine.

*Oxytocin causes contraction myoepithelial cells surrounding sac-like alveoli of the mammary glands to induce milk letdown.

Diabetes Insipidus

- Distinguish from diabetes mellitus.
- Shares in common with diabetes mellitus:
  - Polydipsia.
  - Polyuria (very dilute).
- Different mechanism
  - ↓ ADH (or ADH doesn't work).
  - ↓ tubular reabsorption of H_2O in the kidney.
    - Pass large amount of dilute urine.
    - Hypertonic serum.
      - ↑ thirst.

Causes of Diabetes Insipidus

Central Diabetes Insipidus (↓ ADH)	Nephrogenic Diabetes Insipidus (ADH Normal OR ↑)
↓ ADH to stimulate renal tubule - ↓ activity of posterior pituitary gland - Destruction of supraoptic nuclei (hypothalamus)	Renal tubule does not respond to ADH - Congenital and familial - Drug induced (eg, lithium)

↓ ADH (or ADH doesn't work) = DI (polydipsia, polyuria).

Syndrome of Inappropriate ADH Secretion (SIADH)

- Strong association with small cell lung carcinoma
- Non-osmotically driven (ADH secretion)
- Hyponatremia (↑ Na⁺)
- Hypotonicity
- Concentrated urine
- Elevated urine Na⁺

Anterior Pituitary Hormones

Hormone	Prolactin (Lactogenic or Luteotropic Hormone)	Growth Hormone
Produced	Acidophils of pars distalis/anterior pituitary	Acidophils of pars distalis/anterior pituitary
↑ release	TRH ↓ dopamine, with pregnancy or lactation	GHRH ↓ plasma glucose concentration ↑ plasma level of amino acids (especially arginine) Gigantism Acromegaly
↓ release	↑ dopamine (prolactin inhibitory factor)	Somatostatin Somatomedins Obesity Hyperglycemia Pregnancy Dwarfism
Action	Stimulates milk production by mammary glands (during pregnancy for breast development and after delivery of the child for lactation)	Exerts effect on almost all tissues ↑ all aspects of bone growth ↑ rate protein synthesis in all cells ↑ mobilization of fats; use fat for energy ↓ rate of carbohydrate utilization - Cells shift from using carbohydrates to fat in presence of GH Works by way of IGF-1

GH is released in a pulsatile fashion (rate of GH increases and decreases within minutes).

GH (eg, GH supplements) causes positive nitrogen balance; nitrogen intake exceeds output. Also causes increased protein synthesis.

Lactogenesis is production of milk by mammary glands. Prolactin and oxytocin work together to facilitate breastfeeding: milk production then milk letdown.

Prolactin is under predominant inhibitory control. Normally high level of baseline dopamine is transmitted to the anterior pituitary, allowing for minimal prolactin secretion. Then, with pregnancy or lactation, dopamine formation is suppressed, allowing anterior pituitary to secrete prolactin.

ABNORMALITIES OF GH SECRETION

- **Dwarfism:** ↓ GH (undersecretion) in children.
- **Gigantism:** ↑ GH (oversecretion) in children.
- **Acromegaly:** ↑ GH (oversecretion) in adults (after growth plate fuses).

Somatostatin

- Peptide hormone
- Secreted by:
    - Median eminence of hypothalamus.
    - Delta cells of pancreatic islets.
- Functions to **inhibit** release/secretion of:
    - GH (somatotropin) and thyrotropin (TSH) by anterior pituitary.
    - Insulin (from beta cells of pancreas).
    - Glucagon (from alpha cells of pancreas).
    - Gastrin (by gastric mucosa).

Sex Hormones

- FSH and LH.
- GnRH from hypothalamus stimulates release of both FSH and LH.

Progesterone is made by the ovaries.

All estrogens have an aromatic A ring (unlike other steroid hormones).

COMPARISON OF MAJOR SEX HORMONES

	FSH	**LH**
Males	Sertoli (sustentacular) cells • Sperm production, maturation	Leydig (interstitial) cells • Produce testosterone
Females	Ovary • Graafian follicle development • Steroid production 　• Estradiol (during follicular phase) (granulosa cells) 　• Progesterone (during luteal phase)	Ovary • Steroid production—theca cells • Estrogen-induced LH surge stimulates ovulation 　• Forms corpus luteum

Puberty

See Figures 17–5 and 17–6.

- Age 10–15.
- ↑ GnRH (from the hypothalamus).
    - Stimulates anterior pituitary:
        - ↑ FSH
        - ↑ LH
    - Stimulates gonadal tissue (growth and function)
        - Ovaries
        - Testes
- Secondary sex characteristics appear (see following chart).
- During early childhood, a boy does not secrete gonadotropins and so has little circulating testosterone.
- On completion of puberty a male has full adult sexual capabilities and is capable of reproduction.
- Females reach puberty 1 to 2 years earlier than males. Puberty in females is heralded by menarche (first menses).

Secondary Sex Characteristics

Males (↑ Testosterone)	Females (↑ Estrogens)*
Enlargement of penis, scrotum, testis, hair growth, voice changes	Enlargement of vagina, uterus, uterine tubes; deposition of fat in breasts and hips

*Estrogen is effective at very low concentrations and generates a slowly developing long-term response in target tissues by binding to an intracellular receptor.

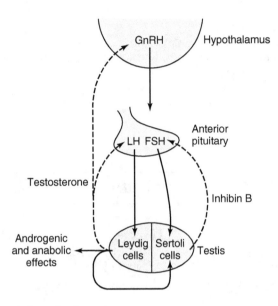

FIGURE 17–5. **Puberty in the male.**

Reproduced, with permission, from Ganong WF. *Review of Medical Physiology,* 22nd ed. New York: McGraw-Hill, 2005.

A decrease in estrogen levels feeds back to hypothalamus to start cycle over again.

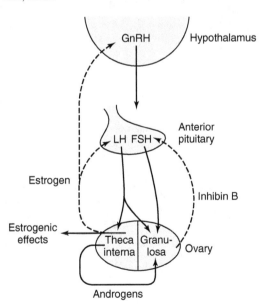

FIGURE 17–6. **Puberty in the female.**

Reproduced, with permission, from Ganong WF. *Review of Medical Physiology,* 22nd ed. New York: McGraw-Hill, 2005.

Granulosa cells convert androgens from theca cells to estradiol by aromatase.

PRECOCIOUS PUBERTY

- Puberty occurs at an abnormally early age.
- Adrenal cortex: ↑ hormones similar to male and female sex hormones.

> ▶ **REPRODUCTION**

Menstruation

See Figure 17–7.

- Average menstrual cycle is 28 days (range 22–34).
- Without estrogen and progesterone, the endometrial lining is shed as menstrual fluid during menstruation/menses.
- Usually lasts about 3–5 days and involves loss of about 50 mL of blood.

	Follicular Phase	Ovulation*	Luteal Phase
Days	1–14	15	16–28

Events	FSH, LH:
	  Stimulate ovarian
	  follicle.
	  ↑ estrogen secretion.
		LH surge:
		  Caused by estrogen
		  ~day 14 or 15.
		  Stimulates ovulation.
			↓ FSH, LH levels.

	Estrogen:
	  Endometrium
	  proliferation.
		Ovulation occurs
		14 days before
		menses (regardless
		of cycle length).
			Corpus luteum forms.
			↑ estrogen and
			progesterone.

	Late in this phase:
	  Estrogen levels ↑ *peak*.
	  FSH secretion ↓.
	  LH secretion ↑.
			If no fertilization:
			  Corpus luteum
			  degenerates.
			  ↓ estrogen and
			  progesterone levels.
			  Feedback to
			  hypothalamus:
			  ↑ GnRH (cycle
			  begins again).

*Oral contraceptive pills (OCPs) contain synthetic estrogen-like and progesterone-like substances that inhibit ovulation. OCPs suppress LHRH (GnRH) (by hypothalamus) → prevent the LH surge (by pituitary) → prevent ovulation.

Ovulation

- Stimulated by estrogen-induced LH surge.
- Ovulation is the discharge of an ovum (oocyte) from the mature follicle (Graafian follicle) of the ovary.

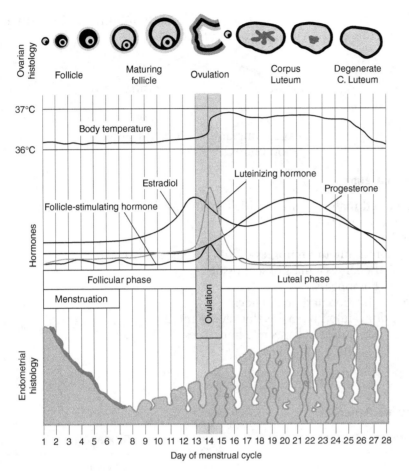

FIGURE 17-7. Female reproductive cycle.

Courtesy of WikiMedia user Lyrl, licensed and distributed under the Creative Commons Attribution ShareAlike 2.5 license (http://creativecommons.org/licenses/by-sa/2.5). Image is available in digital format at: http://commons.wikimedia.org/wiki/Image:MestrualCycle2.png.

Oogonia

- See the embryology section, Chapter 4.
- Source of oocytes
- Primordial follicles
  - Stimulated by FSH (from ant pituitary) to form:
  - *Primary oocytes* (in first meiotic division) and become:
    ↓
- Primary follicles
  - With primary oocytes
  - Form the antrum (cavity) to become:
    ↓
- Secondary follicles
  - Primary oocytes complete first meiotic division.
    ↓
- Mature Graafian follicles
  - With *secondary oocytes* (in second meiotic division).
  - LH surge causes release of secondary oocyte (egg) into abdominal cavity (ovulation).

The LH surge leads to final maturation of the follicle, rupture of follicle, and ovulation. In the absence of LH, even in the presence off large amounts of FSH, the follicle will not progress to ovulation.

Key points of the female sexual cycle:

- Only a single mature ovum is released (normally) from the ovaries each month.
- So only a single fetus can begin to grow at a time.
- Uterine endometrium is prepared for implantation of the fertilized ovum at the time of ovulation.

Oogenesis:
Formation of primary oocytes before birth and secondary oocytes at ovulation.

*Human chorionic gonadotropin (**hCG**), produced by the placenta, stimulates corpus luteum to persist and to secrete/produce progesterone and estradiol.*

Egg swept by fimbraie into infundibulum/ostium of Fallopian tube (uterine tube, oviduct) to be fertilized.

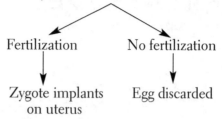

Fertilization   No fertilization

Zygote implants   Egg discarded
on uterus

Corpus Luteum

- Ruptured mature ovarian follicle forms a yellow mass of cells after ovulation (egg release).
- **No** fertilization:
  - Corpus luteum retrogresses into corpus albicans.
    - Becomes a mass of scar tissue.
    - Disappears.
- **Yes** fertilization and pregnancy:
  - Corpus luteum persists (for several months).
    - Granulosa cells secrete hormones.
      - Progesterone > estrogen.

FSH and LH work together to cause ovulation and formation of corpus luteum.

▶ **PANCREAS**

Endocrine Pancreas

Hormone	Insulin	Glucagon

Secreted	Pancreas
	Beta cells of islets
	  of Langerhans
		Pancreas
		Alpha cells in islets
		  of Langerhans

↑ release	**↑ BGL (hyperglycemia)**
	major stimuli.
	↑ amino acids, especially
	  arginine, lysine, leucine.
	Glucagon.
	GH.
	Cortisol.
	Parasympathetic
	  stimulation.
		↓ BGL (hypoglycemia).
		↓ amino acids (especially
		  arginine).
		Cholecystokinin secretion.
		Sympathetic stimulation.
		  Epinephrine, NE
		  secretion.

↓ release	↓ BGL (hypoglycemia). Sympathetic stimulation.	↑ BGL. Insulin. Somatostatin. Free fatty acids. Ketoacids.

Action	↓ BGL.
	  ↑ glucose uptake and utilization.
	  ↑↑ GLUT transporters.
	↑ glycogenesis in liver.
	  ↑ glucose → glycogen.
	↑ synthesis of triglycerides,
	  proteins.
		↑ BGL.
		↑ glycogenolysis in liver.
		  Glycogen → glucose.
		↑ free fatty acids.
		↑ amino acids.
		↑ urea production.
		It does not stimulate
		  glycogen breakdown
		  in the muscle.

Insulin conserves proteins, carbohydrates, and fats in the body: ↑ protein synthesis (inhibits protein breakdown), ↑ glycogenesis (inhibits glucose breakdown), and ↑ triglyceride synthesis (inhibits lipolysis).

Removal of anterior lobe of pituitary gland results in ↑ sensitivity to insulin.

Diabetes Mellitus

- Metabolic syndrome characterized by hyperglycemia.
- Secondary to either or both
  - Insulin deficiency.
  - Reduced effectiveness of insulin.
- Most common endocrine disorder involving the pancreas.
  - Pancreas itself may be entirely normal in cases of insulin resistance.

Diabetes Insipidus

- Distinguish from diabetes mellitus.
- Not a problem with the pancreas and insulin, but rather with ADH secretion or action.

Polyuria in diabetes mellitus (DM) is a result of osmotic diuresis, secondary to sustained hyperglycemia. (Distinguish from polyuria in DI).

Normal blood glucose level (BGL) = 80–100 mg/dL.

Histologic layers of the adrenal cortex, from outermost to innermost:

- *Salt (aldosterone) = Glomerulosa.*
- *Sugar (cortisol) = Fasciculata.*
- *Sex (androgens) = Reticularis.*

▶ ADRENAL GLAND

Adrenal Cortex

- Steroid hormones
- Cholesterol core

CRH–ACTH–Cortisol Axis

- Hypothalamus

CRH acts on (travels via portal system)
↓
Anterior pituitary (basophils of pars distalis)
ACTH acts on
↓
Adrenal cortex (zona fasciculata)
Cortisol (travels via bloodstream → systemic effects)

Negative Feedback Loop

- CRH → ACTH → cortisol.
- Cortisol feeds back and inhibits both the hypothalamus and anterior pituitary.
- **ACTH**
  - Controls production and secretion of cortisol.
  - Secretion is controlled by hypothalamus.
  - Secreted in bursts, causing cortisol levels to rise and fall.
  - Bursts are most frequent in the early morning; ~ 75% of the daily production of cortisol occurs between 4 am and 10 am.

Corticosteroids = aldosterone (mineralocorticoid) + cortisol (glucocorticoid).

Action of cortisol is to help deal with stressors and provide the brain with adequate energy sources.

Cortisol is produced in the body (endogenous). Hydrocortisone is a synthetic corticosteroid (exogenous). Other synthetic forms: decadron, methylprednisolone.

Cortisol

Secreted	Adrenal cortex (zona fasiculata)
↑ release	▪ Stress ▪ Illness ▪ Trauma ▪ Surgery ▪ Temperature extremes ▪ Psychological ▪ Cushing's syndrome or disease (See Figure 17–8)
↓ release	Adrenal axis suppression (eg, pharmacologically induced) Addison's disease Waterhouse–Frederickson ▪ Disease of adrenal glands caused by *N. meningitidis*, leads to hemorrhage into adrenal glands, low bp, shock, DIC, adrenal insufficiency
Action	▪ ↑ BGL (blood glucose level) ▪ ↑ glucagon and epinephrine action; ↓ insulin action. ▪ ↑ gluconeogenesis (induces synthesis of PEPCK) ▪ ↓ glucose uptake ▪ ↑ lipolysis ▪ ↑ fatty acids ▪ ↑ proteolysis (protein breakdown) ▪ ↑ amino acids Anti-inflammatory action Effects on immune system, bone, calcium absorption from GI, CNS

Patients taking exogenous cortisol for a long time suppress the adrenal–ACTH (pituitary) axis. Lack of stimulation from ACTH causes atrophy of adrenal cortex. Adrenal insufficiency occurs when exogenous therapy is ceased.

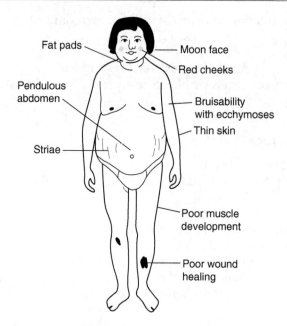

FIGURE 17–8. Cushing's syndrome.

Reproduced, with permission, from Ganong WF. *Review of Medical Physiology,* 22nd ed. New York: McGraw-Hill, 2005.

Cushing's Syndrome vs. Cushing's Disease

	Cushing's Syndrome	Cushing's Disease
Cause	↑ cortisol Exogenously administered glucocorticoids (cortisol-like medications) Endogenous ↑ cortisol (cortisol-secreting adrenalcortical tumor) Ectopic ACTH production (eg, oat cell carcinoma, small cell carcinoma)	↑ cortisol Secondary to ACTH (ACTH-secreting pituitary tumor)

Symptoms	Usually no ↑ pigmentation
	Central obesity
	Moon facies
	Buffalo hump
	Exophthalmos (retroorbital fat)
	Skin atrophy
	Striae
	(Hyperpigmentation if ↑ ACTH)
	Proximal muscle wasting/weakness
	Bone loss
	Glucose intolerance/DM-2 picture
	HTN
	  ▪ ↑ sensitivity to catecholamines, ↑ angiotensinogen, ↑ aldosterone receptors
	  ▪ Cortisol can exhibit mineral corticoid activity in increased concentrations
	  ▪ Cortisol enhances epi effects (both of these effects can lead to HTN)
	Thromboembolism
	Irritability, anxiety, panic attacks
	Depression, insomnia
	↑ Infection
		Hyperpigmentation

ADDISON'S DISEASE

- Adrenocortical insufficiency.
- ↓ corticosteroids (glucocorticoids and mineralocorticoids).
- Can occur with any age and M = F.
- In primary Addison's, cutaneous pigmentation tends to disappear following therapy, but oral pigmentation usually persists.

	Primary Addison's Disease	Secondary Addison's Disease
Cause	↓ cortisol Destruction of adrenal cortex ▪ >90% cortex must be destroyed before symptoms ▪ 70% unknown ▪ Likely autoimmune ▪ 30% identifiable cause ▪ Infection (eg, TB) Cancer/neoplasm Amyloidosis Hemorrhage in the gland	↓ cortisol ↓ or lack of ACTH ▪ Abruptly stopping chronic exogenous corticoids (eg, prednisone); usually temporary ▪ ↓ pituitary function: surgical removal, apoplexy, tumor, infection
Symptoms	↑ skin pigmentation (bronzing of skin) ↓ BP (hypotension) ↓ Na⁺, Cl⁻, HCO₃⁻ ↑ K⁺ ↓ BGL Malaise Weight loss Depression	**No ↑ skin pigmentation**
Oral signs	Diffuse intraoral pigmentation ▪ Gingiva ▪ Tongue ▪ Hard palate ▪ Buccal mucosa	**No oral pigmentation**
Treatment	Cortisol (exogenous, as hydrocortisone or prednisone)	

The adrenal medulla is a neural crest derivative.

NE can be released in two ways:

▪ By adrenal medulla into bloodstream.
▪ Directly within an organ:
  ▪ Via sympathetic innervation.
  ▪ Postganglionic sympathetic (adrenergic) neuron that stores NE.

Note: Effects are more widespread when NE is released into bloodstream by adrenal medulla than within an organ from a postganglionic sympathetic nerve ending.

Adrenal Medulla

See Figure 17–9.

▪ Specialized ganglion of sympathetic nervous system
▪ Preganglionic sympathetic fibers (cholinergic)
▪ Synapse directly on chromaffin cells in the adrenal medulla
▪ Chromaffin cells then secrete into the circulation:
  ▪ Epinephrine (80%)
  ▪ Norepinephrine (NE) (20%)

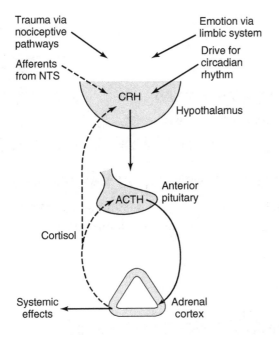

FIGURE 17-9. Adrenal medulla.

Reproduced, with permission, from Ganong WF. *Review of Medical Physiology,* 22nd ed. New York: McGraw-Hill, 2005.

EPINEPHRINE AND NOREPINEPHRINE

- Direct-acting adrenergic agonists
- Biosynthesized from tyrosine (amino acid)
- Released from adrenal medulla from storage vesicles in response to:
  - Sympathetic stimulation (fright, startle)
  - Exercise
  - Cold
  - ↓ BGL
- Function: (regulators of carbohydrate and lipid metabolism, cardiovascular effects)
  - ↑ Fatty acids
    - ↑ Triacylglycerol breakdown (lipolysis)
    - NE on α₂ inhibits lipolysis
  - ↑ BGL
    - ↑ Glycogen breakdown (glycogenolysis)
      - Activates muscle glycogen phosphorylase. (Remember McArdle's syndrome)
    - ↑ Gluconeogenesis
  - ↑ CO (especially epinephrine)
    - ↑↑ rate, force, and amplitude of heart beat
  - ↑ BP
    - ↑ Vasoconstriction in skin, mucous membranes, kidneys
  - Bronchodilation
    - ↑ Relaxes bronchiolar smooth muscle

Catecholamines (epinephrine, norepinephrine, and dopamine) are products of tyrosine metabolism.
Pathway:
Tyrosine → DOPA → dopamine → norepinephrine → epinephrine.

See Figure 17–10.

Hypothalamic–Pituitary–Thyroid Axis

▫ TRH-TSH-thyroid hormone axis

Hypothalamus: TRH released (travels via portal system).
↓
Anterior pituitary (basophils of pars distalis): TSH acts on
↓
Thyroid gland (TSH receptor): Thyroid hormones (T_3, T_4) (travel via bloodstream → systemic effects).

Negative Feedback Loop

Stress can inhibit TSH secretion secondary to neural influences that inhibit secretion of TRH from hypothalamus.

See Figure 17–10.

▫ TRH → TSH → thyroid hormones.
▫ Thyroid hormones feedback and inhibit both the hypothalamus and anterior pituitary.
  ▫ ↑ thyroid hormones: ↓ both TRH and TSH secretion.
  ▫ ↑ TSH: ↓ TRH secretion.

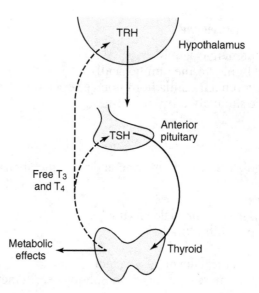

FIGURE 17–10. **Thyroid gland.**

Reproduced, with permission, from Ganong WF. *Review of Medical Physiology*, 22nd ed. New York: McGraw-Hill, 2005.

Thyroid Gland

- Well vascularized gland.
  - One of highest rates of blood flow per gram of tissue of any organ.
- Composed of follicles, filled with colloid.
  - Colloid contains thyroglobulin (tyrosine-containing glycoprotein).
    - Thyroglobulin contains thyroid hormones within its molecule.

Thyroid Cells (Follicular Cells)

Three functions:

- Collect and transport iodine.
- Synthesize and secrete (into colloid) thyroglobulin.
- Remove thyroid hormones from thyroglobulin and secrete them into the circulation.

Thyroglobulin

- Glycoprotein hormone (10% carbohydrate).
- Contains many tyrosine residues (incorporated into thyroid hormones).
- Synthesized by thyroid follicular cell.
- Secreted/stored in colloid region of follicles.

Thyroid Hormone Production

- Thyroglobulin is iodinated (within the colloid).
  - Iodine attaches to tyrosine molecules.
  - Thyroid hormones (T_3, T_4) remain part of the thyroglobulin molecules until secreted.

Thyroid hormones are lipophillic hormones. They exert effect via gene transcription.

T_4 acts as pro-hormone to T_3 (enzymatic removal of one iodine atom) in the peripheral tissues. T_3 is a more potent hormone.

Thyroid Hormone Secretion

Colloid is taken up into the cytoplasm of the thyroid follicular cells (small globules of colloid are endocytosed).
↓
Peptide bonds between iodinated residues and thyroglobulin are hydrolyzed.
↓
Thyroglobulin releases thyroid hormones as free T_4 and T_3.
↓
T_4 (mostly) and T_3 are discharged into the bloodstream/capillaries (systemic effects).

Thyroid Hormones

- Necessary for normal growth and development.
  - ↑ cellular metabolism, growth.
  - ↑ differentiation of tissues, especially brain, neural tissues.
- Affect many metabolic processes and metabolic rate ↑ HR, ↑ cardiac contractility.
- ↑ O_2 consumption and heat production.
- ↑ glycogenolysis.
- ↑ gluconeogenesis.
- ↑ GI carbohydrate absorption.
- ↑ lipolysis.
- ↑ protein breakdown.

Hypo- and Hyperthyroidism

	HYPOTHYROID	HYPERTHYROIDISM
Diseases	Cretinism (children)	Grave's disease*
	Myxedema (adults)	Plummer's disease
	Hashimoto's thyroiditis	Solitary toxic adenoma
		Toxic multinodular goiter
		TSH-secreting pituitary tumor
Symptoms	Weight gain	Restlessness, irritability
	Cold intolerance	Fatigue
	Low-pitched voice	Heat intolerance (sweating)
	Mental and physical slowness	$\uparrow$ temperature
	Constipation	Tachycardia
	Dry skin	Fine hair
	Coarse hair	Diarrhea
	Puffiness of face, eyelids, hands	Tremor (shakiness)
		$\uparrow$ Basal metabolic rate
		Weight loss
		Generalized osteoporosis
		Oral manifestations:
		If hyperthyroid in childhood, can get:
		▪ Premature eruption of teeth
		▪ Loss of deciduous dentition

*Grave's disease is the most common form of hyperthyroidism; 50% get exophthalmos (secondary to TSH-receptor antibodies in circulation).

GRAVE'S DISEASE

▪ Most common form of hyperthyroidism.
▪ Caused by binding of immunoglobulin antibodies to TSH receptors in the thyroid.
  ▪ Stimulates production of thyroxin.
▪ Typical signs
  ▪ Goiter (enlarged thyroid)
  ▪ Exophthalmos (bulging eyes) (hypertrophy of eye muscles in response to IgG)

PLUMMER'S DISEASE

▪ Toxic multinodular goiter.
▪ Multiple secreting thyroid nodules (adenomas) within gland.
▪ Uncommon in adolescents and young adults ($\uparrow$ with age).
▪ Exophthalmos is rare.

	Normal Serum Value	
Regulation	**Calcium**	**Phosphorus**
PTH	8.5–10.5 mg/dL ↑ Ca^{2+} ↑ bone resorption ↑ renal tubular reabsorption	3.0–4.5 mg/dL ↓ P ↓ renal tubular reabsorption ↑ renal P excretion
Vitamin D	↑ Ca^{2+} ↑ GI absorption of Ca^{2+}	

↓ *calcium in diet* = ↑ *PTH secretion,* ↑ *bone resorption (to compensate).*

	Hypocalcemia	**Hypercalcemia**
Effect	Irritability/excitability nerves and muscles Tetany	Cardiac and CNS depression

Hormones and Calcium Regulation

Hormone	Parathyroid Hormone	Calcitonin
Secreted	Parathyroid gland (chief cells)	Thyroid gland (parafollicular [C-cells])
↑ release	▪ ↓ plasma Ca^{2+}	▪ ↑ plasma Ca^{2+}
↓ release	▪ ↑ plasma Ca^{2+}	▪ ↓ plasma Ca^{2+}

Action	↑ plasma Ca^{2+}
	▪ ↑ bone resorption
	▪ Directly
	▪ By osteoclasts
	   ↑ Ca^{2+} reabsorption in kidney
	   ↑ GI absorption of Ca^{2+}
	   (via vitamin D)
	   ↓ plasma phosphate
	▪ ↑ phosphate excretion in urine
	   (via vitamin D)
		Plasma Ca^{2+}
		▪ ↑ Ca^{2+} deposition in bone
		▪ ↓ bone resorption
		   ↓ GI absorption of Ca^{2+}
		   ↑ Ca^{2+} renal excretion
		   ↓ plasma phosphate
		▪ ↑ phosphate renal excretion

▪ PTH is the most important hormone in Ca^{2+} metabolism (principal controller of Ca^{2+} and phosphate metabolism) and is involved in remodeling of bone. Plasma Ca^{2+} is major controller of PTH secretion.

▪ PTH stimulates 1-alpha hydroxylase in the kidneys.

▪ Compared to PTH, calcitonin has only a minor role in regulating blood calcium (in fact, calcitonin is not required in adult humans). Calcitonin is important during bone development.

	Hypoparathyroidism	Hyperparathyroidism
Example(s)	Congenital (DiGeorge syndrome). Iatrogenic (surgery) Infiltration/destruction (sarcoidosis) Idiopathic ▪ ↓ bone resorption ▪ ↓ renal Ca^{2+} reabsorption ▪ ↑ renal phosphate reabsorption ▪ ↓ 1, 25-dihydroxycholecalciferol*	Parathyroid adenoma Parathyroid carcinoma (rare) Multiple endocrine neoplasm (MEN) von Recklinghausen's disease ▪ ↑ bone resorption ▪ ↑ renal Ca^{2+} reabsorption ▪ ↓ renal phosphate reabsorption ▪ ↓/↓ 1, 25-dihydroxycholecalciferol
Calcium	↓ plasma Ca^{2+} (↑ Ca^{2+} in bone)	↑ plasma Ca^{2+} (↓ Ca^{2+} in bone)
Phosphate symptom(s)	↑ plasma phosphate Tetany Mental status changes (MS Δ's) seizures ↓ Cardiac contractility Vomiting	↓ plasma phosphate Bone pain Pathologic fractures Osteitis fibrosa cystica Brown tumors of bone Nephrolithiasis Muscular weakness

*1, 25-dihydroxycholecalciferol = active form of vitamin D.

Hormones and Calcium Regulation

See Chapter 15, "Gastrointestinal Physiology."

▶ **HORMONES AND THE KIDNEY**

See Chapter 14.

Erythropoietin

▪ Released by kidneys.
▪ Stimulates RBC production.

	Erythropoietin
Secreted	Kidney (peritubular capillary interstitial cells)
↑ release	↓ PO$_2$ (hypoxemia) ▪ Anemia ▪ Lung disease ▪ Cardiac disease ▪ High altitudes
↓ release	Normal PO$_2$ ↑ RBC volume
Action	↑ RBCs ▪ EPO receptors on erythroid progenitors ↑ replication ▪ ↑ maturation

Aldosterone

See Figure 17–11.

▪ Released by adrenal cortex zona glomerulosa.

Hormone	Aldosterone (Mineralocorticoid)
Secreted	Adrenal cortex (zona glomerulosa)
↑ release	↑ K^+
↓ release	↑ AT-II (via ↑ renin) ↓ K^+ ↓ AT-II (via ↓ renin)

Action	Site of action is distal nephron—DCT, collecting ducts
	  ▪ ↑ plasma volume (↑ H_2O reabsorption)
	  ▪ ↑ plasma Na^+ (↑ Na^+ reabsorption)
	  ▪ ↓ plasma K^+ (↓ K^+ reabsorption; ↑ K^+ excretion)

↓ Na^+ → juxtaglomerular (JG) cells secrete renin → renin cleaves angiotensinogen into AT-I → AT-I (converted by ACE) → AT-II. AT-II then stimulates adrenal cortex to release aldosterone.
In Addison's disease there is hyposecretion of both aldosterone and cortisol.

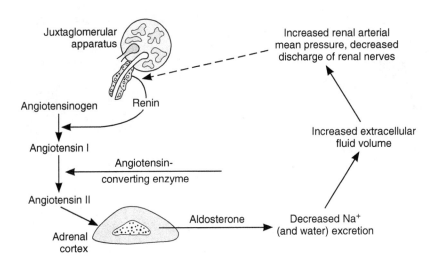

FIGURE 17–11. **Adrenal cortex.**

Reproduced, with permission, from Ganong WF. *Review of Medical Physiology,* 22nd ed. New York: McGraw-Hill, 2005.

Microbiology-Pathology

CHAPTER 18

Microbiology

Cell Types

See Table 18–1.

- Prokaryotes
- Eukaryotes

Microorganisms

See Table 18–2.

- Bacteria
- Viruses
- Fungi
- Parasites

TABLE 18-1.   **Comparison of Prokaryotic and Eukaryotic Cells**

CELL TYPE	MEMBRANE-ENVELOPED NUCLEUS	MEMBRANE-BOUND ORGANELLES	RIBOSOME SIZE	NUCLEIC ACID LOCATION	DNA TYPE	REPLICATION
Prokaryote	No	No	70S	Nucleoid (cytoplasm)	Circular	Binary fission
Eukaryote	Yes	Yes	80S	Nucleus	Linear	Mitosis

TABLE 18-2.   **Comparison of Major Microorganisms Implicated in Infectious Diseases**

MICRO-ORGANISM	CELL TYPE	OUTER SURFACE	NUCLEIC ACID	RIBOSOMES	MITOCHONDRIA	REPLICATION
Bacteria	Prokaryotic	Cell wall of peptidoglycan	RNA and DNA	70S	No	Binary fission
Viruses	Noncellular	Protein capsid and lipoprotein envelope	RNA or DNA	None	No	Assembly within host cells
Fungi	Eukaryotic	Cell wall of chitin	RNA and DNA	80S	Yes	Budding (yeasts) Mitosis (molds)
Parasites	Eukaryotic	Cell membrane	RNA and DNA	80S	Yes	Mitosis

Infections

EPIDEMIOLOGY

- An **endemic** infection occurs at minimal levels within a population.
- An **epidemic** infection occurs more frequently than normal within a population.
- A **pandemic** infection occurs worldwide.

443

BACTERIAL AND VIRAL INFECTIONS

- **Bacteremia:** The presence of bacteria in the bloodstream. Leads to **sepsis.**
- **Viremia:** The presence of viruses in the bloodstream. Leads to disseminated infections.

INFECTIOUS STATES

- **Acute:** Short-term active infection with symptoms.
- **Chronic:** Long-term active infection with symptoms.
- **Subclinical:** Infection is detectable only by serological tests.
- **Latent:** No active growth of microorganisms but potential for reactivation.
- **Carrier:** Active growth of microorganisms with or without symptoms.

Pus is a creamy substance that contains dead neutrophils, necrotic cells, and exudate.

SYMBIOTIC ASSOCIATIONS

- **Symbiosis:** The essential association between two *different* organisms that live close to each other with or without mutual benefit.
    - **Mutualism:** Both organisms derive benefit from each other.
    - **Commensalism:** One organism benefits, whereas the other is neither harmed nor helped.
    - **Parasitism:** One organism benefits, whereas the other is harmed.

INFECTIOUS SWELLINGS

Ludwig's angina is a rapidly occurring cellulitis involving the submandibular, sublingual, and submental fascial spaces, bilaterally. Because it can cause airway obstruction, emergency treatment is critical.

- **Abscess:** An *acute inflammatory lesion* consisting of a localized collection of **pus** surrounded by a cellular wall.
- **Granuloma:** A *chronic inflammatory lesion* consisting of **granulation tissue:** fibrosis (fibroblasts), angiogenesis (new capillaries), and inflammatory cells (macrophages, lymphocytes, plasma cells, epithelioid cells, and multinucleated giant cells).
- **Cyst:** An epithelial-lined sac filled with fluid or air.
- **Cellulitis:** An acute, diffuse swelling along fascial planes that separate muscle bundles.

SEPSIS

- Infection of bloodstream by toxin-producing bacteria.
- Common signs and symptoms of sepsis:
    - Fever
    - Fatigue/weakness
    - Nausea/vomiting
    - Chills
    - Diarrhea

Sepsis is most commonly caused by Staph. aureus, Klebsiella sp., and E. coli.

▶ STERILIZATION AND DISINFECTION

Sterilization

See Table 18–3.

Spore tests (with Bacillus stearothermophilus) are recommended on a weekly basis.

- The killing of *all* microorganisms, including bacterial spores.
- Heat sterilization (moist heat and dry heat) is the most reliable mode of sterilization because it can be easily biologically tested.
- **Ultrasonic cleaning** of instruments *before* sterilization helps to minimize microbial concentrations and maximize sterilization efficacy.

TABLE 18-3.   **Common Sterilization Techniques**

STERILIZATION TECHNIQUE	MECHANISM OF ACTION	COMMON USE	CHARACTERISTICS
Moist heat (autoclaving)	Coagulates and denatures proteins	**Normal cycle** heats to **121°C (250°F) for 15–20 minutes,** yielding 15 lb/in² of vapor pressure **Fast cycle** heats to 134°C (270°F) for 3 minutes, yielding 30 lb/in² of vapor pressure	Most common form of sterilization Can corrode or dull carbon-steel instruments
Dry heat	Denatures proteins	Heats to 160°C (320°F) for 2 hours, or 170°C (340°F) for 1 hour	Does *not* corrode or dull instruments
Chemical vapor (chemiclave)	Denatures and alkylates nucleic acids and proteins	Heats to 132°C (270°F) for 20–30 minutes, yielding 25 lb/in² of vapor pressure	Uses a combination of alcohol and formaldehyde Does *not* corrode or dull instruments
Ethylene oxide gas	Alkylates nucleic acids and proteins	Sterilization is slow, taking 8–10 hours	Requires an appropriate chamber and ventilation system (toxic to humans) Used mostly in hospitals for heat/moisture-sensitive materials
Formaldehyde	Alkylates nucleic acids and proteins Cross-links proteins	Commonly used as a 37% solution in water (formalin)	Toxic fumes Less efficacious compared to other methods of sterilization
Glutaraldehyde (2%) ▪ Broadest antimicrobial spectrum of activity	Alkylates nucleic acids and proteins Cross-links proteins	Sterilization is slow, taking 10 hours	Most potent chemical germicide Used mostly for heat-sensitive materials Associated with hypersensitivity
Filtration	Physically and electrostatically traps microorganisms larger than the pore size	Commonly uses a nitrocellulose filter with a 0.22 μm pore size	The preferred method of sterilizing **liquid solutions**

MICROBIOLOGY–PATHOLOGY

MICROBIOLOGY

Disinfection

- The killing of many, but not all, microorganisms.

Disinfectant effectiveness is determined by killing activity against **Mycobacterium tuberculosis.**

DISINFECTANTS

See Table 18–4.

- Disinfectants are used only on *inanimate objects* such as countertops and chairs.

ANTISEPTICS

See Table 18–5.

- Chemicals that kill microorganisms on the surface of *skin and mucous membranes.*
- Many antiseptics can also be used as disinfectants.

HIV is relatively easy to kill on most environmental surfaces.

Pasteurization

- A method of heat-killing milk-borne pathogens such as *Mycobacterium tuberculosis, Salmonella, Streptococcus, Listeria,* and *Brucella.*
- Heats milk to 62°C for 30 minutes, then cools rapidly.

TABLE 18–4. **Common Disinfectants**

DISINFECTANT	FAMILY	MECHANISM OF ACTION	CHARACTERISTICS
Phenols	Phenol	Disrupts cell membranes and denatures proteins	Rarely used today because they are extremely caustic
Quarternary ammonium compounds	Cationic detergent	Disrupts cell membranes and denatures proteins	Also used as antiseptics
Chlorine	Chlorine	Oxidation of sulfhydryl enzymes and amino acids	Most common form is sodium hypochlorite (household bleach)

TABLE 18-5. Common Antiseptics

ANTISEPTIC	FAMILY	MECHANISM OF ACTION	CHARACTERISTICS
Iodophors	Iodine	Oxidation of sulfhydryl enzymes and amino acids	Most effective skin antiseptics Associated with hypersensitivity
Ethanol and isopropyl alcohol (70–90%)	Alcohol	Disrupts cell membranes and denatures proteins Poor activity against viruses in dried blood and saliva	Most widely used skin antiseptic Evaporates quickly Used on skin prior to venipuncture or immunizations Isopropyl alcohol can be used as a waterless handwash
Hydrogen peroxide	Peroxide	Oxidation of sulfhydryl enzymes and amino acids	Effective only against *catalase-negative* organisms
Chlorhexidine gluconate	Bis-biguanide	Disrupts cell membranes (due to its cationic properties)	Highly substantive Used as a handwash and a mouthrinse
Triclosan	Bis-phenol	Disrupts cell membranes	Used as a handwash and as an ingredient in some toothpastes

Sanitization

- A method of treating public water supplies to reduce microbial loads.

Infection Control

REGULATIONS VS RECOMMENDATIONS

- The **Centers for Disease Control and Prevention (CDC)** is the major agency responsible for infectious disease epidemiology, surveillance, and prevention. It provides *recommendations* and *guidelines* for infection control procedures used by healthcare workers.
- The **Occupational Safety and Health Administration (OSHA)**, a division of the U.S. Department of Labor, is responsible for composing and enforcing infection control *laws* and *regulations* that must be followed by healthcare workers. OSHA may use CDC recommendations and guidelines in drafting its mandates.

MICROBIOLOGY–PATHOLOGY

MICROBIOLOGY

*The greatest risk for bloodborne infection among healthcare workers is **HBV**.*

***Handwashing** is the most important infection control practice for reducing nosocomial infections and must be performed after removal of PPE.*

UNIVERSAL PRECAUTIONS

- **Universal precautions:** All human blood (and other body fluids that contain visible blood) are treated as infectious. Emphasizes prevention of bloodborne diseases (HIV, HBV, etc).
- **Standard precautions:** Any body fluid (excretion or secretion) except sweat, regardless of the presence of blood, is treated as infectious. Emphasizes prevention of bloodborne, as well as airborne, droplet, and contact transmitted diseases.
- **Engineering controls** (sharps disposal containers, etc) and **work practice controls** (prohibiting food storage near potentially contaminated material, etc) must be used to eliminate or minimize exposure.
- All reusable equipment and instruments that contact a patient's blood, saliva, or mucous membranes must be sterilized.
- All environmental and working surfaces must be cleaned and disinfected after contact with a patient's blood or other potentially infectious materials.
- All disposable sharps (needles, blades, etc.) must be discarded in closable, puncture-resistant containers.
- Extracted teeth are considered to be potentially hazardous materials, and should be disposed of in medical waste containers.
- All other regulated wastes (disposable equipment, gauze, etc.) must be discarded in closable containers.
- All containers of sharps, regulated wastes, and potentially infectious material must be labeled "biohazard."
- Dental unit waterlines should not exceed a bacterial concentration of 500 CFU/mL.
- Appropriate **personal protective equipment (PPE)**, including gloves, face shields or masks, eye protection, long-sleeve gowns/coats, surgical caps, and shoe covers must be worn (depending on the degree of exposure risk).
- Gloves are required during the handling and cleaning of blood-soiled equipment.
- Latex-free gloves *(vinyl* or *nitrile)* must be provided for patients or employees with rubber latex hypersensitivity.

PREEXPOSURE PROTOCOL

- Dentists *must* offer the HBV vaccine to their employees at no cost.
- If the employee declines, a declination form must be signed.
- The employee must be given the vaccine at no cost if he or she changes his mind.

POSTEXPOSURE PROTOCOL

- If someone is exposed to or comes into contact with infectious material, *immediate* aggressive washing and first aid of the site is required.
- The dentist *must* provide **confidential** medical evaluation and follow-up at no cost to the employee.
- The medical evaluation includes blood collection and testing from the source individual and the employee.
- The follow-up includes postexposure prophylaxis, counseling, and evaluation.
- The employee has the right to decline blood collection and testing.
- The dentist does *not* have the right to know the test results of the employee or the source individual.

Bacteria

- Prokaryotic cells of various shapes and sizes.
- All bacteria (except *Mycoplasma* sp.) contain a selectively permeable **plasma membrane** surrounded by a **peptidoglycan cell wall** of differing thicknesses.
- A gelatinous **polysaccharide capsule** surrounds the cell wall, which functions in virulence (prevents opsonization and phagocytosis), antigenicity, and bacterial adhesion.

Pathogenesis

BACTERIAL GROWTH CURVE

See Figure 18–1.

- **Lag phase:** Increased metabolic activity in preparation for division.
- **Log phase:** Exponential growth and division.
- Cidal antibiotics work best in this phase.
- **Stationary phase:** Cell growth plateaus as the number of new cells balances the number of dying cells due to the depletion of required nutrients.
- **Death phase:** Exponential increase in bacterial cell death.

BACTERIAL GENETIC EXCHANGE

- Genetic information is exchanged *between* bacteria in three ways (conjugation, transduction, and transformation), creating genetic variability and antibiotic resistance (Table 18–6).
- **Plasmids:** Extrachromosomal DNA that replicates independently within bacteria. They determine traits not essential to their viability, but allow them to adapt (eg, antibiotic resistance).
- **Transposition:** Transfer of DNA *within* a bacterial cell occurs via **transposons,** which are portions of DNA that "jump" from plasmid → chromosome and vice versa.
- Regardless of the mode of exchange, the DNA becomes integrated in the host cell chromosome by **recombination**.

Peptidoglycan is a cross-linked polysaccharide consisting of alternating N-acetylmuramic acid and N-acetylglucosamine residues.

Salivary **lysozyme** cleaves the glycosidic bonds of the peptidoglycan molecule.

All bacterial capsules are polysaccharides except that of Bacillus anthracis, which is a protein containing D-glutamate.

Bacteria reproduce by **binary fission**, in which one parent cell divides into two progeny cells. Bacterial growth is thus exponential.

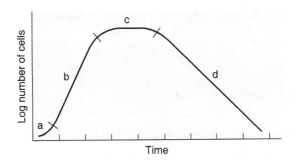

FIGURE 18–1. Bacterial growth curve.

Reproduced, with permission, from Levinson W. *Medical Microbiology and Immunology,* 8th ed. New York: McGraw-Hill, 2004.

TABLE 18-6. Bacterial Genetic Exchange

GENETIC EXCHANGE	DNA TRANSFER BY	CHARACTERISTICS

Transformation	Uptake	DNA transfer from environment
		Only a few natural transformers:
		  • *Streptococcus* sp.
		  • *Haemophilus* sp.
		  • *Neisseria gonorrhoeae*

Conjugation
  • Transfers largest amount
  of genetic information
	Conjugation tube (sex pilus)	Bacterial DNA is transferred as a separate
		F plasmid (fertility factor):
		  • F⁺ cell → F⁻ cell (plasmid only)
		Or, the F plasmid can be incorporated into
		the bacterial chromosome:
		  • Hfr cell → F⁻ cell (plasmid and chromosomal
		  genes)

Transduction	Virus (bacteriophage)	Can occur via lytic or lysogenic bacteriophage replication pathways

Bacterial Virulence Factors

MEDIATORS OF BACTERIAL ADHESION/ATTACHMENT

- Capsule: Polysaccharide (except in *Bacillus anthracis*)
- Glycocalyx: Polysaccharide (allows adhesion to teeth, heart valves, catheters)
- Fimbriae/pili: Glycoproteins (shorter appendages)
- Adhesins: Surface proteins

MEDIATORS OF EVASION OF HOST DEFENSES

- Capsule
  - Prevents opsonization and phagocytosis.
- Surface proteins
  - **M protein:** Prevents phagocytosis (from group A streptococci).
  - **Protein A:** Prevents opsonization and phagocytosis (from *Staph. aureus*).
- Enzymes
  - **Coagulase:** Promotes fibrin clot formation.
  - **IgA protease:** Degrades IgA (from *Strep. pneumoniae*, *H. influenzae*, *Neisseria* sp.).
  - **Leukocidins:** Destroy polymorphonuclear neutrophils (PMNs) and macrophages.

MEDIATORS OF HOST TISSUE DESTRUCTION

- Enzymes
  - **Collagenases (metalloproteinases):** Degrade collagens.
  - **Hyaluronidase:** Degrades hyaluronic acid.
  - **Lecithinase:** Hydrolyzes lecithin to destroy plasma membranes. Causes gas gangrene.
  - **Streptodornase (DNase):** Depolymerizes DNA.
  - **Streptolysin O:** Causes β-hemolysis (oxygen-labile).
  - **Streptolysin S:** Causes β-hemolysis (oxygen-stable).

- **Pneumolysin:** Causes β-hemolysis.
- **Streptokinase:** Activates plasminogen to dissolve clots.
- **Staphylokinase:** Activates plasminogen to dissolve clots.
- **Exfoliatin:** Epidermolytic protease that cleaves desmoglein. Causes scalded skin syndrome.
- Toxins (Tables 18–7 and 18–8)
  - Exotoxin
  - Endotoxin (See Figures 18–2 and 18–3.)

Enterotoxins: Exotoxins that affect intestinal endothelial cells.

TABLE 18–7. Exotoxin vs Endotoxin

Toxin	Location	Bacteria	Structure	Toxicity	Heat Stable	Characteristics
Exotoxin	Outside cell wall	G (+) G (−)	Polypeptides	High	No	Include **enterotoxins** Detected by ELISA
Endotoxin	Within cell wall	G (−) *Listeria*	LPS <ul><li>**Lipid A:** most toxic portion</li></ul>	Low	Yes	Not secreted, but released when bacteria die

TABLE 18–8. Bacterial Exotoxins

Classification	Exotoxin	Mode of Action	Bacteria
ADP-ribosylation	Diphtheria toxin	Inhibits protein synthesis	*Corynebacterium diphtheriae*
	Cholera toxin	↑ adenylate cyclase activity	*Vibrio cholerae*
	Pertussis toxin	↑ adenylate cyclase activity	*Bordetella pertussis*
	Anthrax toxin (edema factor)	↑ adenylate cyclase activity	*Bacillus anthracis*
	Heat-labile toxin	↑ adenylate cyclase activity	*E. coli*
Superantigens	TSST	Binds to both class II MHC and T-cell receptors, stimulating release of cytokines from T_H-cells	*Staph. aureus*
	Erythrogenic toxin	Binds to both class II MHC and T-cell receptors, stimulating release of cytokines from T_H-cells	*Strep. pyogenes*
Proteases	Tetanus toxin	Neurotoxin: inhibits glycine NT	*Clostridium tetani*
	Botulinum toxin	Neurotoxin: inhibits Ach at synapse	*Clostridium botulinum*
	Anthrax toxin (lethal factor)	Cleaves phosphokinase	*Bacillus anthracis*
	Exfoliatin	Cleaves desmoglein	*Staph. aureus*
Lecithinase	α-toxin	Cleaves lecithin in cell membrane	*Clostridium perfringens*

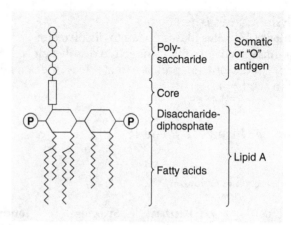

FIGURE 18-2. Endotoxin (LPS) structure.

Reproduced, with permission, from Levinson W. *Medical Microbiology and Immunology*, 8th ed. New York: McGraw-Hill, 2004.

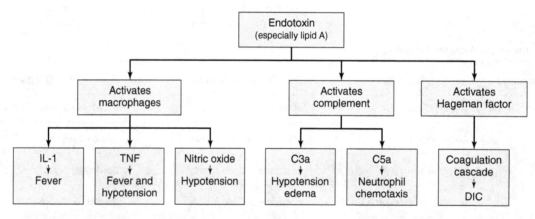

FIGURE 18-3. Mode of action of endotoxin.

Reproduced, with permission, from Levinson W. *Medical Microbiology and Immunology*, 8th ed. New York: McGraw-Hill, 2004.

SPECIALIZED BACTERIAL STRUCTURES

- **Flagella:** Long appendages that provide bacterial motility.

Classification

See Figure 18–4.

- By shape:
  - **Cocci:** Round
    - **Diplococci:** Pairs
    - **Streptococci:** Chains
    - **Staphylococci:** Clusters
  - **Bacilli:** Rods
  - **Spirochetes:** Spiral
  - **Pleomorphic:** Multiple shapes

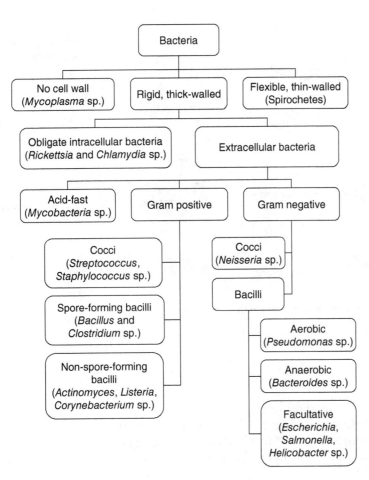

FIGURE 18-4. **Classification of bacteria.**

- By diagnostic stain (based on cell wall type) (see Table 18–9).
    - **Gram stain:** Separates almost all bacteria into two categories (see Figure 18–5):
        - Gram positive.
        - Gram negative.
    - **Acid-fast stain:** Stains *Mycobacteria* sp.

TABLE 18-9. **Comparison of Gram-Positive and Gram-Negative Bacteria**

GRAM STAIN	STAIN COLOR	PEPTIDOGLYCAN WALL	MAJOR WALL CONSTITUENT	PERIPLASMIC SPACE	ENDOTOXIN
Gram (+)	Purple	Thick	Lipoteichoic acid (LTA)	No	No
Gram (−)	Pink	Thin	Lipopolysac-charide (LPS)	Yes	Yes (LPS)

Mycobacteria *cell walls contain mostly* **mycolic acid,** *and very little peptidoglycan.*

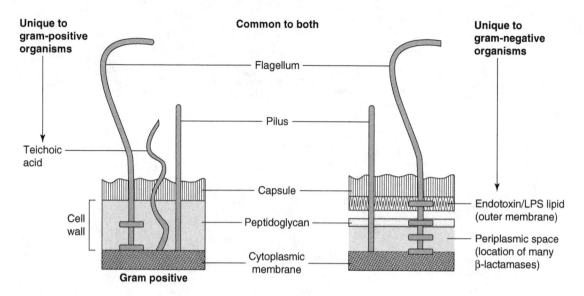

Unique to gram-positive organisms

Teichoic acid

Cell wall

Gram positive

Common to both

Flagellum

Pilus

Capsule

Peptidoglycan

Cytoplasmic membrane

Unique to gram-negative organisms

Endotoxin/LPS lipid (outer membrane)

Periplasmic space (location of many β-lactamases)

FIGURE 18–5. Comparison of Gram-positive and Gram-negative cell walls.

Adapted, with permission, from Levinson W, Jawetz E. *Medical Microbiology and Immunology: Examination and Board Review.* 9th ed. New York: McGraw-Hill, 2006.

- By oxygen requirements:
  - **Obligate aerobic:** Require oxygen for growth.
  - **Obligate anaerobic:** Cannot grow in oxygenated environments because they lack *superoxide dismutase* (rids O_2 radicals) and/or *catalase* (rids H_2O_2).
  - **Facultative anaerobic:** Grow aerobically when oxygen is present, but use fermentation pathways in its absence.

Bacteria	Superoxide Dismutase	Catalase	Peroxidase
Obligate aerobes Most facultative anaerobes	+	+	–
Most aerotolerant anaerobes	+	–	+
Obligate anaserobes	–	–	–

Only sterilization procedures (autoclaving, ethylene oxide gas, etc) are sporicidal.

- By spore production:
  - **Spores** are thick-walled cells produced only by certain **gram-positive rods:** *Bacillus* (aerobic) and *Clostridium* (anaerobic) species.
  - They are formed in low-nutrient states (during the **stationary phase** of bacterial cell growth) and remain dormant, often in soil.
  - When nutrients are restored, they germinate to form new bacteria.
  - Spores are extremely **heat resistant.**
- By pH Range
  - Acidophiles: Thrive in acidic environment (pH < 2).
  - Neutrophiles: Thrive in neutral pH environment.
  - Alkaliphiles: Thrive in basic environment (pH > 9).

Medically Relevant Bacteria

Gram-Positive Bacteria (Figure 18–6)

Gram-positive lab algorithm

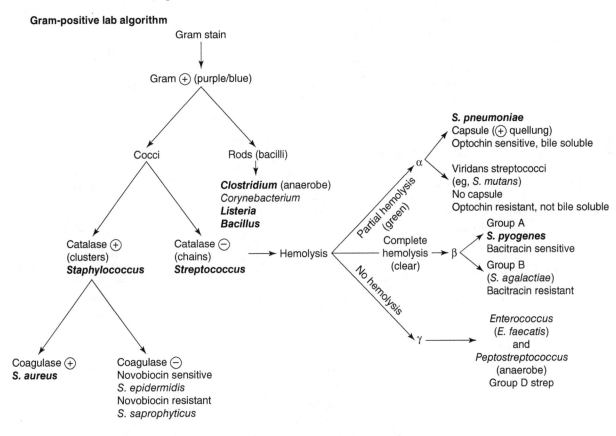

Important pathogens are in **bold type.**
Note: *Enterococcus* is either α- or γ-hemolytic.

FIGURE 18-6. Gram-positive bacteria.

Reproduced, with permission, from Le T, Bhushan V, Vasan N. *First Aid for the USMLE Step 1* 2011. 21st ed. New York: McGraw-Hill, 2011.

GRAM-POSITIVE COCCI

- *Streptococci*
  - Grow in pairs or chains.
  - Many are part of the normal human flora.
  - Catalase (–).
  - Classified by lysis of erythrocytes (hemolysis) when plated on blood agar. (See Tables 18–10 and 18–11.)
  - Beta-hemolytic *Strep* are further classified by **Lancefield groups** (Group A, B, C, F, G, etc.). Many group D *Strep* have since been reclassified as enterococci.
- *Staphylococci*
  - Grow in grapelike clusters.
  - Produce pyogenic (suppurative) infections.
  - Catalase (+): rids H_2O_2.

See Table 18–12.

Streptococci hemolysis:

Alpha: **A**lmost (incomplete)
Beta: **B**est (complete)
Gamma: **G**arbage (none)

*Lancefield group is determined by the **C carbohydrate** composition of the cell wall.*

TABLE 18–10. Hemolytic Classification

CLASSIFICATION	HEMOLYSIS	BLOOD AGAR APPEARANCE
Alpha	Incomplete	Green ring around colonies
Beta	Complete	Clear area of hemolysis
Gamma	None	No hemolysis

TABLE 18–11. Comparison of the Major *Streptococci*

HEMOLYSIS	SPECIES	MAJOR VIRULENCE FACTORS	DISEASE

Alpha	S. pneumoniae
	  Lancet-shaped
	  diplococcus
		Capsule
		Pneumolysin
		IgA protease
			Meningitis
			Otitis media (children)
			Pneumonia
			Sinusitis

Alpha	Viridans group: S. mutans S. sanguis	Normal flora of oropharynx	Caries Endocarditis
Beta (Group A)	S. pyogenes	**M protein** Hyaluronidase Streptokinase Erythrogenic toxin Streptolysin O and S Exotoxin A and B	Pyogenic infections Pharyngitis Cellulitis Impetigo Scarlet fever Rheumatic fever Glomerulonephritis
Beta (Group B)	S. agalactiae	Capsule	Neonatal pneumonia Neonatal meningitis Neonatal sepsis
Gamma (Group D)	S. bovis	Normal colon flora	Subacute endocarditis (assoc. with colon cancer)
Gamma (Group D)	Enterococci: E. faecalis E. faecium	Normal colon flora	UTI Subacute endocarditis

Spores contain dipicolinic acid in their core. Killed by autoclave sterilization.

GRAM-POSITIVE BACILLI

See Table 18–13.

- Spore-forming.
- Non-spore-forming.

TABLE 18-12. Comparison of Major *Staphylococci*

Species	Coagulase	Hemolysis	Major Virulence Factors	Disease

S. aureus	+	Beta	**Protein A**
			 β-lactamase
			 Enterotoxin
			 TSST
			 Exfoliatin
			 Hyaluronidase
			 Staphylokinase
				Abscess
				 Pneumonia
				 Toxic shock
				   syndrome
				 Scalded skin
				   syndrome
				 Food poisoning
				 MRSA
				 Endocarditis
				 Osteomyelitis

S. epidermidis	–	Gamma	Normal skin flora	Infection of IV
				   catheters and
				   prosthetic devices

S. saprophyticus	–	Gamma	Normal vaginal flora	UTI

TABLE 18-13. Comparison of Major Gram-Positive Bacilli

Bacterium	Oxygen Requirement	Major Virulence Factors	Disease
Spore-forming			

Bacillus anthracis	Aerobic	Anthrax toxin
		 Polypeptide capsule
		 (has D-glutamate)
			Anthrax
			 ▪ Cutaneous: black eschar
			   (painless ulcer)
			 ▪ Pulmonary: inhalation
			   of spores

Bacillus cereus	Facultative	Enterotoxins	Food poisoning ▪ Ingestion of reheated grains and rice (fried rice)

Clostridium botulinum	Anaerobic	Botulinum toxin
		 (neurotoxin)
		 ▪ Most potent
		   bacterial toxin
		 ▪ Botox
		   derives from
		   exotoxin A
			Botulism
			 ▪ CN/muscle paralysis
			 ▪ Respiratory failure
			 ▪ Ingestion of undercooked
			   canned foods, fish,
			   ham, pork

(Continued)

TABLE 18–13. Comparison of Major Gram-Positive Bacilli (Continued)

Bacterium	Oxygen Requirement	Major Virulence Factors	Disease
Clostridium tetani	Anaerobic	Tetanus toxin (neurotoxin)	Tetanus ▪ Associated with puncture wounds ▪ Spastic paralysis ▪ Trismus (lockjaw)
Clostridium perfringens	Anaerobic	Alpha toxin (lecithinase)	Gas gangrene ▪ Necrotizing faciitis ▪ Myonecrosis Food poisoning ▪ Ingestion of reheated meats
Clostridium difficile	Anaerobic	Exotoxin A and B	Pseudomembranous colitis ▪ Often secondary to antibiotic use (clindamycin)
Non-spore-forming			
Corynebacterium diphtheriae ▪ Club-shaped	Aerobic	Diphtheria toxin	Diphtheria ▪ Pseudomembranous pharyngitis (grayish-white membrane on tonsils)
Listeria monocytogenes ▪ Motile via actin rockets	Facultative	Listeriolysin O Endotoxin	Neonatal meningitis ▪ Vaginal transmission during birth Gastroenteritis ▪ Ingestion of unpasteurized milk/cheese and deli meats
Actinomyces israelii	Anaerobic	Normal oral flora	Actinomycosis ▪ Slow-growing, lumpy orofacial abscesses ▪ Characteristic **sulfur granules** in colonies

Gram-Negative Bacteria (Figure 18–7)

Gram-negative lab algorithm

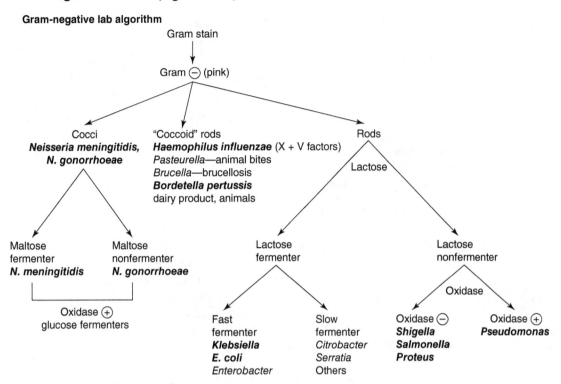

Important pathogens are in **bold type**.

FIGURE 18-7. **Gram-negative bacteria.**

Reproduced, with permission, from Le T, Bhushan V, Tolles J. *First Aid for the USMLE Step 1 2011.* 20th ed. New York: McGraw-Hill, 2010.

GRAM-NEGATIVE COCCI

See Table 18–14.

TABLE 18-14. **Comparison of Major Gram-Negative Cocci**

BACTERIUM	OXYGEN REQUIREMENT	MAJOR VIRULENCE FACTORS	DISEASE
Neisseria meningitidis ▪ Vaccine ▪ Low prevalence ▪ High mortality	Aerobic	Capsule Endotoxin (LPS) IgA protease	Meningitis (adolescents) Waterhouse–Friderichsen syndrome
Neisseria gonorrhoeae ▪ No vaccine ▪ High prevalence ▪ Low mortality	Aerobic	Endotoxin (LOS) Fimbriae IgA protease	Gonorrhea (STD): ▪ Urethritis: burning sensation during urination ▪ ♀: Vaginal discharge, PID ▪ ♂: Epididymitis ▪ Symptoms start 2–10 days after intercourse Pelvic inflammatory disease (PID) Neonatal conjunctivitis Septic arthritis

GRAM-NEGATIVE BACILLI

See Table 18–15.

- Enteric
- Respiratory
- Zoonotic

TABLE 18-15. Comparison of Major Gram-Negative Bacilli

BACTERIUM	OXYGEN REQUIREMENT	MAJOR VIRULENCE FACTORS	DISEASE
Enteric bacilli (associated with the enteric tract)			
Escherichia coli	Facultative	Heat-labile toxin Enterotoxin Endotoxin	UTI Dysentery Traveler's diarrhea Neonatal meningitis Septic shock
Salmonella sp. ■ Flagella	Facultative	Endotoxin	Enterocolitis ■ Transmission: animals (eggs, poultry, pets) Typhoid fever ■ Septicemia → osteomyelitis ■ Often in patients with sickle cell anemia
Shigella sp.	Facultative	Enterotoxin Endotoxin	Enterocolitis Dysentery ■ Bloody diarrhea
Vibrio cholerae ■ Comma-shaped	Facultative	Cholera toxin Enterotoxin Endotoxin	Cholera ■ Watery diarrhea
Campylobacter jejuni ■ Comma-shaped	Facultative	Enterotoxin Endotoxin	Enterocolitis (children)
Helicobacter pylori	Facultative	Endotoxin	Gastritis Peptic ulcers Gastric carcinoma (associated)
Klebsiella pneumoniae	Facultative	Capsule Endotoxin	Pneumonia ■ Assoc. with chronic respiratory disease, alcoholism, or diabetes UTI (nosocomial)

(Continued)

TABLE 18-15. Comparison of Major Gram-Negative Bacilli (Continued)

BACTERIUM	OXYGEN REQUIREMENT	MAJOR VIRULENCE FACTORS	DISEASE
Pseudomonas aeruginosa ▪ Produces a blue-green pigment in culture	Aerobic	Exotoxin A Endotoxin	**P**neumonia (cystic fibrosis) **S**epsis (burn infections) **E**xternal otitis (swimmer's ear) **U**TI **D**iabetic **o**steomyelitis
Bacteroides sp.	Anaerobic	Endotoxin Fimbriae	Abscess Periodontitis (associated)
Respiratory bacilli (associated with respiratory tract)			
Haemophilus influenzae	Facultative	Capsule Endotoxin IgA protease	Epiglottitis Meningitis (children) Otitis media Pneumonia
Haemophilus aegyptius ▪ Koch-Weeks bacillus	Facultative	Endotoxin (LOS)	Acute conjunctivitis (**pink eye**) ▪ Transmission: hand-to-hand contact Brazilian purpuric fever
Legionella pneumophila ▪ Silver stain > Gram stain	Facultative	Endotoxin	Legionnaires' disease ▪ Pneumonia and fever ▪ Transmission: environmental water sources (air conditioners) ▪ Patients tend to be older, smokers, and alcoholics
Bordetella pertussis ▪ Fimbriae	Aerobic	Pertussis toxin Tracheal cytotoxin Endotoxin	Pertussis (whooping cough)
Zoonotic bacilli (transmitted by animals)			
Brucella sp.	Facultative	Endotoxin	Brucellosis (undulant fever) ▪ Transmission: dairy products; contact with animals (goats, sheep, pigs, cattle)
Francisella tularensis	Facultative	Endotoxin	Tularemia ▪ Transmission: ticks; contact with wild animals (rabbits, deer)
Yersinia pestis	Facultative	Exotoxin Endotoxin F-1, V, and W antigens	Plague ▪ Transmission: fleas; rodents (prairie dogs, rats)
Pasteurella multocida	Facultative	Endotoxin	Cellulitis ▪ Transmission: animal bites (cats, dogs)

MICROBIOLOGY–PATHOLOGY

MICROBIOLOGY

If PPD(+): Indicates current TB infection, past exposure, or BCG vaccinated.

If PPD(–): Indicates no infection, or anergic.

MYCOBACTERIA

- Aerobic, nonmotile bacilli.
- Cell wall constituents:
  - Peptidoglycan: Prevents osmotic lysis.
  - **Mycolic acid:** Impedes chemical entry; resists phagocytosis. Waxy coating.
  - Surface proteins: Adhesins.
  - Periplasm: Contains enzymes for nutrient breakdown.
- Stain with **acid-fast** stain (carbolfuchsin): Red against blue background.

See Table 18–16.

OTHER BACTERIAL TYPES

(See Table 18–17.)

- *Mycoplasma* sp.: Lack a cell wall.
- *Chlamydia* sp.: Obligate intracellular bacteria (cannot make own ATP).
- *Rickettsia* sp.: Obligate intracellular bacteria (need host CoA and NAD^+).
- Spirochetes: Spiral-shaped.

TABLE 18–16. Comparison of Major *Mycobacteria* Species

	MAJOR VIRULENCE FACTORS	CHARACTERISTICS	DISEASE
Mycobacterium tuberculosis	Cord factor Tuberculoproteins	Inhalation of airborne droplets Treatment: rifampin, isoniazid, and pyrazinamide **PPD skin test** elicits type IV (delayed) hypersensitivity reaction	Tuberculosis: <ul><li>Fever, night sweats, weight loss, hemoptysis</li></ul> **1° TB:** granulomatous lesions and hilar lymphadenopathy (**Ghon complex**) in lungs **2° TB:** caseous granulomas which may lead to miliary or disseminated infection
Mycobacterium leprae	Lepromin proteins	Reservoir in US: armadillos Treatment: dapsone, rifampin	Leprosy: **Tuberculoid type:** Cell-mediated immune response and granulomas in nerves **Lepromatous type:** Foam cells containing bacteria in skin

TABLE 18-17. **Comparison of Wall-Less, Obligate Intracellular, and Spirochete Bacteria**

BACTERIUM	CHARACTERISTICS	DISEASE
Wall-less bacteria		
Mycoplasma pneumoniae	**Smallest bacterium** No cell wall; cell membrane contains **cholesterol**	Atypical "walking" pneumonia
Obligate intracellular bacteria		
Chlamydia trachomatis	Cannot make its own ATP Cell wall lacks muramic acid Forms cytoplasmic inclusions Most common cause of preventable blindness (can be contracted in a swimming pool) Most common cause of STDs	Trachoma: ▪ Chronic infection ▪ Inclusion conjunctivitis (IC) ▪ **Blindness** Chlamydia (STD): ▪ Urethritis/PID ▪ Neonatal conjunctivitis
Rickettsia rickettsii	Need host CoA and NAD$^+$ Causes vasculitis, headache, fever Positive Weil-Felix reaction Transmission: ticks	Rocky Mountain spotted fever ▪ Rash: palms and soles
Rickettsia prowazekii	Need host CoA and NAD$^+$ Causes vasculitis, headache, fever Positive Weil-Felix reaction Transmission: lice	Epidemic typhus ▪ Rash: central → peripheral (no palms/soles)
Coxiella burnetii	An atypical rickettsia Need host CoA and NAD$^+$ Negative Weil-Felix reaction Transmission: inhaled aerosols	Q fever ▪ Pneumonia
Spirochetes		
Treponema pallidum	Visualized by dark-field microscopy Congenital syphilis: CN VII deafness, Hutchinson's incisors, mulberry molars Treatment: penicillin	Syphilis: 1°: Painless chancre (ulcer) at site of local contact 2°: Highly infectious maculopapular rash, condylomata lata, mucous patch 3°: Gummas (granulomas) often on tongue or palate; neurosyphilis; Argyll-Robertson pupil
Borrelia burgdorferi	Visualized using aniline dyes (Wright's or Giemsa stain) with light microscopy Transmission: ticks (require deer) Most often occurs in CT, NY, PA, NJ Treatment: doxycycline	Lyme disease: **Stage 1:** Erythema migrans ("bull's eye" rash) **Stage 2:** Neuropathies (Bell's palsy) **Stage 3:** Arthritis and CNS disease

Bacterial Vaccines

Bacterial vaccinations can confer two types of acquired immunity. (See also Chapter 21, "Immunology and Immunopathology.")

Vaccine Type	Conferred Immunity	Treated Diseases
Live attenuated	Active	TB Typhoid fever Tularemia
Killed bacteria ▪ Whole bacteria	Active	Cholera Typhus Plague Q fever
Toxoid ▪ Inactivated endotoxin	Active	**D**iphtheria **P**ertussis **T**etanus
Capsular polysaccharide	Active	Pneumonia (*Strep. pneumoniae*) Meningitis (*N. meningitidis* and *H. influenzae*)
Purified protein	Active	Pertussis Lyme disease Anthrax
Antitoxin ▪ Preformed antibody to endotoxin	Passive	Diphtheria Tetanus Botulism

Concomitant administration of bacteriocidal and bacteriostatic antibiotics has an antagonistic effect because each interferes with the other's mechanism of action.

The DPT vaccine is given to all children in the US. It is a toxoid vaccine.

Most antibacterial activity occurs during the log phase of bacterial growth.

Toxoid: *inactivated bacterial exotoxin.*

Antitoxin: *antibody to bacterial exotoxin.*

Antibiotic Drugs

See Table 8–18.

CLASSIFICATION

▪ By spectrum:
  ▪ Broad: Effective against several types of bacteria.
  ▪ Narrow: Effective against only one or a few types of bacteria.
▪ By activity:
  ▪ Bacteriocidal: Kills bacteria.
  ▪ Bacteriostatic: Inhibits bacterial growth (host immune cells kill bacteria).

PENICILLINS

▪ Inhibit peptidoglycan cross-linking by blocking transpeptidase during last stage of cell wall synthesis
▪ Bacteriocidal
▪ Contain β-lactam rings, which are cleaved by bacterial β-lactamase (penicillinase), inactivating the drug

TABLE 18-18. Comparison of Common Antibiotics

DRUG CLASS	MECHANISM OF ACTION	ACTIVITY	SPECTRUM	PREGNANCY SAFE
Vancomycin	Inhibits peptidoglycan cross-linking by binding to D-alanyl-D-alanine during cell wall synthesis	Cidal	Narrow	Yes
Penicillins	Inhibit peptidoglycan cross-linking by blocking transpeptidase during last stage of cell wall synthesis	Cidal	Narrow ↓ Broader	Yes
Cephalosporins	Inhibit peptidoglycan cross-linking by blocking transpeptidase during last stage of cell wall synthesis	Cidal	Narrow ↓ Broader	Yes
Metronidazole	Inhibits DNA synthesis	Cidal	Narrow	No
Fluoroquinolones	Inhibit DNA gyrase (topoisomerase)	Cidal	Broader	No
Aminoglycosides	Inhibit protein synthesis by binding to 30S ribosomal subunits (block the formation of the initiation complex)	Cidal	Broader	No
Macrolides	Inhibit protein synthesis by binding to 50S ribosomal subunits (block the release of tRNA)	Static	Narrow	Yes
Clindamycin	Inhibit protein synthesis by binding to 50S ribosomal subunits (blocks the release of tRNA)	Static	Narrow	Yes
Chloramphenicol	Inhibits protein synthesis by binding to 50S ribosomal subunits (blocks peptidyl transferase)	Static	Broad	No
Tetracyclines	Inhibit protein synthesis by binding to 30S ribosomal subunits (block aminoacyl-tRNA binding)	Static	Broad	No
Sulfonamides	Inhibit folic acid synthesis by competing with p-aminobenzoic acid (PABA)	Static	Broad	No

Buy AT 30, CCELL at 50:
30S: Aminoglycocides, Tetracyclines
50S: Clindamycin, Chloramphenicol, Erythromycin, Lincomycin, Linezolid

MICROBIOLOGY–PATHOLOGY

MICROBIOLOGY

- 10% risk of hypersensitivity
  - First generation
    - Narrow spectrum: G(+) cocci/bacilli and some G(–) aerobic cocci
      - Penicillin G (IV)
      - Penicillin V (PO)
  - Second generation (β-lactamase resistant)
    - Narrow spectrum: Target G (+) β-lactamase-producing staphylococci (especially *S. aureus*)
      - Methicillin
      - Nafcillin
      - Oxacillin
      - Cloxacillin
      - Dicloxacillin
  - Third generation (extended spectrum)
    - Broader spectrum: Also include some G(–) bacilli.
      - Ampicillin (IV)
      - Amoxicillin (PO)
  - Combinations
    - An extended spectrum penicillin with a β-lactamase inhibitor.
    - Broader spectrum: Target more G(+) bacilli including β-lactamase staphylococci (especially *S. aureus*)
      - Amoxicillin and clavulanic acid
      - Ampicillin and sublactam

CEPHALOSPORINS

- Inhibit peptidoglycan cross-linking by blocking transpeptidase during last stage of cell wall synthesis
- Bacteriocidal
- Contain β-lactam rings
- 10% cross-hypersensitivity with penicillins
  - First generation
    - Narrow spectrum: G(+) cocci (but not enterococci) and some G(–) bacilli
      - Cefazolin
      - Cephalexin
      - Cefadroxil
  - Second generation
    - Broader spectrum: Fewer G(+) cocci, but more G(–) bacilli.
      - Cefaclor
      - Cefprozil
      - Cefoxitin
  - Third generation
    - Broader spectrum: Fewer G(+) cocci (except some enterococci), but more G(–) bacilli, and anaerobes
      - Cefpodoxime
      - Cefixime
  - Fourth generation
    - Broader spectrum: Fewer G(+) cocci (except more enterococci), but more G(–) bacilli, and anaerobes
      - Cefepime

VANCOMYCIN

- Inhibits peptidoglycan cross-linking by binding to D-alanyl-D-alanine during cell wall synthesis

- Bacteriocidal
- Treatment of choice for MRSA
- Narrow spectrum: Mostly G(+) cocci and bacilli (especially penicillinase-resistant *S. aureus*)

MACROLIDES

- Inhibit protein synthesis by binding to 50S ribosomal subunits (block the release of tRNA)
- Bacteriostatic
- Associated with GI upset
  - Erythromycin
    - Narrow spectrum: G(+) cocci/bacilli, some G(–) anaerobes, and *Mycoplasma* sp.
    - Inhibits cytochrome P450
  - Clarithromycin
    - Broader spectrum: Targets more anaerobes
  - Azithromycin
    - Broader spectrum: Targets more anaerobes

CLINDAMYCIN

- Inhibit protein synthesis by binding to 50S ribosomal subunits (blocks the release of tRNA)
- Bacteriostatic (in low doses)
- Narrow spectrum: G(+) and some G(–) anaerobes (*Bacteroides* sp.)
- Associated with diarrhea and **pseudomembranous colitis** (caused by an overgrowth of *Clostridium difficile*)

TETRACYCLINES

- Inhibit protein synthesis by binding to 30S ribosomal subunits (block aminoacyl-tRNA binding)
- Bacteriostatic
- Broad spectrum: G(+) and G(–) aerobes/anaerobes, spirochetes, *Mycoplasma* sp., *Chlamydia*, and *Rickettsia*
- Divalent and trivalent cations inhibit absorption
- Associated with staining of teeth during their calcification
  - Tetracycline
  - Doxycycline
  - Minocycline

METRONIDAZOLE

- Inhibits DNA synthesis
- Bacteriocidal
- Narrow spectrum: Targets anaerobes and some protozoa
- Disulfuram-like reaction with alcohol
- Often used to treat pseudomembranous colitis

FLUOROQUINOLONES

- Inhibit DNA gyrase (topoisomerase)
- Bacteriocidal
- Disulfuram-like reaction with alcohol
- Broader spectrum: G(+) and G(–) aerobes/facultatives and mycobacteria, but not anaerobes

    ■ Divalent and trivalent cations inhibit absorption
       ■ Ciprofloxacin
       ■ Ofloxacin

AMINOGLYCOSIDES

■ Inhibit protein synthesis by binding to 30S ribosomal subunits (block the formation of the initiation complex)
■ Bacteriocidal (in clinical doses)
■ Broader spectrum: G(+) and G(−) aerobes; ineffective against anaerobes
■ Associated with ototoxicity and nephrotoxicity; teratogens
    ■ Streptomycin
    ■ Gentamycin

SULFONAMIDES

■ Inhibit folic acid synthesis by competing with p-aminobenzoic acid (PABA)
■ Bacteriostatic
■ Broad spectrum: Targets G(+), many G(−), *Actinomyces* sp., and *Chlamydia* sp.
■ Associated with hypersensitivity, renal toxicity, and hematopoietic toxicity
    ■ Sulfadiazine
    ■ Sulfamethoxazole
    ■ Trimethoprim

CHLORAMPHENICOL

■ Inhibits protein synthesis by binding to 50S ribosomal subunits (blocks peptidyl transferase)
■ Bacteriostatic
■ Broad spectrum: Some G(+) cocci, G(−) aerobes/anaerobes, spirochetes, *Rickettsia* sp., *Chlamydia* sp., *Mycoplasma* sp., and *Salmonella* sp.
■ Associated with bone marrow toxicity, gray baby syndrome

TOPICAL ANTIBIOTICS

■ Neomycin: An aminoglycoside
■ Polymyxin B: Alters cell membrane permeability
■ Bacitracin: Inhibits cell wall synthesis

ANTIBIOTIC PROPHYLAXIS PRIOR TO DENTAL TREATMENT

See Table 18–19.

■ Prophylaxis is recommended for all dental procedures that involve manipulation of gingival tissues or periapical regions of the teeth, or perforation of the oral mucosa.
■ Prophylaxis recommendations are for patients with:
    ■ Heart conditions that may predispose them for infective endocarditis (IE).
    ■ Total joint replacement that may be at risk for infection at the site of the prosthesis.
■ The American Dental Association (ADA) has standardized the current guidelines for IE prevention in conjunction with the American Heart Association (AHA).
■ The ADA and the American Association of Orthopedic Surgeons (AAOS) do not have a joint recommendation at this time.

TABLE 18-19. Guidelines for Antibiotic Prophylaxis

SITUATION	DRUG	DOSAGE
Standard prophylaxis	Amoxicillin	Adults: 2 g PO 1 h before procedure. Children: 50 mg/kg PO 1 h before procedure.
Unable to take oral medications	Ampicillin	Adults: 2 g IM or IV within 30 min before procedure. Children: 50 mg/kg IM or IV within 30 min before procedure.
Allergic to penicillins	Clindamycin	Adults: 600 mg PO 1 h before procedure. Children: 20 mg/kg PO 1 h before procedure.
	Azithromycin or Clarithromycin	Adults: 500 mg PO 1 h before procedure. Children: 15 mg/kg PO 1 h before procedure.
	Cephalexin or Cefadroxil	Adults: 2 g PO 1 h before procedure. Children: 50 mg/kg PO 1 h before procedure.
Allergic to penicillins and unable to take oral medications.	Clindamycin	Adults: 600 mg IM or IV within 30 min before procedure. Children: 20 mg/kg IM or IV within 30 min before procedure.
	Cefazolin	Adults: 1 g IM or IV within 30 min before procedure. Children: 50 mg/kg IM or IV within 30 min before procedure.

Patient Selection

See Table 18–20.

TABLE 18-20. Antibiotic Prophylaxis for Patients at Risk for IE

PROPHYLAXIS NECESSARY	PROPHYLAXIS NOT NECESSARY
Artificial heart valves	Mitral valve prolapse
History of previous IE	Rheumatic heart disease
Heart transplant that develops a valve problem	Calcified aortic stenosis
Unrepaired or incompletely repaired cyanotic congenital heart disease, including those with palliative shunts and conduits	Congenital ventricular septal defect
Repaired congenital heart defect with a prosthetic device during the first 6 months after the procedure	Congenital atrial septal defect
Any repaired congenital heart defect with residual defect at the site of or adjacent to the site of a prosthetic device	Congenital hypertrophic cardiomyopathy

All viruses are haploid (1 copy of RNA/DNA) except retroviruses, which are diploid.

All RNA viruses (except retrovirus and orthomyxovirus) replicate in the cytoplasm using their own RNA polymerase.

All DNA viruses (except poxvirus) replicate in the nucleus using host RNA polymerase.

Viruses

See Figure 18–8.

■ **Virion:** Infectious; complete virus particle (DNA/RNA + proteins).
■ Characterized by single- or double-stranded DNA or RNA (never both) surrounded by a protein **capsid.**
  ■ Repeating polypeptide subunits (capsomeres).
  ■ Protects viral genome from extracellular nucleases.
  ■ Essential for infectivity of virus.
  ■ Antigenic; provokes host immune response.
  ■ Serves as attachment protein in nonenveloped viruses.

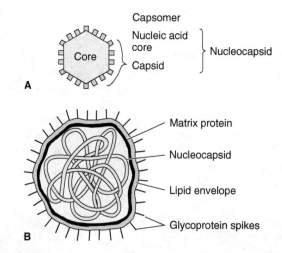

FIGURE 18–8. **Comparison of nonenveloped and enveloped viruses.**

Reproduced, with permission, from Levinson W. *Medical Microbiology and Immunology*, 8th ed. New York: McGraw-Hill, 2004.

Viroid: *Single molecule of circular RNA without a protein envelope. Causes plant diseases.*

■ **Nucleocapsid:** nucleic acid core + protein capsid.
■ Some viruses have an outer membrane called an **envelope**, which is composed of plasma membrane **lipoproteins** and glycoproteins obtained as the virus leaves its host cell (**budding**).
■ Do *not* contain mitochondria or ribosomes; must replicate within living host cells.
■ Not visible by light microscopy.

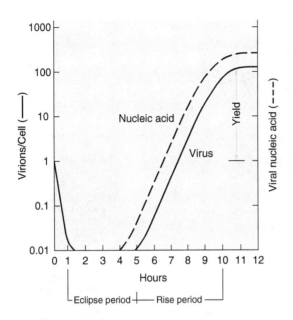

FIGURE 18-9. Viral growth curve.

Reproduced, with permission, from Levinson W. *Medical Microbiology and Immunology*, 8th ed. New York: McGraw-Hill, 2004.

Pathogenesis

VIRAL GROWTH CURVE

See Figure 18–9.

- **Latent phase:** Viral penetration → viral release 10–12 hours.
- **Eclipse phase:** Viral penetration → viral assembly within host cell.
  - No virus can be detected during this phase.
- **Rise phase:** Viral assembly → viral release.

VIRAL REPLICATION

See Figure 18–10.

- **Attachment:** Determined by the specificity of viral proteins to host cells.
- **Penetration:** Via receptor-mediated endocytosis (eg, pinocytosis).
- **Uncoating:** Viral nucleic acid is spilled into the cytoplasm.
- **Transcription and Translation:**
  - All **DNA viruses** (except poxviruses) replicate in the *nucleus* using host cell RNA polymerase.
  - All **RNA viruses** (except retroviruses and orthomyxoviruses) replicate in the *cytoplasm* using their own RNA polymerase. Transcription is only necessary for viruses whose RNA has *negative polarity* (a virus's RNA that has positive polarity serves as the mRNA itself).
  - All **retroviruses** use their own **reverse transcriptase** for transcription.
- **Assembly:** The new viral nucleic acid and capsid proteins are packaged.
- **Release:** Either by *budding* through the host plasma membrane (creating a viral envelope) or by host plasma membrane *rupture*.

One virion can replicate to form hundreds of progeny viruses.

*The host cellular morphologic and functional changes associated with viral replication and release are known as the **cytopathic effect (CPE)**. CPE is often specific for a particular virus. Not all viruses cause CPE.*

*Poliovirus, coxsackieviruses, and hepatitis A virus are **enteroviruses**.*

***Roboviruses** are rodent-borne viruses (rodent excrement): hantavirus (Sin Nombe virus).*

***Arboviruses** are arthropod-borne viruses (mosquitoes, ticks): West Nile virus, yellow fever virus, Dengue virus, Colorado tick fever virus, and Eastern/Western encephalitis virus.*

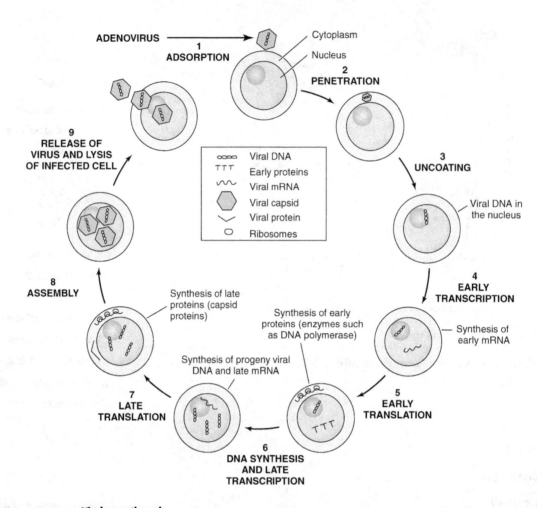

FIGURE 18–10. Viral growth cycle.

Reproduced, with permission, from Levinson W. *Medical Microbiology and Immunology*, 8th ed. New York: McGraw-Hill, 2004.

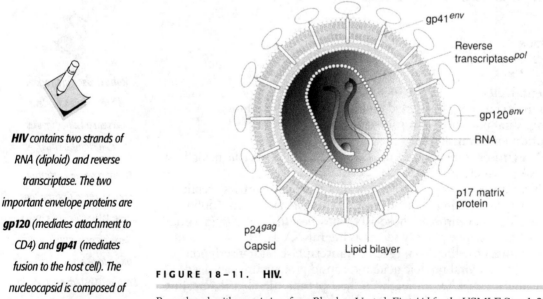

*HIV contains two strands of RNA (diploid) and reverse transcriptase. The two important envelope proteins are **gp120** (mediates attachment to CD4) and **gp41** (mediates fusion to the host cell). The nucleocapsid is composed of p24 and p7. (See Figure 18–11.)*

FIGURE 18–11. HIV.

Reproduced, with permission, from Bhushan V, et al. *First Aid for the USMLE Step 1*: 2006. New York: McGraw-Hill, 2006.

VIRAL ANTIGENIC CHANGES

- Antigenic changes contribute to the cause of epidemics and pandemics.
- Commonly associated with **influenza viruses** (orthomyxoviruses).
- There are two modes of antigenic change:
  - **Antigenic drifts:** Minor changes caused by genomic mutations.
  - **Antigenic shifts:** Major changes caused by genomic re-assortment.

Classification

RNA NONENVELOPED VIRUSES

See Table 18–21.

*Influenza viruses have two envelope glycoprotein spikes, **hemagglutinin** and **neuraminidase**, which exhibit the majority of antigenic changes.*

TABLE 18–21. RNA Nonenveloped Viruses in Order of Increasing Size

FAMILY	NUCLEIC ACID	VIRUS	DISEASE	ANTIVIRAL TREATMENT	VACCINE
Picornavirus ■ Smallest RNA virus	Single, Linear	**P**oliovirus	Polio	None	Yes ■ Salk ■ Sabin
		Echovirus	Aseptic meningitis	None	No
		Rhinovirus	Common cold	None	No
		Coxsackie A virus	**Herpangina:** ■ Soft palate, posterior pharynx **Hand-foot-and-mouth disease:** ■ Palms, soles, anterior oral mucosa Acute lymphonodular pharyngitis Aseptic meningitis	None	No
		Coxsackie B virus	Pleurodynia Myocarditis Pericarditis Aseptic meningitis	None	No
		HAV	Hepatitis A	None	Yes
Calicivirus	Single, Linear	Norwalk virus	Gastroenteritis (adults)	None	No
Hepevirus	Single, Linear	HEV	Hepatitis E	None	No
Reovirus	**Double,** Linear	Rotavirus	Gastroenteritis (infants)	None	No
		Coltivirus ■ Only virus transmitted by ticks	Colorado tick fever	None	No

- Picornavirus
- Calicivirus
- Hepevirus
- Reovirus

*Poliovirus, coxsackieviruses, echoviruses, and HAV are **enteroviruses:** they primarily infect the enteric tract.*

RNA-ENVELOPED VIRUSES

See Table 18–22.

- Deltavirus
- Flavivirus
- Togavirus
- Orthomyxovirus
- Retrovirus
- Paramyxovirus
- Rhabdovirus
- Filovirus
- Coronavirus
- Bunyavirus

TABLE 18–22. RNA-Enveloped Viruses in Order of Increasing Size

FAMILY	NUCLEIC ACID	VIRUS	DISEASE	ANTIVIRAL TREATMENT	VACCINE
Deltavirus	Single, circular	HDV	Hepatitis D	α-interferon	Yes
Flavivirus	Single, linear	Japanese encephalitis virus	Encephalitis	None	Yes
		Yellow fever virus	Yellow fever	None	Yes
		West Nile virus	Encephalitis	None	No
		Dengue virus	Dengue fever	None	No
		HCV	Hepatitis C Hepatocellular carcinoma (associated)	α-interferon Ribavirin	No
Togavirus	Single, linear	Rubella virus	**Rubella:** (German, "3-day" measles) Truncal rash Teratogen	None	Yes
		Eastern/Western encephalitis virus	Encephalitis	None	No

(Continued)

FAMILY	NUCLEIC ACID	VIRUS	DISEASE	ANTIVIRAL TREATMENT	VACCINE
Orthomyxovirus ▪ Exhibit various **antigenic changes** ▪ Replicate in nucleus	Single, linear	Influenza viruses	Influenza Reye's syndrome (association)	Amantidine Rimantidine Zanamivir Oseltamivir	Yes
Retrovirus ▪ Uses reverse transcriptase ▪ Replicate in nucleus ▪ Diploid	Single, linear	HTLV	Adult T-cell leukemia/ lymphoma Chronic progressive myelopathy	None	No
		HIV ▪ Infects CD4 T-helper cells ▪ Diagnosis confirmed by Western blot	AIDS	Zidovudine (AZT) Lamivudine Stavudine Indinavir Ritonavir	No
Paramyxovirus	Single, linear	**M**easles virus	**Measles (rubeola)** ▪ Nonpruritic maculopapular brick-red rash ▪ Multiple white lesions (Koplik's spots) are often seen on the buccal mucosa	None	Yes
		Mumps virus	**Mumps** ▪ Parotitis, orchitis, deafness	None	Yes
		RSV ▪ Infants only	Bronchiolitis Pneumonia	Ribavirin	No
		Parainfluenza viruses	**Croup** Bronchiolitis Common cold	None	No
Rhabdovirus	Single, linear	Rabies virus	Rabies	None	Yes
Filovirus	Single, linear	Ebola virus	Ebola Hemorrhagic fever	None	No
Coronavirus	Single, linear	Coronavirus	Common cold SARS	None	No
Bunyavirus	Single, circular	Hantavirus (Sin Nombre virus)	Hantavirus Hemorrhagic fever	None	No

MICROBIOLOGY-PATHOLOGY

MICROBIOLOGY

DNA Nonenveloped Viruses

See Table 18–23.

- Parvovirus
- Papillomavirus
- Polyomavirus
- Adenovirus

TABLE 18–23. Major DNA Nonenveloped Viruses in Order of Increasing Size

Family	Nucleic Acid	Virus	Disease	Antiviral Treatment	Vaccine
Parvovirus • Smallest DNA virus	**Single,** linear	B19 virus	Aplastic anemia • Sickle cell disease associated Erythema infectiosum (fifth disease) Fetal infections	None	No
Papillomavirus*	Double, circular	HPV	Papillomas (warts) Condyloma acuminatum (genital warts) Verruca vulgaris Cervical cancer	Podophyllin α-interferon Cidofovir	Yes
Polyomavirus*	Double, Circular	JC virus	Progressive multifocal leukoencephalopathy (PML) • HIV associated	None	No
Adenovirus	Double, linear	Adenovirus	Pharyngitis Conjunctivitis Pneumonia Common cold	None	Yes

* Formerly classified as papovaviruses.

DNA-Enveloped Viruses

See Table 18–24.

- Hepadnavirus
- Herpesvirus
- Poxvirus

Reye's syndrome is a potentially deadly disease that typically occurs in children aged 4–12 years. It is associated with the use of **aspirin** to treat influenza or varicella (chickenpox).

TABLE 18-24. **Major DNA-Enveloped Viruses in Order of Increasing Size**

FAMILY	NUCLEIC ACID	VIRUS	DISEASE	ANTIVIRAL TREATMENT	VACCINE
Hepadnavirus ▪ Has reverse transcriptase	Double, circular	HBV	Hepatitis B ▪ Hepatocellular carcinoma (associated)	α-interferon Lamivudine	Yes
Herpesvirus ▪ Lies dormant in **sensory nerve ganglia**, esp. trigeminal ganglion ▪ Obtains envelope from host nuclear membrane (not plasma membrane) ▪ **Tzanck test** assay for HSV-1, HSV-2, and VZV	Double, linear	HSV-1	Herpes labialis Keratoconjunctivitis Gingivostomatitis Recurrent encephalitis	Acyclovir Penciclovir Valacyclovir Famciclovir	No
		HSV-2	Herpes genitalis Neonatal encephalitis Aseptic meningitis	Acyclovir Penciclovir Valacyclovir Famciclovir	
		VZV	**Varicella**—primary ▪ Chickenpox ▪ Pruritic, macular lesions that become pustular and crusted ▪ Reye's syndrome (associated) **Zoster**—recurrent ▪ Shingles ▪ Usually localized to a single dermatome	Acyclovir Famciclovir Valacyclovir	Yes
		CMV	Congenital abnormalities ▪ Primary viral cause of mental retardation Cytomegalic inclusion disease	Ganciclovir Valganciclovir Foscarnet	No
		EBV	**Infectious mononucleosis** ▪ Transmission via saliva ▪ Splenomegaly, necrotizing pharyngitis ↑ abnormal lymphocytes ▪ Heterophile test used for screening Burkitt's lymphoma (association) Nasopharyngeal carcinoma (association) B-cell lymphoma (association) Hairy leukoplakia (association)	None (self-limiting in 2–3 weeks)	No
		HHV-8	Kaposi's sarcoma	None	No

(Continued)

TABLE 18–24. Major DNA-Enveloped Viruses in Order of Increasing Size (Continued)

Family	Nucleic Acid	Virus	Disease	Antiviral Treatment	Vaccine
Poxvirus ■ Largest DNA virus ■ Replicates in cytoplasm	Double, linear	Variola virus	Smallpox ■ Eradicated	None	Yes
		MCV	Molluscum contagiosum	None	No

Hepatitis Viruses

CLASSIFICATION

See Table 18–25.

SIGNS AND SYMPTOMS OF VIRAL HEPATITIS

Hepatitis viruses are extremely heat resistant (more so than HIV). Proper autoclaving kills all hepatitis viruses.

- Fatigue
- Myalgia
- Loss of appetite
- Nausea
- Diarrhea
- Constipation
- Fever
- Jaundice

TESTS OF LIVER FUNCTION

Viral hepatitis: ALT > AST
Alcoholic hepatitis: AST > ALT

- Bilirubin
- ALT (alanine aminotransferase)
- AST (aspartate aminotransferase)

SEROLOGY

See Figure 18–12 and Table 18–26.

TABLE 18–25. Comparison of Major Hepatitis Viruses

Virus	Nucleic Acid	Viral Class	Envelope	Transmission	Characteristics	Vaccine
HAV	ss RNA	Picornavirus	No	Fecal-oral	Usually self-limiting; recovery within 4 months.	Yes
HBV	ds DNA	Hepadnavirus	Yes	Bloodborne	Increased incidence of chronic liver disease, cirrhosis, HCC.	Yes
HCV	ss RNA	Flavivirus	Yes	Bloodborne	Increased incidence of chronic liver disease, cirrhosis, HCC.	No
HDV	ss RNA	Deltavirus	Yes	Bloodborne	Requires presence of HBsAg for replication.	Yes
HEV	ss RNA	Calicivirus	No	Fecal-oral	Causes occasional epidemics in underdeveloped countries.	No

HCC: hepatocellular carcinoma.

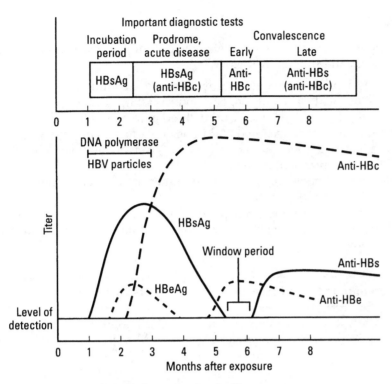

FIGURE 18–12. **Serologic findings associated with acute HBV.**

Reproduced, with permission, from Bhushan V, et al. *First Aid for the USMLE Step 1: 2006.* New York: McGraw-Hill, 2006.

TABLE 18–26. **Serological Profiles of Hepatitis Infections**

VIRUS	ACUTE INFECTION	CHRONIC DISEASE	IMMUNITY	PERCENT CHRONICITY
HAV	IgM Anti-HAV	None	Anti-HAV	None
HBV	**IgM Anti-HBc** HBsAg HBeAg	IgG Anti-HBc HBsAg	**Anti-HBs**	10% (adults) 30–90% (infants)
HCV	Anti-HCV	Anti-HCV	Anti-HCV	80%
HDV	IgM Anti-HDV	Anti-HDV	Anti-HDV	6%
HEV	IgM Anti-HEV	None	Anti-HEV	None

HCV is the most common reason for liver transplantation in the United States.

An individual vaccinated for HBV will show serology positive only for anti-HBs.

Viral Vaccines

Vaccinations can confer two types of acquired immunity. (See also Chapter 21, "Immunology and Immunopathology.")

- Viral vaccinations can confer two types of acquired immunity.
- Live attenuated vaccines provide longer-lasting and broader range of immunity than killed vaccines, but they have the potential to revert to virulence, or can be excreted and transmitted to nonimmune individuals.
- Live attenuated vaccines should not be given to immunocompromised individuals or pregnant women.
- Preformed antibody vaccines provide immediate protection, but only for a few weeks-months.
- Most viral vaccines are given pre-exposure; however, vaccines for rabies and hepatitis B may be given post-exposure since their incubation periods are so long.

Vaccine Type	Conferred Immunity	Protection	Treated Diseases
Live attenuated	Active - IgA - IgG - T$_C$-cell	Slow onset Longest lasting	Measles Mumps Rubella Polio (Sabin): oral Chickenpox Smallpox
Killed virus	Active - IgG	Slow onset Long lasting	Rabies Influenza Polio (Salk): injection Hepatitis A
Purified viral protein subunits	Active	Slow onset Long lasting	Hepatitis B - via HBsAg
Preformed antibody	Passive	Fast onset Short life span	Rabies Hepatitis B Shingles

Antiviral Drugs

INTERFERONS

- Glycoproteins that originate from infected host cells to protect other non-infected host cells.
- Do not directly affect viruses, but instead **nonspecifically prevent their replication** within host cells.
- Block various stages of viral RNA/DNA synthesis.
- INF-α: Treats chronic hepatitis B and C.
- Toxicity: neutropenia.

Bacteriophages (Phages)

- Viruses that infect bacterial cells.
- Replication can occur by two pathways (see Figure 18–13).
  - **Lytic cycle:** The process by which some phages replicate within the host cell, producing hundreds of new progeny phage. The host cell is ultimately destroyed.

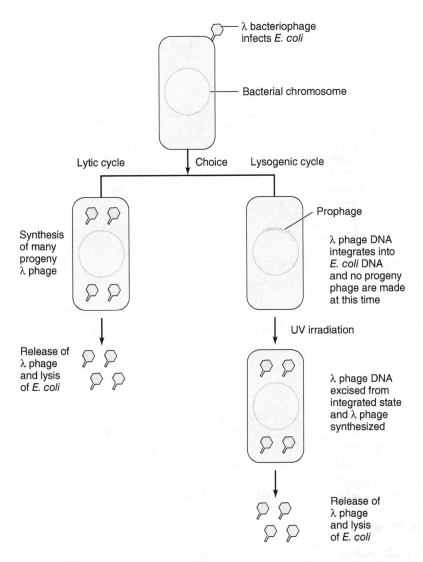

λ bacteriophage
infects *E. coli*

Bacterial chromosome

Lytic cycle Choice Lysogenic cycle

Prophage

Synthesis
of many
progeny
λ phage

λ phage DNA
integrates into
E. coli DNA
and no progeny
phage are made
at this time

UV irradiation

Release of
λ phage
and lysis
of *E. coli*

λ phage DNA
excised from
integrated state
and λ phage
synthesized

Release of
λ phage
and lysis
of *E. coli*

FIGURE 18–13. **Bacteriophage replication.**

Reproduced, with permission, from Levinson W. *Medical Microbiology and Immunology*, 8th ed. New York: McGraw-Hill, 2004.

- **Lysogenic cycle:** The process by which some phages incorporate their DNA in the host cell chromosome. The integrated viral DNA is called a **prophage**. Replication occurs only when the host DNA is damaged, excising the viral DNA. The host cell is usually not destroyed.

Lysogenic Conversion

- Alteration of the host bacterium to a pathogenic strain via expression of the integrated prophage genes (Figure 18–14). Eg, *Corynebacterium diphtheriae* producing diphtheria toxin.

Prions

- Infectious agents composed entirely of protein (no nucleic acid).
- Do *not* elicit inflammatory or antibody responses.
- Cause **transmissible spongiform encephalopathy:**
  - Creutzfeldt–Jakob disease (in humans).
  - Mad cow disease (in cows).

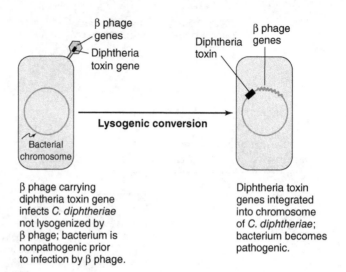

β phage carrying diphtheria toxin gene infects *C. diphtheriae* not lysogenized by β phage; bacterium is nonpathogenic prior to infection by β phage.

Diphtheria toxin genes integrated into chromosome of *C. diphtheriae*; bacterium becomes pathogenic.

FIGURE 18-14. Lysogenic conversion.

Reproduced, with permission, from Levinson W. *Medical Microbiology and Immunology*, 8th ed. New York: McGraw-Hill, 2004.

Fungi

- Gram (+), eukaryotic microorganisms.
- All are either obligate (the majority) or facultative **aerobes**.
- Cell membranes: lipid bilayer contains **ergosterol**.
- Cell walls: carbohydrate and protein (**chitin**).
- Capsule (if present): polysaccharide coating.
- Laboratory diagnosis by **KOH preparation**.

FUNGAL REPRODUCTION

- **Sexual:** Mating and formation of **spores**.
    - **Zygospores:** Single, large spores with thick walls.
    - **Ascospores:** Formed in a sac (ascus).
    - **Basidiospores:** Formed on the tip of a pedestal (basidium).
- **Asexual:** Budding and formation of **conidia** (asexual spores).
    - **Arthrospores:** Formed by fragmentation of the ends of hyphae.
    - **Chlamydospores:** Rounded, thick-walled, and highly resistant.
    - **Blastospores:** Formed by budding process.
    - **Sporangiospores:** Formed on a stalk within a sac (sporangium).

Pathogenesis

- **Fungal infection:** Leads to a largely **cell-mediated immune response** (type IV hypersensitivity reaction) and **granuloma** formation.
- **Mycotoxicosis:** Induced by ingestion of fungal toxins.
- **Allergic response:** Type I hypersensitivity reactions to inhalation of fungal spores.

Classification

See Table 18–27.

- Yeasts
- Molds

Most fungal spores and conidia are killed at temperatures > 80°C for 30 minutes.

Most antifungal drugs target the ergosterol component of fungal cell membranes, altering their permeability.

***Aflatoxins** are hepato-carcinogenic toxins produced by **Aspergillus flavus**, generally found in contaminated grains and peanuts.*

*Some fungi are **dimorphic**— they exist as molds at ambient temperatures but as yeasts at warmer (body) temperatures.*

TABLE 18–27.   Comparison of Yeasts and Molds

FUNGUS	MORPHOLOGY	REPRODUCTION
Yeasts	Single cells	Asexual budding
Molds	**Hyphae** (long filaments), which form a mat-like structure (**mycelium**)	Cell division

MEDICALLY RELEVANT FUNGI

- Systemic fungal infections. (See Table 18–28.)
- Cutaneous fungal infections (See Table 18–29).
- Opportunistic fungal infections. (See Table 18–30.)

*Most systemic mycoses can mimic TB infection – they form **granulomas**.*

TABLE 18–28.   Major Systemic Fungal Infections

FUNGUS	DISEASE	TYPE	CHARACTERISTICS	TREATMENT
Blastomyces dermatitidis	Blastomycosis	Dimorphic	Endemic in eastern US and Central America. Inhalation of microconidia produces granulomatous nodules in lungs and respiratory infection.	Itraconazole Amphotericin B
Coccidioides immitis	Coccidioidomycosis (desert valley fever) (San Joaquin fever)	Dimorphic	Endemic in southwest US and Latin America. Inhalation of **arthrospores** produces respiratory infection.	Amphotericin B Itraconazole Ketoconazole Fluconazole
Histoplasma capsulatum	Histoplasmosis	Dimorphic	Endemic in Ohio and Mississippi River valleys. Found in soil often contaminated by **bird/bat droppings**. Inhalation of microconidia produces respiratory infection. **Yeast cells located within host macrophages.**	Itraconazole Amphotericin B Fluconazole

TABLE 18–29.   Major Cutaneous Fungal Infections

FUNGUS	DISEASE	TYPE	CHARACTERISTICS	TREATMENT
Trichophyton sp. *Epidermophyton* sp. *Microsporum* sp.	Dermatophytosis	Molds	Tinea corporus (**ringworm**) Tinea capitis (scalp itch) Tinea cruris (jock itch) Tinea pedis (athlete's foot) Tinea unguium (nail fungus)	Miconazole Clotrimazole Tolnaftate **Griseofulvin**

TABLE 18-30. **Major Opportunistic Fungal Infections**

FUNGUS	DISEASE	TYPE	CHARACTERISTICS	SUSCEPTIBILITY
Aspergillus fumigatus	Aspergillosis	Mold	Inhalation of conidia causes respiratory infection and aspergilloma (**fungus ball**) formation in lungs.	AIDS Organ transplantation
Candida albicans	**Candidiasis** Vaginitis Angular cheilitis Median rhomboid glossitis	Yeast	Part of normal human flora of mouth, vagina, GI tract, and skin. Appears as budding yeasts or **pseudohyphae.**	AIDS Prolonged use of antibiotics
Cryptococcus neoformans	Cryptococcosis	Yeast	Heavily encapsulated. Inhalation of spores causes respiratory infection, meningitis, and pneumonia.	AIDS
Mucor sp. *Rhizopus* sp. *Absidia* sp.	Mucormycosis	Molds	Inhalation of conidia causes respiratory, skin, **paranasal sinus, and brain infections.**	**Diabetes (ketoacidosis)** Leukemia Burns

Opportunistic infections

induce disease in immunocompromised patients, such as those with AIDS or who take immunosuppressive medications.

Antifungal Drugs

See Table 18–31.

- The vast majority of the antifungal drugs prescribed by dentists are used to treat *candidiasis*, the major fungal infection that affects the oral cavity.

TABLE 18-31. **Common Antifungal Drugs to Treat Candidiasis**

DRUG	MECHANISM OF ACTION	COMMON FORMS
Nystatin	Binds to ergosterol.	Topical Oral suspension
Amphotericin B	Binds to ergosterol.	Topical Oral suspension Intravenous
Clotrimazole	Inhibits ergosterol synthesis.	Troche
Ketoconazole	Inhibits ergosterol synthesis. Blocks fungal cytochrome P450.	Tablet
Fluconazole	Inhibits ergosterol synthesis. Blocks fungal cytochrome P450.	Tablet

Parasites

CLASSIFICATION

- Protozoa
  - *Unicellular*, eukaryotic microorganisms that lack a cell wall and largely infect blood cells, intestinal and urogenital tissue, and meninges.
- Metazoa (helminths)
  - *Multicellular* worms that often infect the intestines, brain, liver, and other tissues.

PHYLOGENY

See Figure 18–15.

*Parasitic infections generally elicit an **IgE-mediated** host immune response accompanied by marked **eosinophilia**.*

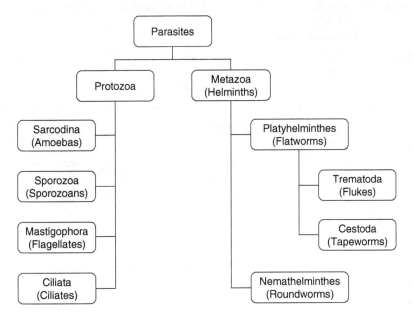

FIGURE 18–15. Phylogeny of parasites.

Reproduced, with permission, from Levinson W. *Medical Microbiology and Immunology*, 8th ed. New York: McGraw-Hill, 2004.

MICROBIOLOGY–PATHOLOGY

MICROBIOLOGY

MEDICALLY RELEVANT PARASITES

- Protozoa. (See Table 18–32.)
- Metazoa (helminths). (See Table 18–33.)

TABLE 18-32. Common Protozoa Associated with Human Infection

PROTOZOAN	DISEASE	TRANSMISSION	MORPHOLOGY	TREATMENT
Entamoeba histolytica	**Amebiasis:** Dysentery Liver abscess	Fecal-oral	Motile **trophozoite** (intestinal). Nonmotile **cyst** (contaminated food/water).	Metronidazole
Giardia lamblia	**Giardiasis:** Diarrhea Flatulence	Fecal-oral	Motile **trophozoite** (intestinal). Nonmotile **cyst** (contaminated food/water). Common in US.	Metronidazole
Cryptosporidium parvum	**Cryptosporidiosis:** Diarrhea	Fecal-oral	Associated with immuno-suppression (AIDS)	Preventive
Trichomonas vaginalis	**Trichomoniasis:** Vaginitis (♀) Urethritis (♂)	STD	Motile **trophozoite.**	Metronidazole
Plasmodium vivax *Plasmodium ovale* *Plasmodium malariae* *Plasmodium falciparum* (most fatal)	**Malaria** (influenza-like onset): Fever Headache Anemia Splenomegaly	Female **mosquitoes** (*Anopheles*) Infected blood products	**Sporozoite.** **Merozoite** (liver). **Hypnozoite** (latent). Causes lysis of **erythrocytes.**	Chloroquine Mefloquine Primaquine
Toxoplasma gondii	**Toxoplasmosis:** CNS infection Encephalitis Seizures Associated with AIDS	Fecal-oral **Transplacental**	Motile **trophozoite** (intestinal). Nonmotile **cyst** (uncooked meat and **cat feces**).	Sulfadiazine Pyrimethamine
Pneumocystis jiroveci (formerly *P. carinii*)	**Pneumonia**	Inhalation	**Fungus** (originally classified as protozoan). Associated with immuno-suppression (AIDS). Found in oral cavity, but not pathologic.	Trimethoprim Sulfamethoxazole Pentamidine

TABLE 18-33. **Common Metazoa (Helminths) Associated with Human Infection**

METAZOAN	DISEASE	TRANSMISSION	CHARACTERISTICS	TREATMENT
Taenia solium	Taeniasis (tapeworm)	Ingestion of undercooked **pork.**	**Cysticercosis** (muscle cysts). **Neurocysticercosis** (brain cysts).	Praziquantel Albendazole
Taenia saginata	Taeniasis (tapeworm)	Ingestion of undercooked **beef.**	Does not cause cysticercosis.	Praziquantel
Enterobius vermicularis	Enterobiasis (pinworm)	Ingestion of worm eggs.	**Most common worm** in US. Associated with **perianal pruritis.**	Mebendazole
Trichinella spiralis	Trichinosis (roundworm)	Ingestion of undercooked meat (pork, wild game).	Larvae only grow in **striated muscle.** Associated with muscle pain, **periorbital edema,** fever.	Mebendazole

CHAPTER 19

Oral Microbiology and Pathology

Periodontal health is characterized by the predominant inhabitants of the oral cavity, mostly gram-positive facultative species such as Streptococcus sanguis, Streptococcus mitis, Streptococcus salivarius, Actinomyces viscosus, Actinomyces naeslundii, and a few beneficial gram-negative species such as Veillonella parvula and Capnocytophaga ochracea.

Streptococcus salivarius is the microorganism most commonly found on the surface of the tongue.

As a plaque biofilm extends from a supragingival to a subgingival environment, there is a shift in the microbial flora from mostly gram-positive, facultative cocci to predominantly gram-negative, anaerobic bacilli and spirochetes.

- Even though the oral cavity harbors more than 300 species of bacteria, most are part of the normal oral flora. A few, however, are heavily associated with both dental and periodontal diseases.

Plaque

- An organized **biofilm** consisting of 80% water and 20% solids: 95% microorganisms; and 5% organic components (polysaccharides, proteins, glycoproteins), inorganic components (calcium, phosphorus), desquamated cells (epithelial cells, leukocytes), and food debris.
- It adheres to teeth, dental prostheses, and oral mucosal surfaces and is also found in the gingival sulcus and periodontal pockets.
- Dental plaque is classified as *supragingival* and *subgingival* based on its position along the tooth surface. (See Table 19–1.)
- As plaque matures, there is a transition from the early aerobic environment characterized by gram-positive facultative species to an exceedingly oxygen-deprived milieu in which gram-negative anaerobes predominate.
- It is the key etiologic agent in the initiation of both caries and periodontal diseases.

PLAQUE FORMATION

- **Pellicle formation:** Salivary and GCF **glycoproteins** bind to oral mucosal, tooth, and dental prosthesis surfaces *almost immediately* via electrostatic and van der Waals forces. It prevents tissue desiccation and provides surface lubrication, but also promotes bacterial adherence.
- **Bacterial colonization:** Occurs within a few hours of pellicle formation. Gram-positive facultative species (*Streptococcus* sp., *Actinomyces* sp., *Lactobacillus* sp.) are the first to colonize through the binding of their adhesins and fimbriae to the pellicle.

TABLE 19–1. Comparison of Supragingival and Subgingival Plaque

PLAQUE	LOCATION	FORM	DOMINANT BACTERIAL SPECIES	AFFECTED BY DIET AND SALIVA
Supragingival	At or coronal to the gingival margin	Attached to gingival epithelial and tooth surfaces	Gram-positive facultative cocci	Yes
Subgingival	Apical to the gingival margin	Attached to gingival epithelial and tooth surfaces, but also loosely adherent within the sulcus	Gram-negative anaerobic bacilli and spirochetes	No

- **Maturation:** Multiplication and coaggregation of bacterial species that do not initially colonize tooth and gingival epithelial surfaces.
- **Mineralization:** Calculus formation. Plaque becomes 50% mineralized in about 2 days, and 90% mineralized in about 12 days.

Calculus

- Calcified bacterial plaque that forms on teeth and dental prostheses.
- 70–90% of calculus is composed of inorganic components (calcium, phosphorus), the majority of which are crystalline (**hydroxyapatite**).
- The remaining 10–30% of calculus is organic, consisting of protein— **carbohydrate** complexes, desquamated cells (epithelial cells, leukocytes), and microorganisms.
- **Saliva** is the main mineral source for *supragingival calculus*, but **GCF** provides most of the mineral for *subgingival calculus*.
- The most common locations for supragingival calculus are the lingual of mandibular anterior teeth and the buccal of maxillary molars (due to their proximity to salivary ducts).

*Calculus does **not** directly cause gingival inflammation, but provides a rough surface for the continued accumulation of perio-pathogenic bacterial plaque.*

CALCULUS FORMATION

- **Epitactic concept:** The predominant theory of calculus formation, which suggests that seeding agents (protein–carbohydrate complexes or bacteria) induce small foci of mineralization, which ultimately enlarge and coalesce to form a calcified mass.

Materia Alba

- Loosely adherent matter largely composed of desquamated cells, food debris, and other components of dental plaque that is easily washed away.

▶ ORAL PATHOLOGY

Caries

CHARACTERISTICS

- Cariogenic bacteria synthesize glucans (dextrans) and fructans (levans) from their metabolism of dietary sucrose (via *glucosyltransferase*), which contribute to their adherence to tooth surfaces.
- As a consequence, **lactic acid** is formed, reducing salivary pH and creating sites of enamel demineralization and cavitation.

Caries formation needs:
- *Cariogenic bacteria*
- *A susceptible surface*
- *A fermentable carbohydrate source*

STEPHAN CURVE

See Figure 19–1.

- Rapid drop in salivary pH within a few minutes after fermentable carbohydrate (eg, sucrose) intake.
- Enamel demineralization occurs once the pH falls below 5.5.
- Recovery to a normal salivary pH can take 15–40 minutes.
- The *frequency* of carbohydrate intake is more detrimental than the *quantity* because it maintains a prolonged decrease in pH.

- **Streptococcus sp.**
  (S. mutans, S. sanguis, S. salivarius) *generally cause pit and fissure, smooth-surface, and root caries.*
- **Lactobacillus sp.**
  (L. casei, L. acidophilus) *generally cause pit and fissure caries.*
- **Actinomyces sp.**
  (A. viscosus, A. naeslundii) *generally cause root caries.*

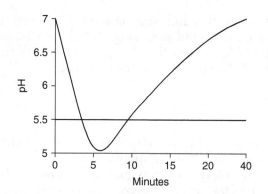

FIGURE 19-1. The Stephan curve.

Recurrent caries *occurs around an existing restoration. It may occur on the crown or the root.*

Gingivitis associated with sex steroid fluctuations (pregnancy, puberty, menstrual cycle, oral contraceptive use) is associated with elevated proportions of **Prevotella intermedia,** *which uses these steroids as growth factors.*

CLASSIFICATION

- Pit and fissure
- Smooth-surface
- Root
- Recurrent

PREDOMINANT MICROBIAL FLORA

- Generally **gram-positive, facultative cocci and bacilli.**
- They are acidogenic (make acid) and aciduric (tolerate living in acid).
- *Streptococcus mutans* is the primary etiologic agent of caries.

Plaque-Induced Gingivitis

CHARACTERISTICS

- Presence of plaque.
- Absence of attachment loss.
- Gingival inflammation, starting at the gingival margin.
- Can be modified by systemic factors, medications, or malnutrition.
- *Reversible* with removal of plaque (and modifying factor).

PREDOMINANT MICROBIAL FLORA

- Variable microbial pattern containing predominantly **gram-positive and gram-negative facultative and anaerobic cocci, bacilli, and spirochetes** such as *Streptococcus sanguis, Streptococcus mitis, Actinomyces viscosus, Actinomyces naeslundii, Peptostreptococcus micros, Fusobacterium nucleatum, Prevotella intermedia,* and *Campylobacter rectus.*

Chronic Periodontitis

- Formerly known as **adult periodontitis.**

CHARACTERISTICS

- Presence of plaque.
- Presence of attachment loss.
- Amount of periodontal destruction is *consistent* with presence of microbial deposits (subgingival plaque and calculus).
- Most prevalent in adults but can occur in children and adolescents.
- Generally progresses at a slow to moderate rate but may have periods of rapid progression.
- Can be modified by other local factors, systemic factors, medications, smoking, or emotional stress.

PREDOMINANT MICROBIAL FLORA

- Variable microbial pattern containing predominantly **gram-negative, anaerobic bacilli and spirochetes** such as *Porphyromonas gingivalis, Tanerella forsythensus* (formerly *Bacteroides forsythus*), *Treponema denticola, Prevotella intermedia, Fusobacterium nucleatum, Eikenella corrodens,* and *Campylobacter rectus.*

Recurrent periodontitis describes a recurrence of periodontitis after successful treatment.
Refractory periodontitis *describes periodontitis that does not respond to treatment.*

Aggressive Periodontitis

- Formerly known as **juvenile periodontitis** or **early-onset periodontitis**.

CHARACTERISTICS

- Presence of plaque.
- Presence of attachment loss.
- Amount of periodontal destruction is generally *inconsistent* with presence of microbial deposits.
- *Familial* aggregation.
- Usually affects individuals younger than 30 years but can occur in older patients.
- Generally progresses *rapidly* but may be self-arresting.
- Phagocyte abnormalities are common.
- Hyper-responsive monocyte/macrophage phenotype is common.
- Can be modified by other local factors, systemic factors, medications, smoking, or emotional stress.

CLASSIFICATION

- **Localized:** Localized to *first molars* and/or *incisors*. Typically a circumpubertal onset. Often self-limiting ("burns out") in 20s.
- **Generalized:** Affects at least three permanent teeth other than first molars and incisors. Usually affects people <30 years old, but patients may be older. Often associated with systemic diseases (neutropenias, leukemias, etc).

PREDOMINANT MICROBIAL FLORA

- Similar to chronic periodontitis with often elevated proportions of *Aggregatibacter actinmomycetemcomitans* (formerly *Actinobacillus actinomycetemcomitans*) and/or *Porphyromonas gingivalis.*

493

Necrotizing Periodontal Diseases

- Formerly known as **trench mouth** or **Vincent's disease**.

CHARACTERISTICS

- Presence of plaque.
- Interproximal gingival necrosis ("punched-out" papillae).
- Marginal gingival pseudomembrane formation.
- Attachment loss may or may not be present.
- Gingiva bleeds easily.
- Pain when brushing or eating.
- Bad breath (fetor oris).
- Commonly associated with emotional stress, malnutrition, smoking, or immunosuppression (HIV).

CLASSIFICATION

Spirochetes have been shown to invade the sulcular connective tissue in cases of NUG.

- **Necrotizing ulcerative gingivitis (NUG):** No attachment loss.
- **Necrotizing ulcerative periodontitis (NUP):** Attachment loss present.

PREDOMINANT MICROBIAL FLORA

- Variable microbial flora with elevated proportions of **spirochetes** (*Treponema* sp.), *Prevotella intermedia*, *Fusobacterium* sp., and *Selenomonas* sp.

Candidiasis

CHARACTERISTICS

- An opportunistic fungal infection.
- Commonly associated with immunosuppression (HIV), ill-fitting dentures, chronic xerostomia (Sjögren's syndrome), or prolonged use of antibiotics.

CLASSIFICATION

- **Pseudomembranous candidiasis (thrush):** Whitish patches of desquamative epithelium, which can be easily wiped off, leaving a slightly bleeding surface. Most common form.
- **Atrophic (erythematous) candidiasis:** Painful bright-red, smooth, "beefy" lesions on the tongue, palate, or other mucosal surfaces, usually associated with ill-fitting dentures.
- **Chronic hyperplastic candidiasis:** Asymptomatic whitish plaques commonly found on the buccal mucosa near the commissures that cannot be removed, resembling oral leukoplakia.

PREDOMINANT MICROBIAL FLORA

- *Candida albicans.*

Mechanical

- Toothbrushing and flossing are proven methods to remove plaque.
- However, they cannot remove subgingival plaque in pockets >3 mm deep (as in cases of periodontal disease).
- Dental professionals must scale teeth and root plane in order to remove the subgingival plaque and calculus.

Chemical

- Chemical means of plaque control is often used as an *adjunct* to mechanical cleaning.
- See Table 19–2 for commercially available products for chemical plaque control.

Two mouthrinses are ADA approved for the treatment of gingivitis: Rx-only chlorhexidine gluconate and an OTC phenolic/essential oil compound.

TABLE 19-2. **Commercially Available Products Used for Chemical Plaque Control**

CHEMICAL	FORMULATION	INHIBITS	CHARACTERISTICS
Chlorhexidine gluconate	Rinse	Plaque Gingivitis **(most potent inhibitor)**	Side effects: extrinsic staining, altered taste perception, and supragingival calculus formation
Phenolic/essential oil compound	Rinse	Plaque Gingivitis	Contains highest alcohol content (up to 26.9%)
Triclosan	Paste Gel	Plaque Gingivitis	
Stannous fluoride	Rinse Gel	Plaque Gingivitis	Side effects: extrinsic staining Anti-caries properties
Cetylpyridinium chloride	Rinse	Plaque	

Chlorhexidine gluconate is the most effective antiplaque mouthrinse due to its substantivity.

Reactions to Tissue Injury

Cell Injury

MODES OF CELL INJURY

Heart, brain, and lungs are very vulnerable to hypoxia. Results from:

- Vascular ischemia.
- ↓ blood oxygen (eg, anemia, pulmonary disease).
- ↓ tissue perfusion (eg, shock, cardiac failure).
- CO poisoning.

- Hypoxia and ischemia.
- Physical trauma: Burns, frostbite, radiation, electric shock, etc.
- Microorganisms: Bacteria, viruses, fungi, parasites, etc.
- Immunologic reactions: Autoimmunity and anaphylaxis.
- Chemical / pharmacologic insult: Poisons, drugs, alcohol, etc.
- Nutritional imbalances: Vitamin deficiency, obesity, etc.
- Genetic defects: Hemoglobinopathies, storage diseases, etc.
- Aging: ↑ telomerase activity, inaccurate repair of DNA, etc.

CHEMICAL INJURY

See Table 20–1.

TABLE 20–1. Chemical-Induced Cell Injury

CHEMICAL	FINDINGS
Carbon monoxide (CO)	Systemic hypoxia
Carbon tetrachloride (CCl_4)	Hepatocellular damage ("fatty liver")
Mercury	Renal tubular necrosis Pneumonitis GI ulceration Gingival lesions
Cyanide	Prevents cellular oxidation Odor of bitter almonds
Methanol	Blindness
Lead	Basophilic stippling of RBCs

FREE RADICAL INJURY

- Induced by activated oxygen species.
- Initiate autocatalytic reactions.
- Cellular damage:
    - Membrane lipid peroxidation
    - Nucleic acid denaturation
    - Cross-linking of proteins
- Generated from:
    - Redox reactions
    - Radiation (UV light)
    - Drugs and chemicals
    - Reperfusion injury
- Antioxidants:
    - Superoxide dismutase ($2O_2 + 2H^+ \rightarrow H_2O_2 + O_2$)
    - Catalase ($2H_2O_2 \rightarrow O_2 + 2H_2O$)

- Vitamin E
- Ceruloplasmin: Carries copper in blood

TYPES OF CELL INJURY

- Reversible cell injury
  - Cellular and organelle swelling (due to Ca^{2+} influx).
  - Bleb formation.
  - Ribosomal detachment from ER.
  - Clumping of chromatin (due to ↓ pH).
  - Increased lipid deposition (due to ↓ protein synthesis).
- Irreversible cell injury
  - Extensive plasma membrane damage.
  - Massive Ca^{2+} influx.
  - Diminished oxidative phosphorylation within mitochondria (due to accumulation of Ca^{2+}-rich densities).
  - Release of lysosomal enzymes into the cytoplasm (due to lysosomal rupture).
  - Nuclear fragmentation (**karyorrhexis**).
  - Cell death (necrosis).

The outcome of cell injury depends largely on the severity and duration of the insult, but also on the cell type and its adaptive mechanisms.

CELLULAR REACTIONS TO INJURY

See Table 20–2.

TABLE 20–2. **Cellular Reactions to Injury**

CELLULAR REACTION	DEFINITION	RESULTS
Atrophy	Decrease in cell size	Decrease in tissue or organ size (usually secondary to decreased workload, neurovascular supply, nutrition, endocrine stimulation, and increase in age)
Hypertrophy	Increase in cell size	Increase in tissue or organ size (usually secondary to increased tissue workload or endocrine stimulation)
Aplasia	Complete lack of cells	**Agenesis** (tissue or organ absence)
Hypoplasia	Decrease in cell numbers	Decrease in tissue or organ size
Hyperplasia	Increase in cell numbers	Increase in tissue or organ size (eg, glandular breast proliferation associated with pregnancy)
Metaplasia	Reversible, morphological change from one cell type to another	Usually occurs in response to stress (eg, conversion of columnar epithelium to stratified squamous)

Hypertrophy and hyperplasia can occur simultaneously (eg, uterine enlargement during pregnancy).

Gingival overgrowth is often drug related:

- Phenytoin (Dilantin)
- Ca^{2+} channel blockers (eg, nifedipine)
- Cyclosporin

ENZYMATIC CELLULAR DEGRADATION

■ **Autolysis:** Cellular degradation caused by *intracellular* enzymes indigenous to the cell itself.
■ **Heterolysis:** Cellular degradation caused by enzymes *extrinsic* to the cell.

ENDOGENOUS PIGMENTATION

See Table 20–3.

TABLE 20–3. Comparison of Endogenous Pigments

PIGMENT	CHARACTERISTICS	ASSOCIATED PATHOLOGY
Lipofuscin	Yellow-brown color "Wear-and-tear" pigment Derived from lipid peroxidation Has no effect on cell function Accumulates in heart, liver, brain	Brown atrophy Age
Bilirubin	Yellowish color Major bile pigment Derived from heme **Jaundice:** Bilirubin accumulation	Biliary tree obstruction Hepatocellular injury Hemolytic anemias

Hemosiderin (see Table 20–4)	Golden brown color
	Derived from heme
	Aggregates of ferritin micelles (iron storage sites)
	Identified with Prussian blue stain
	Accumulates in phagocytes of:
	  Bone marrow
	  Liver
	  Spleen
		Hemosiderosis
		Hemochromatosis

Melanin	Brown-black color
	Derived from *tyrosine*
	Synthesized in melanocytes
	Accumulates in skin, eyes, hair
		Increased melanin:
		  Physiologic pigmentation
		  Suntan
		  Addison's disease
		Decreased melanin:
		  Albinism
		  Vitiligo

Ceroid	Derived from lipofuscin (via auto-oxidation) Accumulates in hepatic Kupffer cells	Hepatocellular injury

TABLE 20–4. Hemosiderin Accumulation

PROCESS	DEFINITION	ASSOCIATIONS	TISSUE INJURY
Hemosiderosis	Increased hemosiderin accumulation (in tissue macrophages)	Hemorrhage Thalassemia	No
Hemochromatosis (Bronzed disease)	More extensive hemosiderin accumulation (throughout body)	↑ Iron absorption ↓ Iron utilization Hemolytic anemias Blood transfusions	Yes

Hemosiderin is an insoluble, iron-containing protein derived from ferritin. It is detected histologically by Prussian blue stain.

PATHOLOGIC CALCIFICATIONS

See Table 20–5.

- Abnormal deposition of calcium salts in normally noncalcified tissues.
- Types of calcifications:
  - Dystrophic
  - Metastatic

TABLE 20–5. Types of Pathologic Calcification

CALCIFICATION TYPE	DEFINITION	SERUM CA²⁺	PATHOGENESIS	COMMON LOCATIONS
Dystrophic	Calcification of degenerate or necrotic tissue	Normal	Enhanced by *collagen* and *acidic phosphoproteins* (eg, osteopontin)	Hyalinized scars Degenerated leiomyoma foci Caseous nodules (Tb) Damaged heart valves Atherosclerotic plaques
Metastatic	Calcification of normal tissue	Abnormal	Precipitation caused by tissue *acidity* and increased Ca²⁺ concentration *Associated with:* Hyperparathyroidism Vitamin D intoxication Bone destruction (eg, metastatic cancer) Sarcoidosis	Stomach Lungs Kidneys

Eggshell calcification:
- Thin layer of calcification around intrathoracic lymph nodes.
- Seen on chest X-ray.
- Associated with silicosis.

Calcinosis:
- Calcification in or under the skin.
- Associated with *scleroderma* and *dermatomyositis.*

Sialolithiasis:
- Formation of salivary stone (sialolith) within salivary gland or duct.
- Pain more severe when eating.

Cell Death

NECROSIS

See Table 20–6.

- Most common form of cell death resulting from irreversible injury.
- Characterized histologically by a vacuolated cytoplasm, calcification, and nuclear changes.
- Cellular degradation:
    - **Autolysis:** Caused by intracellular enzymes of necrotic cell.
    - **Heterolysis:** Caused by enzymes outside the necrotic cell.
- Three major forms of necrosis:
    - Coagulative
    - Liquefactive
    - Caseous

Coagulative necrosis is the most common form of necrosis.

Infarction: *Tissue death secondary to ↓ O₂ supply (↓ blood supply).*

TABLE 20-6. Major Types of Necrosis

NECROSIS	CHARACTERISTICS	EXAMPLE
Coagulative	Ischemia	Myocardial infarction
	Protein denaturation	
	Tissue architecture preserved	
	Infarct area is triangular shaped	
Gangrenous	Ischemic coagulation	Gangrene
	Putrefaction	
Liquefactive	Enzymatic digestion	Brain abscess
	Suppuration	
	Loss of tissue architecture	
Fat	Adipose liquefaction	Acute pancreatitis
	Fatty acids released	
Caseous	Granulomatous inflammation	Tuberculosis
	Clumped cheesy material	

NUCLEAR CHANGES ASSOCIATED WITH CELL DEATH

See Table 20–7.

TABLE 20-7. Irreversible Nuclear Changes Associated with Cell Death

NUCLEAR CHANGE	DESCRIPTION
Pyknosis	Nuclear shrinkage and chromatin condensation
Karyolysis	Nuclear dissolution and chromatin fading (basophilia)
Karyorrhexis	Nuclear fragmentation; completely disappears in 1–2 days

APOPTOSIS

- Programmed cell death that occurs in both physiologic and pathologic states.
- Does *not* result in an inflammatory response.
- Induced by several cytosolic proteases.
- There is no breakdown in the mechanisms that supply cellular energy.
- Leads to nuclear pyknosis and karyorrhexis, cell shrinkage, and ultimately phagocytosis by macrophages or neighboring parenchymal cells.
- There is no rupture of the cell membrane.
- Normal cell volume is maintained.

Inflammation

- A *vascular* and *cellular* response to tissue injury, resulting in the isolation of the causative agent, elimination of necrotic cells and tissues, and host tissue repair.
- There are two basic types of inflammatory response:
  - Acute
  - Chronic

ACUTE INFLAMMATION

See Table 20–8 for two stages of acute inflammation.

- The initial response to tissue injury, largely consisting of leukocyte infiltration, which rids the affected area of infectious agents (mostly bacteria) and degrades necrotic tissues resulting from the damage.
- **PMNs** are the first leukocytes to respond.
- Will elicit increased antibody titer.
- The presence of *monocytes* and *macrophages* marks the transition from acute to chronic inflammation.
- Its outcome may include the following (see also the section "Wound Repair" later in this chapter):
  - **Regeneration:** Complete resolution of affected tissues.
  - **Repair:** Fibrosis (scarring) of affected tissues.
  - **Abscess:** Formation of *pus* (neutrophils, necrotic cells, and exudate).
  - **Chronic inflammation:** See the section "Chronic Inflammation."

Acute inflammation generally precedes chronic inflammation, although some types of injury can directly induce a chronic inflammatory response.

The five classic signs of acute inflammation:

- **Redness (rubor):** From vasodilation and ↑ vascular permeability.
- **Heat (calor):** From vasodilation and ↑ vascular permeability.
- **Swelling (tumor):** From edema.
- **Pain (dolor):** From inflammatory mediators and pressure due to edema.
- **Loss of function (functio laesa):** From swelling and pain.

TABLE 20–8. The Two Stages of Acute Inflammation

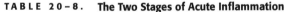

STAGE	EVENTS	CHARACTERISTICS
Vascular	Vasodilation and increased vascular permeability, predominantly mediated by **histamine-producing cells** (mast cells, basophils, and platelets)	Formation of an exudative **edema** (a straw-colored *protein-rich exudate* of extravascular fluid) Increased blood flow (hyperemia) may lead to vascular *congestion*
Cellular	Margination, adhesion, diapedesis, and chemotaxis of leukocytes (predominantly polymorphonuclear neutrophils [**PMNs**]) toward the site of injury	Phagocytosis and leukocyte degranulation leads to *microbial cell lysis*, but also host tissue damage

EDEMA

Edema Type	Cause	Characteristics
Exudate	*Inflammatory* increase in vascular permeability	Cell-rich (WBCs, cellular debris) High plasma protein High specific gravity Flushes away foreign material
Transudate	*Noninflammatory* alteration of vascular hydrostatic or osmotic pressures	Few cells Low plasma protein Low specific gravity

CHRONIC INFLAMMATION

- A prolonged inflammatory response consisting of *continuous* inflammatory cell infiltrates, tissue injury, and wound healing.
- Can be caused by *persistent* infections, foreign bodies, immune reactions, or unknown reasons.

The Three Stages of Chronic Inflammation

Stage	Events
Mononuclear cell infiltration	Migration of macrophages, lymphocytes, plasma cells, and eosinophils
Granulation tissue formation	Healing tissue consisting largely of fibrosis (fibroblasts), angiogenesis (new capillaries), and inflammatory cells
Host tissue destruction	Mediated by cytokines of host leukocytes

COMPARISON OF ACUTE AND CHRONIC INFLAMMATION

Inflammation	Duration	Predominant Cells	Response	Maximum Healing Potential	Example
Acute	Days	Neutrophils Mast cells	Exudative	Regeneration	Pulpal abscess
Chronic	Weeks to years	Macrophages Lymphocytes Plasma cells	Proliferative	Repair (fibrosis)	Chronic periodontitis

GRANULOMATOUS INFLAMMATION

- A specific type of *chronic inflammation* characterized by macrophages that have been transformed into **epithelioid cells** and are surrounded by lymphocytes, fibroblasts, and local parenchymal cells.

- Associated with tuberculosis, leprosy, sarcoidosis, syphilis, blastomycosis, histoplasmosis, coccidioidomycosis, Crohn's disease, and foreign body containment (eg, sutures).

SYSTEMIC EFFECTS OF INFLAMMATION

- Fever
- Leukocytosis
    - Neutrophilia: Largely associated with *bacterial* infections.
    - Eosinophilia: Largely associated with *parasitic* infections.
    - Lymphocytosis: Associated with some *viral* infections (mumps, rubella).

Inflammatory Mediators

CYTOKINES

See Table 20–9 for inflammatory cytokines.

- Small peptides secreted by many cell types.
- Most are involved in host defense and immunity.
- There are four major categories of cytokines:
    - **Interleukins (IL):** Largest group of cytokines. Regulate leukocyte activity.
    - **Interferons (INF):** Interfere with *viral* replication. Anti-proliferative effects (protect cells that haven't been infected yet). Associated with nonspecific immune system.
    - **Tumor necrosis factors (TNF):** Regulate tumor suppression.
    - **Colony stimulating factors (CSF):** Regulate differentiation and growth of bone marrow elements.

Neurons **(CNS)**, alveolar **(lung)**, cardiac **(heart)**, and skeletal and smooth **(muscle)** cells do not have potential to regenerate.

A **granuloma** consists of granulation tissue (fibrosis, angiogenesis, and inflammatory cells) frequently containing epithelioid cells and multinucleated giant cells.

Lymphokines: Cytokines secreted by T cells.

TABLE 20–9. Important Inflammatory Cytokines

CYTOKINE	SECRETED BY	FUNCTION
IL-1	Monocytes	Produces fever
	Macrophages	Stimulates T$_H$ cells
	PMNs	Stimulates osteoclasts
	Fibroblasts	
	Epithelial cells	
	Endothelial cells	
IL-2	T$_H$-1 cells	Stimulates other T$_H$ cells and T$_C$ cells
IL-3 (CSF)*	T$_H$ cells	Stimulates hematopoietic stem cells
	NK cells	
IL-4	T$_H$-2 cells	Stimulates B cells and IgE
IL-5	T$_H$-2 cells	Stimulates B cells and IgA
		Stimulates eosinophils
IL-6	Monocytes	Produces fever
	Macrophages	Stimulates B cells
	Fibroblasts	Stimulates T$_H$ cells
	T$_H$ cells	Stimulates osteoclasts

(Continued)

Hot **T-B**one st**EA**k:

IL-1: Fever (*"hot"*)
IL-2: **T** cell activation
IL-3: **B**one marrow stimulation
IL-4: Ig**E** stimulation
IL-5: Ig**A** stimulation

Activated macrophages secrete:

- IL-1
- IL-6
- IL-8
- IL-12
- TNF-α

TABLE 20–9. Important Inflammatory Cytokines (Continued)

CYTOKINE	SECRETED BY	FUNCTION
IL-8	Monocytes Macrophages	Chemotaxis of PMNs
IL-10	T_H-2 cells	Inhibits T_H-1 cells
IL-12	Monocytes Macrophages	Stimulates T_H-1 cells
INF-γ	T_H-1 cells	Stimulates monocytes, macrophages, NK cells, and PMNs
TNF-α TNF-β	Monocytes (α) Macrophages (α) T cells (β)	Stimulates adhesion molecules Stimulates T_H cells Stimulates osteoclasts Cachexia (wasting syndrome)
TGF-β	Monocytes Macrophages T cells B cells	The "anti-cytokine" Inhibits T cells, B cells, PMNs, monocytes, macrophages, NK cells Stimulates collagen formation and wound healing

* IL-3 is also known as colony stimulating factor (CSF)

INFLAMMATORY MEDIATORS

See Table 20–10 and "Eicosanoids" section (pg. 273).

TABLE 20–10. Major Inflammatory Mediators

MEDIATOR	SECRETED BY	VASCULAR RESPONSE	BRONCHIAL RESPONSE	DERIVE FROM	MAJOR FUNCTION
Histamine	Mast cells Basophils	Dilation	Constriction	Histidine	Vasodilation Vascular permeability Primary mediator of **anaphylaxis**
Prostaglandins	Many tissues	Dilation	Variable	Arachidonic acid	Vasodilation Pain Fever
Leukotrienes (SRS-A)	Leukocytes Lung Endothelium Mast cells	Dilation	Constriction	Arachidonic acid	Vascular permeability Chemotaxis (LT-B$_4$) Primary mediator of **asthma**

TABLE 20–10. **Major Inflammatory Mediators**

MEDIATOR	SECRETED BY	VASCULAR RESPONSE	BRONCHIAL RESPONSE	DERIVE FROM	MAJOR FUNCTION
Cytokines	Leukocytes Endothelium	None directly	None directly	Various	Fever (IL-1, IL-6, TNF-α) Chemotaxis (IL-8)
Serotonin	Platelets Gastric mucosa	Constriction	No effect	Tryptophan	Vascular permeability
Bradykinin	In plasma	Dilation	Dilation	Kininogen	**Pain** Vascular permeability
Nitric oxide	Endothelium Macrophages	Dilation	Variable	Arginine	Vasodilation Tissue damage
Complement proteins	In plasma	Dilation	Constriction	Hepatocytes	Vascular permeability (C3a, C5a) Chemotaxis (C5a)
Lysosomal enzymes	Neutrophils Macrophages	No effect	No effect	Various	Bacterial killing Tissue damage
f-met-leu-phe (FMLP)	Bacterial cells	No effect	No effect	Various amino acids	Chemotaxis

Hageman factor (factor XII) is necessary in the production of bradykinin.

Wound Repair

STAGES OF WOUND REPAIR

- Inflammatory stage
    - Starts immediately after tissue injury and lasts 3–5 days.
    - The vascular and cellular phases of acute inflammation are activated. (See the section "Inflammation" earlier in this chapter.)
    - Fibrin clot formation.
    - Epithelial migration starts from opposing wound margins.
    - Local mesenchymal cells differentiate into fibroblasts.
- Fibroplastic stage
    - Starts 3–4 days after tissue injury and lasts 2–3 weeks.
    - Epithelial migration is completed and its thickness increases.
    - Collagen formation occurs as fibroblasts migrate across the fibrin network.

Although there are three sequential stages, they are not mutually exclusive; their events commonly overlap.

*During epithelialization, the free edges of the wound epithelium migrate toward each other until they meet, signaling a stop in lateral growth. This is known as **contact inhibition**.*

The tensile strength of a healing wound is dependent on collagen fiber formation.

Liver is a very uncommon site for infarction because of its regenerative capacity; can remove as much as 70% of hepatic tissue. Hepatocyte mitosis peaks at 33 hours.

- Angiogenesis and new capillary formation starts from the wound margins.
- Fibrinolysis occurs as more connective tissue is formed.
- Remodeling stage
  - Starts 2–3 weeks after tissue injury and continues indefinitely.
  - Epithelial stratification is restored.
  - Collagen remodeling, re-orienting the fibers to provide better tensile strength.
  - Wound contraction and scar formation.

METHODS OF WOUND HEALING

Method	Definition	Characteristics	Examples
Primary intention	Occurs when wound margins are closely re-approximated	Faster healing with minimal scarring and risk of infection	Well-approximated surgical incisions or lacerations Well-reduced bone fractures Replaced periodontal flaps
Secondary intention	Occurs when there is a gap between the wound margins because close re-approximation cannot occur	Slower healing with granulation tissue formation and scarring More prone to infection	Extraction sockets Large burns and ulcers Poorly reduced bone fractures External-bevel gingivectomies

REGENERATION

- Adaptive mechanism for restoring a tissue or organ.
- Occurs in several tissue types:
  - Liver
  - Bone
  - Cartilage
  - Intestinal mucosa
  - Surface epithelium
- Does *not* occur in several tissue types:
  - Skeletal muscle
  - Cardiac muscle
  - Neurons

CHAPTER 21

Immunology and Immunopathology

The Immune System

- Its primary purpose is to prevent microbial infection.
- Once infection occurs, the combined effects of the immune system elicit an inflammatory response, targeting the microbial antigens.

LINES OF DEFENSE

- Skin and mucous membranes
- Innate (natural) immunity
  - Functions *immediately* after microbial infiltration.
  - **Nonspecific** targeting of antigens.
  - **No memory**: Does *not* arise from previous infection or vaccination.
    - Natural killer (NK) cells
    - Polymorphonuclear neutrophils (PMNs)
    - Macrophages
    - Complement system
    - Nonspecific enzymes (cytokines, lysozyme, etc)
- Acquired (adaptive) immunity
  - Functions *days* after microbial infiltration.
  - **Specific** targeting of antigens.
  - **Exhibits diversity**: Responds to millions of unique antigens.
  - **Memory**: Improves on multiple exposure to microorganisms.
  - Two types of acquired immunity (see table below):
    - Cell-mediated: T cells
    - Antibody-mediated (humoral): B cells, antibodies

CLASSIFICATION OF ACQUIRED IMMUNITY

Type	Mediators	Occurs	Onset	Duration	Example
Active	Antibodies T cells	After exposure to foreign antigens	Slow (days)	Long (years)	Previous microbial infection Vaccination with live attenuated or killed antigens
Passive	Antibodies	After exposure to preformed antibodies from another host	Immediate	Short (months)	Pregnancy (IgG) Breast feeding (IgA) Vaccination with antibodies

ANTIGENS

Many drugs, such as penicillin, are haptens.

- Most are **proteins**, but many are also polysaccharides, lipoproteins, and nucleoproteins.
- **Immunogens**: Molecules that react with antibodies to induce an immune response. All immunogens are antigens, but not all antigens are immunogens.
- **Hapten**: An antigen that cannot elicit an immune response on its own (can't activate T_H cells); it must be bound to a carrier protein.
- **Superantigen**: Activates a large number of T_H cells at one time. Eg, TSST.
- **Epitope**: The specific antibody-binding site on an antigen.

- **Adjuvant**: A molecule that enhances the immune response to an antigen.
  - Added to vaccine to ↓ absorption and ↑ effectiveness.
  - Elicits stronger T- and B-cell response.
  - Eliminates need for repeated boosters.

Cell-Mediated vs Antibody-Mediated Immunity

Immunity	Host Defense	Mediators	Example
Cell mediated	Viruses Bacteria (intracellular) Fungi Protozoa	T cells NK cells Macrophages	Intracellular infections Granulomatous infections Tumor suppression Organ transplant rejection Graft versus host reactions Type IV (delayed) hypersensitivity
Antibody mediated (humoral)	Bacteria Some viruses Helminths	B cells Antibodies	Bacterial toxin-induced infections Autoimmune reactions Type I, II, III hypersensitivity

Cellular Components of the Immune System

T CELLS

See Table 21–1.

- Differentiate in the **thymus.** See Figure 21–1.
- Long life span, ranging from months to years.
- Have a **CD3-associated T-cell receptor (TCR),** which recognizes a unique antigen *only* in conjunction with MHC proteins.

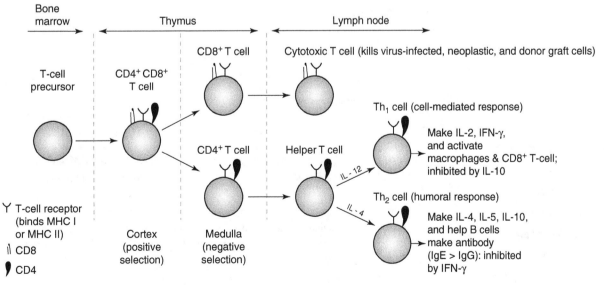

FIGURE 21–1. T-cell differentiation.

Reproduced, with permission, from Le T, Bhushan V, Tolles J. *First Aid for the USMLE Step 1 2011.* 20th ed. New York: McGraw-Hill, 2010.

511

CD8 lymphocytes function in two ways:

- Release perforins (disrupt cell membranes).
- Induce apoptosis (programmed cell death).

*The process by which an antigen binds to a specific TCR (T cell) or Ig (B cell), activating that immune cell to clonally expand into cells of the same specificity is called **clonal selection.***

TABLE 21–1.   T cells

T Cell	Function	Characteristics
CD4 lymphocytes, helper T cells (T$_H$ cells)		Respond to antigen associated with **class II MHC** proteins
▪ T$_H$-1 cells	Signal CD8 cells to differentiate into cytotoxic T cells Signal macrophages in type IV (delayed) hypersensitivity reactions	Secrete IL-2 and INF-γ
▪ T$_H$-2 cells	Signal B cells to differentiate into plasma cells, producing antibodies	Secrete IL-4 and IL-5
CD8 lymphocytes, cytotoxic T cells (T$_C$ cells)	Kill virus-infected, tumor, and allograft cells	Respond to antigen associated with **class I MHC** proteins
Memory T cells	Activated in response to re-exposure to antigen	Exist for years after initial exposure

B Cells

See Table 21–2.

- Differentiate in the **bone marrow.**
- Short life span, ranging from days to weeks.

__Class I MHC__ surface proteins: On __all nucleated cells.__ Recognition of self vs non-self.
__Class II MHC__ surface proteins: Only on __antigen-presenting cells (APCs).__ Present antigen to T$_H$ cells.

TABLE 21–2.   Major Types of B cells

B Cell	Function	Characteristics
Plasma cells	Synthesize immunoglobulins (antibodies)	*Only* **monomeric IgM** and **IgD** are expressed on their surfaces as antigen receptors
Mature B cells	Antigen presentation	Express class II MHC proteins
Memory B cells	Activated in response to re-exposure to antigen	Exist for years after initial exposure

Natural Killer (NK) Cells

- Lack a CD3-associated TCR and surface IgM or IgD.
- Are *not* specific to any antigen and do not need to recognize MHC proteins.
- **No memory:** Do *not* require previous exposure to antigen.
- Activated by IL-12 and INF-γ.
- Functions:
  - Kill virus-infected cells and tumor cells (induce apoptosis via perforins and granzymes).

Monocytes and Macrophages

- *Agranular* leukocytes.
- Derived from bone marrow histiocytes.
- Exist in plasma (monocytes) and in tissues (macrophages).
- Activated by bacterial LPS, peptidoglycan, and DNA, as well as T_H-1 cell-mediated INF-γ.
- Functions:
  - Phagocytosis: Via Fc and C3b receptors.
  - Antigen presentation: Express class II MHC proteins.
  - Cytokine production: IL-1, IL-6, IL-8, INF, and TNF.

Dendritic Cells

- *Agranular* leukocytes.
- Located primarily in the skin and mucous membranes.
- Functions:
  - Antigen presentation: Express class II MHC proteins.

Polymorphonuclear Neutrophils

See Table 21–3.

- *Granular* leukocytes. Cytoplasmic granules (lysosomes) contain several bacteriocidal enzymes.
- Functions:
  - Phagocytosis
  - Cytokine production.

IgG antibodies enhance NK cell effectiveness via antibody-dependent cellular cytotoxicity (ADCC).

Other phagocytes:

- **Histiocytes:** *CT*
- **Microglia:** *CNS*
- **Dust cells:** *lung*
- **Kupffer cells:** *liver*

Monocytes and macrophages are major components of the **reticuloendothelial system,** *which includes all phagocytic cells except for granulocytes (PMNs).*

Langerhans cells *are the major dendritic cells of the gingival epithelium.*

TABLE 21-3. Major Contents of PMN Cytoplasmic Granules

Granule Type	Enzymes
Primary (azurophilic)	Hydrolase
	Myeloperoxidase
	Neuraminidase
Secondary	Collagenase
	Lysozyme
	Lactoferrin

EOSINOPHILS

- *Granular* leukocytes.
- Bind antigen-bound IgG or IgE, subsequently releasing cytoplasmic granules.
- Do *not* present antigen to T cells.
- Functions:
  - Defense against **parasitic infections** (especially nematodes).
  - Mediate hypersensitivity diseases: Release histaminase, leukotrienes, and peroxidase.
  - Phagocytosis.

BASOPHILS AND MAST CELLS

- *Granular* leukocytes.
- Exist in plasma (basophils) and in tissues (mast cells).
- Bind antigen-bound **IgE**, subsequently releasing cytoplasmic granules (histamine, heparin, peroxidase, and hydrolase) and inflammatory cytokines.
- Function:
  - Mediate immediate hypersensitivity reactions such as **anaphylaxis**.

Opsonization and Phagocytosis

OPSONIZATION

- Enhances phagocytosis of *encapsulated* microorganisms.
- Antibody (**IgG**) or complement protein (**C3b**) coat the outer surface of microorganisms, allowing phagocytes to bind and engulf them more efficiently.

PHAGOCYTOSIS

See Table 21–4.

- The process by which microorganisms, cell debris, dead or damaged host cells, and other insoluble particles are taken up and broken down by phagocytes.

Antigen-presenting cells (APCs) express class II MHC proteins and present antigen to CD4 T cells. The predominant APCs of the immune system are monocytes and macrophages, dendritic cells (Langerhans cells), and B cells.

Chemokines (IL-8, C5a, LT-B$_4$, FMLP) are chemotactic cytokines for PMNs and macrophages.

The two major opsonins are IgG and C3b.

TABLE 21–4. Stages of Phagocytosis

STAGE	EVENTS	CHARACTERISTICS
Adhesion	Plasma phagocytes (PMNs, monocytes) bind to vascular endothelium	Mediated by *selectins* and *cellular adhesion molecules (CAMs)*
Migration	Phagocytes migrate toward the microorganisms	**Diapedesis** is the movement of the phagocyte through the vascular endothelium. Mediated by *chemokines* (IL-8, C5a, LT-B$_4$, FMLP)
Ingestion	The phagocyte cell membrane forms *pseudopods*, which surround and engulf the microorganism	**Phagosome** formation occurs when the internalized endosome fuses with lysosomes. Mediated by *opsonization* (C3b, IgG)
Lysosomal degranulation	The lysosome empties its hydrolytic enzymes into the phagosome, killing the microorganism	Mediated by *lysosomal enzymes*

LYSOSOMAL CONTENTS

- Superoxide radicals (O_2^-)
  - $O_2 + e^- \rightarrow O_2^-$
- Superoxide dismutase
  - Produces **hydrogen peroxide** (H_2O_2).
  - $2O_2^- + 2H^+ \rightarrow H_2O_2 + O_2$.
- Myeloperoxidase
  - Produces **hypochlorite ions** (ClO^-), which damage cell walls.
  - $Cl^- + H_2O_2 \rightarrow ClO^- + H_2O$.
- Lactoferrin
  - Chelates iron from bacteria.
- Lysozyme
  - Degrades bacterial cell wall peptidoglycan.
- Proteases
- Nucleases
- Lipases

Immunoglobulins (Antibodies)

See Table 21–5.

- Y-shaped glycoproteins secreted by plasma cells. (See Figure 21–2.)
- Contain two identical **light polypeptide chains** (κ or λ), and two identical **heavy polypeptide chains** (α, γ, δ, ε, or μ) linked by **disulfide bonds**.

Lysosomes are membrane-bound vesicles that contain hydrolytic enzymes necessary for intracellular digestion.

Catalase and other peroxidases (enzymes that break down H_2O_2) are located in membrane-bound organelles called **peroxisomes (microbodies)**. Bacteria that contain **catalase** (Staphylococci *sp.*) are able to resist the cidal effects of H_2O_2.

TABLE 21–5. Immunoglobulin Isotypes

ISOTYPE	SUBUNITS	LOCATION OF ACTION	FUNCTION	CHARACTERISTICS
IgA	1 or 2	Blood plasma (monomer) Exocrine secretions (dimer)	Prevents microbial attachment to mucous membranes	*2nd most abundant* antibody
IgD	1	B cells	Uncertain	*Least abundant* antibody
IgE	1	Mast cells Basophils Eosinophils	Mediates type I hypersensitivity reactions **(anaphylaxis)**	Main host defense against **parasites** (especially helminths)
IgM	1 or 5	B cells (monomer) Plasma (pentamer)	Main antimicrobial defense of **primary response** Activates complement Opsonizes B cells	*Largest* antibody Most potent activator of complement Has highest avidity of all antibodies
IgG	1	Plasma	Main antimicrobial defense of **secondary response** Opsonizes bacteria Activates complement Neutralizes bacterial toxins and viruses	*Most abundant* antibody Crosses the **placenta** Has four subclasses (IgG$_{1, 2, 3, 4}$)

IgA and *IgM* are the only antibodies that can exist as polymers, as a dimer, and a pentamer, respectively. Only the polymeric forms contain a *J chain*, which initiates the polymerization process.

Secretory IgA (sIgA) differs from serum IgA in that it is more resistant to proteolytic degradation. It always exists as a dimer.

IgM and IgG are the only antibodies that can activate complement.

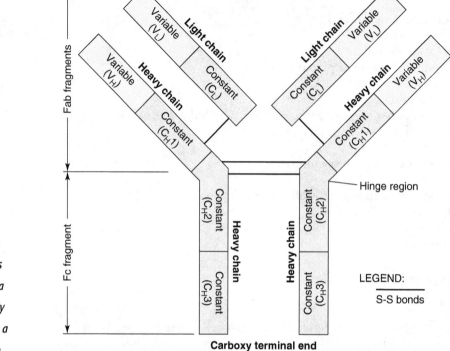

FIGURE 21–2. **Immunoglubulin structure.**

Reproduced, with permission, from Levinson W. *Medical Microbiology and Immunology*, 8th ed. New York: McGraw-Hill, 2004.

- The *constant regions* of the two heavy chains form the **F$_c$ site**, which binds to APCs or C3b. They define the immunoglobulin class **(isotype)**.
- The two *variable regions* of the heavy and light chains form the **F$_{ab}$ sites**, which are specific for binding antigen and determine the **idiotype**.
- Can be bound to plasma membrane of B cells, or free in extracellular fluid.
- Functions:
  - Neutralize bacterial toxins and viruses.
  - Opsonization (enhances phagocytosis).
  - Activate complement via the *classical pathway*.
  - Inhibit microbial attachment to mucosal surfaces.

Complement

See Tables 21–6 and 21–7 and Figure 21–3.

- Consists of about 20 plasma proteins.
- Mostly synthesized in the **liver.**
- Augment the humoral immune system and inflammation.
- All modes of activation lead to the production of C3.

TABLE 21–6. **Pathways of Complement Activation**

PATHWAY	CHARACTERISTICS
Classic	Primarily activated by **antigen–antibody complexes** with **IgG$_{1, 2, 3}$** or **IgM**
Alternative	Primarily activated by bacterial **LPS (endotoxin)**
Lectin	Primarily activated by microorganisms containing cell-surface **mannan** (a polymer of mannose)

FUNCTION	MEDIATORS
Viral neutralization	C1, C2, C3, C4
Opsonization	**C3b**
Chemotaxis	**C5a**
Anaphylaxis	C3a, C5a (most potent)
Cell lysis (cytolysis)	**Membrane attack complex (MAC)** disrupts cell membrane permeability (composed of **C5b** and **C6–9**)

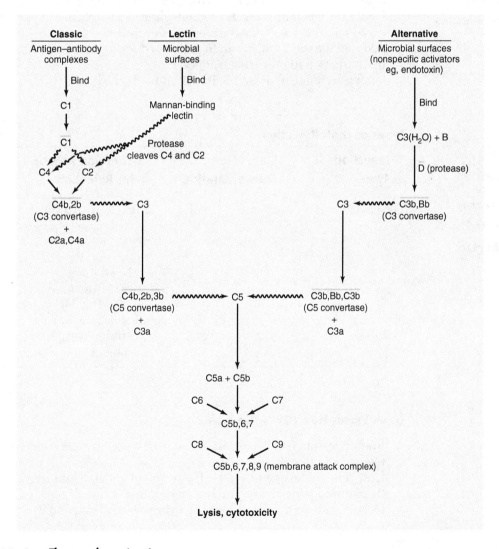

F I G U R E 2 1 - 3 . The complement system.

Reproduced, with permission, from Levinson W. *Medical Microbiology and Immunology*, 8th ed. New York: McGraw-Hill, 2004.

Transplantation

TYPES OF GRAFT

- **Autograft:** Transplantation of tissue from one site to another within the same individual.
- **Isograft:** Transplantation of tissue between two genetically *identical* individuals in the same species.
- **Allograft:** Transplantation of tissue between two genetically *different* individuals in the same species.
- **Xenograft:** Transplantation of tissue between two different species.

GRAFT REJECTION

CD8 T$_C$ cells elicit most of the destruction in graft rejection.

- **T-cell-mediated** (mostly CD8 T$_C$ cells) immune response against donor alloantigens.
- The severity and rapidity of graft rejection is determined by the degree of differences between donor and recipient class I and II MHC proteins.
- If a *second* graft from the same donor is given to a sensitized recipient, an accelerated rejection response occurs due to the presence of presensitized T$_C$ cells.
- Allografts are the most common grafts used for organ transplantation, blood transfusions, and other tissue grafts.
- Graft rejection can occur at different time intervals.

Types of Graft Rejection

The most common types of hyperacute rejection are ABO blood mismatches.

Rejection Type	Time after Transplantation	Common Reason for Rejection
Hyperacute	Minutes	Preformed antibody-mediated immune response to graft antigens
Acute	Weeks	T-cell-mediated immune response to foreign class I and II MHC proteins
Chronic	Months to years	Antibody-mediated necrosis of graft vasculature

GRAFT-VERSUS-HOST (GVH) REACTION

- Immunocompetent T cells **from the graft** recognize the recipient's cells as foreign, eliciting their destruction.
- Host cells are targeted because the recipient generally undergoes radiation therapy, inducing severe immunocompromise.
- Occurs most commonly after *bone marrow transplants* and can be fatal.

Hypersensitivity

See Table 21–8.

- Hypersensitivity reactions elicit exaggerated immune responses, which are damaging and destructive to the host.
- See Chapter 20 for a list of the major inflammatory mediators.

TABLE 21-8. Hypersensitivity Reactions

HYPERSENSITIVITY TYPE	MAJOR MEDIATOR	REACTION	EXAMPLE
Type I: Immediate (anaphylactic)	IgE	Antigen-bound IgE activates the release histamine and other mediators from mast cells and basophils	Atopic allergy Angioedema Anaphylaxis Prausnitz-Küstner reaction
Type II: Cytotoxic	IgM IgG	IgM or IgG bind to host cell surface antigens, activating complement and producing MAC-mediated cell destruction	Hemolytic anemia ADCC Goodpasture's syndrome Erythroblastosis fetalis
Type III: Immune-complex	Antigen–antibody complexes	Antigen–antibody complexes (IgG, IgM, and IgA) are deposited in various tissues, activating complement and eliciting PMN/macrophage-mediated tissue destruction	Arthus reaction Serum sickness Glomerulonephritis RA SLE
Type IV: Delayed (cell-mediated)	T cell	Macrophages present antigen, activating T cells and producing lymphokine-mediated tissue destruction Starts hours-days after contact with antigen	Contact dermatitis Tuberculin (PPD) test Tuberculosis Sarcoidosis Leprosy GVHD

Atopic allergies are common type I hypersensitivity reactions that have a strong genetic predisposition for excessive IgE production. Clinical manifestations include asthma, edema, and erythema ("wheal and flare"), and urticaria (hives). Common allergens include pollens, animal danders, foods (shellfish and peanuts), drugs (penicillin), bee venom, and latex.

Angioedema is a more generalized version of type I hypersensitivity. It involves larger areas and deeper tissues beneath the skin and underlying tissues, causing a more diffuse swelling. May involve the hands, feet, lips, eyelids, genitals, oral mucosa, and airway. Rapid (immediate) onset.

HYPERSENSITIVITY REACTIONS

See Figures 21–4 to 21–7.

- Type I: Immediate (anaphylactic).
- Type II: Cytotoxic.
- Type III: Immune-complex.
- Type IV: Delayed (cell-mediated).

ACID: **A**naphylactic + Atopic
Cytotoxic
Immune complex
Delayed

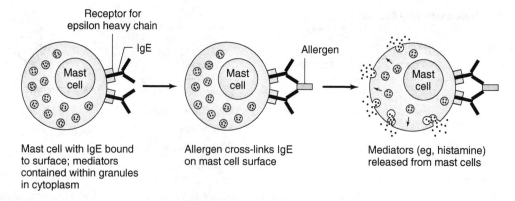

Receptor for epsilon heavy chain
IgE
Mast cell
Allergen
Mast cell
Mast cell
Mast cell with IgE bound to surface; mediators contained within granules in cytoplasm
Allergen cross-links IgE on mast cell surface
Mediators (eg, histamine) released from mast cells

FIGURE 21-4. Type I: Immediate (anaphylactic) hypersensitivity.

Reproduced, with permission, from Levinson W. *Medical Microbiology and Immunology*, 8th ed. New York: McGraw-Hill, 2004.

Antigen
RBC
IgG
RBC
+ Complement
Cell death
Red blood cell with antigens (△) on cell membrane
IgG binds to antigens on membrane
Membrane attack complex of complement lyses red cell

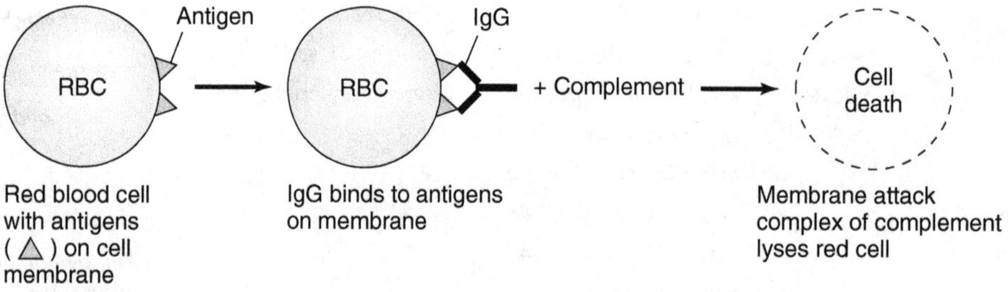

FIGURE 21-5. Type II: Cytotoxic hypersensitivity.

Reproduced, with permission, from Levinson W. *Medical Microbiology and Immunology*, 8th ed. New York: McGraw-Hill, 2004.

Antigen
+
IgG
RBC
Antigen–antibody complexes form in blood
Immune complexes are deposited on blood vessel wall, complement is activated, and C3a and C5a are released
Neutrophils are attracted by C5a; they release enzymes that destroy the endothelium and red cells escape from within the blood vessels

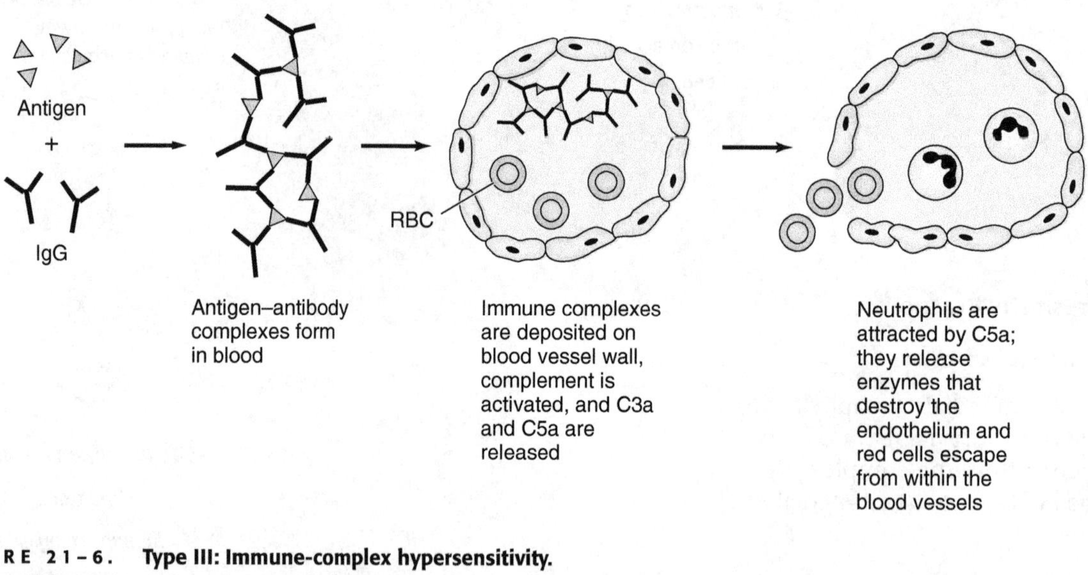

FIGURE 21-6. Type III: Immune-complex hypersensitivity.

Reproduced, with permission, from Levinson W. *Medical Microbiology and Immunology*, 8th ed. New York: McGraw-Hill, 2004.

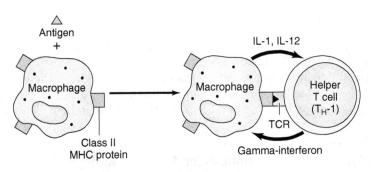

FIGURE 21-7. Type IV: Delayed (cell-mediated) hypersensitivity.

Reproduced, with permission, from Levinson W. *Medical Microbiology and Immunology,* 8th ed. New York: McGraw-Hill, 2004.

Laboratory Tests

See Table 21–9.

■ There are several methods for the detection and diagnosis of infectious diseases, autoimmune diseases, and blood typing.

TABLE 21-9. Common Antigen–Antibody Laboratory Tests

Test	Function	Common Use
Agglutination	Antibody cross-links with a **particulate** antigen, creating visible clumping if positive.	ABO blood typing.
Precipitation	Antibody cross-links with a **soluble** antigen, creating visible precipitates if positive.	Detection of serum antigen or antibody.
Radioimmunoassay (RIA)	Radio-labeled antibodies cross-link with unlabeled (unknown) antigen, creating measurable radioactive complexes if positive.	Detection of serum antigen or hapten.
Enzyme-linked immunosorbent assay (ELISA)	Enzyme-labeled antibody binds to serum antibody–antigen complexes. A substrate is then added, activating the enzyme, and eliciting a color reaction (determined by spectrophotometry) if positive.	Detection of antigen or antibody in patient specimens.
Immunofluorescence (IF)	Fluorescent-labeled antibodies bind to unlabeled (unknown) antigen, creating visible fluorescence in UV light if positive.	Detection of antigen in histologic sections or tissue specimens.

*Anaphylaxis is the most severe form of type I hypersensitivity, leading to bronchoconstriction and hypotension (shock); can be life-threatening without treatment. Its treatment is **epinephrine** 0.3 mg (1:1,000) IM or 0.1 mg (1:10,000) IV. Once vital signs are stabilized, antihistamines or corticosteroids can be administered.*

ABO Blood Typing

- All erythrocytes have alloantigens of the ABO type, which are important for blood typing and transfusions.
- Although there are only two genes (A and B) that encode for these antigens, there are four possible antigenic combinations: A, B, AB, or O.
- *Hemagglutination* occurs when blood types are mismatched.

Blood Type	Antigen (on RBC)	Antibody (in Plasma)
A	A	Anti-B
B	B	Anti-A
AB (universal recipient)	Both A and B	Neither anti-A nor anti-B
O (universal donor)	Neither A nor B	Both anti-A and anti-B

► **IMMUNOPATHOLOGY**

Immunodeficiency Diseases

See Table 21–10.

TABLE 21-10. Immunodeficiency Diseases

DISEASE	CELLULAR PATHOLOGY	CAUSE	IMMUNOLOGICAL FINDINGS	CLINICAL FINDINGS
Bruton's X-linked agammaglobulinemia	B cells	Pre-B-cells do not differentiate into mature B cells (*tyrosine kinase* mutation)	Absence of B cells, plasma cells, and Ig T-cells are normal	Increased bacterial infections Affects young boys after 6 months of age (maternal IgG initially protects) Lymphoma, leukemia, myeloma
Isolated IgA deficiency	B cells	Mature B cells do not differentiate into IgA-secreting plasma cells	Absence of IgA Other Ig isotypes are normal	Most common inherited B-cell defect Increased infection at mucosal surfaces
Common variable immunodeficiency (CVID)	B cells	Mature B cells do not differentiate into plasma cells	Absence of various Ig isotypes	Hemolytic anemias Lymphoid tumors

TABLE 21–10. Immunodeficiency Diseases (Continued)

DISEASE	CELLULAR PATHOLOGY	CAUSE	IMMUNOLOGICAL FINDINGS	CLINICAL FINDINGS
DiGeorge's syndrome	T cells	Thymic aplasia (undeveloped thymus and parathyroids)	Absence of T cells B cells are normal	Defective development of 3rd and 4th pharyngeal arches Increased viral and fungal infections **CATCH 22**: **C**ardiac defects, **A**bnormal facies, **T**hymic aplasia, **C**left palate, **H**ypocalcemia (tetany), microdeletion of chromosome **22**
Job's syndrome	T cells	T_H cells do not produce INF-γ (poor PMN chemotaxis)	Elevated IgE levels	**FATED**: Abnormal **F**acies, *Staph aureus* **A**bscesses, retained primary **T**eeth, ↑ Ig**E**, **D**ermatologic problems (eczema)
Severe combined immunodeficiency disease (SCID)	B cells and T cells	X-linked (defective IL-2 receptor) Autosomal recessive (*adenosine deaminase* deficiency)	Absent or diminished lymphoid tissue	Most severe inherited immunodeficiency Increased viral, bacterial, fungal infections Death generally before 2 y old
Wiskott–Aldrich syndrome	B cells and T cells	Defective IgM response to bacterial LPS	Decreased IgM levels Elevated IgA levels Normal IgE levels	X-linked (male infants) Clinical triad: ▪ Infections ▪ Eczema ▪ Thrombocytopenia
Ataxia-telangiectasia	B cells and T cells	Defective DNA repair (often by *ionizing radiation*)	Decreased IgA levels	**Ataxia**: Cerebellar problems (uncoordinated gait) **Telangiectasias**: Dilation of capillaries (sclera, ear, nose) Graying of hair Irregular skin pigmentation to sun-exposed areas Increased infections and malignancies

Autoimmune Diseases (Table 21–11)

- Caused by immune reactions versus self (host tissues).
- Usually involves auto-antibodies.
- HLA antigen association.
- Mechanisms:
  - Hypersensitivity reactions
  - Disordered immunoregulation
    - $\uparrow$ T_H-cell function
    - $\downarrow$ T_S-cell function
    - Nonspecific B-cell activation
- Examples:
  - Graves' disease
  - Hashimoto's thyroiditis
  - Pernicious anemia
  - Sjögren's syndrome
  - Systemic lupus erythematosus
  - Scleroderma
  - Polyarteritis nodosa
  - Rheumatoid arthritis
  - Reiter's syndrome
  - Ankylosing spondylitis
  - Myasthenia gravis
  - Multiple sclerosis

Thymus gland:

- Important for development of the immune system, beginning prenatally.
- Involved in T cell development and differentiation.
- Located behind the sternum.
- Functions in childhood then gradually atrophies with age.

TABLE 21–11. Autoimmune Diseases Affecting Oral Mucosa

DISEASE	AUTOANTIBODY	HISTOPATHOLOGY	IF	CLINICAL
Lichen planus	Unknown	Epithelial acanthosis with "sawtooth" rete pegs Dense accumulation of T cells in underlying CT and into epithelium	Fibrinogen in a "shaggy" linear pattern along BM	Oral lesions on buccal mucosa, tongue, and gingiva Types: **Reticular** (with Wickham's striae), **erosive, plaque** Certain medications can cause lichenoid reactions Skin lesions appear as clusters of **p**ruritic **p**urplish **p**apules with a white keratotic "cap"
Mucous membrane pemphigoid	Anti-BP-1 (of hemidesmosomes)	Separation of epithelial basal cells from BM	IgG and C3 in linear pattern along BM	Erythematous and erosive lesions on gingiva precede other oral areas: buccal mucosa, palate, FOM Can extend to other mucosa: nasopharynx, esophagus, vaginal, eye conjunctiva (**symblepharon** formation), and skin

(Continued)

TABLE 21-11. Autoimmune Diseases Affecting Oral Mucosa (Continued)

Disease	Autoantibody	Histopathology	IF	Clinical
Pemphigus vulgaris	Anti-desmoglein (of desmosomes)	Suprabasilar acantholysis with Tzanck cells	IgG antibody in "fishnet" pattern within spinous layer	Oral lesions often precede skin lesions Erosive lesions on soft palate, buccal mucosa, gingiva, lateral tongue High mortality rate
Erythema multiforme	Immune complexes	Intraepithelial pooling of eosinophilic amorphous coagulum Perivascular infiltrate of mononuclear cells within lamina propria	IgM and C3 in perivascular pattern within lamina propria	Causative agents include infections (HSV), medications, GI diseases (Crohn's, UC) Bullous "target" lesions on skin and oral mucosa (25% prevalence), which may collapse and crust over (**Stevens-Johnson syndrome**) Severe form is toxic epidermal necrolysis (TEN)

Systemic Pathology

Teratogenesis

- Induction of nonhereditary congenital malformations (birth defects) in a developing fetus by exogenous factors:
  - Physical
  - Chemical
  - Biologic agents
- Teratogens = Teratogenic agents
- **Physical agents**
  - Radiation
  - Hypoxia
  - CO_2
  - Mechanical trauma
- **Maternal infection**
  - TORCH complex (**T**oxoplasmosis, **O**ther agents, **R**ubella, CMV, and HSV)
- **Hormones**
  - Sex hormones
  - Corticosteroids
- **Vitamin deficiencies**
  - Riboflavin
  - Niacin
  - Folic acid
  - Vitamin E
- **Drugs**
  - Mitomycin
  - Dactinomycin
  - Puromycin

- Effects of teratogens:
  - Death
  - Growth retardation
  - Malformation
  - Functional impairment
- Mechanism of teratogens:
  - Specific for each teratogen: inhibit, interfere, or block metabolic steps critical for normal morphogenesis.
  - Most are site or tissue specific.
- Susceptibility to teratogens is
  - Variable.
  - Specific for each developmental stage.
  - Dose dependent.

Chromosomal Abnormalities

AUTOSOMAL ABNORMALITIES

Syndrome	Chromosomal Abnormality	Findings
Down syndrome	Trisomy 21	Mental retardation Epicanthal folds Large protruding tongue Small head, low-set ears Broad flat face Simian crease **Complications** ↑ leukemia ↑ infection Alzheimer-like brain Δ
Edward syndrome	Trisomy 18	Mental retardation Small head Micrognathia (small lower jaw) Pinched facial appearance Low-set, malformed ears Rocker bottom feet Heart defects Prognosis: months
Patau syndrome	Trisomy 13	Mental retardation Microcephaly Microphthalmia Brain abnormalities Cleft lip and palate Polydactyly Heart defects Prognosis: < 1 y

Chromosomal abnormalities in decreasing order of incidence:

- Down's = 1:700.
- Edward's = 1:3000.
- Patau's = 1:5000.

SEX CHROMOSOME ABNORMALITIES

Syndrome	Chromosomal Abnormality	Findings
Klinefelter syndrome	XXY	1:500 men Manifests at puberty Hypogonadism, atrophic testes Tall stature Gynecomastia Female pubic hair distribution. Low IQ Associated with ↑ maternal and ↑ paternal age
Turner syndrome	XO	1:3000 live female births Diagnose at birth or puberty Female hypogonadism Primary amenorrhea Short stature Webbed neck Wide-spaced nipples Coarctation of aorta

Lysosomal Storage Diseases

LYSOSOMAL STORAGE DISEASES

Lysosomal storage diseases are most common in people of Eastern European ancestry.

- Hunter's
- Tay–Sachs
- Gaucher
- Neimann–Pick
- Fabry
- See also Chapter 6, Biological Compounds.

Autosomal Recessive	X-linked
Tay–Sachs	Fabry
Gaucher	Hunter's
Niemann–Pick	

Other Childhood Genetic Disorders

CYSTIC FIBROSIS

Cystic fibrosis
- Problem with Cl⁻ transporter
- Findings
  - Bronchiectasis
  - Meconium ileus

- Most common fatal genetic disease in white children.
- Occurs in both males and females (M = F).
- Life expectancy = 28 years.
- Generalized exocrine gland dysfunction. Problem with Cl^- transporter.
- Multiple organ systems.
  - Characterized by respiratory and digestive problems.
- **Pathogenesis:** Chromosome 7q.
  - Gene encodes CFTR (cystic fibrosis transmembrane regulator).
  - Regulates Cl^- and Na^+ transport across epithelial membranes.
- Affects Na^+ channels, especially mucous and sweat glands.
- **Test:** Sweat chloride test.
- **Findings**
  - Chronic pulmonary disease.
    - From thick mucous in airways:
      - Lung infections.
      - Bronchiectasis.
  - Pancreatic exocrine insufficiency.
  - Meconium ileus.
    - Intestinal obstruction in infants/newborns.

The most common cause of cystic fibrosis is a deletion causing loss of phenylalanine at position 508 in the CFTR gene.

VON HIPPEL–LINDAU DISEASE

- Autosomal dominant
  - Chromosome 3
  - VHL gene
- **Findings**
  - Hemangiomas
    - Retina
    - Cerebellum

- Cysts and adenomas
  - Liver
  - Kidney
  - Adrenal glands
  - Pancreas

MARFAN'S SYNDROME

- Uncommon hereditary connective-tissue disorder:
  - Fibrillin gene mutation.
- **Findings**
  - Skeletal
    - Tall and thin patients.
    - Abnormally long legs and arms.
    - Spiderlike fingers.
  - Cardiovascular
    - Cystic medial necrosis of aorta.
      - Risk aortic incompetence, dissecting aortic aneurysms.
    - Distensible mitral valve.
  - Ocular: Lens dislocation.

Disorders of Skin Pigmentation

HYPOPIGMENTATION

- Albinism
  - Failure in pigment production from otherwise intact melanocytes.
  - Usually tyrosinase problem; can't convert tyrosine to DOPA (in the pathway to form melanin).
- Vitiligo
  - Acquired loss of melanocytes.
  - Discrete areas of skin with depigmented white patches.
  - May be autoimmune.

HYPERPIGMENTATION

- **Freckle** (ephelis): Increased melanin pigment within basal keratinocytes.
- **Lentigo:** Pigmented macule caused by melanocytic hyperplasia in epidermis.
- **Pigmented nevi:** (See the section "Benign (Nonneoplastic) Skin Lesions" later in this chapter.)
- **Lentigo maligna** (See the section "Benign (Nonneoplastic) Skin Lesions" later in this chapter.)
- Café au lait spots
  - Increase in melanin content with giant melanosomes.
  - Conditions with café au lait spots include:
    - Neurofibromatosis type 1 (most frequent neurocutaneous syndrome).
    - McCune–Albright syndrome (See the section "Fibrous Dysplasia" later in this chapter).
    - Tuberous sclerosis (rare disease that causes nonmalignant tumors in the brain and organs).
    - Fanconi anemia (rare disease resulting in loss of DNA repair with increased risk of cancer and endocrine problems).
- Diffuse hyperpigmentation with **Addison's disease.**
  - Secondary to ↑ melanocyte-stimulating hormone.

Skin Infections

VIRAL SKIN ERUPTIONS

- Molluscum contagiosum (Poxvirus)
- Verruca vulgaris (common wart) (human papilloma virus [HPV])
- Herpes simplex
- Roseola (exanthema subitum) (herpes virus 6 and 7)
- Rubella
- Measles (rubeola) (paramyxovirus)

BACTERIAL SKIN ERUPTIONS

IMPETIGO

- Common skin infection.
  - Common in preschool age children (2–5 years old).
  - Especially during warm weather.
- Etiology
  - Invasion of epidermis by *Staphylococcus aureus* or *Streptococcus pyogenes*.
  - Similar to cellulitis, but more superficial.
  - Highly infectious.
- Signs/symptoms
  - Starts as itchy, red sore.
  - Blisters → breaks → oozes.
  - Ooze dries; lesion becomes covered with a tightly adherent crust.
  - Grows and spreads circumferentially (not deep); rarely impetigo forms deeper skin ulcers
  - Contagious; carried in the oozing fluid.
- Treatment
  - Topical antimicrobial (eg, bactroban).
  - Oral antibiotic (eg, erythromycin or dicloxacillin); rapid clearing of lesions.
- Course/prognosis
  - Impetigo sores heal slowly and seldom scar.
  - Cure rate is extremely high.
  - Recurrence is common in young children.

Note: Acute glomerulonephritis (renal disease) is an occasional complication (poststreptococcal glomerulonephritis [GMN]).

Immunologic Skin Lesions

HIVES

- Urticaria = wheals.
- Type I hypersensitivity.
- (See section on hypersensitivity in Immunology, Chapter 21.)

PEMPHIGUS VULGARIS

- Ages 30–60.
- Clinical
  - Oral mucosal lesions (often first sign).
  - Skin lesions follow.
  - Bullae rupture, leaving raw surface susceptible to infection.

- Etiology
  - Autoimmune: IgG antibodies against desmosome proteins.
- Histology
  - Formation of intradermal bullae
    - Acantholysis: Tzanck cells.
    - Basal layer intact.
- Immunofluorescence shows encircling of epidermal cells.

Tzanck cells are multinucleate giant cells caused by a variety of skin pathologies.

BULLOUS PEMPHIGOID

- Resembles pemphigus vulgaris.
- Clinically less severe.
- Etiology
  - Autoimmune: IgG antibodies against hemidesmosome proteins.
- Histology
  - Subepidermal bullae.
  - Characteristic inflammatory infiltrate of eosinophils in surrounding dermis.
  - Immunofluorescence shows linear band.

Pemphigus vulgaris = Intraepidermal bullae.
Bullous pemphigoid = Subepidermal bullae.

ERYTHEMA MULTIFORME

- Peak incidence second and third decades.
- Etiology
  - Type III hypersensitivity
  - Response to:
    - Medications:
      - Sulfa drugs
      - Penicillins
      - Barbiturates
    - Infections
    - HSV
    - Mycoplasma
    - Other illnesses
- Damage to blood vessels of skin (because of immune complexes).
- Clinical
  - Classic "target," "bull's-eye," or "iris" skin lesion.
    - Central lesion surrounded by concentric rings of pallor and redness.
    - Dorsal hands.
    - Forearms.
  - No systemic symptoms.

STEVENS–JOHNSON SYNDROME

- Variant, more severe form of erythema multiforme.
- Severe systemic symptoms.
- Extensive skin target lesions
  - Involve multiple body areas, especially mucous membranes.

TOXIC EPIDERMAL NECROLYSIS

- Also called TEN syndrome and Lyell's syndrome.
- Multiple large blisters (bullae) that coalesce, sloughing of all or most of skin and mucous membranes.

Benign (Nonneoplastic) Skin Lesions

ACANTHOSIS NIGRICANS

A hamartoma is disorganized growth composed of tissue normally found in a given location.
A choristoma is a growth composted of histologically normal tissue found at a site where it is not normally found in the body.

- Cutaneous finding of velvety hyperkeratosis and pigmentation.
  - Flexural areas, most often.
    - Axilla.
    - Nape of neck.
    - Other flexures.
    - Anogenital region.
- Often a marker of visceral malignancy.
  - > 50% have cancer.
    - Gastric carcinoma.
    - Breast, lung, uterine cancer.
- Seen in diabetes.
- **Histology**
  - Acanthosis.
  - Hyperkeratosis.
  - Hyperpigmentation.

HEMANGIOMA

- Hamartoma (not true neoplasm).

XANTHOMA

- Associated with hypercholesterolemia.
- **Clinical**
  - Most common sites:
    - Eyelids (xanthelasma).
    - Nodules over tendons or joints.
- **Histology**
  - Yellowish papules or nodules composed of
    - Focal dermal collections of lipid-laden histiocytes.

► CARDIOVASCULAR PATHOLOGY

Edema

- Abnormal accumulation of fluid in interstitial spaces or body cavities.
- Fluid moves out of intravascular space.
- Results from some combination of:
- ↑ capillary permeability (as with histamine).
- ↑ capillary hydrostatic pressure.
- ↑ interstitial fluid colloid osmotic pressure.
- ↓ plasma colloid osmotic pressure.

(See also Chapter 20, Reactions to Tissue Injury.)

Types of Edema

Transudate	Exudate
More watery (serous) edema fluid	More protein-rich edema fluid
Usually noninflammatory	Usually inflammatory
From altered intravascular hydrostatic or osmotic pressure	From ↑ vascular permeability (with inflammation)

EXAMPLES OF TRANSUDATE

- **Anasarca:** Generalized edema.
- **Hydrothorax:** Excess serous fluid in pleural cavity.
- **Hydropericardium:** Excess watery fluid in pericardial cavity.
- **Ascites (hydroperitoneum):** Excess serous fluid in peritoneal cavity.

Remember: Right-sided CHF results in peripheral edema; left-sided CHF results in pulmonary edema.

CLINICAL EXAM OF EDEMA

- **Pitting:** Press finger for 5 s and quickly remove; an indentation is left that fills slowly.
- **Nonpitting:** No indentation left when finger is removed.

Edemas and Causes

Process	Cause
Congestive heart failure	↑ plasma/capillary hydrostatic pressure
Nephrotic syndrome	↓ plasma oncotic pressure
Cirrhosis	↑ capillary hydrostatic pressure
	↓ plasma oncotic pressure
Elephantiasis	↑ plasma/capillary hydrostatic pressure
	Secondary to ↓ lymphatic return

Shock

- ↓ tissue perfusion.
- Hemodynamic changes result in:
  - ↓ blood flow, thereby.
  - ↓ oxygen and metabolic supply to tissues.
- Can result in multiple organ damage or failure.
- **Symptoms**
  - Fatigue
  - Confusion
- **Signs**
  - Cool pale skin (pallor)
  - Weak rapid pulse (tachycardia = ↑ HR)
  - ↓ BP (hypotension)
  - ↓ urine output
- Shock requires immediate medical treatment and can worsen rapidly.

↓ cardiac output is the major factor in all types of shock (because either ↓ HR, ↓ SV, or both).

MAJOR CATEGORIES OF SHOCK

- Hypovolemic
- Cardiogenic
- Distributive
  - Septic
  - Neurogenic
  - Anaphylactic

Type	Cause	Examples
Hypovolemic	↓ blood volume	Hemorrhage Dehydration Vomiting Diarrhea Fluid loss from burns
Cardiogenic	Pump failure Usually LV failure Sudden ↓ CO	Massive MI Arrhythmia
Septic	Infection (endotoxin release) Gram-negative bacteria Causes vasodilation	Severe infection
Neurogenic	CNS injury Causes vasodilation	CNS injury
Anaphylactic	Type I hypersensitivity Histamine release Vasodilation	Anaphylactic allergic reaction (eg, insect sting)

STAGES OF SHOCK

Nonprogressive (Early)	Progressive	Irreversible
= compensated ↑ sympathetic nervous system ↑ CO ↑ TPR Try to maintain perfusion to vital organs	↓ cardiac perfusion Cardiac depression CO ↓ Metabolic acidosis. (Compensatory mechanisms are no longer adequate)	Organ damage ↓ high energy phosphate reserves Death (even if restore blood flow)

Congestion (Hyperemia)

- ↑ volume of blood in local capillaries and small vessels.
- **Active congestion** (active hyperemia): ↑ arteriolar dilation (inflammation, blushing).
- **Passive congestion** (passive hyperemia): ↓ venous return (obstruction, increased back pressure).
    - Two forms:
        - Acute
            - Shock or right-sided heart failure
        - Chronic
            - In lung (usually secondary to left-sided heart failure)
            - In liver (usually secondary to right-sided heart failure)

Thrombosis

- Blood clot attached to endothelial surface (blood vessel or heart [endocardium])
  - Usually a vein.
  - Virchow's triad.
- **Arterial thrombi**
  - Lines of Zahn (morphologically).
  - Alternating red and white laminations.
- **Venous thrombi**
  - Propagate: Enlarge while remaining attached to vessel wall.
  - Embolize.
  - Detach as large embolus.
  - Fragment off as many small emboli; shower emboli.

TYPES OF THROMBUS

Agonal	Intracardiac thrombi – After prolonged heart failure
Mural	Thrombus from endocardial surface (or endothelium of large vessel) protrudes into lumen of heart or large vessel Forms after – MI; damage to ventricular endocardium (LV most often) – Atrial fibrillation – Aortic atherosclerosis Can cause cerebral embolism
White	Thrombus composed mostly of blood platelets
Red	Thrombus composed of RBCs (rather than platelets) Occurs rapidly by coagulation with blood stagnation
Fibrin	Thrombus composed of fibrin deposits Does not completely occlude the vessel

Embolus

- Intravascular mass.
  - Solid
  - Liquid
  - Gas
- Travels within a blood vessel.
  - Lodges at distant site.
  - Occludes blood flow to vital organs.
  - Possibly leads to infarction.
- **Thromboemboli** (most common): Blood clot.
  - Breaks off existing thrombus.
  - Forms and is released downstream in the circulation (eg, from heart chambers in atrial fibrillation).
- **Fat embolism:** Especially in long bone fractures.
- **Gas embolism:** Air into circulation (eg, Caisson disease).

Thrombolysis = Breakdown

of a clot.

Virchow's triad:
- Endothelial injury.
- Alteration in blood flow.
- Hypercoagulability of blood.

Lines of Zahn
1. White (fibrin and platelet) layers alternating with dark (RBC) layers.
2. Indicated thrombosis in aorta or heart before death.

Predisposing factors to thrombosis
- **Arterial thrombosis**
  - Atherosclerosis (major cause)
- **Venous thrombosis**
  - Heart failure
  - Tissue damage
  - Bed rest (immobilization)
  - Pregnancy
  - Oral contraceptive pills
  - Age
  - Obesity
  - Smoking

Pulmonary embolism

- Embolism causing pulmonary artery obstruction.
- Usually arises from
  - Deep vein thrombosis (DVT); usually from lower extremities (above popliteal fossa).
- **Course**
  - Systemic vein.
  - Right heart.
  - Pulmonary artery.
- **Causes**
  - Right heart strain.
  - Possibly infarction in the affected segment.
  - Possibly pleurisy (pleuritic chest pain).
- **Predisposing factors**
- Virchow's triad.
  - Especially immobilization (leading to stagnation).
  - Thrombophlebitis.
  - Hypercoagulable states.

Saddle embolus: *Large pulmonary embolus that obstructs the bifurcation of the pulmonary artery.*

Paradoxical emboli

Begin in the venous system.

End up in the systemic arterial system rather than the pulmonary artery.

Most often allowed by an atrial septal defect.

The only time a DVT can cause a stroke.

- **Amniotic fluid embolism:** With delivery; can activate diffuse/disseminated intravascular coagulation (DIC).
- **Tumor embolism.**

Phlebitis

- Inflammation of the vein.
- **Common sites**
  - Legs.
  - Varicose veins.
- **Common causes**
  - Local irritation (eg, IV).
  - Infection in or near vein.
  - Blood clots.

THROMBOPHLEBITIS

- Inflammation of the vein related to blood clot.
- Associated with
  - **Superficial thrombophlebitis:** Veins near skin surface.
  - **Deep venous thrombosis:** Deeper, larger veins.
  - **Pelvic vein thrombosis.**
- **Clinical symptoms**
  - Tenderness over vein.
  - Pain in body part affected.
  - Skin redness or inflammation.

Arteriosclerosis

- Hardening of the arteries
- General term for several diseases causing changes to artery wall:
  - Thicker
  - Less elastic

ATHEROSCLEROSIS

- Degenerative changes in artery walls
- Most common cause of arteriosclerosis
- Atherosclerotic plaques: Fatty material accumulating under the arterial wall's inner lining
- Occurs in arteries (**not** veins)
- **Risks**
  - Men and postmenopausal women (estrogen may be protective)
  - Smoking
  - Hypertension
  - Heredity (familial hypercholesterolemia)
  - Nephrosclerosis
  - Diabetes
  - Hyperlipidemia
- **Sites**
  - Carotid
  - Coronary

- Circle of Willis
- Renal and mesenteric arteries
- **Pathogenesis**
  - Fatty streak
    - Foam cells in intima (lipid laden macrophages)
  - Atheromas
    - Cholesterol
    - Fibrous tissue
    - Necrotic debris
    - Smooth muscle cells
- **Complications**
  - ↓ elasticity of vessel.
  - Ulceration of plaque; predisposing to thrombus formation.
  - Hemorrhage into the plaque; narrowing lumen, possibly occluding blood flow.
  - Thrombus formation.
  - Embolization; overlying thrombus or plaque material itself.
- **Symptoms**
  - Depend on site.
    - Visual changes, dizziness: Carotid or intracerebral arteries.
    - Angina: Coronary arteries.
    - Leg pain (claudication): Lower extremity arteries.

Hypertension

- Primary (essential).
- Secondary (related to another disease).

PRIMARY (ESSENTIAL) HYPERTENSION

- Accounts for 90–95% of hypertension.
- No identifiable cause; related to ↑ CO, ↑ TPR.
- **Risks**
  - Genetic
    - Family history
    - African Americans
  - Environmental
    - ↑ dietary salt intake
    - Stress
    - Obesity
    - Cigarette smoking
    - Physical inactivity
- **Pathologic findings**
  - Hypertrophy of arteries and arterioles **not** capillaries (because no smooth muscle).
  - ↑ wall-to-lumen ratio.
    - ↑ smooth muscle cell growth (because of ↑ pressure, stretch).
  - ↓ arteriolar and capillary density.
  - ↓ total cross-sectional area of capillaries and arterioles.
- Three organs most often damaged.
  - Heart: 60% die of cardiac complications.
  - Kidneys: 25% die of renal failure.
  - Brain: 15% die of stroke or neurologic complications.

Atherosclerosis

- Most important contributor to arterial thrombosis.
- Most susceptible arteries—aorta and coronary arteries.

Atherosclerosis can lead to:

- Ischemic heart disease (CAD).
- Heart attack (myocardial infarction [MI]).
- Stroke or aneurysm formation.

Familial hypercholesterolemia

- Autosomal dominant disease.
- Anomalies of LDL (low-density lipoprotein) receptors.
- Atherosclerosis and its complications.
  - Xanthomas.
  - MI by age 20.

- Diet, exercise, and antihypertensive medications are used to treat hypertension.
- Untreated (or undertreated) hypertension can result in
  - "wear out" (cardiac failure).
  - "blow out" (CVA).
  - "run out" (renal failure).

Hypertension is the "silent killer"; usually has no symptoms.

Neurologic	Ophthalmologic	Cardiovascular	Renal
Headaches	Retinal hemorrhage	BP >140/90	Polyuria
Nausea/vomiting	and exudates	**Arteriolar**	Nocturia
Drowsiness	▣ Damage to	**constriction**	↓ urine
Anxiety	retinal	↑ resistance	concentration
Mental	arterioles	**Claudication**	**Nephrosclerosis**
impairment		↓ blood supply	Hardening of renal
▣ Intracerebral		to legs	arterioles
vessel		↑ **cardiac workload**	Proteinuria possible
damage		Angina	Hematuria possible
		↓ coronary	
		blood flow	
		Heart failure	
		▣ Dyspnea on	
		exertion (LHF)	
		▣ Peripheral	
		edema (RHF)	

Renal disease is the most common cause of secondary hypertension.

Preeclampsia occurs in pregnant patients:

- Hypertension: >140 systolic, or > 90 diastolic after 20 weeks' gestation.
- Proteinuria.
- Edema.

Eclampsia = Preeclampsia + seizures.

Predisposing conditions for preeclampsia and eclampsia:

- Hypertension
- Diabetes
- Autoimmune diseases (eg, SLE)
- Laboratory findings
- Hyperuricemia
- Thrombocytopenia

SECONDARY HYPERTENSION

- ▣ Hypertension (HTN) from known causes.
  - ▣ 5–10% of HTN cases.
  - ▣ Identifiable, often correctable cause.
- ▣ **Renal disease**
  - ▣ Most common cause of secondary hypertension.
  - ▣ Renin–angiotensin–aldosterone system.
  - ▣ Two categories:
    - ▪ Renal parenchymal diseases.
    - ▪ Renal artery stenosis.
- ▣ **Endocrine disorders**
  - ▣ Hyperaldosteronism (Conn syndrome).
  - ▣ Cushing syndrome.
  - ▣ Hyperthyroidism.
  - ▣ Diabetes.
  - ▣ Pheochromocytoma.
- ▣ **Other causes**
  - ▣ Coarctation of the aorta.
  - ▣ Preeclampsia/eclampsia/toxemia of pregnancy.

MALIGNANT HYPERTENSION

- ▣ Severe form of high blood pressure.
  - ▣ Medical emergency.
  - ▣ Can lead to death in 3–6 months if untreated.
- ▣ Complication of either primary or secondary hypertension.
  - ▣ Most often with secondary hypertension from kidney disease.

- Occurs in
  - African American young adults
  - Women with toxemia of pregnancy (preeclampsia/eclampsia)
  - Patients with renal or collagen vascular disorders
- Findings
  - Sudden rapid ↑ BP, usually without a precipitating event
- Life-threatening consequences to multiple organ systems:
  - Cerebrovascular accident
  - Retinal hemorrhage and papilledema
  - Cardiac failure
  - Renal failure

Aortic Aneurysm

- Abnormal, localized dilation of the aorta
- True aneurysm = dilation of all three layers (intima, media, adventitia)
- Causes
  - Atherosclerosis
  - Cystic medial necrosis
    - Marfan
    - Ehlers–Danlos
  - Infectious aortitis
    - Syphilitic aortitis
  - Vasculitis
- Risk
  - Rupture

Aortic Dissection

- Life-threatening
- Blood into medial layers of aorta
  - "Dissecting" the intima from the adventitia
- Symptoms
  - Ripping/tearing chest pain
  - Different BP measurement in each arm
- Complications
  - Rupture
    - Pericardial tamponade
    - Hemomediastinum or hemothorax
  - Occlusion of aortic branches
    - Carotid (stroke)
    - Coronary (MI)
    - Splanchnic (organ infarction)
    - Renal (acute renal failure)
  - Distortion of aortic valve
    - Aortic regurgitation

Aortic dissection most often ruptures into the pericardial sac (hemopericardium), causing fatal tamponade.

Hemopericardium:
Can occur after MI.

- Ventricular rupture (necrotic myocardium).
- Blood into pericardial space.
- Can cause cardiac tamponade and death.

PATHOLOGY INVOLVING THE PERICARDIUM

Infections of the heart

- Pericardium (pericarditis)
- Myocardium (myocarditis, often viral)
- Endocardium and heart valves (endocarditis, often bacterial or inflammatory)

Pericardial Effusion	Acute Pericarditis	Chronic (Constrictive) Pericarditis
Accumulation of fluid in the pericardial space • Hydropericardium = serous fluid • Hemopericardium = blood Can cause cardiac tamponade	Inflammation of the pericardium: • Serous • Fibrinous • Purulent • Hemorrhagic • Often painful • Can cause cardiac tamponade	Thickening and scarring of the pericardium Tb. ↓ elasticity Can cause tamponade-like picture

CARDIAC TAMPONADE

Beck's triad

1. Distension of jugular veins
2. Decreased blood pressure
3. Muffled heart sounds

- Extrinsic compression of the heart
  - Fluid (accumulating quickly into the pericardial space)
    - Pericardial effusion
    - Acute pericarditis
- Cardiac compression
  - ↓ venous return (↓ filling)
  - ↓ CO
  - Death
- **Signs**
  - Distended neck veins
  - Hypotension
  - ↓ heart sounds
  - Tachypnea
  - Weak/absent peripheral pulses

ENDOCARDITIS

Remember that the tricuspid valve is most often affected in IV drug users.

- Inflammation of endocardium and/or heart valves
- **Symptoms:** Develop quickly (acute) or slowly (subacute):
  - Fever (hallmark)
  - Nonspecific constitutional signs
  - Fatigue
  - Malaise
  - Headache
  - Night sweats
- **Findings**
  - Murmur (secondary to vegetations); may change with time.
  - Splenomegaly
  - Splinter hemorrhages (small dark lines) under fingernails

Infective	Rheumatic	Libmann–Sacks

Usually bacterial
Intrinsic bacteremia
  Dental
  Upper respiratory
  Urologic
  Lower GI tract
  Introduced bacteremia
  IV drug users
	Complication of
	  rheumatic fever
	Occurs in areas with
	  greatest hemodynamic
	  stress
		Occurs in SLE
		
		Nonbacterial
		  endocarditis

Valvular involvement
Vegetations
  Mitral
  Tricuspid (in IVDU)
	Mitral valve most often
	Calcification
	  Stenosis
	  Insufficiency
	  Both
		Mitral valve most often
		Small vegetations
		  on either or both
		  surfaces of valve
		  leaflets

Infective Endocarditis

Acute Endocarditis	Subacute (Bacterial) Endocarditis
Staphylococcus aureus (50%) Usually secondary to infection elsewhere in body IVDUs	*Streptococcus viridans* (> 50%) Patients with preexisting valve disease

Rheumatic Fever

- Acute inflammatory disease.
- Develops after streptococcal infection, usually a URI with group A β-hemolytic strep.
- Most common in children 5–15 years old.
- Onset
  - Usually sudden, often after 1–5 weeks (asymptomatic) after recovery from sore throat or scarlet fever.
- Course
  - Mild cases = 3–4 weeks.
  - Severe cases = 2–3 months.
- Etiology
  - Due to cross-reactivity, not direct effect of the bacteria.
  - Type III hypersensitivity.
- Sites
  - Heart
  - Joints
  - Skin
  - Brain

Antibiotic prophylaxis before dental procedures

- Children with congenital heart disease
- To help prevent subacute bacterial endocarditis (SBE), *Streptococcus viridans,* from a dental/oral source.

Valvular vegetations can be dislodged and send septic emboli to organs:

- Brain
- Lungs
- Kidneys
- Spleen

Mnemonics for rheumatic fever

PECCS

Polyarthritis
Erythema marginatum
Chorea
Carditis
Subcutaneous nodules

FEVERSS

Fever
Erythema marginatum
Valve damage
ESR
Red-hot (polyarthritis)
Subcutaneous nodules
St. Vitus dance (chorea)

MICROBIOLOGY–PATHOLOGY

SYSTEMIC PATHOLOGY

- **Pathology**
  - Aschoff bodies
    - Focal interstitial myocardial inflammation: Fragmented collagen, and fibrinoid material
    - Anitschkow cells: Large unusual cells
    - Aschoff myocytes: Multinucleated giant cells
- **Laboratory**
  - ↑ ASO titers
  - ↑ ESR
- **Findings/criteria for diagnosis** = Jones criteria
  - Diagnose when two major or one major and one minor criteria are met. (See chart.)
- Treatment
  - Penicillin
  - Rest

JONES CRITERIA FOR DIAGNOSIS OF RHEUMATIC FEVER

Major Criteria	Minor Criteria
Carditis	Fever
Arthritis	Arthralgias
Chorea	History of rheumatic fever
Erythema marginatum	ECG changes
Subcutaneous nodules	Leukocytosis

Coronary Artery Disease (CAD)

- CAD = Narrowing of coronary arteries
  - Atherosclerosis plaques
  - ↓ blood supply to myocardium
- **Consequences**
  - Ischemia
  - Infarction
- **Symptoms**
  - Classic symptom of CAD = angina
- **Risks**
  - Same as for atherosclerosis
  - Hypertension
  - Hyperlipidemia
  - Smoking
  - Obesity
  - Inactivity
  - Diabetes
  - Male gender

ANGINA

- Squeezing (tight) substernal chest discomfort; may radiate to
  - Left arm
  - Neck
  - Jaw
  - Shoulder blade

- Caused by ↓ myocardial oxygenation
- Atherosclerotic narrowing
- Vasospasm

Stable Angina	Unstable Angina	Prinzmetal Angina
Most common type CAD/atherosclerotic narrowing Precipitated by exertion	Occurs even at rest More severe CAD Often imminent MI	Intermittent chest pain at rest Vasospasm

MYOCARDIAL INFARCTION (MI)

- Most important cause of morbidity from CAD.
- Prolonged interruption of coronary blood flow to myocardium; coagulative necrosis.
- **Cause:** Usually thrombus formation in the setting of a ruptured, unstable plaque.

Complete Occlusion	Partial Occlusion
Transmural infarction ST elevation MI	Subendocardial infarction Non-ST elevation MI

- Symptoms
    - Angina (that does not remit)
    - Sweating
    - Nausea, stomach upset
- Signs
    - ECG changes (ST elevation, ST depression, T waves, Q waves).
    - Enzyme leak.
- **Prognosis:** Good (if patient reaches hospital).
- Complications
    - Arrhythmia.
    - Myocardial (pump) failure.
    - Cardiac rupture.
    - Papillary muscle rupture.
    - Ventricular aneurysm.

Heart Failure

- Heart's ability to pump does not meet needs of the body.
- Usually a chronic progressive condition.
- Can occur suddenly.
- **Causes:** Secondary to heart muscle damage
    - After MI
    - Cardiomyopathy
    - Valvular diseases

Most deaths from heart attack occur outside hospital; are due to arrhythmias causing ventricular fibrillation.

MICROBIOLOGY-PATHOLOGY

SYSTEMIC PATHOLOGY

Cardiac enzymes elevated after an MI:

- CK–MB (creatine kinase, MB fraction)
- TnT (troponin T)
- Myoglobin

Creatine phosphokinase (CPK): Enzyme found in (↑ when damage to):

- Heart
- Brain
- Skeletal muscle
- Not found in liver

Pulmonary edema: Life-threatening complication of left heart failure.

Two earliest and most common signs of heart failure:

- Exertional dyspnea
- Paroxysmal nocturnal dyspnea

Right heart failure

- Usually caused by left heart failure.
- Isolated right heart failure (RHF) is uncommon.
- When right heart failure does occur: **Corpulmonale.**
  - Lung disease causes pulmonary hypertension, can lead to R heart failure.
  - ↑ pulmonary vascular resistance causing ↑ R heart strain.
- RHF leads to
  - Systemic venous congestion.
  - Peripheral edema (swollen ankles).

Cyanide poisoning poisons oxidative phosphorylation.

Pulmonary hypertension

can lead to RV hypertrophy

and R heart failure

(corpulmonale).

- **Affects**
  - Left heart
  - Right heart
  - Both

SIGNS AND SYMPTOMS OF HEART FAILURE

Left Heart Failure	Right Heart Failure
Exertional dyspnea	Elevated venous pressure
Fatigue	Hepatomegaly
Orthopnea	Dependent edema
Cough	
Cardiac enlargement	
Rales	
Gallop rhythm (S3 or S4)	
Pulmonary venous congestion	

Primary Pulmonary Hypertension	Secondary Pulmonary Hypertension
No known heart or lung disease	Most common form
Unknown etiology	▪ COPD (most often)
	▪ Left to right shunt
	▪ ↑ pulmonary resistance
	▪ Embolism
	▪ Vasoconstriction from hypoxia
	▪ Left heart failure

CV Pulmonary Cross-Correlation

CARBON MONOXIDE (CO) POISONING

- **Symptoms**
  - Cherry-red discoloration of the skin, mucosa, and tissues
  - Mental status changes
  - Coma
  - Ultimately death

PULMONARY EDEMA

- Fluid in alveolar spaces of the lungs.
  - ↓ O$_2$ exchange.
- **Cause**
  - Usually left heart failure.
    - ↑ hydrostatic pressure.
      - Fluid extravasation into lung spaces.
- **Mechanism**
  - Backlog of blood in left heart (↑ volume).
  - ↑ left heart pressure.
  - ↑ pressure in pulmonary veins (transmitted backward from heart).
- **Symptoms**
  - Shortness of breath (SOB)/dyspnea
  - Orthopnea

- Cough
- Tachypnea
- Dependent crackles
- Tachycardia
- Neck vein distention
- **Treatment**
  - $\downarrow$ Vascular fluid
    - Diuretics
  - $\uparrow$ gas exchange and heart function
    - O_2
    - Antihypertensives
    - Positive inotropic agents
    - Antiarrhythmics

▶ RESPIRATORY PATHOLOGY

Asthma

- Chronic reactive airway disorder caused by episodic airway obstruction
- Any age
  - 3–5% of adults (usually < 30 years old)
  - 7–10% of children
  - 50% of asthma cases occur in children (<10 years old)
  - Boys > Girls (2:1)
- **Cause**
  - Bronchospasm (primary cause of airway obstruction)
  - Other contributors ($\uparrow$ airflow resistance)
    - $\uparrow$ mucus secretion
    - Mucosal edema
- **Symptoms**
  - Dyspnea/SOB
  - Expiratory wheezes
  - Chest tightness
  - Cough
- **Pathology**
  - Bronchial smooth muscle hypertrophy
  - $\uparrow$ bronchial submucosal glands
  - Eosinophils
  - Charcot–Leyden crystals

TYPES OF ASTHMA

Extrinsic (Allergic, Atopic, Immune)	Intrinsic (Nonimmune, Idiosyncratic)
Type I hypersensitivity	Exercise
Inhaled allergens (allergy triggers)	Cold air
Pet dander	Tobacco smoke
Dust mites	Respiratory infections
Cockroach allergens	Stress/Anxiety
Molds	Other pollutants
Pollens	Drugs

Mild CO poisoning can present with exhaustion and symptoms similar to a common cold or flu, delaying the diagnosis.

CO = colorless, odorless gas.
Sources: Automobile exhaust; home heating fumes.
Mechanism: Competitive inhibition
- Much higher affinity for Hb than O_2.
- Attaches to Hb and prevents O_2 carrying.

Pulmonary edema from heart failure
- Transudate into lungs
- Heart failure cells (macrophages that have phagocytized red blood cells in the alveoli)

Pulmonary edema can be caused by
- $\uparrow$ intracapillary hydrostatic pressure
  - Heart failure
- $\uparrow$ capillary permeability
  - Acute respiratory distress syndrome (ARDS)

MECHANISMS OF ASTHMA PRECIPITATION

Distinguish between

- Intraalveolar fluid: Pulmonary edema.
- Intrapleural (between visceral and parietal pleura): Pleural effusion.

Status asthmaticus

- Severe asthma attack
  - **Does not** respond to normal measures.
  - Usually requires hospitalization.
- Can lead to death from respiratory acidosis (obstruction).
- Treat with epinephrine.

Allergic (Immune)		Intrinsic (Nonimmune)		
Type I Hypersensitivity	**Direct Bronchoconstrictor Release**	**↑ Vagal Stimulation**	**Cox Inhibitors (NSAIDs, ASA)**
Atopic asthma	Caused by chemical inhalation or medications:	Respiratory threshold to vagal stimulation is lowered by	Cyclooxygenase pathway blocked
▪ IgE vs allergen			▪ Arachidonic acid metabolism
▪ Fc binds mast cell			**Cause**
▪ Reexposure to allergen	▪ Chemicals	▪ Viral infections	▪ ↑ Leukotrienes
▪ IgE cross-linked	▪ Resins	▪ URIs (cold or flu)	▪ Bronchocon-strictors
▪ Mast cells degranulate:	▪ Plastics	Parasympathetic activity causes bronchoconstriction	(as opposed to prostaglandins = bronchodilators)
▫ Histamine	▪ Cotton fibers		
▫ Other substances	▪ Toluene Formaldehyde		
Cause	▪ Penicillin		
▪ Bronchospasm			
▪ More inflammatory cell recruitment			

Nitrous oxide is safe to administer to people with asthma, especially if their asthma is triggered by anxiety.

Asthmatics taking chronic steroids may need corticosteroid augmentation.

In children, asthma symptoms can decrease with time (children can outgrow it).

COPD can overlap with asthma and bronchiectasis.

Cigarette smoking is the greatest cause of COPD.

Secondary pulmonary hypertension is most commonly caused by COPD.

- **Treatment**
  - β_2 agonist inhalers.
    - Preferred treatment for acute asthma attack.
    - Terbutaline.
    - Albuterol.
  - Steroids.
  - Mast cell stabilizers.
  - Epinephrine (sympathetic stimulation for status asthmaticus).

Chronic Obstructive Pulmonary Disease (COPD)

- Group of lung diseases characterized by ↑ airflow resistance.
  - Emphysema.
  - Chronic bronchitis.

Obstructive Lung Diseases	Restrictive Lung Diseases
↑ TLV	**↓ TLV**
Asthma	Intrinsic lung diseases:
COPD	▪ Pneumoconioses
▪ Emphysema	▪ Sarcoidosis
▪ Chronic bronchitis	▪ Idiopathic pulmonary fibrosis
	Extrinsic lung diseases:
	▪ Kyphosis
	▪ Obesity
	▪ Neuromuscular weakness

EMPHYSEMA

- "Pink puffer."
- Adults, usually smokers.

TYPES OF EMPHYSEMA

	Centrilobular	Panlobular
Cause	Cigarette smoking	Familial antiproteinase deficiency ↓ alpha-1 antitrypsin
Region	Upper lobes of lungs	Upper and lower lobes

- **Pathophysiology**
  - Destruction of elastic fibers in alveolar walls (distal to respiratory bronchioles).
    - ↓ elastic recoil.
      - Distal airspaces enlarge (dilated alveoli) with inhalation.
      - Lungs overexpand (↑ total lung capacity [TLC]).
    - ↓ radial traction.
      - Airways collapse with exhalation (leaving air behind, air trapping).
    - ↓ functioning parenchyma.
      - ↓ surface area for gas exchange.
- **Microscopic**
  - Enlarged air spaces.
  - Broken septae projecting into alveoli.
    - No fibrosis.
- **Clinical**
  - "Pink puffer."
  - Dyspnea.
  - Labored breathing.
  - No productive cough.
    - Scant clear mucoid sputum production.
    - ↑ infection susceptibility.
- **Findings**
  - PO_2 near normal.
    - No cyanosis (they are "pink").
    - Barrel chest on chest x-ray (CXR) (overexpansion).
    - Quiet chest to auscultation.
    - Adventitious sounds.
- **Pulmonary function tests (PFTs)**
  - ↑ TLC.
  - ↑ residual volume (RV).
  - ↓ FEV1/FVC (forced expiratory volume in 1 second/forced vital capacity).
- **Course**
  - Damage worsens with time.
    - ↑ as continue smoking.

Smoking related diseases:

- COPD
- Carcinoma
  - Oral cavity
  - Larynx
  - Lung
  - Esophagus
  - Pancreas
  - Kidney
  - Bladder
  - Peptic ulcer disease (PUD)
  - Low birth weight infants

Restrictive lung diseases:

- ↓ lung compliance.
- ↓ all lung volumes.
- ↑ FEV1/FVC.

Mechanisms of Airway Obstruction

- Airway hyperreactivity (bronchoconstriction): Asthma.
- ↓ elastic recoil (airways collapse): Emphysema.
- ↑ mucous: Chronic bronchitis.

SYSTEMIC PATHOLOGY

Emphysema has two basic problems:

- Lungs are "fixed" in inspiration: Difficult to exhale (airways collapse, trapping air).
- ↓ gas exchange: ↓ respiratory surface area.

In emphysema, destruction of lymphatic structural support can lead to ↑ pigment deposition in the lungs.

Productive cough

- Cough contains sputum. Sputum can contain
  - Mucus
  - Cellular debris
  - Bacteria
  - Blood
  - Pus
- Common causes of productive cough:
  - Chronic lung abscess
  - Tb
  - Lobar PNA
  - Bronchogenic carcinoma
  - Pulmonary embolism

Atelectasis neonatorum:

Alveolar collapse in newborn, usually due to ↓ surfactant (in premature infants).

CHRONIC BRONCHITIS

- "Blue bloaters"
- Adults with history of cigarette smoking
- **Definition:** Chronic productive cough for at least 3 months of the year for 2 years.
- Microscopic
  - Mucous hypersecretion.
    - Bronchi: Hypertrophy of mucous glands and smooth muscle.
    - Smaller airways: Goblet cell hyperplasia.
  - ↑ Reid index
    - ↑ ratio mucous gland thickness: bronchial wall thickness.
- Clinical
  - Productive cough.
    - ↑ sputum production.
  - Wheezing.
  - Auscultation.
    - Noisy chest.
    - Rhonchi.
- Findings
  - ↓ PO_2.
    - Cyanosis (look blue).
- Complications
  - Pulmonary hypertension.
    - RV overload; Cor pulmonale (R heart failure).
    - Peripheral edema (bloaters).
  - ↑ lung cancer risk (bronchogenic carcinoma).
    - Squamous metaplasia from chronic inflammation.

Bronchiectasis

- Permanent abnormal bronchial dilation.
- Cause
  - Bronchial obstruction.
    - Cystic fibrosis.
    - Lung tumor.
    - Kartagener syndrome (loss of function of the cilia).
    - Chronic sinusitis.
- Clinical
  - Chronic, productive cough.
    - Foul-smelling purulent sputum.
  - Hemoptysis.
  - Recurrent pulmonary infection.

Atelectasis

- Lung collapse (alveolar collapse)
- Causes
  - Failure of expansion
  - Bronchial obstruction
  - External compression

Pneumoconioses

- Caused by prolonged inhalation of foreign material.
- Named for the particle inhaled.

- Symptoms
  - Chronic dry cough
  - Shortness of breath
- Leads to pulmonary fibrosis.

ANTHRACOSIS

- Coal workers pneumoconiosis = black lung disease.
  - Inhalation of carbon dust.
- Two forms
  - Simple: Small lung opacities.
  - Complicated (= progressive massive fibrosis): Masses of fibrous tissue.
- Findings
  - Carbon-carrying macrophages.
  - Progressive nodular pulmonary disease (pulmonary fibrosis).

SILICOSIS

- Most common and most serious pneumoconiosis.
- Inhalation of silica (eg, by miners, glass makers, stone cutters).
- Findings
  - Silica dust in alveolar macrophages.
  - Silicotic nodules (dense, made of collagen, can calcify).
    - Visualized silica within the nodules using polarized light.
  - Thick pleural scars.
  - ↑ susceptibility to Tb.
    - Silicotuberculosis.

ASBESTOSIS

- Inhalation of asbestos fibers.
- Can develop 15–20 years after cessation of regular asbestos exposure.
- **Results in:** Diffuse interstitial fibrosis.
- **Findings**
  - Asbestos in alveolar macrophages.
  - Ferruginous bodies (yellow-brown, rod-shaped).
    - Stain with Prussian blue.
  - Hyalinized fibrocalcific plaques on parietal pleura.
- Course
  - ↑ predisposition to
    - Bronchogenic carcinoma.
    - Malignant mesothelioma of pleura.

Sarcoidosis

- Unknown etiology
- Diagnosis/biopsy; noncaseating granulomas
- Black females
  - Manifests in teen or young adult years
- Findings
  - Interstitial lung disease

Mesothelioma

- Rare tumor.
- Involves parietal or visceral pleura.
- Associated with asbestos exposure; 25- to 45-year latency.
- Diffuse lesion; spreads over lung surface.

Byssinosis: *Pneumoconiosis caused by inhalation of cotton particles.*

Beryliosis

- Inhalation of berylium particle.
- **Causes**
  - Systemic granulomatous disorder.
    - Noncaseating granulomas.
    - Primary pulmonary involvement.
  - Mimics sarcoidosis.

- Enlarged hilar lymph nodes
- Uveitis
- Erythema nodosum
- Polyarthritis
- Hypercalcemia
- **Pathology**
  - Noncaseating granulomas
    - Schaumann and asteroid bodies
- **Clinical**
  - Bilateral hilar lymphadenopathy on CXR
  - Interstitial lung disease (restrictive lung disease)
    - Cough
    - Dyspnea
  - Skin findings

> **Interstitial fibrosis**
>
> - Usually the result of fibrosing alveolitis.
> - Characterized by
>   - Thickening/fibrosis of the alveolar interstitium.
>   - Wall/space between the alveolus and the capillary.
>   - Results in restrictive lung disease.
> - **Causes**
>   - Idiopathic.
>   - Secondary to
>   - Connective tissue disorders: SLE, PAN, RA.
>   - Allergic extrinsic alveolitis.

Idiopathic Pulmonary Fibrosis

- Chronic inflammation and fibrosis of alveolar wall
- **Progression**
  - Alveolitis
  - Fibrosis
  - Fibrotic lung (honeycomb lung)
- Prognosis
  - Death within 5 years

Pneumonia

- Lung infection
  - Bacteria
  - Viruses
  - Fungi
- **Clinical**
  - Fever
  - Chills
  - Productive cough
  - Blood-tinged sputum
  - Dyspnea
  - Chest pain
- **Findings**
  - Hypoxia
  - Infiltrate on CXR
  - Crackles, other noises on auscultation

	Lobar Pneumonia	Bronchopneumonia	Interstitial Pneumonia
Causes	*Pneumococcus*	*Staph. aureus* *H. flu* *Klebsiella* *Strep. pyogenes*	Viruses; RSV, adenoviruses *Mycoplasma* *Legionella*
Findings	Exudate within alveolus Consolidation Lobe or entire lung	Bronchiole and alveolar infiltrates Patchy 1+ lobe	Diffuse patchy infiltrates (within interstitium) 1+ lobe
Age	Middle age	Infants Elderly	Young children

Viral Pneumonia	Bacterial Pneumonia
Most common cause of pneumonia in young children Peaks between age 2 and 3 y	Most serious pneumonias (typically) Pneumococcus (*Strep. pneumo*) is most common cause Most common fatal infection in the hospital

Lung Abscess

- Localized collection of pus in lung
- Causes
  - Aspiration
    - Altered mental status
  - Bronchial obstruction
    - Cancer
    - Pneumonia
    - Bronchiestasis
  - Septic emboli
- Organisms
  - Staphylococcus (most common)
    - Other organisms
      - Pseudomonas
      - Klebsiella (in alcoholics)
      - Proteus
      - Anaerobes
- Clinical
  - Productive cough; large amounts of foul-smelling sputum
  - Fever
  - Dyspnea
  - Chest pain
  - Cyanosis
  - Chest X-ray with fluid-filled cavity

Lung abscess
- Most common predisposing factor = alcoholism.
  - In particular, aspiration.
- Aspiration predisposed by
  - Altered consciousness:
    - Alcoholic stupor.
    - Drug overdose.
    - Seizures.
    - Debilitated, comatose.
  - Neurologic dysfunction:
    - Impaired gag reflex.
    - Impaired swallowing.
  - Contents aspirated.
    - Bacteria (including anaerobes) from
      - Oral secretions.
      - Decayed teeth.
      - Vomitus.
      - Foreign material.

Hemoptysis = *Coughing up blood (or blood-streaked sputum).*

- Respiratory infections (minor URIs)
- Bronchitis
- TB
- Pneumonia
- Bronchogenic carcinoma
- Idiopathic pulmonary hemosiderosis (iron in lungs)

Remember: *Ghon's complex = Calcified primary lesion + lymph node (LN) involvement.*

Clinical presentation of TB

- Usually secondary TB; only 5% patients with primary TB have symptoms.
- Secondary TB = reactivation of the primary Ghon's complex, which has remained quiescent (subclinical) and/or occurred years earlier.

Pott's disease = *TB involving the vertebral body.*

Tuberculosis (TB)

- Worldwide condition
- ↑ in conditions of
  - Poor sanitation
  - Poverty
  - Overcrowding
- Mycobacterium TB
  - Acid-fast bacilli
  - Strict aerobe
- Transmitted by aerosolized "droplets"
- **Pathology**
  - Granulomas
    - Giant cells
    - Caseous necrosis
- **Clinical**
  - Hemoptysis
  - Weight loss
  - Night sweats
  - Malaise
  - Weakness

TYPES OF TUBERCULOSIS

	Primary TB	**Secondary TB**	**Miliary TB**
Site	Between upper and middle lobes Lower part of upper lobe or Upper part of lower lobe	Lung apices High O$_2$ tension	Widely disseminated
Characteristic	Ghon's complex: Parenchymal lesion Hilar LNs	Reactivation of Ghon's complex	Lesions like "millet seed" Multiple extrapulmonary sites

▶ **GASTROINTESTINAL PATHOLOGY**

Esophagus

MALLORY–WEISS SYNDROME

- Mild to major bleeding (usually painless) at the distal esophagus, proximal stomach.
  - Near or involving the LES (lower esophageal sphincter).
  - **Cause:** Longitudinal mucosal lacerations (tear in mucous membrane).
  - Occur because of severe retching or vomiting, especially following alcohol intake.
- Most common in:
  - Men > age 40.
  - Alcoholics.
  - Hiatal hernia.

- Clinical
  - Vomiting of blood (hematemsis).
- Treatment
  - Depends on amount/severity of bleeding.
  - Often stops spontaneously.
  - Tear usually heals in about 10 days without special treatment.
  - Local control.
    - Cautery.
    - Banding.

ACHALSIA

- ↓ propulsion of food down the esophagus (↓ peristalsis).
- Failure of lower esophageal sphincter (LES) to relax.
  - High pressure on manometry.
  - Difficulty opening.
  - Characteristic "bird's-beak appearance" on barium swallow.
- Cause
  - Nerve related.
- Clinical
  - Dysphagia to both solids and liquids.
  - Regurgitation of food.
- Treatment
  - Pneumatic dilation.
  - Botox.
  - Heller myotomy.
  - Calcium channel blockers.

GASTROESOPHAGEAL REFLUX DISEASE (GERD)

- Acid reflux
- Backflow of acidic stomach contents up into esophagus
  - Lower esophageal sphincter leaky
- Risks
  - Hiatal hernia
  - Scleroderma
- Symptoms
  - Heartburn
  - Regurgitation of food
  - Hoarse voice
  - Wheeze
  - Cough
- Treatment
  - Proton pump inhibitors
  - Antacids
- Complications
  - Can lead to *Barrett's esophagus*
    - Premalignant condition

HIATAL HERNIA

- Protrusion of part of the stomach through diaphragm into the thoracic cavity.
- Symptoms
  - Heartburn
  - Dysphagia
  - Belching

ESOPHAGEAL ULCERS

- Erosion on the esophageal lining mucosa.
- Usually caused by repeated regurgitation of stomach acid (HCl) to lower part of esophagus.
- Can also get esophageal infections causing erosion (eg, candidal or viral).

BARRETT'S ESOPHAGUS

- Type of metaplasia.
- Change from squamous cell epithelium to columnar cell epithelium.
- Precancerous condition.
- Complication of chronic heartburn.

Stomach

PEPTIC ULCER DISEASE (PUD)

- Erosion in the lining of the stomach or duodenum.
- Circumscribed lesions in the mucous membrane.
- Occur mostly in men age 20–50 years.
- ~80% are duodenal ulcers.
- **Causes**
    - Imbalance between acid and mucosal protection.
        - NSAIDs ($\downarrow$ mucosal protection: $\downarrow$ prostaglandins).
        - Acid hypersecretion (eg, Zollinger–Ellison).
    - Infection
        - *Helicobacter pylori*
- **Risks**
    - Aspirin, NSAIDs (as above)
    - Cigarette smoking
    - Older age
- **Symptom**
    - Pain
- **Complications**
    - Bleeding
        - When erode deep into blood vessels
        - Bleeding ulcer
    - Perforation
        - Ulcerate transmurally (through the entire wall).
        - Causes acute peritonitis; can lead to death.
        - Most often occurs with duodenal ulcers.
    - Malignant change is uncommon.
- **Treatment**
    - Antibiotics
    - Antacid medications
    - Proton pump inhibitors

Hemorrhage is the most common complication of PUD. It is most likely with duodenal ulcers.

Gastric Ulcer	Duodenal Ulcer
20% of PUD	80% of PUD
Peptic ulcer located in the stomach	Peptic ulcer located in duodenum
More common in middle-aged and elderly men	More associated with *H. pylori*

HEMATEMESIS

- Vomiting bright red blood
- Usually indicates upper GI bleeding
  - Esophageal varices
  - Peptic ulcers

Small and Large Intestines

MECKEL DIVERTICULUM

- Most common congenital anomaly of the small intestine.
- Remnant of the embryonic vitelline duct.
- Located in distal small bowel.
- May contain ectopic gastric and duodenal, colonic, or pancreatic tissue.

INTESTINAL LYMPHANGIECTASIA

- In children, young adults in which lymph vessels supplying lining of small intestine become enlarged; fluid retention is massive

INFLAMMATORY BOWEL DISEASE

- Crohn's and ulcerative colitis (UC)
- Both can present with:
  - Abdominal pain
  - Obstruction
  - Bloody diarrhea (occult or gross)

COMPARISON OF CROHN'S DISEASE AND ULCERATIVE COLITIS

Crohn's Disease	Ulcerative Colitis
Can affect entire GI from mouth to anus Cobblestone appearance Transmural inflammation (giant cells)	Only the colon Inflammation limited to mucosa and submucosa ↑ risk of secondary malignancy

MALABSORPTION SYNDROMES

- Nutrients from food are not absorbed properly.
- Not absorbed across small intestine into the bloodstream.
- Clinical
  - Children
    - Growth retardation
    - Failure to thrive
  - Adults
    - Weight loss

Steatorrhea = Soft, bulky, foul-smelling light-colored stool.

- Occurs when fat is not absorbed.
  - Pancreatic disease (↓ digestive enzymes).
  - Bile obstruction (↓ bile for emulsification).

Malabsorption Syndrome*	Cause	Comments
Celiac disease	Autoimmune disease triggered by gluten protein	Child or adult ↑ risk of GI lymphoma MALToma
Tropical sprue	Unknown Probably infection	Travelers to the tropics Steatorrhea Diarrhea Weight loss Sore tongue (↓ vitamin B)
Whipple's disease	*Tropheryma whippelii*	Middle-aged men Slow onset of symptoms: <ul><li>Skin darkening</li><li>Inflamed painful joints</li><li>Diarrhea</li></ul> Can be fatal without treatment

*For vitamin and mineral deficiencies, see Chapter 16, "Nutrition."

Pancreas

PANCREATITIS

- Inflammation or infection of the pancreas.
- Cause
    - Injury to pancreatic cells.
    - Obstruction of normal pancreatic outflow.
        - Autodigestion/autolysis by pancreatic enzymes.
        - Zymogens prematurely convert into their catalytically active forms.
        - These enzymes then attack the pancreatic tissue itself.
    - In chronic cases, inflammation and fibrosis cause destruction of functioning glandular tissue.
- Symptoms
    - Pain, destruction of pancreas.
- Laboratory
    - ↑ lipase (more important).
    - ↑ amylase.

	Acute Pancreatitis	Chronic Pancreatitis
Causes	Gallstones (#1) Other biliary disease Trauma Cystic fibrosis in children	Alcoholism (most often) Hyperlipidemia Hyperparathyroidism
Symptoms	Abdominal pain Knifelike Radiating to back Nausea and vomiting Jaundice (if gallstone) Pale or clay-colored stools (if bile blockage too)	Abdominal pain Nausea and vomiting Fatty stools
Complications	Enzymatic hemorrhagic fat necrosis with calcium soap formation with resultant hypocalcemia	Pseudocyst* Pancreatic abscess Ascites

*Pancreatic abscesses occur in pancreatic pseudocysts that become infected.

CHOLELITHIASIS

- Stones in the gallbladder = gallstones.
- Almost all gallstones are formed in the gallbladder, where bile is stored after it is produced in liver.
- Bile is composed of
  - Water
  - Bile salts (glycine and taurine)
  - Lecithin
  - Cholesterol
  - Small solutes
- Stone formation
  - Changes in relative concentration of bile components.
  - Precipitation from solution.
  - Nidus, or nest, around which gallstones are formed.
- Stone size
  - Ranges from small as a grain of sand to large as 1-in diameter.
  - Depends on time elapsed since initial formation.
- Stone color
  - Depends on primary precipitated substance:
    - Yellow-white—cholesterol.
    - Red-brown—bilirubin and calcium salts.

CHOLESTEROLOSIS

- Called strawberry gallbladder (GB).
- Small yellow cholesterol flecks against a red background in the lining of the gallbladder.
  - Polyps may form inside the GB.
  - May necessitate GB removal if outflow is blocked.

Choledocholithiasis = Gallstones in the common bile duct (CBD).

Gallstones that block the CBD result in obstructive jaundice, with yellow skin color caused by bile pigments being deposited in skin.

GALLBLADDER DIVERTICULOSIS

- Small fingerlike outpouchings of the GB lining may develop as a person ages; may cause inflammation and require GB removal.

Liver Disease

CIRRHOSIS (OF LIVER)

- Most common chronic liver disease.
- Occurs twice as often in males as in females.
- Third most common cause of death among people aged 45–65 (behind heart disease and cancer).
- Characteristics
  - Scarring/fibrosis
  - Loss of hepatic architecture
  - Formation of regenerative nodules
- Causes
  - Alcoholism (75%)
  - Viral hepatitis (hepatitis B, C)
  - Hemochromatosis
  - Wilson disease
  - Drugs/toxic injury
  - Biliary obstruction
  - Other inborn errors of metabolism:
    - Galactosemia
    - Glycogen storage diseases
    - Alpha-1 antitrypsin deficiency
- Clinical findings/complications
  - Ascites
  - Splenomegaly
  - Jaundice
  - Coagulopathy/bleeding disorders
  - Confusion/hepatic encephalopathy
  - Portal hypertension (and its complications)
  - Esophageal varices (with hematemesis)

Cirrhosis is associated with increase in hepatocellular carcinoma.

Wilson's disease (hepatolenticular degeneration) is the hereditary accumulation of copper in liver, kidney, brain, and cornea. It is characterized by cirrhosis of the liver, degeneration of the basal ganglia in the brain, and deposition of green pigment in periphera of cornea.

PORTAL HYPERTENSION

- Abnormally high blood pressure in the portal vein/system
- Factors ↑ BP in portal vessels
  - ↓ volume of blood flowing through the portal system
  - ↑ resistance to blood flow through the liver
- Causes
  - Cirrhosis of liver—most common cause.
  - Splenic or portal vein thrombosis (prehepatic).
  - Schistosomiasis (intrahepatic).
  - Congestion distal hepatic venous circulation (Budd–Chiari syndrome) (posthepatic).
- Results/complications
  - Development of venous collaterals
    - Esophageal varices (common source of massive hematemesis in alcoholics).

Splenomegaly is the most important sign of portal hypertension.

- ▨ Hemorrhoids
- ▨ Enlarged veins on the anterior abdominal wall (caput Medusae)
- ▨ Spider angiomas
- ▨ Ascites (fluid within abdominal cavity)
- ▨ Splenomegaly (congestive)
- ▨ See Chapter 1 for the anatomy of the portal blood supply.

ASCITES

- ▨ Excess fluid in the space between the membranes lining the abdomen and abdominal organs.
  - ▨ Peritoneal cavity
    - ▨ Visceral peritoneum.
    - ▨ Parietal peritoneum.
- ▨ Ascites can be free serous fluid or protein-laden (like almost pure plasma).
- ▨ Disorders associated with ascites include:
  - ▨ Cirrhosis.
  - ▨ Hepatitis.
  - ▨ Portal vein thrombosis.
  - ▨ Constrictive pericarditis.
  - ▨ CHF.
  - ▨ Liver cancer.
  - ▨ Nephrotic syndrome.
  - ▨ Pancreatitis.

JAUNDICE

- ▨ Yellow discoloration of skin, mucous membranes, eyes.
- ▨ **Mechanism**
  - ▨ ↑ bilirubin in blood.
  - ▨ Dissolves in subcutaneous tissues/fat.
- ▨ **Causes**
  - ▨ ↑ RBC destruction.
    - ▨ Release of bilirubin into blood (unconjugated).
  - ▨ Biliary obstruction.
    - ▨ Inability of bilirubin to be excreted into GI tract (conjugated).
  - ▨ Liver damage.
    - ▨ Bilirubin release into blood.
  - ▨ Any age, either sex.

BILIRUBIN

- ▨ Waste product from hemoglobin breakdown in RBCs.
- ▨ Excreted from body as chief component of bile.
- ▨ **Conjugated bilirubin.**
  - ▨ Bilirubin conjugates with glucuronic acid in the liver.
- ▨ **Free bilirubin** (unconjugated) (converted to conjugated bilirubin in the liver).
  - ▨ Travels in blood bound to albumin.
  - ▨ Toxic.

Hematemesis and bleeding from esophageal varices (dilated tortuous veins in submucosa of the lower esophagus) is often the first sign of cirrhosis and portal hypertension; it requires emergency treatment to control hemorrhage and prevent hypovolemic shock. This is an important cause of death in this group.

Liver disease is the most common cause of ascites.

Jaundice is a leading manifestation of liver disease.

- Kernicterus
  - Newborn infants.
  - High levels of bilirubin accumulate in the brain.
  - Characteristic form of crippling.
    - Athetoid cerebral palsy.

HEPATITIS

- Inflammation of the liver.

TRANSAMINITIS

- Damage to liver cells → release enzymes into blood → ↑ serum levels of enzymes (transaminases = AST, ALT).
- ↑ transaminases used to diagnose liver disease.

VIRAL HEPATITIS

- Liver inflammation caused by a virus.
- See Chapter 16 for virology.

▶ GENITOURINARY PATHOLOGY

Nephrolithiasis

- Renal calculi (kidney stones).
  - Form within renal pelvis, calyces.
  - Pass into urinary system.
- Occurs more often in males than in females (M > F); rare in children.
- Predisposing factors
  - Dehydration
  - Infection
  - Changes in urine pH
  - Obstruction of urine flow
  - Immobilization with bone reabsorption
  - Metabolic factors (eg, hyperparathyroidism with hypercalcemia)
  - Renal acidosis
  - ↑ uric acid
  - Defective oxalate metabolism
- Stone composition
  - Calcium oxalate or calcium phosphate (most common)
  - Struvite (from infection)
  - Uric acid (from metabolic disorder, obesity)
  - Cystine (inborn errors of metabolism)
- Clinical symptoms
  - Usually asymptomatic (until stones pass into the ureter)
  - Renal colic (severe pain)
    - Once stone is in ureter, increased pressure and peristalsis from the ureter
- Complications
  - Obstruction of the ureter (with pressure and pain, renal colic)
  - Pyelonephritis (acute or chronic)
  - Hydronephrosis

STONE FORMATION

- Stones result from different processes or disease.
- But pathogenesis is the same: Supersaturation of the urine with a poorly soluble material.
- Renal stones grow on the surfaces of the papillae.
- Stones detach and flow downstream in the urine.
- Large stones will not fit through narrow conduits.
  Usually >1 cm to as large as staghorn stone.
- Obstruction → renal colic, hydronephrosis.
  Bilateral renal calculi are more apt to cause infection.

Calcium stones account for 80–90% of urinary stones. They are composed of calcium oxalate, calcium phosphate, or both.

HYDRONEPHROSIS

- Abnormal dilation of renal pelvis and calyces of one or both kidneys.
- Caused by urinary tract obstruction.
  - ↓ urine outflow.
  - Pressure ↑ behind the obstruction.
  - Renal pelvis and calyces dilate.
- Physical manifestation.
  - **Not** a disease process itself.
  - Disease = Stone, stricture, benign prostatic hyperplasia, etc.

Pyelonephritis

- Infection of the renal pelvis (kidney and ureters), usually *E. coli*.
- **Cause**
  - Most often from a urinary tract infection (UTI).
  - Retrograde/backflow bacteria-laden urine from bladder into ureters up to kidney pelvis.
    - *Vesicoureteral reflux*
- **Forms**
  - Acute
    - Active infection of the renal pelvis.
    - Abscess can develop; renal pelvis filled with pus (neutrophil rich).
  - Chronic
    - Scarring fibrosis; renal failure is possible.

Kidney infections are usually caused by microorganisms ascending from the lower urinary tract.

Poststreptococcal GMN is the classic cause of blood in urine in children.

Hematuria	Glucosuria	Ketonuria	Proteinuria
Blood in urine **Women** Blood may come from vagina. **Men** Bloody ejaculation may be due to a prostate problem. **Children** Bleeding disorders. Recent strep infection may imply post-strep GMN.	Glucose in urine	Ketones in urine; acetonelike odor	Protein in urine
Kidney or urinary tract disease	Diabetes mellitus	Starvation Uncontrolled DM Alcohol intoxication	Kidney disease

Diabetes Insipidus

See Chapter 17, "Endocrine Physiology."

Polycystic Kidney Disease (PCKD)

- **Adult form (APCKD)**
- Inherited disorder with multiple cysts on the kidneys.
- Caused by mutation in the *PKD* gene.
- Course
  - Early stages
    - Kidney enlargement (as cysts form and grow)
    - Kidney function altered, resulting in:
      - Chronic high blood pressure; hypertension caused by polycystic kidneys is difficult to control.
      - Anemia.
      - Erythrocytosis; if cysts cause ↑ erythropoietin (cause ↑ RBCs).
      - Kidney infections.
      - Flank pain, if bleeding into a cyst occurs.
  - Later
    - Slowly progressive.
    - Ultimately results in **end-stage kidney failure.**
  - APCKD also associated with liver disease and infection of liver cysts.
- **Childhood form**
  - Autosomal recessive form of polycystic kidney disease.
  - More serious form appears in infancy or childhood.
- **Course**
  - Progresses rapidly.
  - Resulting in ESRD.
    - Kidney failure leads to death in infancy or childhood.

Note: Kidney stones are less common in PCKD.

Medullary Cystic Disease

- Cysts in the kidney medulla (deep)
  - Results in kidney failure
- Uncommon
- Affects older children

Medullary Sponge Kidney

- Congenital disorder.
- Kidney tubules are dilated, causing the kidney to appear spongy.

Nephrosclerosis

- Renal impairment secondary to arteriosclerosis or hypertension.
- **Arterial nephrosclerosis.**
  - Atrophy and scarring of the kidney.
  - Due to arteriosclerotic thickenings of the walls of large branches of renal arteries.

- Arteriolar nephrosclerosis
  - Arterioles thicken.
  - Areas they supply undergo ischemic atrophy and interstitial fibrosis.
  - Associated with HTN.
- Malignant nephrosclerosis
  - Inflammation of renal arterioles.
  - Results in rapid deterioration of renal function.
  - Accompanies malignant hypertension.

Arteriosclerosis

- Associated with chronic HTN.
- Reactive changes in the smaller arteries and arterioles throughout the body.

BENIGN NEPHROSCLEROSIS

- Arteriosclerosis affecting renal vessels.
- Result is a loss of renal parenchyma.
  - ↓ kidney function.

Nephrotic Syndrome

- **Not** a disease itself.
  - Glomerular defect underlies the process, indicating renal damage.
- Demographics
  - Any age
    - Children; usually age 18 mo–4 years; boys > girls.
    - Adults; males and females alike (M = F).
- Characterized by
  - **Proteinuria;** ↑↑ loss of protein in the urine (> 3.5 g/d).
  - **Hypoalbuminemia.**
  - **Hyperlipidemia.**
  - **Edema;** ↑ salt and water retention.
- Cause; ↑ glomerular capillary permeability.
  - Leads to ↓ blood protein (albumin).
  - Leads to ↑ protein in urine.
- Associated diseases
  - Malignancy such as leukemia, lymphoma, and multiple myeloma
  - Autoimmune disease such as lupus, Goodpasture's syndrome, and Sjogren's syndrome
  - Infections such as bacterial and HIV
  - Diabetes mellitus
  - Drugs such as NSAIDS
- Clinical symptoms
  - Loss of appetite
  - General sick feeling (malaise)
  - Puffy eyelids
  - Abdominal pain
  - Muscle wasting
  - Tissue swelling/edema
  - Frothy urine (protein-laden)

Primary NS means that the disease is limited to the kidneys. Secondary NS means that the disease affects the kidneys and other organs.

Hyperlipidemia in nephrotic syndrome is secondary to

- ↑ hepatic fat synthesis.
- ↓ fat catabolism.

Lipiduria: Cholesterol, triglycerides, lipoproteins leak into the urine.

Glomerulonephropathies

- Kidney disorders where inflammation affects mainly the glomeruli.
- Varied causes, but glomeruli respond to injury similarly.
- **Acute nephritic syndrome**
  - Example: Acute post-streptococcal glomerulonephritis (acute glomerulonephritis).
    - Most common in boys 3–7; can occur at any age.
    - Starts suddenly and usually resolves quickly.
  - Acute glomerular inflammation.
  - Sudden hematuria.
    - Clumps of RBCs (casts).
    - Protein in urine.
- **Rapidly progressive nephritic syndrome**
  - Example: **Rapidly progressive glomerulonephritis (RPGN).**
    - Uncommon disorder; usually occurs at age 50–60.
    - Starts suddenly and worsens rapidly.
    - Most of the glomeruli are partly destroyed.
    - Results in kidney failure.
    - Idiopathic or associated with a proliferative glomerular disease (eg, acute GN).
- **Nephrotic syndrome**
  - See earlier discussion.
  - Many disease processes can affect the kidney to cause **nephrotic syndrome**
    - **Findings**
      - Proteinuria (loss of large amounts of protein in the urine)
      - Hypoalbuminemia
      - Generalized edema
      - Hyperlipidemia
      - Hypercholesterolemia
- **Chronic nephritic syndrome**
  - Also called chronic glomerulonephritis
  - Examples of diseases causing:
    - SLE
    - Goodpasture's syndrome
    - Acute GN
    - Slowly progressive disease
    - Inflammation of the glomeruli
      - Sclerosis
      - Scarring
      - Eventual renal failure

▶ BLOOD-LYMPHATIC PATHOLOGY

Anemia

- ↓ RBCs and/or hemoglobin (absolute or qualitative).
- ↓ oxygen-carrying capacity.
- ↓ energy.
  - Fatigue
  - Weakness
  - Inability to exercise
  - Lightheadedness

CLASSIFICATION OF ANEMIA

↑ RBC Destruction	↓ RBC Production

▢ Blood loss
▢ Hemolytic (= RBC destruction)
  ▢ Autoimmune hemolytic anemia
  ▢ Erythroblastosis fetalis
▢ Hereditary spherocytosis
▢ G6PD deficiency
▢ Sickle cell anemia
▢ Thalassemia
	▢ Hematopoietic cell damage
	  ▢ Aplastic anemia
	▢ Deficiency of factors
	  ▢ B_{12} deficiency (pernicious anemia)
	  ▢ Folate deficiency
	  ▢ Fe deficiency
	▢ Bone marrow replacement
	  ▢ Leukemia
	  ▢ Myelophthisis
	  ▢ Myelodyplasia

Anemia from ↑ RBC Destruction

BLOOD LOSS ANEMIA

▢ ↓RBCs because of external loss.
▢ Hemorrhage.
▢ Symptoms are related to hypovolemia.

Note: Iron-deficiency anemia can be caused by both blood loss (↑ RBC destruction) and dietary deficiency (↓ RBC production).

HEMOLYTIC ANEMIA

▢ ↓ RBC life span (↑ RBC destruction).

AUTOIMMUNE HEMOLYTIC ANEMIA

▢ IgG antibodies combine with RBC surface antigens.
▢ Fc site of the bound antibody reacts with Fc receptor of phagocytic cells (and reticuloendothelial system).
▢ Antibody coated RBCs are sequestered in the spleen (where hemolysis occurs).
  ▢ Splenomegaly.
▢ Diagnosis: Positive direct Coombs' test.
▢ Features (as with other hemolytic anemias):
  ▢ Unconjugated hyperbilirubinemia.
  ▢ Jaundice.

ERYTHROBLASTOSIS FETALIS

▢ Mother produces antibodies against fetal RBCs.
▢ Destruction of fetal RBCs.
▢ **Mechanism**
  ▢ Occurs in cases where Mom = Rh– and fetus = Rh+.
  ▢ Rh+ is dominant trait (passed from father in this case).
  ▢ Rh– mom forms Abs against Rh+ fetal blood.
  ▢ Antibodies cross placenta into fetus circulation where they attach and lead to destruction of fetal RBCs.
  ▢ Anemia in the fetus.

Other causes of anemia:

▢ **Splenic sequestration**
  ▢ Massive splenomegaly leads to ↑ repository of RBCs.
  ▢ RBCs are sequestered in spleen so there are fewer in the bloodstream.
  ▢ ITP and purpura occur with splenic sequestration too.
    ▢ ↓ usable platelets (as they are sequestered in the spleen).
▢ **Renal failure**
  ▢ ↓ synthesis of erythropoietin.
  ▢ Normocytic, normochromic anemia.
  ▢ Treat with Epo.

The direct Coombs' test looks for autoimmune antibodies to one's own RBCs. The indirect Coombs' test looks for cross-reactivity during pregnancy or before a blood transfusion.

Hemolytic anemias

▢ Hyperbilirubinemia and hemoglobinuria.
▢ Broken down RBC:
  ▢ Hb liberated.
  ▢ Hb in urine.
  ▢ Hb in blood.
    ▢ Bilirubin (breakdown product of Hb).
    ▢ ↑unconjugated bilirubin (water insoluble).
      ▢ Jaundice (yellow under tongue = first sign; yellow sclera).

- Conjugated bilirubin (water-soluble) forms when unconjugated bilirubin combines with glucuronic acid.
  - Secreted with bile into the small intestine.
  - Reduction of bilirubin in intestine to urobilinogen.
  - ↑ uro-bilinogen.

*Toxic accumulation of unconjugated bilirubin in the brain and spinal cord is called **kernicterus**.*

Patients with sickle cell anemia can become functionally asplenic. As a result, they are prone to infections caused by encapsulated organisms (including Strep pneumonia and Hemophilus influenza). Salmonella bone infections/ osteomyelitis can occur.

Healing leg ulcers and recurrent bouts of abdominal and chest pain are characteristic of sickle cell anemia.

Repeated sickle cell crises can damage kidneys, lungs, bones, eyes, and CNS.

Note: Erythroblastosis fetalis can also occur because of ABO incompatibility (eg, Mom = O, fetus = type A or B). However, Rh incompatibility causes the most severe form.

HEREDITARY SPHREROCYTOSIS

- Sphere-shaped RBCs are selectively trapped in the spleen.
  - Sequestration splenomegaly.
  - Unconjugated hyperbilirubinemia.
- Autosomal dominant.
- Abnormality of RBC membrane protein (spectrin protein).
- ↑ erythrocyte fragility to hypotonic saline.

G6PD DEFICIENCY

- X-linked inheritance.
- ↓ activity of RBC G6PD.
- Failure of RBC hexose monophosphate shunt under oxidative stress.
- Leads to hemolysis (with hemoglobinemia, hemoglobinuria).

SICKLE CELL ANEMIA

- Primarily in African Americans.
- Inherited autosomal recessive (inherited HbS from both parents).
- Abnormal type of hemoglobin HbS.
  - Globin portion: Valine substituted for glutamic acid in the sixth position.
- **Heterozygote (AS) (less severe) = Sickle cell trait.**
  - One normal Hb (HbA).
  - One abnormal Hb (HbS).
- **Homozygote (SS) (more severe) = Sickle cell disease.**
  - Two abnormal Hb (HbS).
  - HbS causes Hb instability when exposed to stress (eg, ↓ O_2 [hypoxic conditions]).
  - Lead to formation of fibrous precipitates.
  - Distort erythrocytes into sickle shape (crescent shape).
  - ↓ function.
- **Sickle cell pain crisis**
  - Sickled cells form small blood clots.
  - Clots occlude blood vessels and give rise to painful episodes; usually affect bones of back, long bones, and chest.
  - Episodes can last hours to days.
- **Hemolytic crisis**
  - Life-threatening breakdown of damaged RBCs.
- **Splenic sequestration crisis**
  - The spleen enlarges because sickled RBCs are trapped.
- **Aplastic crisis**
  - Infection causes bone marrow to stop producing RBCs.

THALASSEMIAS (MAJOR AND MINOR)

- Group of inherited Hb synthesis disorders (autosomal recessive).
- ↓ globin chain synthesis (one of the four amino acid chains that make up Hb).

- Abnormal Hb.
  - ↓ RBCs.
- Chronic anemia.

Anemia from ↓ RBC Production

HEMATOPOIETIC CELL DAMAGE

- Aplastic anemia
  - ↓ production of RBCs.
    - Inhibition or destruction of bone marrow.
  - Pancytopenia (↓ levels of all blood elements—cells and platelets).
  - BM biopsy.
    - Normal architecture, **but**
    - ↓ cellularity (< 25% normal).
  - Absolute neutrophil counts are extremely low.
- Causes
  - Hereditary
  - Acquired:
    - Radiation
    - Toxins:
      - Benzene
      - Insecticides
    - Viral infections
      - CMV
      - Parvovirus
      - Hepatitis
    - Medications:
      - Chloramphenicol
      - Anticonvulsants
      - Phenylbutazone

In drug-induced aplastic anemias, the RBCs appear normochromic (normal concentration of Hb) and normocytic (normal size).

↓ FACTORS FOR RBC PRODUCTION

B_{12} DEFICIENCY

- Pernicious anemia
- Autoimmune disorder
  - Caused by **autoimmune gastritis** (failure in production of intrinsic factor).
    - Anti-intrinsic factor and antiparietal cell antibodies.
      - Lack of intrinsic factor (IF needed to absorb B_{12}).
    - Achlorhydria.
- Features
  - Megaloblastic (macrocytic) anemia.
  - Abnormal Schilling test.
    - Impaired absorption of B_{12}; corrected by adding intrinsic factor.
  - Hypersegmented neutrophils on peripheral blood smear.
  - Lemon-yellow skin.
  - Stomatitis and glossitis.
  - Subacute combined degeneration of the spinal cord.
- Symptoms
  - Fatigue, SOB, tingling sensations, difficulty walking, diarrhea.

Intrinsic factor is a protein produced in gastric parietal cells. B_{12} must be bound by IF to be absorbed in the ileum. B_{12} is necessary for RBC formation and is needed by nerves.

*Major causes of B$_{12}$
deficiency with the
resultant megaloblastic
anemia:*

- Pernicious anemia ($\downarrow$
  intrinsic factor because
  of autoimmune
  gastritis).
- Dietary deficiency of
  B$_{12}$ (strict vegetarian).
- Gastric resection
  (remove cells that
  produce IF–parietal
  cells).
- Ileal resection (remove
  intestinal cells that
  absorb B$_{12}$).

Plummer–Vinson syndrome:

Fe deficiency anemia

associated with upper

esophageal web.

- Other causes of vitamin B$_{12}$ megaloblastic anemia:
  - Gastric resection (where IF is produced).
  - Strict vegetarian diet.
  - Distal ileum resection (where B$_{12}$ is absorbed).

Note: Patients with atrophic gastritis are prone to gastric carcinomas.

FOLATE DEFICIENCY

- Megaloblastic (macrocytic) anemia.
  - Hypersegmented neutrophils.
  - Lack of folate results in delayed DNA replication.
- **Causes**
  - Dietary deficiency
  - Malabsorption syndromes (*sprue, Giardia lamblia*)
  - Pregnancy
  - Drugs such as methotrexate and Dilantin

Note: Folate deficiency has no neurologic abnormalities (in distinction to B$_{12}$ deficiency)

IRON DEFICIENCY

- Hypochromic microcytic anemia (pale small RBCs)
- **Causes**
  - Chronic blood loss (major cause of Fe deficiency anemia)
    - Excessive menstrual bleeding
    - GI bleeding
    - Results in:
      - $\downarrow$ or absent bone marrow Fe stores
      - $\downarrow$ serum ferritin
  - Dietary deficiency
    - Rare, except infants, elderly
    - $\downarrow$ Fe requirement
    - Pregnancy
    - Infants, fast-growing adolescents.
- **Findings**
  - Pallor
  - Fatigue
  - Shortness of breath
  - Glossitis, koilonychias

MICROCYTIC VERSUS MACROCYTIC ANEMIA

Microcytic	Macrocytic
Average size of RBC < normal Fe deficiency	Average size of RBC > normal B$_{12}$ deficiency Folate deficiency

Other Causes of ↓ RBC Production

ANEMIA OF CHRONIC DISEASE

- Isolated ↓ RBC proliferation; may resemble Fe deficiency.

MYELODYSPLASTIC SYNDROMES

- Example: Myelodysplasia with myelofibrosis.
- Bone marrow is replaced by abnormal (dysplastic) stem cells or by fibrous tissue.
  - Ineffective hematopoiesis
  - ↑ immature RBCs and WBCs
  - Abnormally shaped RBCs (teardrop shaped)
  - Anemia
  - Splenomegaly
- Myeloproliferative disorders
  - Myeloid stem cells develop and reproduce abnormally in bone marrow
  - Peak incidence in middle age
  - ↓ blood basophils
  - ↑ serum uric acid
  - Splenomegaly

PURE RED CELL APLASIA

- Severe ↓ of RBC lineage only.

Erythrocytes and Polycythemia (↑ RBCs)

RELATIVE POLYCYTHEMIA

- ↓ Plasma volume.
- RBCs are more concentrated.
- Spurious polycythemia = Gaisbock syndrome.

TRUE POLYCYTHEMIA

- ↑ total blood volume
- ↑ RBC mass
- Opposite of anemia

PRIMARY POLYCYTHEMIA

- *Polycythemia vera* (a myeloproliferative disease).
- Genetic predisposition.
- ↓ sensitivity of myeloid precursors to erythropoietin.

Erythropoeitin is used to treat anemia caused by chronic kidney disease.

- **Characteristics**
  - Erythrocytosis.
  - Leukocytosis.
  - Thrombocytosis.
  - Splenomegaly.
  - ↓ erythropoietin.

SECONDARY POLYCYTHEMIA

- ↑ RBCs by conditions other than polycythemia vera.
- Secondary to ↑ erythropoietin.
- **Causes**
  - Renal disease
    - Polycystic kidney disease
    - Renal cell carcinoma
  - Chronic hypoxia
    - Pulmonary disease
    - Heavy smoking
    - High altitude (Oskar's disease)
    - CHF
  - Tumors
    - Renal cell cancer (see above)
    - Hepatocellular carcinoma
    - Meningioma
    - Pheochromocytoma
    - Cerebellar hemangioma
    - Adrenal adenoma
  - Androgen therapy
  - Bartter syndrome
- **Features**
  - Plethora
    - Redness of skin and mucous membranes
  - ↓ blood viscosity
    - ↓ tissue perfusion
    - Propensity for thrombosis
  - No splenomegaly (this is a feature of polycythemia vera)

Remember: In polycythemia vera (primary polycythemia) erythropoietin levels are normal or low. In secondary polycythemia, erythropoietin levels are elevated.

Polycythemia is a myeloproliferative disorder, as is myelofibrosis (see above with anemia).

Remember: Erythropoietin is made by the kidney in the juxtaglomerular apparatus.

Aspirin inactivates cyclooxygenase (COX) by acetylation; causes ↓ production thromboxane A2 (a platelet aggregant). More prone to bleeding secondary to ↓ platelet aggregation.

Bleeding Problems

- Bleeding occurs when there are abnormalities in:
  - Primary hemostasis (platelet plug); quantitative or qualitative platelet disorders.
  - Secondary hemostasis; disorder in the coagulation cascade.
  - Disorders affecting the structural integrity of blood vessels.

Primary Hemostasis (Platelet Plug)	Secondary Hemostasis (Coagulation)	Combined Primary and Secondary Defect	Vessel Damage
Quantitative ↓ *platelet* Thrombocytopenia ▪ Marrow damage ▪ Aplastic anemia ▪ Marrow replacement ▪ Leukemia ▪ Myelophthisis ▪ Splenic sequestration DIC ITP TTP *Qualitative* ↓ *platelet* Aspirin use von Willebrand's disease Bernard–Soulier syndrome Glanzman thrombasthenia	Hemophilias Vitamin K deficiency Anticoagulants ▪ Heparin ▪ Warfarin	von Willebrand's disease DIC Coagulopathy of liver disease	Scurvy Henoch–Schonlein purpura HHT Connective tissue disorders

Disorders in Primary Hemostasis

Quantitative Platelet Deficiencies

THROMBOCYTOPENIA

▪ ↓ platelet count (quantitative ↓ platelets).
▪ ↑ bleeding time.
▪ Features
  ▪ Mucosal oozing
  ▪ Petechial cutaneous bleeding
  ▪ Bruising
  ▪ Hemorrhage into tissues
▪ Causes
  ▪ Marrow damage
    ▪ Aplastic anemia (all blood cell elements, including platelets ↓)
  ▪ Marrow replacement
    ▪ Myelophthisis (marrow replaced by tumor cells)
  ▪ Splenic sequestration
  ▪ Disseminated intravascular coagulation (DIC)
  ▪ Idiopathic thrombocytopenic purpura (ITP)
  ▪ Thrombotic thrombocytopenia purpura (TTP)

Note: *DIC and von Willebrand's disease exhibit problems with both platelets and coagulation cascade.*

Platelets
▪ Primary hemostasis (platelet plug, prior to clotting).
▪ Help maintain the integrity of the capillary lining.

Thrombocytopenia is the most common cause of bleeding disorders.

Petechiae	Ecchymoses
Small purpura spots	Large purpura spots

Purpura

- Purplish spots produced by small bleeding vessels.
  - Skin (cutaneous).
  - Mucous membranes (mouth lining and in internal organs).
- Sign of underlying causes of bleeding.
- Nonthrombocytopenic purpura
  - Normal platelet counts.
- Thrombocytopenic purpura
  - ↓ platelet counts.

TTP = ↓ platelet count due to platelet consumption by thrombosis in the terminal arterioles and capillaries.

von Willebrand's disease and Bernard–Soulier disease are causes of qualitative platelet dysfunction.

von Willebrand's disease = qualitative platelet defect resulting in impaired platelet adhesion. It can also affect coagulation by decreasing function of factor VIII.

Remember, clotting occurs when in the presence of thromboplastin and calcium ions, prothrombin is converted to thrombin, which in turn converts fibrinogen into fibrin. Fibrin threads then entrap blood cells, platelets, and plasma to form a blood clot.

DISSEMINATED INTRAVASCULAR COAGULATION (DIC)

- Life-threatening.
- Coagulation system widespread activation.
- Uncontrolled cycle of bleeding and clotting.
- Consumptive coagulopathy (platelets are depleted).
- Clotting: Extensive microclot formation.
- Bleeding: Accompanying fibrinolysis (see increased D-dimer and other fibrin split products).
- ↑ fibrinolysis = ↑ fibrin split products (eg, D-dimer).
- Important indicators of DIC.
- Laboratory
  - ↓ platelet count.
  - ↑ PT.
  - ↑ PTT.
  - Hypofibrinogenemia (↓ fibrinogen).
  - ↓ levels of all clotting factors.
  - ↓ levels of fibrinolytic proteins.
- Causes
  - Amniotic fluid embolism.
  - Infection (gram-negative sepsis).
  - Malignancy.
  - Major trauma.

IDIOPATHIC THROMBOCYTOPENIC PURPURA

- ITP; immune TP.
- Antiplatelet antibodies coat and lead to destruction of platelets.
  - Platelets are opsonized in the spleen.
- Usually ensues after a viral URI.
- Acute form (usually in children).
  - Explosive but self-limited.
- Chronic form (in adults).
  - May respond to steroid therapy.

THROMBOTIC THROMBOCYTOPENIC PURPURA (TTP)

- Thrombocytopenia.
- Hyaline microthrombi in small vessels.
- Microangioathic hemolytic anemia.
  - Lesions in the microcirculation damage platelets and RBCs (become schistocytes) passing through.

Qualitative platelet disorders = von Willebrand's disease.

Qualitative Platelet Problems

VON WILLEBRAND'S DISEASE

- Autosomal dominant.
- No gender predilection.
- Platelet dysfunction secondary to ↓ von Willebrand factor (vWF).
- vWF
  - Large glycoprotein.
  - Allows adhesion of platelets to collagen.
    - Important in formation of platelet plug.
  - Binding sites for factor VIII.

Disorders in Secondary Hemostasis

- Bleeding caused by problems with the coagulation cascade

HEMOPHILIA

- X-linked bleeding disorder.
  - Strong male predilection.
- ↓ plasma clotting factors.
- **Clinically**
  - Bleeding from larger vessels (unlike small vessel bleeding in platelet disorders).
- **Laboratory**
- ↑ PTT (PT and INR are normal).

	Hemophilia A (Classic Hemophilia)	Hemophila B (Christmas Disease)	Hemophilia C (Rosenthal's Syndrome)
↓ factor	VIII (Antihemophilic factor)	IX (Plasma thromboplastin component)	XI (Plasma thromboplastin antecedent)
Features	X-linked (occurs in males) < 25 y Excessive bleeding from minor cuts, epistaxis, hematomas, hemarthroses.	X-linked Clinically identical to hemophilia A 1/5 – 1/10 as common as hemophilia A	Not sex linked Less severe bleeding

VITAMIN K DEFICIENCY

- ↓ activity of vitamin K dependent factors (II, VII, IX, X)
- ↑ PT
- ↑ PTT
- Normal platelet count
- **Causes**
  - Fat malabsorption (pancreatic or GI disease)
  - Warfarin

Hemophilia is characterized by:

- ↑ PTT.
- Normal PT.
- Normal bleeding time.

All clotting factors are made in the liver. Factors II, VII, IX, X are vitamin K dependent.

Severe liver disease (eg, cirrhosis), bleeding because:

- ↓ clotting factor production.
- ↓ vitamin K (↓ production of factors II, VII, IX, X even more).

Note: ↓ prothrombin (factor II) = hypoprothrombinemia. Prothrombin is formed and stored in parenchymal cells of liver; in cirrhosis there is profuse damage to these cells.

Warfarin (Coumadin) is an anticoagulant that interferes with vitamin K. It inhibits formation of prothrombin in liver. The effect of delayed blood clotting is useful to prevent and treat thromboembolic disease.

Review physiology: Hypothalamus makes ADH (vasopressin); it is then stored and secreted from the posterior pituitary. ADH is a hormone that causes kidneys to conserve water, creating concentrated urine. Absence of ADH results in urinary loss of water, lots of highly dilute urine.

Recall that insulin is produced by the pancreatic beta cells in the islets of Langerhans.

The HbA1c test measures long-term elevated blood glucose. An HbA1c of over 6.5% defined diabetes.

Antidiuretic Hormone (Vasopressin) Deficiency

DIABETES INSIPIDUS

- See also Chapter 17, "Endocrine Physiology."
- Characterized by large volume of dilute urine.
- Central or nephrogenic.
- **Central DI**
  - Damage to hypothalamus; supraoptic nuclei or pituitary (post).
    - Lack or ↓ ADH secretion
      - Surgery
      - Infection
      - Inflammation
      - Tumor
      - Head injury
      - Rarely, idiopathic or genetic
  - Body fluid tonicity remains close to normal as long as patient drinks enough water to make up for ↑ water clearance in the urine.
- **Nephrogenic DI**
  - Kidney tubules are not sensitive to ADH.
  - ADH production and secretion is normal.
    - Resistance of ADH receptors.
  - Same result.
  - Large volumes of dilute urine.
  - **Cause**
    - Genetic; sex-linked congenital DI
      - Affects men.
      - Women can pass it on to their children.
    - Lithium (or other medications).

Insulin Deficiency

DIABETES MELLITUS (TYPE 1)

- Most common pancreatic endocrine disorder.
- Metabolic disease involving mostly carbohydrates (glucose) and lipids.
- **Causes**
  - Absolute deficiency of insulin (type 1) or
  - Resistance to insulin action (type 2)
- Classic symptom triad:
  - Polydipsia (increased thirst)
  - Polyuria (increased urine output)
  - Polyphagia (increased hunger)

Summary of Diabetes Type 1 vs. Type 2

	DM-1	DM-2
Symptoms	Polyuria Polydipsia Polyphagia Blurred vision Paresthesias Weakness/fatigue Weight loss	Polyuria Polydipsia Polyphagia Blurred vision Paresthesias Weakness/fatigue Generally overweight
Incidence	15%	85%
Age of onset	Childhood	Adulthood
Obese?	No	Usually
Insulin production	Minimal or none	May be normal or supranormal
Cause	Viral or immune destruction B cells	$\uparrow$ insulin resistance (reduced sensitivity at target cells)
Genetic predisposition	Weak	Strong
Ketoacidosis	Common	Rare
Classic symptoms of polyuria, polydipsia, thirst, weight loss	Common	Sometimes
Rapidity of sexual development	Rapid	Slow
Treatment	Insulin injection Diet	Diet Weight loss Oral hypoglycemic drugs

12 hour fasting blood glucose level
<70 mg/dL (4 mmol/L) = hypoglycemia
80–100 mg/dL (4–6 mmol/L) = normal
>125 mg/dL (7 mmol/L) = hyperglycemia.

Glycosuria occurs when BGL > 160–180 mg/dL.

Blood insulin

- Absent in DM-1.
- Normal or $\uparrow$ in DM-2 (eg, insulin resistance).

Ketoacidosis

- Accumulation of ketone bodies.
- Synthesized from free fatty acids
  - In cases of starvation or severe insulin deficiency.
  - Usually in DM-1.
  - (Rare in DM-2 unless advanced or improperly treated).

Blood ketones

- Acetoacetic acid
- Beta-hydroxybutyric acid

Increased Growth Hormone

ACROMEGALY

- $\uparrow$ secretion of GH by anterior pituitary gland.
  - Usually secondary to a benign secreting pituitary tumor.
  - Ages 35–55.
  - After end plates/growth plates of bone have fused/closed.
  - After completion of skeletal growth.
    - Bones become deformed.
    - Long bones do not elongate.
- **Common findings**
  - Gradual marked enlargement of
    - Head/skull
    - Face

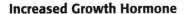

- Jaw
- Hands
- Feet
- Chest
- Excessive perspiration and an offensive body odor.
- Prognathism.
- Enlarged tongue.
- Deep voice.

Causes	↑ GH	↑ GH	↓ GH
	Before end plates closed	After end plates closed	Before end plates closed
Disease process	**Gigantism**	**Acromegaly**	**Dwarfism**
Findings	Abnormally large height, limbs, features	Enlargement of skin, soft tissue, viscera, bones of face	Arrested growth Small limbs and features

Thyroid Hormone

Hashimoto's thyroiditis (autoimmune) is the most common cause of primary hypothyroidism. But remember early in the disease Hashimoto's causes hyperthyroidism.

	Hypothyroidism	Hyperthyroidism
Causes	Primary-Hashimoto's thyroiditis (late) Secondary-pituitary, decreased TSH Tertiary-hypothalamus, decreased TRH	Iodine deficiency Graves' disease Thyroid adenoma Pituitary adenoma (secondary hyperthyroidism) Hashimoto's thyroiditis (early)
Findings	Mental slowing, mental retardation Cold intolerance Weight gain Low-pitched voice Constipation Face, eyelid, hand edema Dry skin Hair loss, brittle hair	Restlessness, irritability Heat intolerance Weight loss, muscle wasting Tremor Diarrhea Sweaty, warm moist skin Fine hair

MYXEDEMIA

- Extreme hypothyroidism.
- Affects females more than males.
- **Risks**
  - Age > 50 y
  - Female
  - Obesity
  - Past thyroid surgery or neck exposure to XRT
- **Causes**
  - Thyroid surgery, XRT.
  - Hashimoto's disease.

- Idiopathic
- Iodine deficiency.
- **Symptoms**
  - Slow basal metabolic rate.
    - Mental and physical sluggishness.
    - Fatigue
  - Puffiness of face and eyelids.
  - Swelling of tongue and larynx.
  - Dry, rough skin.
  - Sparse hair.
  - Poor muscle tone.
- **Treatment**
  - Exogenous thyroid hormone.

Myxedema = extreme hypothyroidism in adults;
Cretinism = extreme hypothyroidism in child. (during development)

CRETINISM

- Severe hypothyroidism in a child due to lack of thyroid hormone.
- **Findings**
  - Growth retardation.
  - Abnormal development of bones.
  - Mental retardation because of improper development of CNS.
- **Treatment**
- Thyroid hormone; recognized and treated early, cretinism can be markedly improved.

See physiology section in Chapter 17 for discussion of TSH, TRH, T_3 (triiodothyronine), and T_4 (thyroxine).

Dental findings in child with hypothyroidism:

- Underdeveloped mandible.
- Delayed tooth eruption.
- Retained deciduous teeth.

HASHIMOTO'S DISEASE

- Autoimmune disease.
- Form of chronic thyroiditis.
  - Slow disease onset (months–years).
- Most common cause of hypothyroidism.
  - Affects 0.1–5% of adults in Western countries.
- Can occur at any age.
  - Often middle-aged women.
- **Risks**
  - Female
  - Family history of Hashimoto's disease
- **Clinical**
  - Typical symptoms of hypothyroidism:
    - Fatigue
    - Slowed speech
    - Cold intolerance
    - Dry skin
    - Coarse hair
    - Edema, etc

HYPERTHYROIDISM

- Thyrotoxicosis.
- ↑ thyroid hormone production
- Role of thyroxine:

Dental findings (few, unless presents in childhood) are premature eruption of teeth and loss of deciduous dentition.

- ↑ cellular metabolism, growth, and differentiation of all tissues
- ↑ basal metabolism
  - Fatigue
  - Weight loss
  - Excitability
  - ↑ temperature
  - Generalized osteoporosis

GRAVES' DISEASE

- Most common form of hyperthyroidism; 85% of cases.
- Women aged 20–40 most often affected.
- Autoimmune disease.
- Onset often after infection or physical or emotional stress.
- **Clinical**
  - Symptoms of hyperthyroidism +
  - **Exophthalmos**
    - Eyeballs protrude; retrobulbar tissue buildup
    - Irritation
    - Tearing

PLUMMER'S DISEASE

- Toxic nodular goiter.
- Usually arises from long-standing simple goiter.
- Most often in elderly.
- **Risks**
  - Female
  - Age > 60 y
  - Never seen in children
- **Symptoms**
  - Typical symptoms of hyperthyroidism
  - No exophthalmos

Parathyroid Hormone

HYPERPARATHYROIDISM

- ↑ PTH

PRIMARY HYPERPARATHYROIDISM

- Common
- Usually caused by secreting adenoma
  - Benign productive tumor of parathyroid glandular epithelium
- **Clinical**
  - Cystic bone lesions
    - Osteitis fibrosa cystica (with giant cells)
    - von Recklinghausen's disease of bone
  - Nephrocalcinosis
    - Kidney stones (renal calculi)
  - Metastatic calcifications

- **Laboratory**
  - ↑ PTH.
    - ↑ Ca^{2+} (hypercalcemia)
    - ↓ phosphorus
    - ↑ alkaline phoshatase

SECONDARY HYPERPARATHYROIDISM

- Feedback for ↓ Ca^{2+} (hypocalcemia)
- Chronic renal disease
  - ↑ loss of calcium in urine
  - ↓ serum Ca^{2+}
  - ↑ parathyroid gland function (chief cells)
    - Hyperplasia
- Clinical
  - ↑ Same as primary hyperparathyroidism
  - Cystic bone lesions
  - Metastatic calcifications
- Laboratory
  - ↑↑ PTH
  - ↓ Ca^{2+} or normal
  - ↓ phosphorus

HYPOTHYROIDISM

- ↓ PTH
- ↓ Ca^{2+} (hypocalcemia)
- Causes
  - Excision of parathyroid glands; usually accidental during thyroidectomy
  - DiGeorge's syndrome
- Clinical
  - Neuromuscular excitability
  - Tetany

TETANY

- Irritability of central and peripheral nervous system.
- Occurs when blood Ca^{2+} falls from 10 mg% (normal) to 6 mg% (4 mg% is lethal).
- Causes
  - ↓ Ca^{2+} = usual cause
    - Hypoparathyroidism
    - ↓ vitamin D
  - Alkalosis
- Characterized by
  - Muscle twitches
  - Cramps
  - Carpopedal spasm
  - Laryngospasm and seizures (if severe)
- Tests for acute hypocalcemia and tetany
  - Chvostek's sign
    - Tap facial nerve above mandibular angle (next to earlobe).
    - Upper lip twitches; facial nerve causes muscle spasm.
    - Confirms tetany.

Symptoms of hyperparathyroidism: bones, stones, moans, abdominal groans (mostly the result of PTH acting at the bone to liberate calcium [↑ Ca^{2+}], by activating osteoclasts: bone lesions, kidney stones, pain, peptic ulcers).

Hyperparathyroidism can be associated with MEN I and MEN IIa.

Remember: The parathyroid glands are located on the sides and posterior surface of thyroid gland.

Hypoparathyroidism is associated with congenital thymic hypoplasia (DiGeorge's syndrome).

- **Trousseau's sign**
  - BP cuff applied to arm and inflated for 3 minutes.
  - Carpopedal spasm (thumb adduction and phalangeal extension).
  - Confirms tetany.

Cortisol

- Adrenal glands

Adrenal Cortex

↑ Cortisol	↓ Cortisol
Cushing's disease*	Addison's disease*
Cushing's syndrome	Waterhouse–Friderichsen syndrome

*See Chapter 17, "Endocrine Physiology," for discussion of Cushing's and further discussion of Addison's.

ADDISON'S DISEASE

- Primary adrenal hypofunction or adrenal insufficiency
  - Partial or complete failure of adrenocortical function
- ↓ Cortisol from adrenal cortex
  - Primary: Caused by damage to adrenal cortex (outer layer of the gland, zona fasiculata especially)
    - Autoimmune
    - Infection
    - Neoplasm
    - Hemorrhage within the gland
  - Secondary: Caused by ↓ ACTH from pituitary
- **Clinical findings**
- ↓ adrenocortical function by > 90% before obvious symptoms occur
  - Symptoms, insidious onset of
    - Weakness
    - Fatigue
    - Depression
    - Hypotension
    - Skin bronzing (with primary adrenocortical insufficiency)
    - Feedback to pituitary causing ↑ ACTH causes ↑ MSH to be released also
- **Laboratory**
  - ↓ cortisol
  - ↓ serum Na$^+$
  - ↑ serum K$^+$

PRIMARY VS. SECONDARY ADDISON'S DISEASE

- Primary Addison's
  - ↑ ACTH : ↓ cortisol.

Remember, the adrenal cortex also produces aldosterone and weak androgens (sex hormones).

- ↑ Aldosterone = Conn's syndrome.
  - HTN.
  - ↑ Na$^+$.
  - ↑ H$_2$O.
  - ↓ K$^+$.
- ↑ androgens = adrenal virilism (adrenogenital syndrome).

Oral signs of Addison's disease (secondary Addison's): *Diffuse mucosal pigmentation:*

- Gingiva
- Tongue
- Hard palate
- Buccal mucosa

Note: Cutaneous pigmentation usually disappears following therapy, but the oral mucosal pigmentation tends to persist.

Waterhouse–Friderichsen syndrome: *Hemorrhagic necrosis of the adrenal cortex; usually associated with meningococcal infection; catastrophic adrenal insufficiency and vascular collapse.*

- Secondary Addison's
  - ↓ cortisol : ↓ ACTH.
- ACTH stimulation test (helps distinguish primary from secondary).
  - Administer exogenous ACTH.
  - Cortisol level ↑ (if adrenal cortex works).
    - Indicates primary Addison's.
  - Cortisol level does not change (adrenal cortex is damaged).
    - Indicates secondary Addison's.
- Treatment
  - Administer cortisol (as hydrocortisone).

▶ MUSCOLOSKELETAL PATHOLOGY

Collagen Vascular Diseases

- Autoimmune in origin
- ANA association (antinuclear antibodies)
- Collagen vascular diseases include:
  - Rheumatoid arthritis, Still's disease
  - Systemic lupus erythematosus (SLE)
  - Scleroderma
  - Dermatomyositis
  - Polyarteritis nodosa

> **Collagen vascular diseases** *are characterized by*
> - Inflammatory damage to connective tissues and blood vessels.
> - Deposition of fibrinoid material.

SYSTEMIC LUPUS ERYTHEMATOSUS (SLE)

- Prototypical autoimmune connective tissue disease.
- Women = > 90% SLE patients.
- Age of onset = late teens to 30s.
- Cause
  - Autoimmune
    - Mechanism poorly understood.
    - Hypersensitivity reactions (type III mostly).
- Clinical
  - Affects many organs (skin, tendons, joints, kidneys, heart, blood cells, and CNS).
  - Butterfly rash
    - Characteristic rash in 50% SLE patients.
    - Erythematous rash over cheeks and bridge of nose; worsened by sunlight
  - Diffuse skin rash
    - Other sun-exposed areas
  - Joint pain and arthritis
  - Raynaud's phenomenon (vasospasm in small vessels in finger)
    - Acrocyanosis
  - Pulmonary fibrosis
  - Immune complex vasculitis
  - Glomerulonephritis (from immune complexes)
    - Renal failure occurs and = usual cause of death
  - CNS involvement

See section on bone diseases and arthritis for discussion of rheumatoid arthritis (RA).

Drug-induced lupus can be caused by certain drugs phenytoin and quinidine. It usually reverses when the medication is stopped.

Anti-DNA and anti-Sm

antibodies are specific for SLE.

CREST syndrome

- Variant of scleroderma.
- Positive anti-Scl-70.

Characterized by

- Calcinosis.
- Raynaud's phenomenon.
- Esophageal dysfunction.
- Sclerodactyly.
- Telangiectasia.

- **Course**
  - Often begins with one organ system.
    - Later, other organs become involved.
  - Periods of remission and exacerbation.
  - Symptom severity ranges from mild and episodic to severe and fatal.
- **Laboratory**
  - Positive antinuclear antibody test (ANA).
    - Positive anti-double-stranded DNA; rim pattern on immunofluorescence.
    - Positive anti-Sm.
- **Treatment**
  - Immunosuppressive therapy.
  - Corticosteroids

SCLERODERMA

- Progressive systemic sclerosis
- Common in young women
- Widespread connective tissue fibrosis
- **Clinical**
  - Subcutaneous collagen hypertrophy
    - Fixed facial expression
  - Sclerodactyly
    - Clawed hands
  - Raynaud's phenomenon
  - Visceral fibrosis
    - Esophageal dysmotility
    - GERD; ↑ Barrett's esophagus

POLYARTERITIS NODOSA

Polyarteritis nodosa is the

only autoimmune disease and

only connective tissue disease

to occur more often in men.

- Most common in men.
- Blood vessel disease.
  - Small and medium-sized arteries become inflamed and damaged.
    - Immune complex vasculitis mechanism.
    - ↓ blood supply to organs.
- Antigen implicated
  - Hepatitis B (30% of cases).
  - Drugs: Sulfa, PCN (penicillin).

POLYMYALGIA RHEUMATICA AND TEMPORAL ARTERITIS

- Other inflammatory diseases of unknown cause.
- Closely related and occur together in 25% of cases.

Polymyalgia Rheumatica	Temporal Arteritis
Pain and stiffness around muscles of the neck, shoulders, and hips. Fatigue and anemia	Inflammation of large arteries (giant cells), especially temporal artery. Causes headache, visual changes.

ANKYLOSING SPONDYLITIS

- Type of spondyloarthropathy.
- Inflammation of the spine and large joints.
  - Stiffness
  - Pain
- Associated with HLA-B27.
- More common in men.

REITER'S SYNDROME (REACTIVE ARTHRITIS)

- Arthritis triggered by an infection in another part of the body
- Associated with HLA-B27
- **Triad**
  - Arthritis: Inflammation of joints, tendon attachments
  - Eye inflammation: Conjunctivitis and uveitis
  - Urethritis

SJÖGREN'S SYNDROME

- Second most common autoimmune rheumatic disorder (RA is first.)
- 90% = women.
- Mean age = 50 y.
- **Clinical triad**
  - Xerostomia (dry mouth)
  - Keratoconjunctivitis sicca (dry eyes)
  - Presence of other autoimmune disorder (eg, SLE or RA)
- Glands ultimately become fibrotic and atrophy
  - Decrease salivation can cause rampant caries because of shift to more acidogenic microflora

BEHÇET'S SYNDROME

- Most common in Turkey and Japan.
- Immune mediated vasculitis.
- **Clinical**
  - Aphthous ulcers
  - Skin blisters
  - Genital sores
  - Swollen joints
  - Hypopyon: Puslike fluid in the anterior chamber of the eye.
  - Pyodermas: Pus-producing disease of skin.
  - CNS involvement.

Osseous Pathology

OSTEOPOROSIS

- ↓ bone mass.
- Bone thinning (↓ bone density over time) from
  - ↑ bone resorption (osteoclastic)
  - ↓ bone formation (osteoblastic)
  - Both
- **Occurs in**
  - Females > males (F > M)
  - Age approximate 50 y

Clinical triad with Reiter's = "Can't pee, can't see, can't climb a tree."

Uveitis = Inflammation of uveal tract of the eye (including iris, ciliary body, and choroids).

Sicca complex =

- Dry eyes (↓ lacrimal secretion).
- Dry mouth (↓ salivary secretion).
- Lymphocytic exocrine gland infiltration.
- Diagnose with two of these three symptoms.

Bisphosphonates are used to treat osteoporosis by decreasing osteoclasts. Long-term IV bisphosphonate use can increase risk of a bone infection with invasive dental surgery.

Dental findings in children with Rickets:

- Delayed eruption.
- Malocclusion.
- Dentin and enamel defects; ↑ caries.

Bone softening from vitamin D deficiency =

- Rickets (children).
- Osteomalacia (adults, growth plates fused).

- **Clinical**
  - Weak, brittle, fragile bones; subject to pathologic fractures (fxs), even in absence of trauma.
- **Cause**
  - ↓ estrogen in postmenopausal women.
  - ↓ testosterone in men.
- **Risks**
  - Postmenopausal.
  - Bed rest, immobilization.
  - Hypercoticism.
  - Hyperthyroidism.
  - ↓ calcium.

OSTEOMALACIA

- F > M.
- Bone softening secondary to ↓ vitamin D.
  - Osteoid matrix does not calcify without vitamin D.
- Causes of ↓ vitamin D:
  - ↓ dietary intake.
  - Hyperparathyroidism
  - ↓ absorption (malabsorption).
  - ↓ sunlight exposure.
  - Hereditary or acquired disorders of vitamin D metabolism.
  - Kidney failure and acidosis.
  - Medication side effects.
  - ↓ phosphate intake.
- **Radiologic findings**
  - Diffuse radiolucency; mimics osteoporosis.
- **Bone biopsy**
  - Difficult to distinguish osteoporosis from osteomalacia.
- **Clinical**
  - Diffuse bone pain, especially hips.
  - Muscle weakness.
  - Fractures with minimal trauma.

RICKETS

- Osteomalacia in children (before growth plates fuse).
- More widespread effects.

Renal osteodystrophy = Osteomalacia secondary to renal disease.

	Ca^{2+}	Phosphorus	Alkaline Phosphate
Osteoporosis	–	–	–/↓
Brown tumor	↑	↓	↑
Rickets/osteomalacia	↓/–	↓/–/↑	↑/–
Paget's disease	–	–	↑↑

Osteitis Fibrosa Cystica

- Brown tumor = von Recklinghausen disease of bone.
- Bone lesion in hyperparathyroidism.
- Osteolytic lesions.
- Cystic spaces with multinucleated osteoclasts, fibrous stroma, brown discoloration from hemorrhage.
- **Laboratory**
  - ↑ PTH.
  - ↑ Ca^{2+}
  - ↓ Phosphorus.
  - ↑ Alkaline phosphatase.

Paget's Disease

- Osteitis deformans
- Metabolic bone disease
- Occurs mostly in the elderly
- Etiology unknown
  - Viral infection
    - Possibly with mumps, measles, paramyxovirus
    - Intranuclear osteoclast inclusions
  - Genetic
- **Findings**
  - Cycle of bone destruction and regrowth of abnormal bone.
  - New bone is structurally enlarged, but weakened, filled with new vessels.
- **Sites**
  - Widespread.
  - Localize to one or two areas of skeleton.
    - Pelvis
    - Femur
    - Tibia
    - Vertebrae
    - Clavicle
    - Humerus
    - Skull
      - ↑ head size
      - Foraminal constriction (with CN compression, eg, hearing loss).
      - Teeth displacement intraorally
- **Laboratory**
  - Anemia.
  - ↑↑ alkaline phosphatase.
  - ↑ urinary hydroxyproline.
- **Risks**
  - ↑ osteosarcomas.

Fibrous Dysplasia

- Normal bone being replaced by fibrous tissue.
- Unknown etiology.
- **Clinical**
  - Bone enlargement (can be deforming)
  - Pain
  - Fractures

Alkaline phosphatase is a marker of ↑ osteoblastic activity and bone formation.

Hydroxyproline is a marker of ↑ osteoclastic hyperactivity.

***Note:** ↑ serum acid phosphatase level with prostate cancer.*

Café au lait spots are associated with

- Neurofibromatosis.
- McCune–Albright syndrome.
- Fanconi's anemia.
- Tuberous sclerosis.

- Three classifications (depending on involvement):
  - **Monostotic:** One bone.
  - **Polyostotic:** Multiple sites (> one bone).
  - **McCune–Albright:** Polyostotic fibrous dysplasia + endocrine abnormality.
    - Precocious puberty.
    - Café au lait spots.
    - Short stature.

OSTEOGENESIS IMPERFECTA

> **Prominent clinical findings of osteogenesis imperfecta:**
>
> - Blue sclera.
> - Multiple childhood fractures.

- "Brittle bones."
- Hereditary: Autosomal dominant is most common type.
- Defective Type I collagen synthesis.
  - ↓ osteoid production.
  - General connective tissue abnormalities.
- Clinical
  - Skeletal fragility.
  - Thin skin.
  - Weak teeth: Malformation of dentin = dentinogenesis imperfecta.
  - Blue sclera.
  - Macular bleeding tendency.
  - Joint hypermobility.

OSTEOCHONDROSES

All osteochondroses occur M = F, except Freiberg's disease (F > M).

- Groups of diseases in children that cause areas of bone necrosis.
- Cause
  - Rapid bone growth/turnover during childhood.
    - ↓ Blood supply to bone (usually epiphyses, growing ends of bones).
      - Avascular necrosis of bone, usually near joints.
  - Necrotic areas self-repair over a period of weeks to months because bone is turning over rapidly (continually rebuilding).
- Cycle of
  - Necrosis.
  - Regeneration.
  - Reossification.
- Three common variants and locations:
  - **Articular**
    - Legg–Calvé-Perthes disease: At joints or articulations (eg, hip).
    - Kohler's disease: Foot.
    - Freiberg's disease: Second toe.
    - Panner's disease: Elbow.
  - **Nonarticular**
    - Osgood–Schlatter disease: Tibia.
  - **Physeal**
    - Scheuermann's disease: Spine of intervertebral joints (physes) (especially chest/thoracic region)

Remember: Achondroplasia (dwarfism) is an autosomal dominant disorder manifesting with short limbs and normal-sized head and trunk.

OSTEOPETROSIS

- Albers–Schonberg disease.
- Autosomal dominant or recessive inheritance.

- **Types**
  - Adult type (mild).
  - Intermediate type.
  - Infantile (severe, often fatal).
- **Findings**
  - ↑ bone density.
    - Overgrowth and sclerosis of bone.
    - Thickening of the cortex.
    - Narrowing or even obliteration of the medullary cavity.
  - Brittle bones.
    - Trivial injuries may cause fractures due to abnormalities of the bone.
  - Skeletal abnormalities, sometimes.
- **Other symptoms**
  - Hepatosplenomegaly
  - Blindness
  - Progressive deafness
- **Cause**
  - Failure of osteoclastic activity

OSTEOMYELITIS

- Bone infection.
- Acute or chronic
- Usually caused by *Staph. aureus*.

ACUTE OSTEOMYELITIS

- Pyogenic bone infection
  - ↓ blood supply to bone
  - Abscess can develop
    - Pus
    - Pyogenic organisms (usually *Staph. aureus*)
  - Sequestrum (necrotic bone)
  - Involucrum (new bone formation surrounding sequestrum)

Etiology of Osteomyelitis

Hematogenous	Direct Spread
Infection in other parts of body spreads via blood to bone.	Direct inoculation after trauma, surgery, or nearby soft-tissue infection.

Sites Affected

Children	Adults
Long bones	Vertebra, pelvis

Salmonella osteomyelitis is seen commonly in sickle cell patients.

Osteomyelitis of the vertebra with TB is called Pott's disease.

Condensing osteitis

(sclerosing osteitis) = Periapical bone reaction/inflammatory response from a low-grade pulpal infection.

Fat embolism is a complication of bone fractures (usually long bones). Fat in the marrow is mechanically disrupted and enters bloodstream. Can be fatal.

Bisphosphonate medications have been associated with osteonecrosis of the jaws.

- **Symptoms**
  - Pain
  - Redness
  - Swelling of affected area
  - Fever
  - Malaise
- **Risks**
  - Trauma
  - Diabetes
  - Hemodialysis
  - Intravenous drug users (IVDU)
  - Splenectomy
  - Sickle cell disease

CHRONIC OSTEOMYELITIS

- Longstanding osteomyelitis results in
  - Loss of blood supply.
  - Necrosis of bone tissue.
- Chronic infection can persist for years

FRACTURES

- Break in bone.
- Most common bone lesion.
- Force exerted overcomes bone strength.
  - Often with some surrounding tissue injury
- **Fracture classifications**
  - Complete: Bone broken into two pieces.
  - Greenstick: Bone cracks one side only (not all the way through).
  - Single: Bone broken in one place.
  - Comminuted: Bone is crushed into two or more pieces.
  - Bending: In children; bone bends but doesn't break.
  - Open: Bone pierces the skin.
- **Fracture healing**
  - Three phases:
    - Inflammatory phase: Formation of blood clot.
    - Reparative phase: Characterized by formation of cartilage callus; replaced by bony callus (compact bone).
    - Remodeling phase: Cortex is revitalized.
- Nonunion: Fracture fails to heal.
  - Associated with
    - Ischemia: ↓ bone vascularity in some site subject to coagulation necrosis after a fracture.
      - Navicular bone of the wrist.
      - Femoral neck.
      - Lower third of tibia.
    - Excessive mobility: Pseudoarthrosis or pseudojoint may occur.
    - Interposition of soft tissue between the fractured ends.
    - Infection; more likely with compound fractures.
- Malunion
  - Bone heals/unites, but in abnormal position.

Arthritis

OSTEOARTHRITIS (OA)

- Degenerative joint disease.
- Most common form of arthritis.
- F > M.
- Age > 50 y.
- Continual wear and tear (overuse).
  - Chronic inflammation
    - Articular cartilage gradually degenerates
- Overused joints affected:
  - Intervertebral joints
  - Phalangeal joints
  - Knees
  - Hips
- Symptoms
  - Those of inflammation:
    - Pain
    - Swelling
    - Stiffness
- Findings
  - Eburnation: Bone wearing on bone.
    - Polished, ivory-like appearance
  - Osteophytes: Bone spurs.
    - Can break off and float into synovial fluid along with fragments of separated cartilage = *joint mice.*
    - Heberden's nodes: Nodules/bony swellings around DIP joints.
    - Produced by osteophytes at the base of the terminal phalanges.
    - Second or third fingers most often affected.
  - Bouchard's nodes: Nodules affecting the PIP joints.

> **Remember:** Cardinal signs of inflammation:
>
> - Rubor (red)
> - Calor (hot)
> - Tumor (swelling)
> - Dolor (pain)

ACUTE GOUTY ARTHRITIS

- Uric acid deposits in the joints.
  - Causes painful arthritis.
    - Joints of feet, especially big toe.
    - Legs.
  - Overlying skin erythema.

GOUT

- M > F.
- ↑ uric acid.
- ↓ uric acid elimination by kidney.
- Inherited form: Disorder of purine metabolism.
  - Uric acid is product of purine metabolism (specifically xanthine metabolism).
- Other forms of gout associated with
  - DM
  - Obesity
  - Sickle cell anemia
  - Kidney disease
  - Drugs that block uric acid excretion

- Four stages:
  - **Asymptomatic**
  - **Acute**
    - Symptoms develop suddenly.
    - Usually involve one or a few joints.
    - Pain begins at night and is throbbing, crushing, excruciating.
    - Joint appears with signs of inflammation (can be confused with infection).
      - Warmth.
      - Tenderness.
      - Redness (erythema).
      - Painful attack may subside in several days.
      - Recurs at irregular intervals.
      - Subsequent attacks have longer duration.
      - Some progress to gouty arthritis (others may have no further attacks).
  - **Intercritical**
  - **Chronic**
- **Findings**
  - Gouty arthritis.
  - Uric acid kidney stones (in ~25%).

***Gout** = Uric acid deposits in joints.*

***Pseudogout** = Calciumpyrophosphate deposits in joints.*

PSEUDOGOUT

- Mimics acute gouty arthritis.
- Disorder of intermittent painful arthritis.
  - Deposition of calcium pyrophosphate crystals.
- M = F.
- Older people.

Still's disease is type of RA that occurs in young people.

RHEUMATOID ARTHRITIS (RA)

- Chronic inflammatory disease (autoimmune)
- Affects joints and surrounding tissues
  - Synovium
  - Muscles
  - Tendons
  - Ligaments
  - Blood vessels
- *Proliferative inflammation of synovial membranes*
- Can affect organs systems
- **Demographics**
  - ~1–2% of population is affected
  - F 2.5 > M
  - Age = 25–55 y (can occur any age)
    - More often in older people
- **Cause**
  - Likely autoimmune
    - Genetic predisposition (association with HLA-DR4)
- **Course**
  - Gradual onset
    - Fatigue
    - Morning stiffness (lasting >1 h)
    - Diffuse muscle aches
    - Loss of appetite
    - Weakness

***Note:** Osteophytes (bone spur) occur in OA **not** RA.*

***Remember:** Collagen vascular diseases =*

- RA
- SLE
- Polyarteritis nodosa
- Dermatomyositis
- Scleroderma

- Progress to severe joint pain.
- Warmth
- Swelling
- Tenderness
- Stiffness after inactivity
- Ultimate condition
  - Permanent deformity
  - Ankylosis
  - Possible invalidism

▶ NEUROPATHOLOGY

Neurologic Trauma

	Epidural Hematoma	Subdural Hematoma
Site	Overlying dura	Between dura and arachnoid
Vascular structure	Middle meningeal artery	Bridging veins
Time until symptoms develop	Immediate or hours (lucid interval)	Hours or days
CT	Lenticular, biconvex lucency	Crescent-shaped lucency

CONCUSSION

- Diffuse reversible brain injury.
  - Occurs secondary to trauma.
- Immediate and temporary disturbance of brain function.
- Cause
  - Shear strain from inertial force.
    - ↑ brain energy demand.
    - ↓ cerebral function (transient); involves reticular formation.
- Characteristics
  - Mental status change.
    - Loss of consciousness; resolution ranges from near immediate to several hours.
- Signs
  - Confusion
  - Amnesia
  - Headache
  - Visual disturbances
  - Nausea, vomiting
  - Dizziness
  - Lack of awareness of surroundings
  - Cold perspiration

CEREBRAL INFARCTION

- Stroke = Infarction of cerebrum or other brain part.
- Causes

Symptoms with head trauma include:

- Headaches
- Disorientation
- Fluctuating levels of consciousness
- Coma

Epidural hematomas occur in ~1% of head traumas.

Subdural hematomas occur in ~15% head traumas.

Subarachnoid hemorrhage

- Blood in subarachnoid space.
- Usually not traumatic (unlike epidural and subdural hematomas).
  - Most are caused by rupture of a saccular aneurysm.
- Prodromal/warning headache.

- **Postconcussion syndrome:** Can be a complication following concussion.
- Persistence of three of the following symptoms:
  - Headache
  - Dizziness
  - Fatigue
  - Irritability
  - Impaired memory and concentration
  - Insomnia
  - Lowered tolerance for noise and light

- Arterial occlusion.
  - Thrombus or embolism (brain or carotid).
  - Bleed; hemorrhagic stroke from rupture of vessel.
- **Symptoms**
  - Depend on area affected.
    - Often include sudden paralysis (hemiparesis) and numbness on side opposite the stroke.

SEIZURES

Epilepsy = Recurrent seizures.

- Temporary abnormal electrical activity of a group of brain cells.
- Usually manifesting as
  - Changed mental state.
  - Tonic or clonic movements.

Partial Seizures	Generalized (Diffuse) Seizures
Simple partial	Absence (vacant stare)
Complex partial (impaired consciousness)	Myoclonic (muscle twitching) Tonic–clonic (grand mal) Tonic (increased muscle tone) Atonic (decreased muscle tone)

Neurodegenerative Diseases

Degenerative Diseases

Disease	Signs and Symptoms
Alzheimer's	Dementia in elderly Plaques (amyloid) and neurofibrillary tangles
Pick's	Pick bodies
Huntington's	Autosomal dominant Chorea + dementia
Parkinson's	Lewy bodies Depigmentation of substantia nigra
ALS (amyotrophic lateral sclerosis or Lou Gehrig's disease)	Motor neuron disease
Werdnig–Hoffman	Floppy baby Tongue fasciculations
Poliomyelitis	Lower motor neuron
Shy–Drager syndrome (multiple system atrophy)	Symptoms similar to Parkinson's

---

Parkinson's is characterized clinically by

- Resting tremor.
- Cogwheel rigidity.
- Akinesia.
- Shuffling gait

Multiple sclerosis

- Autoimmune, demyelinating disease characterized by
  - Disparate lesions in time and space.
  - ↓ or blocked nerve transmission.
  - Affects 1:1000.
  - F > M.
  - Usually begins age 20–40.
  - ↑ IgG in CSF.
  - IV interferon ↓ the frequency of relapses.
- Triad
  - Scanning speech.
  - Intention tremor.
  - Nystagmus.

Demyelinating Diseases

Disease	Signs and Symptoms
Multiple sclerosis	Damage to white matter Relapsing, remitting Symptoms may include visual changes, hemisensory findings, loss of bladder control
Progressive multifocal leukoencephalopathy (PML)	JC virus Seen in 2–4% of AIDS patients.
Guillain-Barré syndrome (acute idiopathic polyneuritis)	Peripheral nerve demyelination Motor > sensory

Myasthenia Gravis

- MG = Neuromuscular disease.
- Affects 3:10000.
- Any age.
- Common in young women and older men.
- **Characterized by** variable weakness of voluntary muscles.
  - Improves with rest.
  - Worsens with activity.
- **Cause:** Autoimmune.
  - Auto-abs attack Ach receptors on postsynaptic (muscle side) of NMJ.
  - Decreases muscle fiber responsiveness.
- **Note:** Patients with MG have a higher risk of developing other autoimmune disorders.
  - Thyrotoxicosis
  - RA
  - SLE

Myasthenia crisis = Life-threatening weakness in the respiratory muscles; ~ 10% MG patients.

Eaton–Lambert syndrome

- Similar to MG.
- Autoimmune disease.
- Causes weakness.
- Caused by ↓ release of Ach (**not** auto-antibodies versus Ach receptor, like MG).

Thymoma

- Tumor of thymus gland.
- Associated with myasthenia gravis.
- Clinical
  - Dyspnea (difficulty breathing).
    - Secondary to pressure on trachea.
  - Engorgement of deep and superficial neck veins.
    - Secondary to pressure on the SVC.

CHAPTER 23

Neoplasia

- Nonmalignant cellular growth.
- Can be precursor to malignancy (eg, cervical dysplasia).
- Reversible.
- **Causes**
  - Chronic irritation.
  - Chemical agent.
  - Cigarette smoke.
  - Chronic inflammatory irritation.
  - Chronic cervicitis.
- **Characteristics**
  - Disorganized, structureless maturation and spatial arrangement of cells.
  - Atypical cells without invasion.
    - Pleomorphism (variability in size and shape).
    - ↑ mitoses.
  - Acanthosis in epithelium.
    - Abnormal thickening of prickle cell layer.

Neoplasia = Uncontrolled, disorderly proliferation of cells, resulting in a benign or malignant tumor or neoplasm.

- Replacement of one tissue cell type with another.
- Example: Squamous metaplasia.
  - Respiratory epithelium bronchi with long-term smoking.
    - Respiratory epithelium is replaced by squamous epithelium.
  - Barrett's esophagus (squamous to glandular columnar).
- Associated with chronic irritation (helps host adapt to the stress/irritant).
- Can be associated with vitamin A deficiency.
- Often reversible.

- Abnormal growth, independent of host control mechanisms.
- **Classification**
  - Malignant vs benign
  - Well- or poorly differentiated
  - Based on appearance
  - Based on tissue of origin

*Metastasis is most important characteristic distinguishing malignant from benign. Benign tumors do **not** invade or metastasize.*

Benign tumors cause harm by:

- Pressure
- Hormone overproduction
- Hemorrhage following ulcerations of an overlying mucosal surface

They usually do not recur after surgical excision.

Malignant vs Benign Tumors

Benign	Malignant
Well-differentiated	Less well-differentiated (anaplastic)
Slow growth	Rapid growth
Encapsulated/well-circumscribed	Invasion
Localized	Metastasis
Movable	Immovable

Invasion and Metastasis

Malignant tumors spread by local invasion and metastasis. Metastasis is an absolute indicator of malignancy.

- **Invasion**
  - Aggressive infiltration of adjacent tissues by a malignant tumor.
    - Extension into lymphatics and blood vessels.
    - Can lead to metastasis.
  - However, tumor emboli within blood or lymph does **not** = metastasis.
    - Indicates only the penetration of basement membrane.
- **Metastasis**
  - Spread of tumor to secondary site distant and separate from primary site.
  - Implantation of tumor in distal site.
    - Liver
    - Lung
    - Brain
    - Bone marrow
    - Spleen
    - Soft tissue
- **Multiple steps**
  - Growth and vascularization.
  - Invasion (penetrate basement membrane to reach vessels, lymph).
  - Transport of tumor emboli in circulation (and survival).
  - Collection of tumor emboli in target tissue (again pierce basement membrane).
  - Avoid target tissue defense mechanism.
- **Routes of metastasis**
  - Bloodstream (usually venous at first) (hematogenous).
    - Sarcomas.
  - Lymph.
    - Carcinomas.

A malignancy will continue to grow even after removal of the irritating agent, as opposed to a benign lesion of inflammatory origin like an irritation fibroma (it may recede when the irritation is removed).

Immunologic response by the host to malignancy is reflected by lymphocytic infiltration at the tumor edge.

HISTOLOGIC CHARACTERISTICS OF MALIGNANCY

- Anaplasia: Absence of differentiation.
  - Differentiation is a measure of a tumor's resemblance to normal tissue.
- Hyperchromatism.
- Pleomorphism.
- Abnormal mitosis.

Cathepsin D (protease cleaves fibronectin and laminin, high levels associated with greater invasiveness) is involved in invasion and metastasis.

PROGNOSIS OF MALIGNANT TUMORS

- Depends on:
  - **Degree of localization**
    - Most reliable indicator.
  - **Staging**
    - Helps determine treatment.
    - Helps determine chance for cure.
- Factors for staging:
  - Location of tumor
  - Size
  - Growth into nearby structures
  - Metastasis

Tumor Markers

Marker	Associated Cancer
AFP	Hepatoma, hepatocellular carcinoma Yolk sac tumor
CEA (carginoembryonic antigen involved in cell adhesion)	Adenocarcinoma (colon, gastric)
hCG	Choriocarcinoma (usually of the placenta)
Desmin	Rhabdomyosarcoma
LSA	Lymphomas
Enolase	Neuroblastoma

Carcinoma

- Malignant tumor of epithelial cell origin.

SQUAMOUS CELL CARCINOMA

- Originates from stratified squamous epithelium.
- Examples: Skin, mouth, esophagus, vagina, bronchial epithelium (squamous metaplasia).
- Histologically marked by keratin production (keratin pearls).

TRANSITIONAL CELL CARCINOMA

- Arises from transitional cell epithelium of urinary tract.

ADENOCARCINOMA

- Carcinoma of glandular epithelium.
- Examples: GI tract glandular mucosa, endometrium, pancreas.
- **Desmoplasia** (secondary to an insult)
  - Tumor-induced proliferation of nonneoplastic fibrous connective tissue.
  - Especially in breast, pancreatic, prostate adenocarcinomas.

Sarcoma

- Malignant tumor of mesenchymal origin.
- Prefix usually denotes tissue of origin.
- Examples:
  - Osteosarcoma (bone) (most common primary malignant tumor of bone).
  - Leiomyosarcoma (smooth muscle).
  - Rhabdomyosarcoma (skeletal muscle).
  - Liposarcoma (adipose).

Remember: Carcinomas usually spread by lymph. Sarcomas spread hematogenously.

MICROBIOLOGY–PATHOLOGY

NEOPLASIA

Papilloma

- From surface epithelium (eg, skin, larynx, tongue).
- Fingerlike epithelial processes overlying core of connective tissue stroma with blood vessels.
- May also form from transitional epithelium of urinary tract.

Adenoma

- Benign neoplasm of glandular epithelium; several variants.
- **Papillary cystadenoma**
  - Adenomatous papillary processes that extend into cystic spaces (eg, cystadenoma of ovary).
- **Fibroadenoma**
  - Proliferation of connective tissue surrounding neoplastic glandular epithelium (eg, fibroadenoma of the breast).

Benign Tumors of Mesenchymal Origin

- **Leiomyoma** (smooth muscle, eg, uterine fibroid)
  - Most common neoplasm in women
  - **Rhabdomyoma**
  - **Lipoma**
  - **Fibroma**
  - **Chondroma**

Choristoma

- Small benign nonneoplastic mass of normal tissue *misplaced* within another organ.
- Example: Pancreatic tissue in stomach wall.

Hamartoma

- Benign tumorlike overgrowth (nonneoplastic) of cell types regularly found in the affected organ
- Example: Hemangioma (accumulation of blood vessels).

APUD cells: unrelated endocrine cells that share a common function of secreting a low molecular weight polypeptide hormone

APUDoma: endocrine tumor derived from neural crest cells.

Myxoma

- Benign tumor derived from connective tissue.

APUDoma

- Tumor characterized by amine precursor uptake and decarboxylation (converts precursors to amines) (APUD).
- Resultant production of hormonelike substances.

Teratoma

- *Can be malignant or benign.*
- Neoplasm comprised of all three embryonic germ cell layers.
  - Including tissues not normally found in the organ in which they arise.
  - May contain skin, bone, cartilage, teeth, hair, intestinal epithelium.
- Occurs:
  - Ovary (most frequently)
    - Mature teratoma = Dermoid cyst in ovary (benign)—benign because it contains mature tissue.
  - Testes (can be malignant).

Tumors of Mesenchymal Origin

Benign	Malignant
Leiomyoma	Leiomyosarcoma
Rhabdomyoma	Rhabdomyosarcoma
Lipoma	Liposarcoma
Fibroma	Fibrosarcoma
Chondroma	Chondrosarcoma
Osteoma	Osteosarcoma

▶ MUTATIONS AND CARCINOGENESIS

See also Chapter 8, "Molecular Biology."

- Results in alteration in the protein product coded for by the gene.
- Three types of mutation/molecular change:
- **Base substitutions**
  - One base inserted in place of another.
  - Results in either missense *mutation* or a *nonsense mutation.*
- **Frameshift mutations**
  - One or more base pairs are added or deleted.
- **Transposons**
  - Insertion sequences or deletions are integrated into the DNA.

Mutation = Stable, heritable change in the DNA nucleotide sequence.

Causes of Mutagenesis

Cause	Example	Mechanism
Chemicals	Nitrous oxide	Alters existing base
	Alkylating agents	Alter existing base
	Benzpyrene (found in tobacco smoke)	Binds to existing DNA bases and causes frameshift mutations
Ionizing radiation	Gamma and X-rays	Produce free radicals that can attack DNA bases
UV light		Causes cross-linking of adjacent pyrimidine bases to form
Dimers	Thymine dimers	Interfere with DNA replication
Viruses	Bacterial virus Mu (mutator bacteriophage)	Frameshift mutations or deletions

*All neoplasms of muscle are
rare; usually malignant when
they occur.*

*Leukemia in children is usually
acute lymphoblastic leukemia
(ALL).*

*Remember leiomyoma is a
benign process.*

Radiosensitivity

- Cells with high proliferation are more sensitive to radiation.
  - ↑ mutagenesis.
  - ↑ response to therapy (with XRT).
- **High radiosensitive cells:** Cells with high turnover; more radiosensitive.
  - Lymphocytes.
  - Bone marrow blood-forming cells.
  - Reproductive cells (gonads).
  - Epithelial cells of GI tract.
- **Low radiosensitivty cells:** Cells with low turnover; more radioresistant.
  - Nerve cells.
  - Mature bone cells.
  - Muscle cells.

▶ **NEOPLASIA IN CHILDREN**

Neuroblastoma

See also Chapter 17, "Endocrine Pathology."

- Most common malignancy in children.
- Usually affects adrenal medulla.

Rhabdomyosarcoma

- Malignant tumor of muscle; striated muscle/skeletal.
- Infants/children
  - Throat
  - Bladder
  - Prostate
  - Vagina
- Elderly
  - Large muscle groups of the arm or leg.
  - Prognosis is poor.

▶ **NEOPLASIA IN WOMEN**

Leiomyoma

- Uterine fibroid.
- Most common tumor in women.
  - 25% of women older than 30 y during reproductive years.
  - Most common pelvic tumor.
  - 15–20% reproductive-aged women and 30–40% of women > 30 years old.
  - Benign tumor.
  - Derived from smooth muscle.
  - Can occur anywhere in body.
  - Most frequently in uterus (= uterine fibroid).
  - Less often in:
    - Stomach
    - Esophagus
    - Small intestine

- Cause
  - Unknown.
  - Growth depends on regular estrogen stimulation (reproductive age).
  - Menstruation.
    - Continues to grow as long as patient menstruates (though can grow quite slowly).
    - Fibroids are rare before age 20.
    - Shrink after menopause.
  - ↑ size with estrogen therapy.
    - OCPs (oral contraceptive pills).
    - Pregnancy.
- Size
  - Microscopic to macroscopic (eg, weigh several pounds and fill uterine cavity).
  - Prognosis is good.

Malignant Neoplasia in Women

Cancer Incidence (Highest to Lowest)	Cancer Death (Highest to Lowest)
Breast	Lung
Lung	Breast
Colorectal	Colorectal
Uterine	Leukemia and lymphoma

Breast Cancer

- Most common cancer in women.
  - Rare before age 25.
  - ↑ age until menopause (incidence ↓ postmenopausal).
- Cause/history
  - Family history.
    - Strongest association.
    - Specifically in first-degree relatives (mother, sister, daughter).
  - BRCA-1, BRCA-2 genes.
- Clinical
  - Painless mass (in breast) (initially).
  - Breast skin or nipple retraction.
  - Peau d'orange (swollen, pitted surface).
  - Enlargement of the axillary lymph nodes (LNs).
  - Left breast > right.
  - Upper outer quadrant.
- Spread/metastasis
  - Chest wall.
  - Axillary LNs.
  - Distant metastasis (via lymphatic system and bloodstream) to:
    - Other breast.
    - Liver.
    - Bone.
    - Brain.
- Histologic type
  - Usually adenocarcinoma.

Breast cancer
Can present as

- Axillary mass.
- Paget's disease of the nipple: Eczematoid lesion.

Prostate cancer spreads to: bones, lungs

Breast cancer spreads to: liver, bones, brain.

Distinguish breast cancer from fibrocystic disease. The latter is a benign process (but may increase breast cancer risk).

BRCA-1 is associated with both breast and ovarian cancer.

- Prognosis
  - LN involvement (most valuable prognostic predictor).
  - 10-year survival rate (with adjuvant therapy):
    - Node negative = 70–75% will survive 10 years or more.
    - Node positive = 20–25% will survive 10 years.

Fibrocystic Disease (of the Breast)

- **Not** malignant, but may ↑ risk of carcinoma.
- Most common cause of a clinically palpable breast mass in women 28–44 y.
- Signs/symptoms
  - Lumpiness throughout both breasts.
  - Pain (especially prior to menstrual period).

▶ **NEOPLASIA IN MEN**

Lung cancer is the leading cause of cancer death in both men and women.

Distinguish prostate cancer from benign prostatic hyperplasia (BPH). The latter is a benign process, not thought to be premalignant.

Cancer Incidence (Highest to Lowest)	Cancer Death (Highest to Lowest)
Prostate	Lung
Lung	Prostate
Colorectal	Colorectal
Urinary tract	Leukemia and lymphoma

Prostate Cancer

- Common cause of death from cancer in men of all ages.
  - Most common cause of cancer death in men over age 75.
- Rare in men younger than 40.
- Cause
  - Unknown.
  - Possibly ↑ testosterone (hormonally dependent).
    - ↑ dietary fat leads to ↑ testosterone.
- Laboratory
  - ↑ PSA (prostate-specific antigen).
    - PSA testing helps detect prostate cancers prior to development of symptoms.
  - ↑ acid phosphatase.
- Histology
  - Adenocarcinoma
    - Usually arises in gland periphery.
    - May invade entire prostate.
- Metastasis
  - Common sites:
    - Bone
    - Lungs

Benign Prostatic Hyperplasia

- Nodular hyperplasia of the prostate.
- Benign enlargement of the prostate.
  - Hyperplastic nodules of stroma and glands (distorting the prostate).

- This hyperplasia usually occurs in the center of the gland.
  - Compresses the urethra.
  - Causes urinary difficulty or obstruction.
- **Complications**
  - Pyelonephritis.
  - Hydronephrosis.
  - Painful or difficult urination (dysuria).
- **Not** considered premalignant.

Brain Tumors

	Tumor	Signs and Symptoms
Adults	Glioblastoma multiforme	Most common primary brain tumor (most aggressive)
	Meningioma	2nd most common primary brain tumor
		Arises from arachnoid
	Pituitary adenoma	Usually secrete prolactin
		Can present as bitemporal hemianopia
Children	Craniopharyngioma	Benign
		Can cause bitemporal hemianopia
		Derived from Rathke's pouch
	Low-grade astrocytoma	Posterior fossa
	Medulloblastoma	Highly malignant cerebellar tumor
		Form of PNET (primitive neuroectodermal tumor)
	Ependymoma	Often in the 4th ventricle
		Can cause hydrocephalus

Astrocytes: support cell of endothelial cells that make the BBB.

Benign Skin Neoplasms

PIGMENTED NEVI

- **Nevocellular nevus** (common mole) = hamartoma (benign tumor); cluster of nevus cells (derived from melanocytes).
- **Junctional nevus:** Confined to epidermal–dermal junction (usually flat).
- **Compound nevus:** Occurs at epidermal–dermal junction and in the dermis ("beauty mark").
- **Intradermal nevi:** Within the dermis (often not pigmented).

BLUE NEVUS

- Present at birth.
- Nodular foci of dendritic, pigmented melanocytes in dermis.
- Blue appearance (because dermal location) (melanocytes are deep in skin).

SPITZ NEVUS (VARIANT OF THE INTRADERMAL NEVUS) (RAISED AND REDDISH)

- Children
- Benign
- Spindle-shaped cells

DYSPLASTIC NEVUS

- Atypical, irregularly pigmented lesion.
- Disordered proliferation of melanocytes.
- May transform into malignant melanoma, especially in dysplastic nevus syndrome (autosomal dominant).

LENTIGO MALIGNA (MELANOMA IN SITU)

- Precursor to lentigo maligna melanoma.
- Irregular macular pigmented lesion on sun-exposed skin.
- Atypical melanocytes in epidermal–dermal junction.

BASAL CELL CARCINOMA

Incidence of skin cancer is up, partly due to increased sun exposure (increased UV radiation).

Basal cell carcinoma is considered benign, even though "carcinoma" denotes malignancy.

- Most common skin cancer
  - 75% of all skin cancers
  - Most common form of cancer in U.S.
- Derived from basal cells of epidermis
- Clinical
  - > 90% occur on sun-exposed areas of head and neck, including upper face
  - Pearly papule
  - Overlying telangiectatic vessels (often)
  - Locally aggressive
  - Locally invasive and destructive
  - Ulcerate
  - Bleed
  - Nonhealing skin growth
- Histology
  - Clusters of darkly staining basaloid cells with a typical palisade arrangement of the nuclei at the periphery of the tumor cell clusters.
- Prognosis/course
  - Good when found and treated early.
    - Almost never metastasizes (benign).
    - Cured by surgical excision.
    - Radiosensitive if necessary.
  - When diagnosis or treatment is delayed:
    - Disability
    - Disfigurement
    - Destruction
    - Death (rarely)

DERMATOFIBROMA (DISORDERED COLLAGEN LAID DOWN BY FIBROBLASTS—MAY BE A REACTIVE LESION)

- Benign neoplasms.
- Clinical.

- Firm, red-brown nodules.
- Armpit or groin (usually).
- **Histology**
  - Acanthosis (sometimes).
  - Intertwining of collagen bundles and fibroblasts.

ACROCHORDON (CAUSED BY FRICTION)

- Skin tag = fibroepithelial polyp.
- Very common lesion.
- Most common sites:
  - Face (near eyelids).
  - Neck.
  - Armpit (axilla).
  - Groin.

SEBORRHEIC KERATOSIS

- Seborrheic warts.
- Very common benign neoplasm.
- Premalignant epidermal lesion caused by chronic excessive sunlight.
- Older people.
- **Clinical**
  - Rough, scaling, poorly demarcated flesh-colored, brown, or black plaques.
    - "Stuck-on" appearance.
    - Anywhere on the skin, especially, face, neck, upper trunk, or extremities.

▶ MALIGNANT SKIN NEOPLASMS

Squamous Cell Carcinoma (of the Skin)

- Epithelial malignant tumor.
  - More aggressive than basal cell carcinoma.
  - Mean age = 50.
- **Causes**
  - Sun damage: Can arise within actinic keratosis.
  - Radiation
  - X-ray exposure.
  - Chemical carcinogens (eg, arsenic).
- **Clinical:** Can occur in:
  - Normal skin
  - Damaged skin:
    - Burn
    - Scar
    - Site of chronic inflammation (as with skin disorders)
  - Sun-damaged skin areas (eg, preexisting areas of actinic keratosis)
    - Face (lower face unlike basal cell carcinoma)
    - Dorsal hands
- **Lesion**
  - Scaling, indurated, ulcerative nodule.
  - Painless initially.
    - Pain may occur as it enlarges or ulcerates.

Skin cancer is the most common malignancy in the U.S.

Most to least common: Basal cell carcinoma > squamous cell carcinoma > malignant melanoma.

Malignant melanoma is the leading cause of death from skin cancer.

Squamous cell carcinoma (SCC) of the skin resembles cervical cancer in histologic appearance and biologic behavior.

- **Course**
- Usually is locally invasive.
  - May be relatively slow growing.
- Metastasis (unlike basal cell carcinoma).
  - < 5% metastasize (lymph).
  - Lymph nodes, internal organs.
- **Histology**
  - Sheets and islands of neoplastic epidermal cells (keratinocytes) in the middle portion of epidermis.
  - Keratin pearls.
- **Molecular properties**
  - Malignant epithelial cells have:
    - ↑ laminin receptors
    - Laminin (a glycoprotein) = Major component of basement membranes.
    - Biological activities:
      - Cell adhesion
      - Migration
      - Growth and differentiation
- **Treatment**
- Excision usually curative.
- XRT may be used.

Keratoacanthoma

- Common low-grade malignancy.
- Originates in pilosebaceous glands and pathologically resembles SCC.
- Thought to be variant of invasive SCC.
- Was classified as benign, now as malignant.
- **Causes**
  - Sunlight.
  - Chemical carcinogens.
  - Trauma.
  - Human papilloma virus (HPV).
  - Genetic factors.
  - Immunocompromised status.
- **Clinical**
  - Sun-exposed areas:
    - Face.
    - Neck.
    - Dorsum of upper extremities.
- **Lesion**
  - Usually solitary.
  - Firm, roundish, skin-colored, or reddish papules.
  - Rapidly progress to dome-shaped nodules.
    - Smooth shiny surface.
    - Central crateriform ulceration or keratin plug (that may project like a horn).
- **Course**
  - Rapid growth (over weeks to months), then
  - Spontaneous resolution over 4–6 months in most cases.
  - Can progress (rarely) to invasive or metastatic carcinoma.
- **Treatment**
  - Aggressive excision advocated due to possible progression to squamous cell carcinoma.

Malignant Melanoma

- Malignant tumor of melanocytes or nevus cells
- ↑ in incidence
- Median age 53
- Most common in:
  - Fair-skinned persons
  - Those with blue or green eyes
  - Those with red or blonde hair
- Causes
  - Sunlight exposure.
  - Particularly related to sunburns during childhood.
- Clinical
  - May appear on what was
    - Normal skin.
    - Mole (nevus). Some moles present at birth may develop into melanomas.
    - Other skin area that has changed appearance.
- Four major types:
- **Superficial spreading**
  - Most common type.
  - Any age or site.
  - Most common in Caucasians.
  - Usually flat and irregular in shape and color; varying shades of black and brown.
- **Nodular melanoma**
  - Raised/nodular area
  - Blackish-blue or bluish-red (usually), although some lack color
  - Worst prognosis
- **Lentigo maligna melanoma**
  - Elderly (usually).
  - Develops from preexisting lentigo maligna (Hutchinson freckle).
  - Most common in sun-damaged skin (face, neck, arms).
  - Lesion: Large, flat, and tan with intermixed areas of brown.
- **Acral lentiginous melanoma**
  - Least common form.
  - Occurs on palms, soles, or under the nails (usually).
  - Most common in African Americans.
- Histology:
- Course
  - Can spread very rapidly.
  - Most deadly form of skin cancer.
  - **Growth phases**
  - **Radial (initial) phase:**
    - Growth in all directions but predominantly lateral (not invading deep).
    - Does not metastasize in this growth phase.
    - Radial growth is characteristic of spreading types.
  - **Vertical (later) phase:**
    - Growth into reticular dermis or beyond (deep).
    - Metastasis may occur.
    - Prognosis varies with depth of lesion.
    - Vertical growth is characteristic of nodular melanoma.

► LUNG CANCER

Adenocarcinoma

- Less associated with smoking.
- Arises in periphery, usually in upper lobes.
- Develops in sites of prior pulmonary inflammation or injury:
  - Calcified TB granuloma.
  - Scars.
  - Healed infarcts.

Metastatic cancer to the lungs

- Via lymphatics
- Most often from:
  - Breast
  - Colon
  - Prostate
  - Kidney
  - Thyroid
  - Stomach
  - Cervix
  - Rectum
  - Testis
  - Bone
  - Skin
  - Brain

Pancoast tumor

- Tumor in apical segment of upper lung lobe.
- Hoarseness from compression of recurrent laryngeal nerve.
- Horner syndrome:
  - Ptosis
  - Miosis
  - Anhidrosis
  - From compression of cervical sympathetic plexus

- Metastatic
  - Most common.
  - From primary tumors that occur elsewhere, then metastasize to the lung.
- Primary
  - Bronchogenic carcinoma (usually).

Bronchogenic Carcinoma

- Primary malignant neoplasm of the lung.
  - Develops in the wall or epithelium of the bronchial tree.
- M > F (4:1).
  - 50% of cases are inoperable at diagnosis.
  - Most common cause of cancer in men and women.
- Causes
  - Cigarette smoking.
    - Most common etiologic agent.
      - 90% of lung cancers are due to smoking.
      - Especially squamous cell and small cell carcinomas.
    - Benzpyrene (frameshift mutations) is the carcinogen in cigarette smoke.
  - Carcinogenic exposure.
    - Industrial or air pollutants.
  - Familial susceptibility.
- Clinical
  - Persistent cough (smoker's cough).
  - Hemoptysis
  - Hoarseness
  - Wheezing
  - Dyspnea
  - Chest pain
  - Weight loss
  - Digital clubbing (fingers and toes)
    - Associated with chronic low oxygen tension
    - Proliferation of distal tissues; nail beds broaden and curve
  - Symptoms related to metastatic spread, especially to brain
- **Prognosis:** 14% survive 5 years + after diagnosis

Types

Small Cell Carcinoma	Non-Small Cell Carcinoma (NSC)
Oat cell carcinoma (25%)	Squamous cell carcinoma (epidermoid) (35%) Adenocarcinoma (25%) Large cell carcinoma (anaplastic) (15%)

Sites

Peripheral	Central (Smoking-Associated)
Adenocarcinoma	Small cell carcinoma
Large cell carcinoma	Squamous cell carcinoma

Lung Cancers Associated with Smoking; Both Arise Centrally

Squamous Cell Carcinoma	Small (Oat) Cell Carcinoma
Appears as hilar mass. Often undergoes central cavitation. Paraneoplastic; PTH-like hormone with ↑Ca^{2+}	Most aggressive type bronchogenic carcinoma Highly malignant 80% are men 90% are smokers **Pathology** Oat cell: ■ Short, bluntly shaped, anaplastic cell ■ Large, hyperchromatic nucleus ■ Little or no cytoplasm ■ Paraneoplastic syndromes; production of ACTH, ADH

Causes of SVC Syndrome

Malignancy	Infection	Other
Bronchogenic carcinomas Lymphomas Leiomyosarcoma Plasmacytoma	Tuberculosis Syphilis Histoplasmosis	Goiter Thrombus Indwelling IV lines Pacemaker wires

▶ GASTROINTESTINAL CANCER

Esophageal Cancer

■ **Type (in U.S.)**
■ 50% squamous cell carcinoma.
■ 50% adenocarcinoma (related to Barrett's esophagus).
■ **Clinical findings**
  ■ Dysphagia
  ■ Weight loss
  ■ Anorexia
  ■ Pain
  ■ Hematemesis
■ **Course**
  ■ Spreads by local extension.

Gastric Cancer

■ Men > age 50.
■ Japan
■ **Risks**
  ■ *H. pylori*
  ■ Nitrosamines
  ■ Salt intake.

Superior vena cava (SVC) syndrome

■ ↓ Venous return from the head, neck, and upper extremities.
■ Facial swelling.
■ Cyanosis.
■ Dilation of head and neck veins.
■ **Cause:** Compression of SVC
■ > 80% related to malignancy.
  ■ > 80% = bronchogenic carcinomas.
    ■ Those that are located centrally:
      ■ Small cell carcinoma.
      ■ Squamous cell carcinoma.

Hypertrophic pulmonary osteoarthropathy

■ Unknown etiology.
■ Clinical syndrome of
  ■ Clubbing of the fingers and toes.
  ■ Enlargement of the extremities.
  ■ Painful swollen joints.
■ X-ray shows new periosteal bone.
■ Associated with
  ■ Bronchogenic carcinoma (not squamous cell).
  ■ Benign mesothelioma.
  ■ Diaphragmatic neurilemmoma.

MICROBIOLOGY–PATHOLOGY

NEOPLASIA

- Achlorhydria (low HCL in stomach).
- Chronic gastritis.
- **Histology**
  - Adenocarcinoma (most often).
  - Signet-cell rings (mucin pushes nucleus to periphery).
  - Intestinal type.
  - Infiltrating or diffuse carcinoma (linitus plastica).
- **Location**
  - Distal stomach.
    - Antrum, lesser curve, prepylorus.
- **Course**
  - Local spread.
  - LN metastases.
    - Virchow's node (supraclavicular node with metastatic gastric carcinoma).
  - Distant metastasis
    - Krukenberg tumor; metastatic gastric carcinoma to bilateral ovaries.

GASTRIC LYMPHOMA

Colon and rectum are most likely parts of GI to develop cancer.

- 4% malignant gastric tumors.
- Associated with *H. pylori*.
- MALToma
- Better prognosis than adenocarcinoma.

Colorectal Cancer

- Second most common cancer causing death in men.
- Third most common cancer causing death in women.
  - Lung cancer ranks first for both
- Rapidly increasing incidence after age 40.
- **Histology**
  - Adenocarcinoma
- **Cause**
  - No single cause for colon cancer.
  - Tumor progression: Most begin as benign polyps → develop into cancer over many years.
- **Risk factors**
  - Adenomatous polyps.
  - Inherited multiple polyposis syndromes.
  - Long-standing ulcerative colitis.
  - Family history.
  - Low-fiber, high-fat diet.
- **Clinical findings**
  - Rectal bleeding, possibly with diarrhea.
  - Abdominal pain.
  - Weight loss.
- **Site**
  - Sigmoid colon is most common site.
- **Screening and diagnosis**
  - CEA (carcinoembryonic antigen).
  - Colonoscopy (treatable if caught early by colonoscopy).
  - Left (descending) colon cancers are diagnosed earlier (obstructing) than tumors of right colon (ascending) because they present as obstruction (constipation/obstipation).

COLON POLYPS

- Benign polyps.
- Inflammatory polyps.
- Hamartomatous polyps.

PEUTZ–JEGHERS SYNDROME

- Hereditary
- Hamartomatous polyps.
    - Not true neoplasms.
    - Many lumps along GI.
        - Colon and small intestine (especially the jejunum).
- Melanin pigmentation of oral mucosa, especially lips and gingiva.
- **Course**
    - Presence of hamartomatous polyps.
    - Does **not** increase risk of GI cancer.
        - However, increased risk cancer of pancreas, breast, lung, ovary, uterus.

Multiple Polyposis Syndromes

- Associated with ↑ risk malignant transformation

Familial Polyposis	Gardner's Syndrome	Turcot's Syndrome
Autosomal dominant Multiple adenomatous polyps Risk of malignant transformation is near 100%	True hereditary polyposis; autosomal dominant Numerous adenomatous polyps along intestine Osteomas Soft tissue tumors (desmoid tumors) High risk of colon cancer	Adenomatous polyps + CNS tumors – recessive – mismatch repair (MLH1, MSH 2)

▶ NEOPLASIA OF THE GENITOURINARY SYSTEM

Renal Cell Carcinoma

- Most common renal malignancy.
- Originates from renal tubules.
- Men 50–70.
- Associated with
    - Cigarette smoking
    - von Hippel–Lindau (cavernous hemangiomas)
- **Clinical.**
    - Flank pain
    - Palpable mass
    - Hematuria
    - Erythrocytosis
    - Secondary polycythemia

VHL:

Multiple hemangiomas

Spinal cord/cerebellar

hemangioblastomas

Pheochromocytomas

Retinal angiomata

Pancreatic cysts

- Tumor secretes erythropoietin.
  - Erythroid line stimulated in bone marrow.

Bladder Cancer

- Transitional cell carcinoma (usually).
- Hematuria.

Leukemia

Leukemia can modify the inflammatory reaction.

- Leukemia = Group of malignancies that begin in the blood-forming cells of the bone marrow (lymphoid or hematopoietic cell origin).

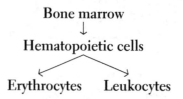

Bone marrow
↓
Hematopoietic cells
Erythrocytes   Leukocytes

Leukemia differs from other cancers by beginning in bone marrow and spreading to major organs (as opposed to beginning in major organs then spreading to bone marrow).

LEUKOCYTES IN LEUKEMIA

- **Normal leukocyte function**
  - Immune cells
  - Fight against infection (viruses and bacteria)
- **Leukemic proliferation of leukocytes**
  - ↑ immature leukemic cells.
  - **Effects**
    - ↓ function of leukocytes.
      - ↑ infection susceptibility.
    - Marrow replacement (↑ leukemic cells = ↓ space for other cell lines in marrow).
    - ↓ RBC (so ↓ O_2-carrying ability).
    - ↓ Platelets (↓ clotting = ↑ bleeding).
    - When ↑↑ leukemic proliferation, overwhelms bone marrow.
    - Leukemic cells into bloodstream.
    - Invade other parts of the body (LNs, spleen, liver, CNS).

The principal organs involved in leukemia = bone marrow, then the spleen and liver.

LEUKEMIA ETIOLOGY

- Exact cause of leukemias remains unknown
- Evidence points to a combination of factors:
  - Familial tendency.
  - Congenital disorders/genetic predisposition.
    - Down's syndrome (↑ acute leukemias).
    - Philadelphia chromosome (in chronic myelogenous leukemia [CML]).
  - Viral infection
    - Herpes-like viral particles have been cultured.
    - High EBV antibody titers have been seen in leukemic patients.
    - HYLV-1 (adult T-cell leukemia) (human T-cell lymphotropic virus-1).
      - CD4 T cells

- Ionizing radiation (usually causes myelogenous).
- Toxin exposures
  - Benzene.
  - Alkylating agents.

LEUKEMIA CLASSIFICATION

- Dominant type cell:
  - Myeloid.
  - Lymphocytic.
- Duration from onset to death.
  - Acute
  - Chronic

LEUKEMIA TYPES

	ALL	AML	CLL	CML
Progression	Rapid	Rapid	Slow	Slow
WBC affected	Lymphocytes	Myelocytes	Lymphocytes	Myelocytes
Age	3–5 y	(children to adults)	> 60	Any age
% diagnosed per year	20	27	31	22
Features	Peak age = 4 y Form of acute leukemia most responsive to therapy	Responds poorly to treatment (vs. ALL)	2–3 × M > F Abnormal small lymphocytes Lymphoid tissue blood Bone marrow ▪ variable course, smudge cells ▪ most common	Young and middle-aged adults Rare in children M > F (slightly) Philadelphia chromosome

Of all cases of leukemia, 50% are acute, 50% are chronic (evenly split). However, in children, ALL (acute lymphocytic leukemia) = two-thirds of cases.

ACUTE LEUKEMIAS

- Rapid onset (few months).
- Fatal unless treated quickly.
  - No treatment = Die within 6 months.
    - Death is usually due to hemorrhage (brain) or superimposed bacterial infection.
  - Intensive treatment can get remissions up to 5 years.
    - Chemotherapy
    - Radiation
    - Bone marrow transplants.
- Immature abnormal cells.
  - ↓ immune system functions.
  - ↓ bone marrow production of erythrocytes, platelets.
  - ↑ leukemic cells spill from bone marrow into peripheral blood and invade:
    - Liver
    - Spleen

AML (acute myelogenous leukemia) and CLL (chronic lymphocytic leukemia) are the most common types of leukemia in adults.

- Lymph nodes
- Other parenchymal organs.
- **Clinical**
  - Anemia (usually severe).
    - Fatigue
    - Malaise
  - ↑ infection.
    - No functioning granulocytes.
    - ↑ bacterial infections are common.
    - ↑ bleeding (thrombocytopenia)
    - Petechiae and ecchymosis (in skin and mucous membranes).
    - Hemorrhage from various sites.
  - Leukemic infiltration of organs.
    - Lymphadenopathy (enlarged LNs)
    - Splenomegaly (enlarged spleen)
    - Hepatomegaly (enlarged liver)
  - Fever
  - Bone and joint pain (common in children).
- **Laboratory**
  - Leukocytosis.
    - Leukocyte counts vary greatly in acute leukemias.
      - 30,000–1 million/mm^3.
      - Immature forms (myeloblasts and lymphoblasts) predominating.
    - ↑ ESR.

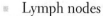

In 75% of cases of ALL, the lymphocytes are neither B- nor T cells and are called "null cells."

CHRONIC LEUKEMIAS

- Slower onset of progression.
- Longer, less devastating clinical course (vs acute leukemias).
  - CML median survival time is 4 years.
    - Death due to hemorrhage or infection.
  - CLL has a variable course.
    - Older patients may survive even without treatment.
- Affected cells are more mature.
  - Perform some of their duties, but not well.
  - These abnormal cells proliferate at a slower rate.
    - Accounts for the slower disease progression.
- **Clinical**
  - Insidious onset (often diagnosed during examination for some other condition)
  - Weight loss
  - Anemia
    - Weakness/fatigue
    - Malaise
    - **Note:** Lymphocytic anemia may be complicated by autoimmune hemolytic anemia.
  - ↑ infection
    - ↑ bacterial infections are common.
  - ↑ bleeding (thrombocytopenia)
    - Petechiae and ecchymosis (in skin and mucous membranes)
    - Hemorrhage from various sites (unexplained)
  - Leukemic infiltration of organs
    - Lymphadenopathy (enlarged LNs) (primary finding in CLL)
    - Massive splenomegaly (enlarged spleen) (characteristic of CML)
    - Hepatomegaly (enlarged liver)

- Laboratory
  - Leukocytosis > 10,000/mm^3.
  - Mature forms on blood smear (granulocytes and lymphocytes predominating).
- CML
  - Philadelphia chromosome.
  - Low levels of leukocyte alkaline phosphatase.

Chronic Myelogenous Leukemia (CML)

- 90% of patients with CML have the Philadelphia chromosome.
- **Philadelphia chromosome** = Remnant of chromosome 22 + small segment of 9.
- Translocation:
  - Long arm of chromosome 22 (*bcr* [oncogene]).
  - Chromosome 9 (*c-abl* [proto-oncogene]).
- **Caused by:**
  - Radiation
  - Carcinogenic chemicals
- **Characterized by:**
  - ↑ granulocytic precursors (myeloblasts and promyelocytes).
    - Bone marrow.
    - Peripheral blood.
    - Body tissues.
  - Most common in young and middle-aged adults.
  - Men > women (slightly).
  - Rare in children.
- **Course**
  - Two distinct phases:
    - Insidious chronic phase: Anemia and bleeding disorders.
    - Blastic crisis or acute phase: Rapid proliferation of myeloblasts (the most primitive granulocyte precursors).
  - CML is invariably fatal.

Lymphomas

- Lymphoid neoplasms.
  - Post germinal centers
- **Hodgkin's lymphoma** (Hodgkin's disease)
- **Non-Hodgkin lymphoma**
  - B-cell neoplasms
  - T-cell neoplasms

Hodgkin's Lymphoma

- Hodgkin's disease (HD).
- Cause unknown.
- **Theories**
  - Inflammatory or infectious process that becomes a neoplasm.
  - Immune disorder primarily.
  - M > F (2:1).
  - Usually between ages 15 and 35.
- **Signs/symptoms**
  - Painless lymph node enlargement (usually first sign) (contiguous spread).
    - Rubbery on exam.
    - Often without obvious/known cause.

Hodgkin's lymphoma is characterized by painless, progressive enlargement of lymphoid tissue. Reed–Sternberg cells are the pathognomonic histological finding and are the actual malignant cells.

Hodgkin's lymphoma is classified as follows:

- Lymphocyte-rich (classical) Hodgkin's lymphoma.
- Mixed cellularity Hodgkin's lymphoma.
- Lymphocyte-depleted Hodgkin's lymphoma.
- Nodular sclerosis Hodgkin's lymphoma.

- Constitutional signs and symptoms may be present:
  - Fever
  - Diaphoresis
  - Anorexia
  - Weight loss
  - Pruritis
  - Low-grade fever
  - Night sweats
  - Anemia
  - Leukocytosis
- Can spread (contiguous spread)
  - Adjacent LNs
  - Extranodal organs
    - Lungs
    - Liver
    - Bones or bone marrow
- Splenomegaly is common
- **Histology**
  - ***Reed–Sternberg cells*** (pathognomonic for HD).
    - Binucleated or multinucleated giant cells.
    - = the actual neoplastic cells.
- Prognosis is favorable with early diagnosis and limited involvement.
  - Lymphocyte predominance is linked with favorable prognosis.

NON-HODGKIN'S LYMPHOMA (NHL)

- Malignant lymphoma.
- Heterogeneous group of malignant disease originating in lymph nodes or other lymphoid tissue.
- Cause is unknown; some suggest a viral source.
- M > F (2–3:1).
- All ages (greatest risk >50–60).
- **Signs/symptoms**
  - Lymph node or other lymph tissue (eg, tonsils or adenoids) (first indication).
  - Painless rubbery nodes in cervical or supraclavicular areas.
  - Symptoms specific to the area involved (as the lymphoma progresses).
- **Systemic signs/symptoms**
  - Fatigue
  - Malaise
  - Weight loss
  - Fever
  - Night sweats
  - Circumscribed solid tumor masses.
    - Composed of primitive cells or cells resembling lymphocytes, plasma cells, or histiocytes
- **Classification:** By cell type.
  - B cell (85%).
    - Hairy cell leukemia
    - MALT lymphoma
    - Follicular lymphoma
    - Mantle cell lymphoma
    - Diffuse large cell lymphoma
    - Burkitt's lymphoma
  - T cell (15%)
    - Adult T-cell leukemia (HTLV1+)

NHLs can also be classified by morphology and clinical behavior as low-, intermediate-, or high-grade.

NHL is similar clinically to HD but Reed–Sternberg cells are not present (also the specific mechanism of LN destruction is different). So, biopsy differentiates NHL (malignant lymphoma) from HD.

- Mycosis fungoides (Sezary syndrome)
  - Cutaneous lymphoma

BURKITT'S LYMPHOMA

- High-grade (aggressive) B-cell lymphoma (classified as a NHL).
  - Defective B lymphocytes.
  - LNs tend to be spared.
- Etiology
  - Closely linked to EBV infection (especially the African variety).
  - Closely related to B-ALL (acute lymphoblastic leukemia).
  - Cytogenic change = t(8; 14).
- African type
  - Middle African regions.
  - Large jaw mass.
  - Closely associated with EBV (95% of cases).
- American type
  - Abdominal mass.
  - Less closely associated with EBV.

There is a relationship between diffuse lymphocytic lymphoma and chronic lymphocytic lymphoma (CLL).

MYCOSIS FUNGOIDES

- Rare persistent slow-growing type of NHL that originates from a mature T lymphocyte and affects the skin.
- Clinical
  - Skin lesions
    - Erythematous, eczematoid, or psoriasiform lesion.
    - Progress to raised plaques then to a tumor stage.
- Histology
  - Atypical CD4+ T cells with cerebriform nuclei.
  - *Pautrier microabscesses:* Small pockets of tumor cells within epidermis.
  - May progress to LNs and internal organs.

Multiple Myeloma

- ~1% of all cancers.
- Mostly in men > 40.
- Cancer of plasma cells.
  - Arises in the bone marrow.
- ↑ Plasma cells
  - Interferes with other bone marrow cell lineages.
    - ↓ RBC: Anemia.
    - ↓ platelets: Bleeding.
    - ↓ WBC: ↑ infection.
  - Abnormally functioning plasma cells: ↑ infection.
- Osteolytic lesions
  - As plasma cell proliferation ↑↑; expand in the bone marrow.
  - X-rays = "Punched-out" appearance.
    - Flat bones
    - Vertebrae
    - Skull
    - Mandible
    - Pelvis
    - Ribs
  - Severe, constant back and rib pain (early diagnostic sign).
    - ↑ with exercise.

Presence of Bence–Jones protein in the urine usually confirms the diagnosis of multiple myeloma. However, absence of Bence–Jones protein does not rule out multiple myeloma (sensitive but not specific).

Death in patients with multiple myeloma is most commonly related to the increased susceptibility to infection.

- ↑ at night.
- Pain is caused when malignant plasma cells create pressure on the nerves in the periosteum.
- Pathologic bone fractures can occur.
- **Renal failure**
  - Hypercalcemia (from bone destruction) leading to hypercalciuria.
  - Bence–Jones proteins (in the urine; is a diagnostic finding).
    - Caused by light chain dimers.
- **Amyloidosis**
  - May be seen in multiple myeloma (overproduction of Ig light chains).
  - Can also contribute to renal failure.

Amyloidosis

Congo red stains amyloid.

Deposits of amyloid (amylin) in islet cells can cause DM-2.

- Rare, chronic disease.
- Affects adults (middle-aged and older).
- Accumulation of abnormal fibrillar scleroprotein (amyloid).
  - Deposited in various organs and tissues of the body.
  - Organ function is eventually compromised (eg, renal disease is a frequent manifestation.)
- Disease states associated with amyloidosis may be
  - Inflammatory
  - Hereditary
  - Neoplastic
- Deposition of amyloid may be
  - Local
  - Generalized
  - Systemic

	Primary Amyloidosis	Secondary Amyloidosis (Overproduction of Acute-Phase Proteins in Chronic Inflammation)	Hereditary Amyloidosis
Cause	Unknown cause Associated w/plasma cell abnormalities Abnormal Ig production Multiple myeloma	Secondary to another disease: TB RA Familial Mediterranean fever Alzheimer's disease DM-2	Autosomal dominant Mutation of transthyretin protein Portugal, Sweden, and Japan
Sites of deposition	Heart Lung Skin Tongue Thyroid gland GI tract Liver Kidney Blood vessels	Spleen Liver Kidneys Adrenal glands Lymph nodes Heart rarely involved	Nerves GI tract

Histiocytosis X

- Langerhans cell histiocytosis, differentiated histiocytosis.
- Group of disorders characterized by abnormal ↑ histiocytes.
- Treatment
  - Radiation
  - Chemotherapy
- Prognosis: Poor

	Eosinophilic Granuloma	Letterer–Siwe Disease	Hand–Schuller–Christian Disease
Epidemiology	Most benign form Males ~20 y	Fatal Infants < 2 y	Early age (< 5 y) Boys > girls
Clinical	Asymptomatic Local pain	Skin rash Persistent fever, malaise	Triad of symptoms: Exophthalmos
	Mouth swelling Mandible most often affected	Anemia Hemorrhage Splenomegaly	DI Bone destruction (skull and jaws affected)
	Mobile teeth Periodontal inflammation	Lymphadenopathy Localized tumefactions over bones Oral lesions uncommon	Oral signs: Halitosis (bad breath) Sore mouth Loose teeth

Histiocytes are immune cells. They include:

- *Monocytes*
- *Macrophages*
- *Dendritic cells*

*Haberman's disease is **not** one of the histiocytosis X diseases. It is a skin condition that manifests as sudden eruption polymorphous skin macules, papules, and occasionally vesicles with hemorrhage.*

▶ NEOPLASIA OF THE ADRENAL GLAND

Adrenal Medulla

- Tumors of the adrenal medulla
  - Pheochromocytoma
  - Neuroblastoma
- Findings
  - ↑ catecholamines

Pheochromocytoma

- Chronic chromaffin-cell tumor
  - Benign, usually
- Uncommon
- Affects men or women of any age
  - Most often ages 30–60
- Results in ↑catecholamines
  - ↑epinephrine and norepinephrine
- Clinical
  - Persistent or paroxysmal HTN (secondary HTN)
  - ↑ metabolism
  - Hyperglycemia

Pheochromocytoma may be associated with:

- *MEN (multiple endocrine neoplasia) syndromes.*
- *Neurofibromatosis (von Reckinghausen's disease).*
- *von Hippel–Lindau disease (multiple hemangiomas).*

Catecholamine-secreting extra-adrenal chromaffin cell tumor = Paraganglioma.

Neuroblastoma

- Most common malignant tumor of childhood and infancy
- Adrenal medulla (most common site)
- **Etiology**
    - *N-myc* oncogene amplification.
- **Clinical presentation**
    - Abdominal mass.
        - Abdominal distention.
        - Sensation of fullness.
        - Abdominal pain.
    - 80% of neuroblastomas are productive of catecholamines.
        - ↑ epinephrine
        - ↑ HR
        - ↑ anxiety
- **Complications**
    - Invasion of abdominal viscera.
    - Direct spread.
    - Metastasis to liver, lung, or bone.

Bone Tumors

Osseous bone tumors arise from bony structure itself. Nonosseous tumors arise most often from hematopoietic, vascular, or neural tissues.

Most common symptom of bone tumor = Bone pain.

- *Dull.*
- *Usually localized.*
- *↑ at night.*
- *↑ with movement .*

Most common type of bone tumors in children are

- *Osteosarcoma (osteogenic sarcoma).*
- *Ewing's sarcoma.*

Primary Bone Tumors	Metastatic Bone Tumors
Rare (<1% all malignant tumors)	Majority of bone tumors
M > F, young men	Secondary; seeds from primary site
<ul><li>Osteosarcoma</li></ul>	<ul><li>Breast</li><li>Lung</li><li>Prostate</li><li>Kidney</li><li>Thyroid</li></ul>

Osseous	Nonosseous
Osteosarcoma	Ewing's (primitive neuroectodermal tumors)
Parosteal osteosarcoma	Chordoma (remnants of notocord, clivus, and coccyx)
Chondrosarcoma (actually from cartilage)	Fibrosarcoma (fibroblasts)
Malignant giant cell tumor (multinucleated giant cells [osteoclast like])	

Osteosarcoma

- Most common primary tumor of bone
- Malignant tumor
- Mesenchymal origin (bone)
    - Arise from osteoblast and osteoclasts

MICROBIOLOGY–PATHOLOGY

NEOPLASIA

- Males 10–30
- **Common sites:**
  - Femur
  - Tibia
  - Humerus
- **Less frequent sites:**
  - Fibula
  - Ileum
  - Vertebra
  - Mandible

PAROSTEAL OSTEOSARCOMA

- Women aged 30–40.
- Most often affects the distal femur.
  - May occur in the humerus, tibia, ulna.
- Develops on bone surface.
  - Not endosseous (interior).
- Progresses slowly.

Chondrosarcoma

- Males aged 30–50.
- Arises from cartilage.
- **Common sites**
  - Pelvis
  - Proximal femur
  - Ribs
  - Shoulder girdle
- **Clinical**
  - Usually painless
- **Course**
  - Grows slowly
  - Locally recurrent and invasive

Malignant Giant Cell Tumor

- Females aged 18–50.
- Arises from benign giant cell tumor.
- **Most common site:** Long bones, especially knee area.

▶ BONE TUMORS OF NONOSSEOUS ORIGIN

Ewing's Sarcoma

- Nonosseous malignant bone tumor.
- Children
  - Usually males aged 10–20 y.
  - Usually develops during puberty when bones are growing rapidly.
- **Sites**
  - Originates in bone marrow; invades long and flat bones.
  - Long bones upper and lower extremities
    - Femur

- Tibia
- Fibula
- Humerus
- Pelvis/innominate bones
- Ribs
- Vertebra
- Skull
- Facial bones
- **Histology**
  - Innominate; difficult to distinguish from neuroblastoma and reticulum cell sarcoma.
- **Symptoms**
  - Few symptoms
  - Pain: ↑ severity and persistence with time
  - Swelling at site
  - Fever
  - Pathologic fractures
- **Course**
  - Metastasis
  - One-third of children have metastases at time of diagnosis.
  - To lungs and other bones.

Ewing's is very radiosensitive.

Metastasize to bone:

- Prostate
- Breast
- Kidney
- Thryoid
- Lung

"Everything" metastasizes to lung, most commonly:

- Breast
- Colon
- Prostate

Fibrosarcoma

- Males 30–40 y
- **Sites:** Originates in fibrous tissue of bone
  - Invades long or flat bones:
    - Femur
    - Tibia
    - Mandible
  - Invades periosteum and overlying muscle.

Chordoma

- Males 50–60 years old.
- Derived from embryonic remnants of notochord.
- Slowly progressive.
- **Sites**
  - End of spinal column
  - Vertebra
  - Sacrococcygeal region
  - Spheno-occipital region
- **Symptoms** (depending on site)
  - Constipation
  - Visual disturbances

Dental Anatomy and Occlusion

CHAPTER 24

Tooth Morphology

Classification of Dentitions

BY MORPHOLOGY

- **Homodont dentition:** All teeth have the same morphology.
- **Heterodont dentition:** Teeth have different morphology (eg, humans).

BY SETS OF TEETH

- **Monophyodont dentition:** One set of teeth.
- **Diphyodont dentition:** Two sets of teeth (eg, humans).
- **Polyphyodont dentition:** Multiple sets of teeth.

Dental Anatomic Terminology

TOOTH LOCATION

- **Anterior teeth:** Incisors and canines. 12 total (6 per arch).
- **Posterior teeth:** Premolars and molars. 20 total (10 per arch).

CROWN TYPES

- **Anatomic crown:** The portion of the tooth that extends from the cementoenamel junction (CEJ) to the incisal edge or occlusal surface (enamel-covered portion of the tooth).
- **Clinical crown:** The portion of the tooth that extends incisally or occlusally from the gingival margin (clinically visible portion of the tooth).

CHEWING SURFACES

- **Incisal edge:** The chewing surface of anterior teeth.
- **Occlusal surface:** The chewing surface of posterior teeth consisting of cusps, ridges, and grooves.
- **Occlusal table:** The occlusal surface within the cusp and marginal ridges.

ENAMEL SURFACE ELEVATIONS

- **Lobe:** The primary center of enamel formation in a tooth. In fully formed teeth, lobes are represented by cusps, mamelons, and cingula, and are separated by developmental depressions (anterior teeth) or developmental grooves (posterior teeth).
- **Mamelon:** A round extension of enamel on the incisal edge of all incisors. (See Figure 24–1.) There are usually three mamelons per incisor (one for each facial lobe). They are often translucent because of a lack of underlying dentin. Mamelons are typically worn down by attrition and mastication; thus, their presence in adults is an indication of malocclusion.
- **Cingulum:** A bulbous convexity of enamel located on the cervical third of the lingual surface of all anterior teeth.
- **Cusp:** A large elevation of enamel located on the occlusal surface of all posterior teeth and the incisal edge of canines.
- **Tubercle:** An extra formation of enamel on the crown of a tooth. Often manifests as a supernumerary cusp, such as the **cusp of Carabelli.**

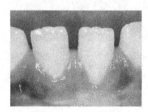

FIGURE 24–1.
Mamelons.

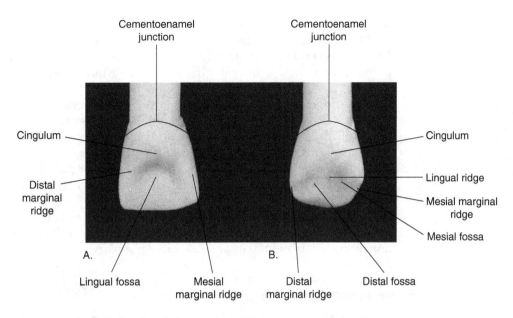

FIGURE 24-2. **Occlusal landmarks of two anterior teeth.**

A. Maxillary right central incisor; B. Maxillary right canine.

RIDGES

See Figures 24–2 and 24–3.

- **Ridge:** A linear elevation on the enamel surface.
- **Marginal ridge:** A ridge on *all teeth* that forms the mesial and distal margins of posterior occlusal surfaces and anterior lingual surfaces.

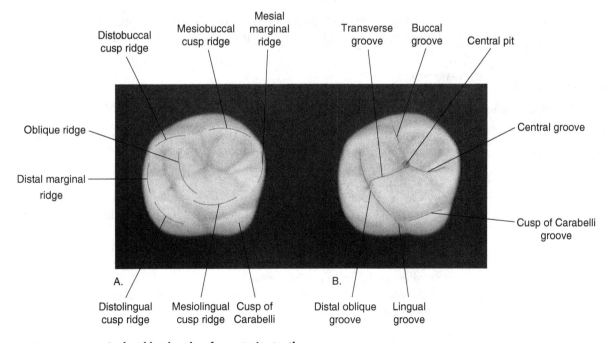

FIGURE 24-3. **Occlusal landmarks of a posterior tooth.**

A. Maxillary right 1st molar—ridges; B. Maxillary right 1st molar—grooves.

- **Labial ridge:** A ridge *only on canines* that runs incisocervically in the center of the facial crown surface. More prominent in maxillary canines.
- **Buccal (cusp) ridge:** A ridge *only on premolars* that runs occlusocervically in the center of the buccal crown surface. More prominent in first premolars.
- **Cervical ridge:** A ridge on *all primary teeth* and *permanent molars* that runs mesiodistally in the cervical third of the buccal surface of the crown.
- **Oblique ridge:** A ridge on *all maxillary molars* that extends from the ML to DB cusps (it separates the MB and DL cusps).
- **Triangular ridge:** A ridge on *all posterior teeth* that extends from the cusp tip to the central groove. The ML cusp of all maxillary molars has two triangular ridges.
- **Transverse ridge:** A ridge on *most posterior teeth* that runs buccolingually and connects opposing buccal and lingual triangular ridges. Most common on maxillary premolars and mandibular molars.

ENAMEL SURFACE DEPRESSIONS

Caries is most likely to occur in pits, fissures, and grooves. The teeth least likely to be lost to caries are mandibular incisors.

- **Sulcus:** A V-shaped depression on the occlusal surface of posterior teeth between ridges and cusps.
- **Fossa:** An irregularly shaped depression in the enamel surface.
- **Developmental groove:** A well-defined, shallow, linear depression in enamel that separates the cusps, lobes, and marginal ridges of a tooth.
- **Fissure:** A narrow crevice at the deepest portion of the developmental groove in enamel.
- **Pit:** A small pinpoint concavity at the termination or junction of developmental grooves.
- **Supplemental groove:** An irregularly defined, short groove auxiliary to a developmental groove that does not separate major tooth parts.

ENAMEL SURFACE JUNCTIONS

- **Line angle:** An angle formed by the junction of *two* surfaces.
- **Point angle:** An angle formed by the junction of *three* surfaces.

*Anterior teeth have **six** line angles. Posterior teeth have **eight** line angles. All teeth have **four** point angles.*

EMBRASURES

- **Contact area:** The location at which the proximal surfaces of two adjacent teeth make contact.
- **Embrasure:** A triangular-shaped space between the proximal surfaces of adjacent teeth which diverges in *four* directions from the contact area.
  - Buccal
  - Lingual
  - Occlusal/incisal
  - Cervical/gingival (**interproximal space**): In health, this space is completely filled with the gingival papilla.
- Largest occlusal embrasure: between max canine and PM1.
- Largest incisal embrasure: between max lateral and canine.
- Smallest incisal embrasure: between mand centrals.
- In general, lingual embrasures > buccal embrasures, *except* Max M1 (buccal embrasures > lingual)

INTERDENTAL SPACES

- **Diastema:** A space between two adjacent teeth in an arch.

INTRADENTAL SPACES

- **Furcation:** The area of a multirooted tooth where the roots diverge.

Innervation

Figure 24–4 illustrates the nerve supply to the teeth and gingiva.

- All dental and periodontal innervation arises from the **trigeminal nerve (CN V).**
- The maxillary nerve (V-2) supplies the maxillary teeth.
- The mandibular nerve (V-3) supplies the mandibular teeth.

Blood Supply

ARTERIAL SUPPLY

- All dental and periodontal arterial supply arises from the **maxillary artery.**
- The arterial supply generally parallels the corresponding nerves.

VENOUS RETURN

- All dental and periodontal venous return drains to the **pterygoid plexus of veins,** which eventually forms as the **maxillary vein.**

Maxillary molars are generally trifurcated; mandibular molars are generally bifurcated.

The DB root of the maxillary first molar is innervated by the posterosuperior alveolar nerve; the MB root receives its nerve supply from the middle superior alveolar nerve.

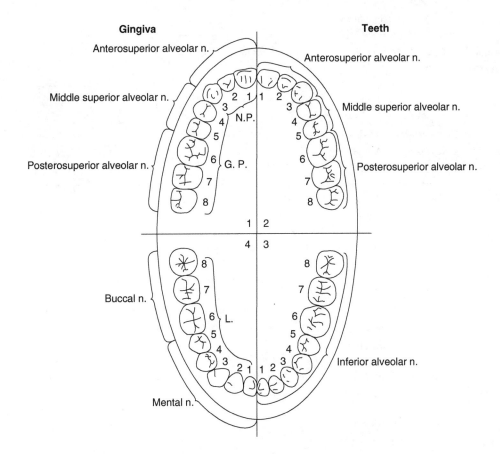

FIGURE 24–4. Nerve supply to maxillary and mandibular dental arches.

Reprinted, with permission, from Liebgott B. *The Anatomical Basis of Dentistry.* Toronto: BC Decker, 1986.

DENTAL ANATOMY AND OCCLUSION

TOOTH MORPHOLOGY

Table 24–1 compares the important characteristics of each permanent tooth.

TABLE 24-1. Comparison of Permanent Tooth Forms

	Inciso-Cervical Direction				Root Length (mm)	Crown Length (mm)	# of Lobes	# of Cusps	# of Roots	# of Root Canals
	Mesial Contact	Distal Contact	Facial HOC	Lingual HOC						
Maxilla										
Central incisor	Incisal 1/3	Junction*	Cervical 1/3	Cervical 1/3 (cingulum)	13	10.5	4	1	1	1
Lateral incisor	Junction*	Middle 1/3	Cervical 1/3	Cervical 1/3 (cingulum)	13	9	4	1	1	1
Canine	Junction*	Middle 1/3	Cervical 1/3	Cervical 1/3 (cingulum)	17	10	4	1	1	1
First premolar	Middle 1/3	Middle 1/3	Cervical 1/3	Middle 1/3	14	8.5	4	2	2	2
Second premolar	Middle 1/3	Middle 1/3	Cervical 1/3	Middle 1/3	14	8.5	4	2	1	1
First molar	Junction*	Middle 1/3	Cervical 1/3	Middle 1/3	12–13	7	5	4 or 5	3	3 or 4
Second molar	Junction*	Middle 1/3	Cervical 1/3	Middle 1/3	11–12	6.5	4	4	3	3 or 4
Third molar	Junction*	N/A	Cervical 1/3	Middle 1/3	11	6	4 or 5	3	3	Variable
Mandible										
Central incisor	Incisal 1/3	Incisal 1/3	Cervical 1/3	Cervical 1/3 (cingulum)	12.5	9	4	1	1	1
Lateral incisor	Incisal 1/3	Incisal 1/3	Cervical 1/3	Cervical 1/3 (cingulum)	14	9.5	4	1	1	1 or 2
Canine	Incisal 1/3	Middle 1/3	Cervical 1/3	Cervical 1/3 (cingulum)	16	11	4	1	1 or 2	1
First premolar	Middle 1/3	Middle 1/3	Cervical 1/3	Middle 1/3	14	8.5	4	2	1	1

(Continued)

TABLE 24-1. Comparison of Permanent Tooth Forms (Continued)

| | INCISO-CERVICAL DIRECTION | | | | ROOT LENGTH (mm) | CROWN LENGTH (mm) | # OF LOBES | # OF CUSPS | # OF ROOTS | # OF ROOT CANALS |
	MESIAL CONTACT	DISTAL CONTACT	FACIAL HOC	LINGUAL HOC						
				Mandible						
Second premolar	Middle 1/3	Middle 1/3	Cervical 1/3	Occlusal 1/3	14.5	8	5	2 or 3	1	1
First molar	Junction*	Middle 1/3	Cervical 1/3	Middle 1/3	14	7.5	5	5	2	3 or 4
Second molar	Junction*	Middle 1/3	Cervical 1/3	Middle 1/3	13	7	4	4	2	3 or 4
Third molar	Junction*	N/A	Cervical 1/3	Middle 1/3	11	7	4 or 5	4 or 5	2	Variable

*Junction of the incisal/occlusal and middle thirds.

General Concepts

TOOTH NUMBERING

See Figures 24–5 through 24–7.

- There are 32 total permanent teeth (16 per arch).

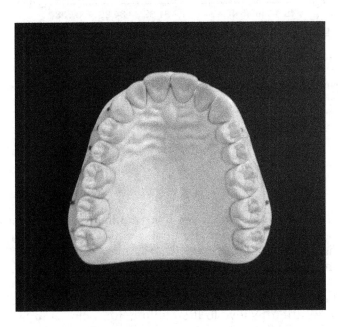

FIGURE 24-5. The maxillary arch.

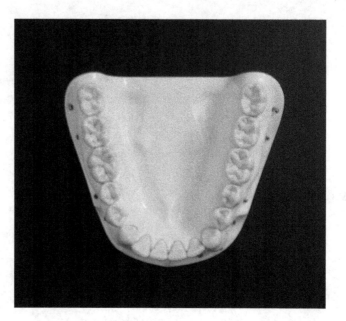

FIGURE 24–6. The mandibular arch.

```
                        Max
        1  2  3  4  5  6  7  8 │ 9 10 11 12 13 14 15 16
Right ──────────────────────────────────────────────── Left
       32 31 30 29 28 27 26 25 │ 24 23 22 21 20 19 18 17
A                       Mand

                        Max
       18 17 16 15 14 13 12 11 │ 21 22 23 24 25 26 27 28
Right ──────────────────────────────────────────────── Left
       48 47 46 45 44 43 42 41 │ 31 32 33 34 35 36 37 38
B                       Mand
```

FIGURE 24–7. Tooth numbering systems.

A. Universal Numbering System of the permanent dentition; B. Federation Dentaire Internationale (FDI) System for the permanent dentition.

- **Universal Numbering System:** Teeth are numbered 1 to 32, starting from the maxillary right 3rd molar and ending with the mandibular right 3rd molar (Figure 24–7A).
- **Federation Dentaire Internationale (FDI) System:** Each tooth is given a two-digit number. The first digit represents the quadrant in which the tooth is located (1, 2, 3, or 4). The second digit indicates the tooth position relative to the midline, from closest to farthest away (1 to 8) (Figure 24–7B).

PROXIMAL CONTACTS (VIEWED FROM THE FACIAL)

See Figures 24–8 and 24–9.

- Generally located increasingly more incisally (occlusally) from the posterior to the anterior.
- The mesial contact is *always* located more incisally than the distal.
- Proximal contacts prevent rotation, mesial drift, and food impaction.

PROXIMAL CONTACTS (VIEWED FROM THE OCCLUSAL)

- All are located in the middle 1/3 of the crown.
- Posterior contacts are positioned slightly buccal.

As one ages, proximal wear (attrition) creates larger contact areas and smaller embrasure spaces.

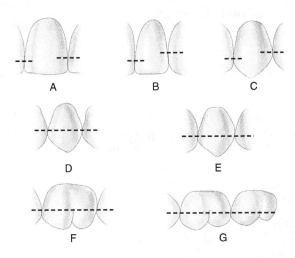

FIGURE 24–8. Proximal contacts of maxillary teeth.

A. Central incisor; B. Lateral incisor; C. Canine; D. First premolar; E. Second premolar; F. First molar; G. Second molar.

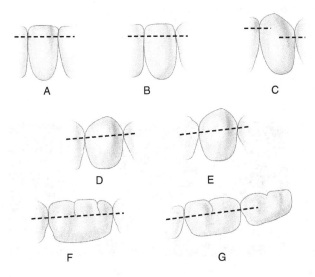

FIGURE 24–9. Proximal contacts of mandibular teeth.

A. Central incisor; B. Lateral incisor; C. Canine; D. First premolar; E. Second premolar; F. First molar; G. Second molar.

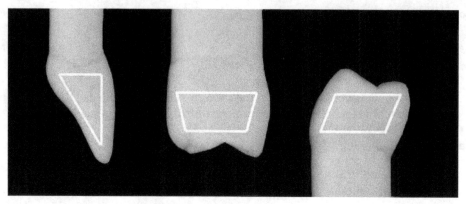

FIGURE 24–10. Proximal surface shapes.

The facial and lingual surfaces of all teeth are trapezoidal.

PROXIMAL SURFACES

See Figure 24–10.

- Triangular: All anterior teeth.
- Trapezoidal: All maxillary posterior teeth.
- Rhomboidal: All mandibular posterior teeth.

HEIGHTS OF CONTOUR (HOC)

- Facial HOC's:
    - Located in the cervical third, *except* mandibular molars (junction of cervical and middle thirds).
    - Most prominent on mandibular posterior teeth.
    - Least prominent on mandibular anterior teeth.
- Lingual HOC's:
    - Anterior teeth: Located in the cervical third (cingulum).
    - Posterior teeth: Located in middle third, *except* mandibular PM2 (occlusal third).
- Help form the mesial and distal contact areas.
- Allow for adequate gingival health.

CEJ CONTOURS

See Figure 24–11.

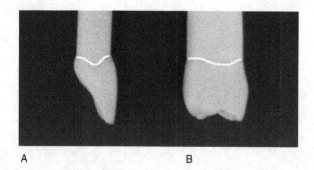

A   B

FIGURE 24–11. Proximal CEJ contours.

A. Maxillary right central incisor; B. Maxillary right 1st molar

- The maximum height of the proximal CEJ contour increases anteriorly.
- The mesial CEJ contour is *always* greater than the distal contour.
- The greatest CEJ contour is on the maxillary central incisor (mesial surface).
- Facial and lingual CEJs curve apically.
- Mesial and distal CEJs curve coronally.

LOBES

- Incisors and canines: 4 lobes (3 labial [mamelons], 1 lingual [cingulum]).
- Premolars: 4 lobes (3 buccal, 1 lingual) *except* mand PM2, which has 5 lobes (3 buccal, 2 lingual).
- First molars: 5 lobes (one for each cusp).
- Second molars: 4 lobes (one for each cusp).
- Third molars: 4 or 5 lobes (one for each cusp, depending on variation).

ARCH LENGTHS

- Maxillary: 128 mm (slightly longer).
- Mandibular: 126 mm.

Maxillary Permanent Teeth

CENTRAL INCISOR

See Figure 24–12.

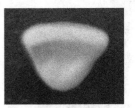

FIGURE 24–12.
Maxillary central incisor.

- Unique characteristics
    - Most prominent tooth.
    - Greatest mesial CEJ contour of all teeth.
    - Second longest crown (next to mandibular canine).
    - Widest (M-D) of all anterior teeth.
- Crown morphology
    - Occlusal shape is triangular; proximal shape is triangular.
    - Has three mamelons and four developmental grooves.
    - MMR > DMR.
    - M-I corner sharper than D-I.
    - Narrowest incisal embrasures of all maxillary teeth.
- Occlusal morphology
    - M-D dimension > F-L (from occlusal).
    - Cingulum: slightly distal.
- Root morphology
    - Least likely to have a divided root canal.
    - Roundest root form; can be rotated during extraction.
    - Blunted apex.
    - Has greatest axial inclination toward the facial.
    - Sits almost vertically (M-D) in alveolar bone.
- Occlusal contacts
    - Occludes with mandibular central and lateral incisors.

For all anterior teeth when viewed from the facial, faciolingual dimension > mesiolingual dimension.

LATERAL INCISOR

See Figure 24–13.

- Unique characteristics
    - Third most common congenitally missing tooth (next to third molars).

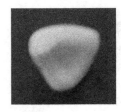

FIGURE 24–13.
Maxillary lateral incisor.

- Third most variable tooth form (next to third molars).
  - Peg lateral (microdont)
  - Dens-in-dente
- Most common tooth to have a **palato-radicular groove** (2–5% prevalence), which can make scaling difficult.
- Crown morphology
  - Occlusal shape is oval; proximal shape is triangular.
  - MMR (straight) > DMR.
  - M-I corner sharper than D-I.
- Occlusal morphology
  - M-D dimension > F-L (from occlusal).
  - Most developed lingual anatomy of all anterior teeth.
  - Lingual surface is the most concave of all incisors.
  - Cingulum: central. Often prominent (**talon cusp**), creating a lingual pit.
- Root morphology
  - Root just as long as maxillary central.
  - Typically curves to the distal.
- Occlusal contacts
  - Occludes with mandibular lateral incisor and canine.

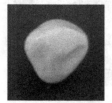

FIGURE 24–14.
Maxillary canine.

CANINE

See Figure 24–14.

- Unique characteristics
  - Longest tooth.
  - Longest cusp.
  - Third longest crown (next to mand canine and max central).
  - Widest (B-L) anterior tooth.
  - Maxillary tooth least likely to be extracted.
- Crown morphology
  - Has prominent facial ridge.
  - Cusp tip centered over root (from facial).
  - Mesial cusp ridge < distal.
  - Mesial surface is straighter (less convex) than the distal.
- Occlusal morphology
  - F-L dimension > M-D (from occlusal).
  - Has a prominent **lingual ridge**, which splits the lingual fossa into mesial and distal fossae.
  - Cusp tip located slightly M-F (from occlusal).
  - Cingulum: central and prominent.
- Root morphology
  - Longest root.
  - Root is oval-shaped and flattened M-D (deeper on distal).
- Occlusal contacts
  - Occludes with mandibular canine and first premolar.

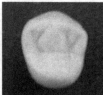

FIGURE 24–15.
Maxillary first premolar.

FIRST PREMOLAR

See Figure 24–15.

- Unique characteristics
  - Largest of all premolars.
- Crown morphology
  - Has a prominent **buccal ridge.**

- Only permanent tooth with mesial cusp ridge > distal cusp ridge.
- Has a prominent **mesial marginal ridge groove**, which can make scaling difficult.
- Occlusal morphology
  - Occlusal shape is **hexagonal**; proximal shape is **trapezoidal**.
  - Occlusal table has long central groove with fewer supplemental grooves. No central pit, but has mesial/distal pits.
  - 2 cusps: buccal (slightly distal), palatal (slightly mesial).
  - Buccal cusp height > palatal.
- Root morphology
  - Only premolar with two roots (B > P).
  - Has a prominent **mesial root concavity**.
  - Sits most vertically (B-L) in alveolar bone.
- Occlusal contacts
  - Occludes with mandibular first and second premolars.

SECOND PREMOLAR

See Figure 24–16.

- Unique Characteristics
  - Shorter and smaller than maxillary first premolar.
- Crown morphology
  - Distal cusp ridge > mesial cusp ridge.
  - Has a **buccal ridge,** but not as prominent as first premolar.
- Occlusal morphology
  - Occlusal shape is **hexagonal**; proximal shape is **trapezoidal**.
  - Occlusal table is more ovoid and symmetrical than maxillary first premolar.
  - Occlusal table has a **short central groove with more supplemental grooves.** Has "wrinkled" appearance.
  - 2 cusps: buccal, palatal (slightly mesial).
  - Buccal cusp height = palatal.
- Root morphology
  - Only premolar without a mesial root depression.
- Occlusal contacts
  - Occludes with mandibular second premolar and first molar.

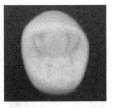

**FIGURE 24–16.
Maxillary second premolar.**

FIRST MOLAR

See Figure 24–17.

- Unique characteristics
  - Largest permanent tooth.
  - Only tooth that is **broader lingually than buccally.**
  - Widest tooth (B-L).
  - First permanent maxillary tooth to erupt.
- Crown morphology
  - Only tooth with a **pronounced distal concavity** at the CEJ, which can make scaling difficult.
  - Has a long buccal groove with a central pit.
  - Has a **distolingual groove** with a pit (on all maxillary molars).
- Occlusal morphology
  - Occlusal shape is **rhomboidal**; proximal shape is **trapezoidal**.
  - 4 cusps: MB, ML (largest), DB, DL (smallest).
  - Sometimes has fifth **cusp of Carabelli** lingual to ML cusp.

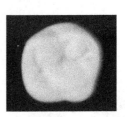

**FIGURE 24–17.
Maxillary first molar.**

- **Primary cusp triangle**: formed by ML, MB, and DB cusps (same for all maxillary molars).
- **Secondary cusp triangle**: formed by DL cusp.
- Cusp heights: ML > MB > DB (primary cusp triangle) > DL (secondary cusp triangle) > Carabelli.
- Only tooth with two triangular ridges on one cusp (ML cusp): form the transverse and oblique ridges.
- Has **most prominent oblique ridge** of all maxillary molars.
- The **transverse groove of the oblique ridge** connects the central and distal fossae (same for all maxillary molars).
- Root morphology
  - 3 roots: MB, DB (shortest), palatal (longest).
  - Distance from furcation entrance to CEJ: Mesial (3.6 mm) < buccal (4.2 mm) < distal (4.8 mm).
  - Apices are closest to **maxillary sinus.**
  - MB and DB roots are often shaped like "plier handles."
  - MB root has more common (94%) and deeper (0.3 mm) concavities than other roots.
- Occlusal contacts
  - Occludes with mandibular first and second molars.

SECOND MOLAR

See Figure 24–18.

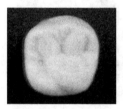

**FIGURE 24–18.
Maxillary second molar.**

- Unique characteristics
  - Similar to maxillary first molar but smaller and more angular.
  - Second most common tooth to have cervical enamel projections (next to mandibular second molar).
  - Closest tooth to the opening of Stenson's (parotid) duct.
- Crown morphology
  - Has a short buccal groove without a pit.
- Occlusal morphology
  - Occlusal table is usually **rhomboidal**, but can be **heart-shaped** if the DL cusp is absent; proximal shape is **trapezoidal.**
  - 4 cusps: MB, ML (largest), DB, DL (smallest).
  - Has smaller oblique ridge with a transverse groove.
- Root morphology
  - Roots are typically longer, closer together, and more distally inclined than the maxillary first molar. Occasionally fused.
  - Longer root trunk than maxillary first molar.
- Occlusal contacts
  - Occludes with mandibular second and third molars.

THIRD MOLAR

See Figure 24–19.

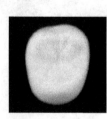

**FIGURE 24–19.
Maxillary third molar.**

- Unique characteristics
  - Most variable shape of any other tooth (with mandibular third molar).
  - Second most congenitally missing tooth (next to mandibular third molar).
  - **Shortest** permanent tooth.
  - Most common tooth to have **enamel pearls** (with mandibular third molars).
- Crown morphology
  - Shortest maxillary crown.

- Occlusal morphology
  - Occlusal table is usually **heart-shaped** since DL cusp has little or no development; proximal shape is **trapezoidal**.
  - Crown tapers lingually.
  - 3 cusps: MB, DB, lingual.
  - Oblique ridge is poorly developed and often absent.
- Root morphology
  - Roots are often fused and distally inclined.
- Occlusal contacts
  - Occludes only with mandibular third molar.

Mandibular Permanent Teeth

CENTRAL INCISOR

See Figure 24–20.

- Unique characteristics
  - Smallest tooth.
  - Narrowest (M-D) tooth.
  - Most symmetrical tooth.
  - Greatest mesial CEJ contour of mandibular teeth.
  - First succedaneous tooth to erupt.
- Crown morphology
  - MMR = DMR.
  - D-I corner is equally as sharp as M-I.
  - Incisal edge lingual to long axis (from proximal).
- Occlusal morphology
  - F-L dimension > M-D (from occlusal).
  - Incisal edge perpendicular to B-L bisector (from occlusal).
  - Cingulum: central and indistinct.
- Root morphology
  - Root has mesial and distal (deeper) concavities (hourglass shaped).
  - Longer than maxillary central.
- Occlusal contacts
  - Occludes with maxillary central incisor.
  - Only anterior tooth to occlude with one tooth.

LATERAL INCISOR

See Figure 24–21.

- Unique characteristics
  - Slightly larger in all dimensions than the mandibular central.
  - Second smallest tooth (next to mandibular central).
  - Not as symmetrical as the mandibular central.
- Crown morphology
  - Crown is tilted distally on the root (from facial).
  - MMR > DMR.
  - Incisal edge lingual to long axis (from proximal).
- Occlusal morphology
  - F-L dimension > M-D (from occlusal).
  - Incisal edge is **twisted disto-lingually** (from occlusal).
  - Cingulum: slightly distal and indistinct.
- Root morphology
  - Longest root of all incisors.
  - Root has mesial (deeper) and distal concavities (hourglass shaped).

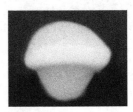

FIGURE 24–20.
Mandibular central incisor.

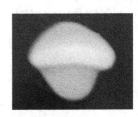

FIGURE 24–21.
Mandibular lateral incisor.

- Occlusal contacts
  - Occludes with maxillary central and lateral incisors.

CANINE

See Figure 24–22.

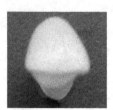

FIGURE 24–22.
Mandibular canine.

- Unique characteristics
  - Longest crown.
  - Second longest tooth (next to max canine). Longest tooth in mandible.
  - Second longest root (next to max canine).
  - Mandibular tooth least likely to be extracted.
- Crown morphology
  - Has a facial ridge, but less prominent than max canine.
  - Mesial cusp ridge < distal.
  - Mesial surface is nearly parallel with the long axis.
  - Cusp tip slightly lingual to long axis (from proximal).
- Occlusal morphology
  - F-L dimension > M-D (from occlusal).
  - Has a lingual ridge, but less prominent than max canine.
  - Cusp tip located slightly distal (from occlusal).
  - Cingulum: slightly distal and less prominent than max canine.
- Root morphology
  - Root is oval-shaped and flattened M-D (deeper on mesial).
  - Anterior tooth most likely to have a bifurcated root.
  - Only root that may be mesially inclined.
- Occlusal contacts
  - Occludes with maxillary lateral incisor and canine.

FIRST PREMOLAR

See Figure 24–23.

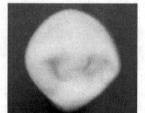

FIGURE 24–23.
Mandibular first premolar.

- Unique characteristics
  - Smallest of all premolars.
- Crown morphology
  - Has a prominent **mesio-lingual groove**.
  - MMR < DMR.
- Occlusal morphology
  - Occlusal shape is **diamond-shaped**; proximal shape is **rhomboidal** (tilted lingually).
  - Only posterior tooth with an **occlusal plane tilted lingually**.
  - Has most prominent **transverse ridge** of all premolars, which splits mesial and distal fossae. No central groove.
  - 2 cusps: buccal (functional), lingual (nonfunctional).
  - Buccal cusp is larger (2/3 of occlusal surface) than the lingual.
- Root morphology
  - Root is broader (B-L), and may have proximal concavities.
- Occlusal contacts
  - Occludes with maxillary canine and first premolar.

SECOND PREMOLAR

See Figure 24–24.

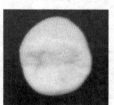

FIGURE 24–24.
Mandibular second premolar.

- Unique characteristics
  - Most congenitally missing premolar.
  - The gingival papilla between the first and second premolar is the shortest.

- Crown morphology
  - Lingual surface is wider (M-D) than that of the mandibular first premolar.
  - Shorter and wider than the mandibular first premolar (from buccal).
  - Mesial marginal ridge has slight concavity.
  - Only premolar with five lobes: three buccal and two lingual.
- Occlusal morphology
  - Occlusal shape is **square**; proximal shape is **rhomboidal** (tilted lingually).
  - Occlusal surface can have three configurations:
    - **Y** (most common configuration): 3 cusps—buccal > ML > DL, with a single **central pit**.
    - **H:** 2 cusps—buccal and lingual with short central groove.
    - **U:** 2 cusps—buccal and lingual with crescent-shaped central groove.
  - Buccal cusp is shorter and blunter than lingual cusps.
  - ML cusp is larger than the DL cusp.
  - Mesial marginal ridge has slight concavity.
- Root morphology
  - Root is longer than the mandibular first premolar.
  - Apex closest to **mental foramen.**
- Occlusal contacts
  - Occludes with maxillary first and second premolars.

First Molar

See Figure 24–25.

- Unique characteristics
  - Largest mandibular tooth.
  - Widest tooth (M-D).
  - First permanent tooth to erupt, and most often restored/extracted.
- Crown morphology
  - Can see all 5 cusps from the buccal.
  - Buccal cusps are shorter and blunter then the lingual cusps.
- Occlusal morphology
  - Occlusal shape is **pentagonal**; proximal shape is **rhomboidal** (tilted lingually 15–20°).
  - 5 cusps: MB (largest), DB, distal (smallest), ML (tallest), DL.
  - Occlusal pattern resembles a +< with a twisted central groove.
  - Has **two transverse ridges**, three fossae with pits, **two buccal grooves** (MB and DB), and a short lingual groove.
- Root morphology
  - Roots are usually widely separated.
  - The mesial root is longer and wider (B-L).
  - Both roots have concavities (mesial slightly more prominent).
  - The root trunk is typically shorter than the mandibular second molar.
- Occlusal contacts
  - Occludes with the maxillary second premolar and first molar.

Second Molar

See Figure 24–26.

- Unique characteristics
  - Most symmetrical molar.
  - Most common tooth to have **cervical enamel projections.**

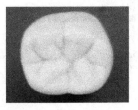

FIGURE 24–25.
Mandibular first molar.

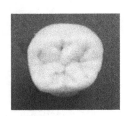

FIGURE 24–26.
Mandibular second molar.

647

- Crown morphology
  - The B-L dimension is greater at the mesial than distal.
  - Cusps are same height when viewed from buccal.
- Occlusal morphology
  - Occlusal shape is **rectangular**; proximal shape is **rhomboidal** (tilted lingually 15–20°).
  - 4 cusps: MB (largest), DB, ML, DL.
  - Occlusal pattern resembles a + with a straight central groove.
  - Has two **transverse ridges,** three fossae with pits, three secondary grooves, **one buccal groove** with a pit, and a short lingual groove.
- Root morphology
  - Roots are closer together than the mandibular first molar and inclined distally.
  - The root trunk is typically longer than the mandibular first molar.
- Occlusal contacts
  - Occludes with the maxillary first and second molar.

THIRD MOLAR

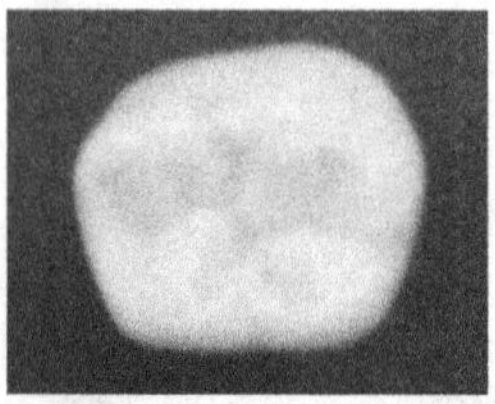

See Figure 24–27.

FIGURE 24–27. Mandibular third molar.

- Unique characteristics
  - Most **variable morphology** (with maxillary third molar).
  - Most common congenitally missing tooth.
  - Most frequently impacted tooth.
  - Most common tooth to have **enamel pearls** (with maxillary third molars).
- Crown morphology
  - Has bulbous crown that tapers distally.
  - Occlusal shape can be similar to mandibular first or second molars; proximal shape is **rhomboidal** (tilted lingually 15–20°).
- Occlusal morphology
  - Occlusal shape can be similar to mandibular first or second molars; proximal shape is **rhomboidal** (tilted lingually 15–20°).
  - 4 or 5 cusps: MB, DB, distal (can be absent), ML, DL.
  - MB cusp > DB cusp.
  - Has an irregular groove pattern.
- Root morphology
  - Roots are usually short, distally inclined, and often fused.
  - Typically has **distally inclined root trunk and apices**.
- Occlusal contacts
  - Occludes with maxillary second and third molar.

▶ PRIMARY (DECIDUOUS) TOOTH FORM

The primary dentition is shown in Figure 24–28.

General Concepts

TOOTH LABELING

See Figure 24–29.

- There are 20 total primary teeth (10 per arch).
- There are no premolars.
- Teeth are labeled A through T.

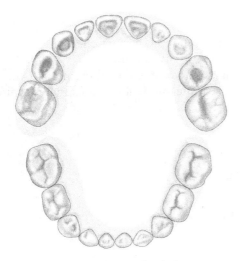

FIGURE 24-28. The primary dentition, occlusal view.

The mesiodistal width of the primary molars is 2–5 mm > the width of the permanent premolars.

```
                    Max
        A B C D E | F G H I J
Right ──────────────────────── Left
        T S R Q P | O N M L K
                    Mand
```

FIGURE 24-29. Tooth labeling of the primary (deciduous) dentition.

Apple Jacks Kill Teeth

PRIMARY VS PERMANENT TEETH

See Table 24–2.

TOOTH STRUCTURE	PRIMARY TEETH ARE/HAVE...COMPARED TO PERMANENT TEETH
Enamel	Lighter (whiter) in color Thinner (only about 1 mm thick) Less calcified (more caries prone) No mamelons (but still develop from lobes) Stops abruptly at the CEJ
Dentin	Thinner (easier to have pulp exposure)
Crowns	More bulbous (larger cervical bulges) Buccal and lingual surfaces are flatter above the HOC Smaller occlusal tables Fewer grooves and pits (shallower and smoother) Anterior crowns: wider M-D and shorter inciso-cervically Posterior crowns: narrower M-D and shorter occluso-cervially
CEJs	More constricted (narrower cervix)
Root trunks	Shorter Narrower
Roots	Longer and more slender relative to crown size Smaller crown:root ratio More tapered (anterior teeth) More divergent (posterior teeth)

PRIMATE SPACE

- Allows for proper alignment of the permanent incisors.
- Occurs in about 50% of primary dentitions.
- Maxillary: Between lateral incisor and canine (mesial to canine).
- Mandibular: Between canine and first molar (distal to canine).

ARCH LENGTHS

- Maxillary: 68.2 mm (longer).
- Mandibular: 61.8 mm.

Maxillary Primary Teeth

See Figure 24–30.

CENTRAL INCISOR

- Straighter incisal edge than permanent maxillary central.
- No mamelons.
- Prominent facial and lingual cervical ridges.
- Occludes with mandibular central and lateral incisors.

LATERAL INCISOR

- Straighter incisal edge than permanent maxillary lateral.
- No mamelons.
- Prominent facial and lingual cervical ridges.
- Occludes with mandibular lateral incisor and canine.

CANINE

- Only primary tooth in which facial shape is pentagonal (not trapezoidal).
- Longer and sharper cusp than permanent maxillary canine.
- Only primary tooth with **mesial cusp ridge > distal cusp ridge**.
- Occludes with mandibular canine and first molar.

FIRST MOLAR

- Smallest primary molar.
- Generally **resembles a permanent maxillary premolar.**
- Occlusal shape is **rectangular.**
- Occlusal surface has **H-shaped** configuration.
- Has a prominent buccal cervical ridge.
- 4 cusps: MB (largest), ML (sharpest), DB, DL (smallest).
- Occludes with mandibular first and second molars.

SECOND MOLAR

- Generally **resembles permanent maxillary first molar** but smaller.
- Occlusal shape is **rhomboidal.**
- Widest (B-L) primary tooth.
- Has a prominent buccal cervical ridge.
- Has an oblique ridge.

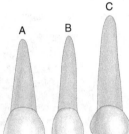
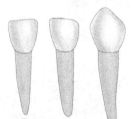
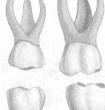
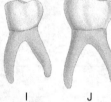

FIGURE 24–30. The primary teeth, facial view.

A. Maxillary central incisor;
B. Maxillary lateral incisor;
C. Maxillary canine;
D. Mandibular central incisor; E. Mandibular lateral incisor; F. Mandibular canine; G. Maxillary first molar; H. Maxillary second molar; I. Mandibular first molar; J. Mandibular second molar.

TABLE 24-2. Comparison of Primary (Deciduous) Tooth Forms

	Root Length (mm)	Crown Length (mm)	Number of Cusps	Number of Roots
Maxilla				
Central incisor	10	6	1	1
Lateral incisor	11.4	5.6	1	1
Canine	13.5	6.5	1	1
First molar	10	5.1	4	3
Second molar	11.7	5.7	5	3
Mandible				
Incisor	9	5	1	1
Lateral incisor	10	5.2	1	1
Canine	11.5	6	1	1
First molar	9.8	6	4	2
Second molar	11.3	5.5	5	2

- 4 cusps: MB (largest), ML (almost as large as MB), DB, DL (smallest).
- May have a fifth cusp of Carabelli.
- Occludes only with mandibular second molar.

Mandibular Primary Teeth

CENTRAL INCISOR

- Straighter incisal edge than permanent mandibular central.
- No mamelons.
- Prominent facial and lingual cervical ridges.
- Occludes only with maxillary central incisor.

LATERAL INCISOR

- Straighter incisal edge than permanent mandibular lateral.
- No mamelons.
- Prominent facial and lingual cervical ridges.
- More exaggerated incisal edge slope than permanent mandibular lateral.
- Occludes with maxillary central and lateral incisors.

CANINE

- Distal cusp ridge > mesial cusp ridge.
- Occludes with maxillary lateral incisor and canine.

DENTAL ANATOMY AND OCCLUSION

TOOTH MORPHOLOGY

First Molar

- **Most unique** primary or permanent tooth.
- Most difficult primary tooth to restore.
- Occlusal shape is **rhomboidal.**
- Has no central fossa (but has mesial and distal triangular fossae).
- Has a prominent buccal cervical ridge.
- Has a well-developed mesial marginal ridge.
- Has a prominent **transverse ridge** (connects MB and ML cusps).
- CEJ curves apically on the mesial (from buccal view).
- 4 cusps: MB (largest), ML (tallest, sharpest), DB, DL (smallest).
- Occludes with maxillary canine and first molar.

Second Molar

- Generally **resembles permanent mandibular first molar.**
- Occlusal shape is **rectangular.**
- Widest (M-D) primary tooth.
- Has a prominent buccal cervical ridge.
- 5 cusps: MB, ML, D (almost as large as MB and DB cusps), DB, DL.
- Occludes with maxillary first and second molars.

CHAPTER 25

Pulp Morphology

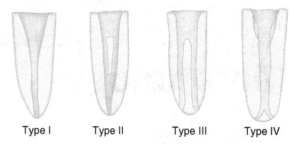

Type I   Type II   Type III   Type IV

FIGURE 25–1. **Pulp canal system classification (Weine).**

Size of pulp cavity is dictated by:

- *Age*
- *Parafunctional activity*
- *Trauma history (caries, abrasion, erosion, etc)*

There are as many pulp horns as there are cusps. In permanent teeth, the size of a pulp horn is directly proportional to the size of its associated cusp.

▶ **CLASSIFICATION**

Pulp Canal System Configuration

See Figure 25–1.

I. Type I: Contains a single canal from the pulp chamber to the apical foramen.
II. Type II: Contains two separate canals leaving the pulp chamber, but later merge together just short of the apical foramen.
III. Type III: Contains two separate canals leaving the pulp chamber which exit the root at two separate apical foramina.
IV. Type IV: Contains a single canal leaving the pulp chamber, but dividing into two separate canals which exit the root at two separate apical foramina.

▶ **PERMANENT DENTITION**

- See Table 25–1 for a comparison of pulpal morphology of the permanent dentition.

Accessory Pulp Canals

- Found in cervical 1/3 of root and furcations.
- Allow pulp to communicate with PDL space.
- Contains pulpal nervous and vascular tissue.

TABLE 25–1. Comparison of Permanent Teeth

TOOTH	# OF ROOTS	# OF CANALS	SHAPE OF PULP CHAMBER AT CEJ	CROSS SECTION AT LEVEL OF CEJ
Maxilla				
Central incisor	1	1	Triangular	
Lateral incisor	1	1	Egg	
Canine	1	1	Oval	
First premolar	2	2	Kidney*	
Second premolar	1	1	Oval	
First molar	3	3† or 4 (55% 2nd in MB)	Rhomboidal	
Second molar	3	3† or 4 (35% 2nd in MB)	Rhomboidal	
Third molar	3	Variable	Rhomboidal	
Mandible				
Central incisor	1	1	Oval	
Lateral incisor	1	1 or 2 (40% 2nd is lingual)	Oval**	
Canine	1	1	Oval	
First premolar	1	1	Oval§	
Second premolar	1	1	Oval	
First molar	2	3‡ or 4 (25% 2nd in D)	Rectangular	
Second molar	2	3‡ or 4 (8% 2nd in D)	Trapezoidal (tapers distally)	
Third molar	2	Variable	Trapezoidal (tapers distally)	

* Often pinched off creating 2 separate canals: B and P.

** Sometimes pinched off creating 2 separate canals: B and L.

§ Oval, but the roundest of all premolars.

† In general, maxillary molars have at least 3 canals, one in each root: MB, DB, and P.

‡ In general, mandibular molars have 3 canals, two in the M root (MB and ML) and one in the D root.

■ See Table 25–2 for a comparison of pulpal morphology of the primary dentition.

TABLE 25–2. Comparison of Primary Teeth

Tooth	# of Roots	# of Canals	Age at Root Completion (y)
Maxilla			
Central incisor	1	1	1.5
Lateral incisor	1	1	1.5–2
Canine	1	1	2–2.5
First molar	3	3 or 4 (MB root may have 2 canals)	3–3.5
Second molar	3	3 or 4 (MB root may have 2 canals)	3
Mandible			
Central incisor	1	1	1.5
Lateral incisor	1	1	1.5–2
Canine	1	1	2–2.5
First molar	2	4 (2 in each root)	3–3.5
Second molar	2	4 (2 in each root)	3

Comparison to Permanent Teeth (Table 25–3)

TABLE 25–3. Comparison to Permanent Teeth

Tooth Structure	Primary Teeth Are/Have...Compared to Permanent Teeth
Pulp horns	More pointed Extend closer to cusp tips (especially on mesial surfaces)
Pulp chambers	Larger More closely approximate shape of crowns

Calcification and Eruption

Only the permanent incisors, canines, and premolars are succedaneous.

Definitions

- **Succedaneous teeth:** Permanent teeth that occupy positions held by primary teeth.
- **Exfoliation:** Shedding of the primary teeth. This is accomplished partly by the resorption of the deciduous roots by odontoclasts.
- **Mixed dentition:** A dentition having both primary and permanent teeth.
- **Active eruption:** Tooth movement from its germinative position until contact is made with opposing and/or adjacent teeth.
- **Passive eruption:** Tooth exposure secondary to the apical migration of the junctional epithelium.

General Concepts

- Teeth erupt in pairs.
- Girls' teeth erupt before boys' teeth.
- Mandibular teeth generally erupt before maxillary teeth.
- Eruption starts once 50% of root formation is complete.

NUMBER OF TEETH

- 20 total primary teeth (10 per arch).
- There are no premolars.

DENTAL FORMULA

- $I\,^2/_2 + C\,^1/_1 + M\,^2/_2$

ERUPTION SEQUENCE AND TIMING

- Same sequence for both arches (months):

I1	I2	M1	**C**	M2
6	9	12	**18**	24

CALCIFICATION (TABLE 26–1)

TABLE 26-1. Calcification of the Primary Dentition

TOOTH	CALCIFICATION STARTS (MO)	CALCIFICATION ENDS
Central incisor	4–6 in utero	6–10 wk
Lateral incisor	4–6 in utero	10–12 wk
First molar	4–6 in utero	6 mo
Canine	4–6 in utero	9 mo
Second molar	4–6 in utero	10–12 mo

DEVELOPMENT

See Table 26–2.

- Begin to develop at 6 weeks in utero.
- Calcification starts at 4–6 months (18 weeks) in utero (2nd trimester).
- Apices are complete 1–$1\frac{1}{2}$ years after eruption (by age 3).

TABLE 26-2. Tooth Development of the Primary (Deciduous) Dentition

| TOOTH | AGE AT ERUPTION | | AGE AT ROOT COMPLETION (y) | AGE AT EXFOLIATION (y) |
	MANDIBULAR (mo)	MAXILLARY (mo)		
Central incisor	6–10	8–12	$1\frac{1}{2}$	6–7
Lateral incisor	10–16	9–13	$1\frac{1}{2}$–2	7–8
First molar	14–18	13–19	2–$2\frac{2}{2}$	9–11
Canine	17–23	16–22	3–$3\frac{1}{2}$	9–12
Second molar	23–31	25–33	3	10–12

▶ MIXED DENTITION

- Occurs from ages 6 through 12 years.
- Starts: Eruption of the permanent 1st molar.
- Ends: Exfoliation of the primary maxillary canine.
- Permanent incisors often erupt *lingual* to their primary counterparts.
- 24 teeth (12 per arch) once the permanent 1st molars erupt.

▶ PERMANENT DENTITION

NUMBER OF TEETH

- 32 total permanent teeth (16 per arch).

DENTAL FORMULA

- $I\,^2/_2 + C\,^1/_1 + PM\,^2/_2 + M\,^3/_3$

ERUPTION SEQUENCE AND TIMING

- Mandibular arch (years):

M1	I1	I2	C	PM1	PM2	M2	M3
6	6–7	7–8	**9–10**	10–12	11–12	12	17–21

- Maxillary arch (years):

M1	I1	I2	PM1	PM2	C	M2	M3
6	7–8	8–9	10–11	10–12	**11–12**	12	17–21

*Permanent mandibular teeth generally erupt before maxillary teeth, **except** the premolars.*

659

CALCIFICATION (TABLE 26–3)

TABLE 26-3 Calcification of the Permanent Dentition

TOOTH	CALCIFICATION STARTS (YR)	CALCIFICATION ENDS (YR)
First molar	Birth	$2^1/_2$–3
Central incisor	<1	$3^1/_2$
Lateral incisor	<1	4–5
Canine	<1	4–7
First premolar	2	5–6
Second premolar	2	$5^1/_2$–7
Second molar	3	6–8
Third molar	7–9	13–16

DEVELOPMENT

See Table 26–4.

- Begin to develop at 4 months in utero.
- Calcification starts at birth (mandibular 1st molar).
- Apices are complete about $2^1/_2$ years after eruption.

TABLE 26-4. Tooth Development of the Permanent Dentition

TOOTH	AGE AT ERUPTION (y)		AGE AT ROOT COMPLETION (y)
	MANDIBULAR	MAXILLARY	
First molar	6–7	6–7	9–10
Central incisor	6–7	7–8	9–$10^1/_2$
Lateral incisor	7–8	8–9	10–11
Canine	9–10	11–12*	12–14
First premolar	10–12	10–11	12–$13^1/_2$
Second premolar	11–12	10–12	$12^1/_2$–14
Second molar	11–13	12–13	14–15
Third molar	17–21	17–21	18–25

*The maxillary canine is the last succedaneous tooth to erupt.

Occlusion and Function

GENERAL TERMS

- **Occlusion:** The contact relationships of the teeth. The contacts are generally edges or points touching other edges, points, or areas.
- **Functional occlusion:** Occlusion during mandibular movement (mastication, swallowing, etc.).
- **Plane of occlusion:** An imaginary plane anatomically related to the cranium that theoretically touches the incisal edges of incisors and the cusp tips of posterior teeth.
- **Occlusal adjustment (equilibration):** Reshaping the occlusal surfaces of teeth to create harmonious contacts between the maxillary and mandibular teeth.

OCCLUSAL DIMENSIONS

- **Vertical dimension:** A vertical measurement of the face between any two arbitrary points (usually in the midline), one above and one below the mouth.
- **Vertical dimension of occlusion (VDO):** The vertical dimension of the face when the teeth are in centric occlusion.
- **Vertical dimension of rest (VDR):** The vertical dimension of the face when the mandible is in the rest position.

OCCLUSAL CURVATURES

- **Curve of Spee:** The anteroposterior curvature of the maxillary and mandibular occlusal surfaces. Concave above the curve; convex below the curve. (See Figure 27–1.)
- **Curve of Wilson:** The mediolateral curvature of the maxillary and mandibular occlusal surfaces. Concave above the curve; convex below the curve. (See Figure 27–2.)
- **Compensating curve:** The anteroposterior curvature (in the median plane) and the mediolateral curvature (in the frontal plane) in the alignment of the occluding surfaces and incisal edges of *artificial teeth* that are used to develop *balanced occlusion.*

OCCLUSAL CONTACTS

- **Functional contacts:** Contacts made during functional occlusion.
- **Parafunctional contacts:** Abnormal contacts; typically result from habits such as bruxism and include *area-to-area contacts.*

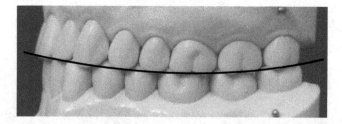

FIGURE 27–1. Curve of Spee.

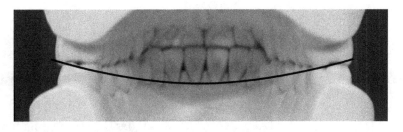

FIGURE 27-2.   Curve of Wilson.

• **Protrusive contacts:** Contacts made when the mandible has moved anteriorly from centric occlusion (protrusive movement). These are usually *edge-to-edge contacts* for anterior teeth.
• **Working side contacts (laterotrusive contacts):** Contacts on the side toward which the mandible has moved from centric occlusion (working side movement).
• **Nonworking side contacts (mediotrusive contacts):** Contacts on the side away from which the mandible has moved from centric occlusion (nonworking side movement).

OCCLUSAL RELATIONSHIPS

• **Overbite:** The *vertical* overlapping of the mandibular incisors by the maxillary incisors when the jaws are in centric occlusion. (See Figure 27–3.)
• **Overjet:** The *horizontal* overlapping of the mandibular incisors by the maxillary incisors when the jaws are in centric occlusion.
• **Open bite:** A condition in which opposing teeth do not occlude.
• **Cross-bite:** An abnormal relation of one or more teeth in one arch to its antagonist in the other arch due to a deviation of tooth or jaw position.
    • **Anterior cross-bite:** One or more maxillary incisors are positioned lingually to the mandibular incisors when in centric occlusion.
    • **Posterior cross-bite:** One or more maxillary posterior teeth are positioned palatally to the mandibular posterior teeth when in centric occlusion.

Occlusal Relationships

FOUR DETERMINANTS OF OCCLUSION

1. The teeth and their occlusal surfaces.
2. The right TMJ.
3. The left TMJ.
4. The neuromusculature of the jaws and TMJs.

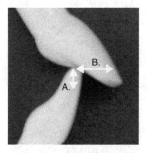

FIGURE 27-3.
Overbite (A) and overjet (B).

In cross-bite occlusions, the working and nonworking cusps are reversed for the affected teeth.

Angle's classification is based on molar and canine relationships.

Chronic thumb sucking can cause:

- *Anterior open bite*
- *Flaring/rotation of maxillary incisors*
- *Crowding of mandibular incisors*
- *Constriction of maxillary arch*
- *High palatal vault*
- *Class II, div I malocclusion*

Angle's Class	Molars	Canines	Characteristics
I (See Figure 27–4)	MB cusp of max M1 occludes with MB groove of mand M1	Max canine occludes between mand canine and PM1	70% of population
II ■ Division I: All max incisors proclined (flared) (See Figure 27–5) ■ Division II: Max centrals retroclined; laterals proclined (See Figure 27–6)	MB cusp of max M1 occludes **mesially** to MB groove of mand M1	Max canine occludes **mesially** to the distal surface of mand canine	25% of population Retrognathic
III (See Figure 27–7)	MB cusp of max M1 occludes **distally** to MB groove of mand M1	Max canine occludes **distally** to the distal surface of mand canine	5% of population Prognathic

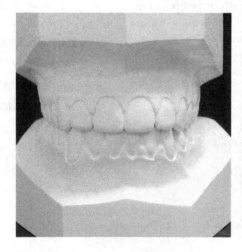
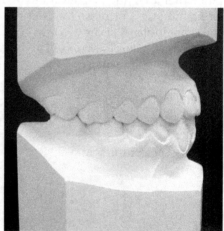

FIGURE 27-4. Class I occlusion.

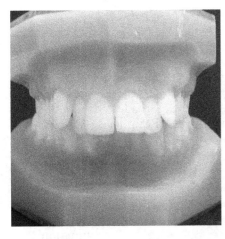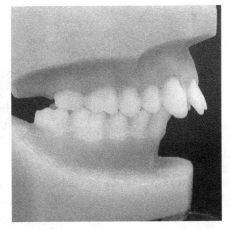

FIGURE 27-5. Class II, division I occlusion.

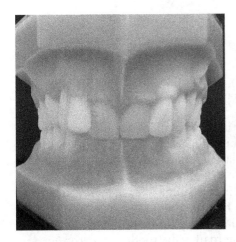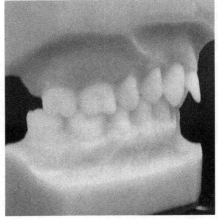

FIGURE 27-6. Class II, division II occlusion.

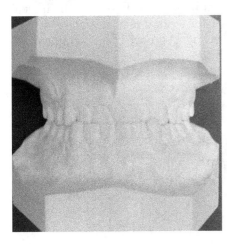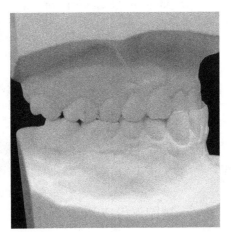

FIGURE 27-7. Class III occlusion.

Cusp Type	Location	Oppose	Shape	Function
Working, supporting, holding	Max lingual Mand buccal	Central fossae Marginal ridges	Broader Rounder	Support vertical dimension of the face
Nonworking, balancing, guiding	Max buccal Mand lingual	Embrasure spaces Grooves	Sharper	Guide movements during function

IDEAL OCCLUSION

See Figure 27–8.

*An **ideal occlusion** is a class I occlusion with a smooth plane of occlusion.*

In ideal CO, every tooth in one arch contacts two teeth in the opposite arch, EXCEPT:

- *Max 3rd molars*
- *Mand central incisors*

- Supporting (lingual) cusps of maxillary posterior teeth occlude with the distal marginal ridge of their mandibular counterpart + the mesial marginal ridge of tooth distal, *except:*
  - ML cusp of molars, which occlude in the central fossa of their counterpart.
- Supporting (buccal) cusps of mandibular posterior teeth occlude with the mesial marginal ridge of their maxillary counterpart + the distal marginal ridge of the tooth mesial, *except:*
  - DB cusp of molars, which occlude in the central fossa of their counterpart,
  - D cusp of M1, which occludes in the triangular fossa of max M1.
- Nonworking (buccal) cusps of maxillary posterior teeth oppose the buccal embrasures of their mandibular counterpart + the tooth distal, *except:*
  - MB cusp of molars, which oppose the buccal groove of their counterpart,
  - DB cusp + oblique ridge of M1, which oppose the DB groove of mand M1.
- Nonworking (lingual) cusps of mandibular posterior teeth oppose the lingual embrasures of the maxillary counterpart + the tooth mesial, *except:*
  - DL cusp of molars, which oppose the lingual groove of their counterpart,
  - L cusp of PM1, which opposes nothing.

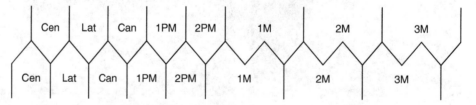

FIGURE 27-8. Ideal occlusion.

Factors of Mandibular Movement

1. Initiating position:
   - CR: Most stable and reproducible position
2. Two types of motion:
   - Rotation
   - Translation
3. Three directions of movement:
   - Frontal
   - Sagittal
   - Horizontal
4. Degree of movement
5. Clinical significance of movements

The mandible acts as a class III lever.

Mandibular Positions

- **Centric occlusion (CO):** The maximum intercuspation of the opposing arches. It is a purely *tooth-guided* position. This creates the **vertical dimension of occlusion (VDO).**
- **Centric relation (CR):** The most anterior and superior position of the mandibular condyles within the glenoid fossae (**terminal hinge position**). By maintaining this position, only rotational movements around a horizontal (hinge) axis can occur. It is a purely *ligament-guided* position.
- **Rest (postural) position (RP):** The position of the mandible when it is in a physiologic rest position. There are no tooth contacts in this position; it is a purely *muscle-guided* position. This creates the **vertical dimension of rest (VDR).** The resulting space between the teeth in this position (about 1–3 mm) is called the **freeway space (FS).**
- **Maximum opening (MO):** The maximum separation of the opposing arches. Creates the greatest amount of space between the teeth (about 40–50 mm).

VDR = VDO + FS

During the act of swallowing, the mandible meets the maxilla in centric occlusion and the tongue touches the palate.

Posselt's Envelope of Motion

See Figure 27–9.

- Sagittal plane
- Horizontal plane
- Frontal (coronal) plane

*Posselt's envelope of motion illustrates the range of motion of the mandible in **three** planes.*

Mandibular Movement and Guidance

- **Protrusive movement:** The anterior movement of the mandible. As the mandible moves anteriorly, the posterior teeth disarticulate. This is known as **anterior guidance.** The maximum posterior disarticulation occurs when the anterior teeth are edge-to-edge. Anterior guidance depends largely on the horizontal and vertical relationship of the maxillary and mandibular incisors and canines. Cusp length varies on the extent of this relationship.
- **Lateral movement:** The lateral movement of the mandible. The side toward which the mandible moves is the **working side;** the side away from which the mandible moves is the **nonworking side.** Lateral movements occur via two types of guidance:

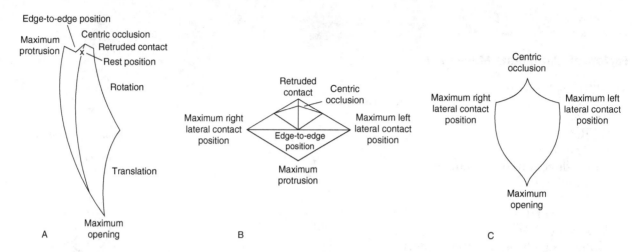

FIGURE 27–9. Three planes of Posselt's envelope of motion.

A. Sagittal; B. Horizontal; C. Frontal.

Mastication involves:

- *Incision: incisors*
- *Prehension: canines*
- *Trituration: premolars + molars*

- **Canine guidance:** The contact between the opposing canines on the working side disarticulates all posterior teeth. Any premature contacts on the working or nonworking sides are working and nonworking interferences, respectively.
- **Group function:** The contact between the opposing canines and posterior teeth on the working side disarticulates the posterior teeth on the nonworking side. Any contacts on the nonworking side are nonworking interferences.

Effects of Occlusal Relationships on Cusp Height

Occlusal Relationship	If...	Then...
Articular eminence	Steeper eminence	Taller cusps
Anterior guidance	Increased overbite Increased overjet	Taller cusps Shorter cusps
Curve of Spee	More concave curve	Shorter cusps
Lateral movement	Greater movement More superior movement of rotating condyle Greater Bennett shift	Shorter cusps

Eliminating nonworking contacts is important because:

- *They are damaging*
- *They are difficult to control due to mandibular flexure*
- *They deliver more force than other contacts*

Occlusal Interferences

- **Occlusal interference:** Any contact that inhibits the remaining occlusal surfaces from achieving harmonious contacts.
- **Protrusive interference:** Premature contact between the mesial aspects of mandibular posterior teeth and the distal aspects of maxillary posterior teeth.
- **Working interference:** Premature contact on the working side during lateral mandibular movement.
- **Nonworking interference:** Premature contact on the nonworking side during lateral mandibular movement.

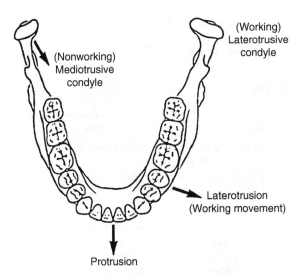

FIGURE 27-10. Condylar movements.

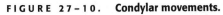

Reprinted, with permission, from Carranza FA. *Clinical Periodontology*, 8th ed., page 176, copyright 1996 by Elsevier.

Condylar Movements

See Figure 27–10.

- **Protrusive movement:** Both right and left condyles rotate and translate anteriorly simultaneously (downward along the articular eminence).
- **Right working movement:** The left condyle rotates and translates anteriorly (downward along the articular eminence) and medially (to the right). The right condyle rotates forward and translates slightly laterally (to the right).
- **Left working movement:** The right condyle rotates and translates anteriorly (downward along the articular eminence) and medially (to the left). The left condyle rotates forward and translates slightly laterally (to the left).

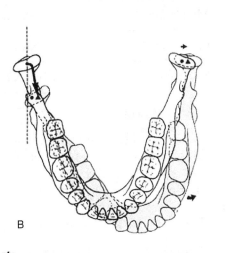

FIGURE 27-11. Lateral condylar movements.

A. Pure left lateral rotation. B. Left lateral movement incorporating a Bennett shift. Reprinted, with permission, from Carranza FA. *Clinical Periodontology*, 8th ed., page 177, copyright 1996 by Elsevier.

Occlusal Musculature and Ligaments

See Chapter 1 for details of oral musculature.

MUSCLES OF MASTICATION

*The **buccinator** is considered the accessory muscle of mastication. It compresses the cheeks, holding food in.*

Empty mouth swallowing occurs throughout the day:
- *Mandible braces in intercuspal position*
- *Masseters contract*
- *Tip of tongue touches palate*

Muscle	Action on Mandible	Excursive Movement	Innervation
Temporalis	Elevation Retrusion	Ipsilateral	CN V3
Masseter	Elevation Retrusion	Ipsilateral	CN V3
Medial pterygoid	Elevation Protrusion	Contralateral	CN V3
Lateral pterygoid	Depression Protrusion (when both contract)	Contralateral	CN V3

SUPRAHYOID MUSCLES

- Elevate the hyoid, especially during swallowing
- Assist in depression of mandible

The suprahyoid muscles generally act to elevate the hyoid, especially during swallowing.

Muscle	Function	Innervation
Digastric (anterior)	Elevates hyoid	CN V3
Digastric (posterior)	Elevates hyoid	CN VII
Mylohyoid	Elevates hyoid, FOM	CN V3
Geniohyoid	Elevates hyoid	C1 fibers via CN XII
Stylohyoid	Elevates hyoid	CN VII

INFRAHYOID MUSCLES

Tooth-tooth contacts are of longer duration during swallowing than during mastication.

- Depress the hyoid and larynx, especially after swallowing
- Assist in depression of mandible

Muscle	Function	Innervation
Omohyoid	Depresses hyoid + larynx	Ansa cervicalis
Sternohyoid	Depresses hyoid + larynx	Ansa cervicalis
Sternothyroid	Depresses larynx	Ansa cervicalis
Thyrohyoid	Depresses hyoid	C1 fibers via CN XII

EXTRINSIC MUSCLES OF THE TONGUE

▪ Move the tongue bodily

Muscle	Action on Tongue	Innervation
Genioglossus	Protrusion	CN XII
Hyoglossus	Depression	CN XII
Styloglossus	Elevation Retrusion	CN XII
Palatoglossus	Elevation (posterior tongue) Closes oropharyngeal isthmus	CN X (pharyngeal plexus)

If the hypoglossal nerve becomes paralyzed or injured, the tongue will always deviate to the same side as the muscle injury.

INTRINSIC MUSCLES OF THE TONGUE

▪ Change shape of tongue

Muscle	Action on Tongue	Innervation
Longitudinal	Shortens, curls tip	CN XII
Transverse	Narrows	CN XII
Vertical	Flattens, broadens	CN XII

LIGAMENTS

Ligament	Location	Function
Temporomandibular (Lateral)	Articular eminence (lateral aspect) of zygomatic process → condyle of mandible (posterior aspect)	Prevents posterior and inferior displacement of condyle Provides direct support to TMJ capsule
Sphenomandibular	Spine of sphenoid bone → lingula of mandible	Accessory ligament
Stylomandibular	Styloid process of temporal bone → angle of mandible	Accessory ligament

Tooth Anomalies

Size

- **Microdontia:** Having one or more teeth that are smaller than normal.
- **Macrodontia:** Having one or more teeth that are larger than normal.

The most common

congenitally missing teeth:

- *3rd molars*
- *Maxillary lateral incisors*
- *Second premolars*

Number

- **Complete anodontia:** Congenital absence of teeth; generally due to developmental abnormalities such as ectodermal dysplasia.
- **Partial anodontia:** Congenital absence of one or more teeth.
  - **Hypodontia:** Congenital absence of a few teeth.
  - **Oligodontia:** Congenital absence of a large number of teeth.
- **Supernumerary teeth:** Teeth in excess of the normal number. Most common in maxilla.
- **Mesiodens:** A supernumerary tooth located between the maxillary central incisors.

Morphology

- **Ankylosis:** Fusion of the tooth and alveolar bone.
- **Dilaceration:** A bend in the root of a tooth.
- **Taurodontism:** A molar with an elongated root trunk. Generally occurs in patients with amelogenesis imperfecta, Klinefelter's syndrome, or Down's syndrome.
- **Dens invaginatus (dens in dente):** Developmental abnormality of *maxillary lateral incisors* in which the focal crown is invaginated for various distances.
- **Dens evaginatus:** Developmental abnormality in which a focal portion of the crown projects outward, creating an extra cusp. A prominent dens evaginatus often seen on *maxillary lateral incisors* is called a **talon cusp.** (See Figure 28–1.)
- **Hypercementosis:** Excessive deposition of cementum.

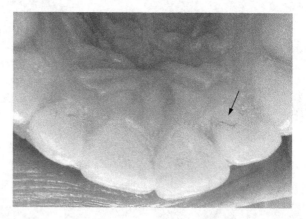

FIGURE 28–1.   Talon cusp.

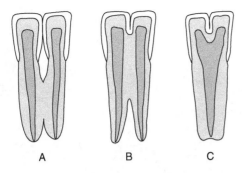

FIGURE 28-2. (A) Concrescence, (B) fusion, and (C) gemination.

- **Cervical enamel projection:** An apical extension of enamel usually located at furcation entrances on molar teeth.
- **Enamel pearl:** A small, focal mass of enamel formed apical to the CEJ.
- **Concrescence:** Fusion of two completely formed teeth at their roots; must have *confluent cementum*.
- **Fusion:** Fusion of two unique tooth buds; must have *confluent dentin*. Its severity depends on the stage of tooth development at which the fusion occurs.
- **Gemination:** Development of two crowns from one tooth bud; *share a single root and root canal.* (See Figure 28–2.)

▶ **ACQUIRED ANOMALIES**

Dental Injuries

Acquired Dental Injuries

Acquired Injury	Definition	Common Cause
Attrition	Loss of tooth structure due to physiologic *tooth-to-tooth contact*, creating **wear facets**	Parafunction (bruxism)
Abrasion	Loss of tooth structure due to abnormal *mechanical* means	Overzealous use of oral hygiene aids Detrimental oral habits (fingernail biting)
Erosion	Loss of tooth structure due to abnormal *chemical means*	Consumption of acidic foods and drinks (facial/ buccal surfaces) Bulimia, GERD (lingual/ palatal surfaces)
Abfraction	Loss of tooth structure due to abnormal *mechanical stresses*	Occlusal trauma Parafunction (bruxism)

Wear facets usually develop at:

- *L-I edge of max. centrals and canines*
- *F-I edge of mand. canines*

INDEX

Note: Page numbers followed by *f*, *t*, and *b* indicate figures, tables, and boxes, respectively.

A

A band, skeletal muscle and, 339, 339*b*
A fibers, 171
α-Amylase, 259
α-globulins, function of, 269
α-ketoacids, oxidative deamination and, 287
abdomen, 81–86
  regions of, 83
abdominal aorta, 92, 94
abdominal muscles, 84
abdominal viscera, 86–110, 143
  pelvic splanchnic nerves and, 143
abducens nerve (CN VI), 24, 121–124, 122*f*
  pituitary tumor and, 25
abfraction, 675
ABO blood typing, 522
abrasion, 675
abscess, 444
  acute inflammation and, 503
absolute refractory period, 321
  heart and, 358, 359*f*
absorption, and digestion, 401–402
acanthosis nigricans, 536
accessory canals, 207
accessory hemiazygos vein (superior
    hemiazygos vein), 95
accessory muscles, 371
accessory nerve (CN XI-accessory),
    schematic illustration, 143*f*
accessory pulp canals, 654
accommodation, pupillary light reflex and,
    124
acetone, ketone bodies and, 286
acetylcholine metabolism, 327
acetyl-CoA fate, metabolic fates of, 286
ACh metabolism, enzymes in, 327*b*
achalasia, 557
achlorhydria, pernicious anemia and, 571
achondroplasia (dwarfism), 471, 590
acid–base balance, 387–388
  control of, 388
  respiratory changes and, 380
acidophiles, 454
acquired dental injuries, 675
acquired immunity, 510
  classification of, 510
acral lentiginous melanoma, 613
acrochordon, 611
acromegaly, 421, 579–580
  GH and, 580
acrosome, egg fertilization and, 220
ACTH, negative feedback loop and,
    427

actin, 157, 338
  skeletal muscle contraction and, 340,
    340*f*
Actinomyces species
  root caries and, 492*b*
action potential, 321
  of cardiac muscle, 343
activation energy, 253
  reaction rate, 253, 254*t*
active cells, 156
active eruption, 658
active immunity, 464, 510
  viruses and, 480
acute gouty arthritis, 593
acute hypocalcemia, Chvostek's sign and,
    583
acute infection, 444
acute inflammation
  chronic inflammation v., 504
  signs of, 503*b*
  stages of, 503, 503*t*
acute leukemias, 619–620
acute lymphoblastic leukemia (ALL), 606
acute myelogenous leukemia (AML), 619
acute nephritic syndrome, 568
acute osteomyelitis, 591–592
acute pancreatitis, 561
acute pericarditis, 544
Addison's disease, 429–430, 437, 584–585
  cortisol and, 584
  hyperpigmentation, 533
  oral signs of, 584*b*
adenine, 292*b*
adenocarcinoma, 603, 614, 615
  prostate cancer and, 608
  smoking and, 614*b*
adenohypophysis, 177
adenoma, 604
adenomatous polyps, colorectal cancer, 616
adenovirus, 476*t*
adenylate cyclase, 416
ADH. *See* antidiuretic hormone
adipose tissue, lipids and, 275
adjuvants
  immunity and, 511
  vaccines and, 480
ADP-riboslation exotoxins, host tissue
    destruction and, 451*t*
adrenal cortex, 107, 431*f*, 437*f*, 584–585,
    584*b*
  aldosterone and, 437
  atrophy of, ACTH and, 428
  histologic layers, 427*b*

precocious puberty, 424
  zones of, 179*b*
adrenal glands, 107, 179, 584–585
  neoplasia of, 625–626
adrenal hormones, 415
adrenal insufficiency, 428
adrenal medulla, 107, 430, 431*f*
  tumors of, 625
adrenal–ACTH axis, exogenous cortisol
    and, 428
adrenergic agonists, 431
adrenergic neurons, 311
adrenergic receptors, 313
adult periodontitis, 492
adult polycystic kidney disease (APCKD),
    566
adults, brain tumors, 609
aerotolerant anaerobic, bacteria, 454
afferent nerves, 338
aflatoxins, 482
afterload, 354
ageusia, 333
aggressive periodontitis
  characteristics of, 493
  classification, 493
  microbial flora in, 493
aging
  cementum and, 210
  dentin and, 204
  enamel matrix and, 207
  PDL and, 214
  presbycusis and, 138–139
  pulp and, 209
agranular leukocytes, 513
agranulocytes, 172
air embolism, 539
airway, CN XII paralysis and, 143
airway obstruction, mechanisms of, 551*b*
Albers–Schonberg disease, 590
albinism, 533
albumin, function of, 269
albuterol, asthma and, 550
alcoholism, lung abscess and, 555, 555*b*
aldoses, 258*f*
aldosterone (mineralocorticoid), 437
  kidney function and, 394
alkaline phosphatase
  bone formation and, 589
  bone mineralization and, 166
alkaliphiles, 454
ALL (acute lymphoblastic leukemia), 606
allantois, formation, 224
allergic response, fungi and, 482

cholesterol
derivatives of steroid hormones, 415
membranes and, 303
as steroid, 273
synthesis, liver and, 403–404
cholesterolosis, 561
choline, 273
choline deficiency, 273
cholinergic neurons, 311
chondroblasts, 164
chondrocytes, 164
chondrosarcoma, 627
chorda tympani nerve
components of, 31
course of, 31
lingual nerve and, 128
chordoma, 628
choristoma, 536, 604
choroid, 192
choroid plexus, intracranial pressure and, 25
Christmas disease, 577
chromatin, 157, 296
DNA, 295
chromosomal disorders, 531, 531*b*
chronic bronchitis, 552
chronic hyperplastic candidiasis, 494
chronic infection, 444
chronic inflammation
acute inflammation and, 503, 504
stages of, 504
chronic leukemias, 620–621
chronic lymphocytic lymphoma (CLL), 619, 623
chronic myelogenous leukemia (CML), 621
chronic nephrotic syndrome, 568
chronic obstructive pulmonary disease (COPD), 550–552
hypoxemia in, 377
chronic osteomyelitis, 592
chronic pancreatitis, 561
chronic pericarditis, 544
chronic periodontitis
characteristics, 493
predominant microbial flora in, 493
Chvostek's sign, tetany, 583
chylomicrons, 402
chyme, 400
segmentation, 400–401
cigarette smoking
adenocarcinoma, 614*b*
COPD and, 550
emphysema and, 551
lung cancers and, 615
related diseases, 551*b*
cilia, 157
ciliary body, 192
of eyeball, 328
ciliary zone, 193*f*
cingulum, 632
circle of Willis, 27, 28*f*
arteries of brainstem and, 28*f*
of brainstem, 28*f*
middle cerebral artery v., 29
circuit, pulmonary circulation, systemic circulation v., 351

circulation, blood vessels in, arrangement of, 173
circumferential fibers, 201
circumpulpal dentin, 203
formation, 203
circumvallate papillae, 32, 333
cirrhosis
edema and, 537
proteins and, 367
cirrhosis (of liver), 562
cisterna chyli, 98
citrate–malate shuttle, fatty acid synthesis, 285
citric acid cycle, 282, 283*f*, 287*f*
clarithromycin, 469*t*
class I MHC surface proteins, nucleated cells and, 511
class II MHC proteins, immune system and, 514
classic hemophilia, 577
clavicle, 81
cleavage stages, morula and blastula embryology and, 223*f*
cleft lip, 241*f*–242*f*, 244
cleft palate, 243–244
climbing fibers, 112
clindamycin, 465*t*, 467, 469*t*
clinical crown, 632
CLL (chronic lymphocytic lymphoma), 619, 623
clonal selection, 512
Clostridium, 454
clotting factors, liver and, 577
CML (chronic myelogenous leukemia), 621
CN I (olfactory nerve), 17
CN II (optic nerve), 120–121, 121*f*
CN III injury, lesions and, 124
CN IX. *See* glossopharyngeal nerve
CN V. *See* trigeminal nerve
CN VI. *See* abducens nerve
CN VII (orbicularis oculi), 131*b*
CN VIII. *See* vestibulococholear nerve
CN X. *See* vagus nerve
CN XI-accessory, 143*f*
CN XII. *See* hypoglossus nerve
CNs (central nerves), taste sensation, tongue and, 30
CNS. *See* central nervous system
CO. *See* centric occlusion; *See* cardiac output
CO₂. *See* carbon dioxide
coagulase, 450
coagulation, intrinsic and extrinsic pathways, 367, 367*f*
coagulation factor XII (Hageman factor), 507
coagulation factors, 367
coagulative necrosis, 502
coal workers pneumoconiosis, 553
codons, 298
coenzyme, 251
coenzyme A, in fatty acid synthesis and catabolism, 285
coenzyme Q, ubiquinone as, 284
cold caloric test, 139, 139*b*
collagen, 165
structure, 267*f*

synthesis, 267*f*, 268
type I, dentogingival connective tissue and, 200
type II, 164
types of, 268
collagen remodeling, wound repair and, 508
collagen vascular diseases, 585–587, 585*b*
types, 594*b*
collagenases (metalloproteinases), host tissue destruction and, 450
collapsing forces, lung and, 371
colloid osmotic pressure (oncotic pressure), 385
colon
blood supply and description, 106
GI cancer and, 616
colon polyps, 617
colony stimulating factors (CSFs), 505, 505*t*–506*t*
colorectal cancer, 616–617
columnar epithelial cells, 161
commensalism, 444
common bile duct, 104
choledocholithiasis and, 561
common carotid, 93
common central vein, 103
common facial vein, 69
common iliac artery
pelvic kidney and, 96
ureter and, 108
common variable immunodeficiency (CVID), 522*t*
communicating–obstruction, in subarachnoid space, 26*b*
compensating curve, 662
compensatory hypertrophy, cardiac demand and, 343
competitive inhibition, 254, 254*f*, 304
complement protein system, 517*f*
complement proteins, 515–518
activation, pathways of, 516*t*
function of, 269, 517*t*
complete anodontia, 674
complete bilateral cleft, 244
complex carbohydrates, 263
compliance
pulmonary circulation, systemic circulation v., 351
venus return and, 355
compound nevus, 609
concrescence, 675, 675*f*
concussion, 595
condensing osteitis, 592
conducting zone, lung and, 372
conduction velocity, 324*b*
conductive loss, 139
condylar movements, 669, 669*f*
condyle, 20
of mandible, 50
cones, 194, 329
confluent cementum, concrescence and, 675, 675*f*
congenital syphilis, enamel and, 207
congestion (hyperemia), 538
congestive heart failure (CHF), edema and, 537

dermatopathology, 533–536
dermis, 191
descending colon, 105
descending motor tracts
       (efferent/descending pathways), 319
desmin, 157
desmoplasia, 603
desmosome (macula adherens), 158
  cardiac muscle and, 343
detoxification, 103
developmental groove, 634
developmental pathology, 530–533
dextran, 262
dextrins, 259
D-form isomerism, monosaccharides,
       258
ΔG. *See* Gibbs free energy change
diabetes insipidus, 427, 578
  causes of, 420
  diabetes mellitus v., 420
diabetes mellitus, 427
  pancreas and, 427
  type 1, 578–579
     v. diabetes type 2, 579
diabetic coma, 286
diapedesis, 514*t*
diaphragm muscles, 82, 98
diaphragma sella, 22
diarrhea, clindamycin and, 467
diarthrosis, 167
diastema, 634
diastole
  cardiac cycle and, 356
  fibrous pericardium and, 353*b*
diastolic pressure, 352
DIC. *See* disseminated intravascular
       coagulation
dicloxacillin, 466
  impetigo and, 534
diencephalon, 112, 307. *See also* posterior
       pituitary
diffuse lymphocytic lymphoma, 623
DiGeorge's syndrome, 523*t*
  hypoparathyroidism and, 583
digestion, absorption and, components,
       401–402
dilaceration, teeth and, 674
Dilantin (phenytoin), gingival overgrowth
       and, 499*b*
dimorphism, molds and, 482
diphtheria toxin, host tissue destruction and,
       451*t*
diphyodont dentition, 632
diploic veins, 24
dipolar ions (Zwitterions), 388
disaccharide absorption, 401
disaccharides, 258
disease. *See specific type disease i.e.*
       degenerative diseases
disinfectants, 446, 446*t*
disinfection, 446
disseminated intravascular coagulation (DIC)
  causes, 576
  laboratory indications, 576
  platelet disorders and, 575
disulfide bonds, 265
  immunoglobulins and, 515

DNA
  backbone structure of, 294*f*
  base pairing and, 292–293, 292*f*
  gyrase, DNA synthesis and, 297
  ligases, 299
     DNA synthesis and, 297, 297*f*
  metronidazole and, 467
  organization, 295–296, 296*f*
  polymerase, 299
     DNA synthesis and, 297, 297*f*
  synthesis, 296–297, 297*f*
  transduction and, 450*t*
  transfer, bacteria and, 449
  transformation and, 450*t*
  viruses, 470
     viral replication and, 471
domains, protein structures and, 267
dorsal column system, pathway, 317
dorsal root ganglion, afferent/sensory nerves
       and, 146
dorsal scapular artery, 77*f*
Down syndrome, 531
  chromosomal disorders and, 531*b*
drug-induced
  aplastic anemia, 571
  lupus erythematosus, 585
drugs
  antiviral, 480
  teratogenesis and, 530
duct of Wirsung, 107
ductus deferens, 110
duodenal ulcer, 558
duodenum, 93, 182
  blood supply and description of, 105
dura mater, dural folds of, 22, 23*f*
dural folds, of dura mater, 22, 23*f*
dural sinuses, 23*f*
  list of, 23
  tributaries of, 24
dust cells, 181, 513
dwarfism, 421, 590
dysarthria, hypoglossus nerve and, 143
dysgeusia, 333
dysosmia, 335
dysplasia, 601
dysplastic nevus, 610
dyspnea, 382
dystrophic calcifications, 209

E
ear, anatomy, 137–138, 138*f*, 331
early-onset periodontitis, 493
Eaton–Lambert syndrome, 597*b*
eburnation, osteoarthritis and, 593
ecchymoses, petechiae v., 576
eclampsia, secondary hypertension and,
       542, 542*b*
ECM (extracellular matrix), 164–165
ectomesenchyme, tooth type and, 216
edemas, 386–387, 504, 536–537
  cause of, 386, 537
  clinical exam of, 537
  nephrotic syndrome and, 537
  types of, 536–537
Edward syndrome, 531
  chromosomal disorders and, 531*b*
EFC. *See* extracellular fluids

effective renal plasma flow (ERPF), 393
efferent nerves, 338
efferent pathways (descending motor tracts),
       319
egg, stages of meiosis in, 219*f*
eggshell calcification, 501*b*
eicosanoids, 273–274
ejaculatory duct, 110
ejection fraction, 353
elastic arteries, 174
elastic cartilage, 165
elastin, hydroxylysine and, 268
electrical synapse, 170, 325, 326
electrocardiogram (ECG), 360–361
  leads, 360
  waves, 361, 361*f*
electron transport chain, 282–283, 283*f*
elephantiasis, edema and, 537
Embden–Meyerhof pathway, 280–281
embolus, 539–540
embrasures, 634, 639
embryo development
  pituitary gland, 418, 418*f*
  week 1, 222*f*
  week 4, 229*b*
embryology, 219–246
  brain, 230
  of face, 236–246
  forebrain, 230
  gametogenesis, 219–228, 219*f*–221*f*
  heart, 233*f*
  kidney, stages of, 235*f*
  pancreas, 236*f*
  patent foramen ovale, 231*b*
  of pharyngeal arches, 236–246
  of renal system, 234–236, 235*f*, 236*f*
  tongue and, 30
embryonic body axis, 225–228, 226*f*
emissary veins, 24
emphysema
  problems with, 552*b*
  types of, 551
empty mouth swallowing, 670
enamel
  aging effects on, 207
  amelogenesis of, 205–206
  cross-striations and incremental lines, 206
  deformities of, 207
  formation, 206*f*, 217*b*
enamel hypoplasia, 207
enamel knot, 217
enamel matrix formation, defect, 207
enamel maturation defect, 207
enamel organ, 216
enamel pearl, 675
enamel surface depression, 634
enamel surface elevations, 632
enamel surface junctions, 634
encapsulated joint receptors, types
       of, 315*b*
endemic infection, 443
endocarditis, 544–545
  types of, 545
endocardium, 174
endochondral ossification, 166
endocrine disorders, secondary hypertension
       and, 542

endocrine glands, 177–179, 186
  function and excretions of, 163
endocrine pancreas, 186
endocrine pathology, 578–585
endogenous pigments, 500
  comparison of, 500t
endomysium, CT and, 340
endopeptidases, 268
endosomes, 157
endosteum, 167
endothelium, 161
endotoxin
  host tissue destruction and, 451, 451t
  mode of action, 452t
  structure, 452f
  v. exotoxin, 451t
end-stage kidney disease, APCKD, 566
enolase, fluoride and, 281
enteric nervous system, 398
entero gastrone, 398–399
enterogastric reflex, 398b
enterohepatic circulation, lipoproteins and, 275
enteroviruses, 471
Entner–Doudoroff pathway, 289
envelope, viruses and, 470
enzymatic cellular degradation, 500
enzyme(s), 250–256
  in ACh metabolism, 327b
  biomechanics, induced-fit model, 251–252, 252f
  classification of, 251
  concentration, reaction rate influencing factors, 254t
  definitions, 251
  digestion and absorption, 401
  host tissue destruction and, 450–451
  inhibition, 254–255
  in intestinal villi, 105b
  kinetics, 252–254
    ΔG and, 252–253, 253t
    reaction equilibrium, 253
    reaction rate, 253
  rate-limiting, 279t
  regulation of, 186
    covalent modification and, 255
  triglycerides and, digestion and, 402
enzyme inhibition, 254–255
  competitive, 254, 254f
  irreversible, 255
  noncompetitive, 255, 255f
  uncompetitive, 255
enzyme kinetics, 252–254. See also enzymes
  Gibbs free energy change (ΔG), 252–253, 253t
  substrate concentration, 252, 253f
enzyme mechanics, 251–252, 252f
enzyme regulation, 255–256
  allosteric regulation, 256
  covalent modification, 255
  protease activity, 256, 256f
eosinophilia, parasitic infections and, 505
eosinophilic granuloma, clinical symptoms, 625
eosinophils, 514

ependymal cells
  cerebrospinal fluid and, 26
  ventricular system and, 25
ependymoma, 609
epidemic infection, 443
epidermal cells, specialized, 191
epidermal layers, of skin, mnemonic for, 191
epidermis, 191
epididymis, 189
  sperm and, 222
epidural hematoma, 22b, 595
epiglottis, 73
epilepsy, 596
epimysium, CT and, 340
epinephrine, 313, 431
  adrenal medulla and, 266
  asthma and, 550
  gluconeogenesis and, 285
  smooth muscle and, 343
  status asthmaticus and, 550b
epiploic foramen of Winslow, 99b
epistaxis (nosebleed), 66
  Kiesselbach's plexus and, 18
epitactic concept, in calculus formation, 491
epithalamus, 112
epithelial cells
  of alveolar wall, 373
  lining microvilli, 182
  specialized, 196
epithelial intercellular junctions, 159f
epithelial malignant tumor, 611
epithelial migration, wound repair and, 507
epithelial rests of Malassez, 212
  root formation and, 218, 218f
epithelial rests of Serres, 217
epithelial types, 160t
epithelium, 160–161
epitope, immunity and, 510
ergosterol
  fungal cell membranes and, 482
  fungi cells and, 482
erosion, 675
ERPF (effective renal plasma flow), 393
ERV (expiratory reserve volume), 370, 370f
erythema multiforme, 525t, 535
erythematous candidiasis, 494
erythroblastosis fetalis, 569–570
erythrocytes, 172
  and polycythemia, 573–574
  red pulp and, 176
erythrogenic toxin, host tissue destruction and, 451t
erythromycin, 467
  impetigo and, 534
erythropoietin, 366, 436, 573
  kidney and, 574
  polycythemia, 574
Escherichia coli, sepsis and, 444
esophageal cancer, 615
esophageal plexus, vagus nerves and, 141
esophageal ulcers, 558
esophageal varices, hematemesis and, 563
esophagus, 101, 181
  disorders of, 556–558
estradiol, hCG and, 425
estrogens, 422, 423

ethanol metabolism, 405
ethmoid bones, 6
  components and functions of, 12
ethmoid sinuses, 18
  location of drainage, 19
euchromatin, 157
eukaryotic cells, 80s ribosomes and, 297
eustachian tube, 138
EV (residual volume), 370, 370f
Ewing's sarcoma, 627–628
excitable cells, 322b
excitatory neurotransmitters, 323
excretion rate, 394
exercise, physiologic response to, 364
exfoliatin, host tissue destruction and, 451, 451t
exfoliation, 658
exocrine glands
  classification of, 163, 164f
  function and excretions of, 163
exocrine pancreas, 186, 402
exogenous cortisol, adrenal-ACTH axis and, 428
exonuclease, 299
  DNA synthesis and, 297
exotoxins
  classification of, 451t
  mode of action, 451t
  v. endotoxin, 451t
expanding forces, lung and, 371
expiration, lung mechanics and, 371
expiratory reserve volume (ERV), lung volumes, 370, 370f
external basal lamina, 200
external capsule, of spleen, 176
external carotid artery, 65–69, 65f
  branches of, mnemonic for, 66
  course of, 65
  supply, 66
external ear, 137, 138f
  anatomy, 331
  innervation of, 63, 131f
  sensation of, nerves for, 131
external jugular vein, 68–69
external nose, 20, 20f
external oblique fibers, 84
external thorax, 81–86
exteroreceptors, CNS and, 315
extracellular fluids (EFC), 384
  expansion, edema and, 386
extracellular matrix (ECM), cartilage, 164–165
extracellular spaces, paracrine glands, 163
extrafusal fibers, 341
extraocular movements, muscles and nerves in, 121
extrapyramidal system, 319
extra-testicular duct system, 189
extrinsic asthma, 549
extrinsic muscles of tongue, 671
exudate, 504
exudate edema, 536
eye, 192–194
  layers, 192
  ophthalmic artery and, 12
  structures, 193f
eye chambers, 192

guanine, 292*b*
　cytosine and, 292*b*
Guillain-Barré syndrome, 597
gustatory nucleus, 134
gut-associated lymphatic tissue (GALT), 184
GVE (general visceral efferent) motor
　　system, 149

H

H band, skeletal muscle and, 339, 339*b*
H₁ receptors, type I hypersensitivity and,
　266
H₂ receptors, pepsin secretion, 266
Haberman's disease, 625
Hageman factor (factor XII), 507
hair, 192
hair cells, 316
hair follicle receptors, 315
Haldane effect, 374–375
haloenzyme, 251
hamartoma, 536, 604
Hand–Schuller–Christian disease, clinical
　　symptoms, 625
handwashing, infection control and, 448
hapten, immunity and, 510
hard palate, 16
　composition of, 37
　lateral, 17*f*
Hashimoto's thyroiditis, 434, 580, 581
haustra, 106, 183
Haversian canal, 166
Haversian systems, 166
HbA1c (glycosylated Hb), 578, 580*b*
HBV. *See* hepatitis B virus
hCG (human chorionic gonadotropin), 425
HCL, as gastric secretion, 399
HCT (hematocrit), 171, 347, 364
HCV. *See* hepatitis C virus
head and neck
　arteries of, 65*f*
　sympathetic ganglia, 313
　vagus nerve branches in, 116*t*–120*t*, 141,
　　142*f*
　veins of, 68*f*
head, cranial anatomy and osteology of,
　　6–29
head injury
　diabetes insipidus and, 578
　symptoms, 595*b*
hearing, 331–332
　cranial nerve sensory nuclei and, 114
　hair cells and, 316
hearing loss, 138–139
hearing pathway, 332
heart
　autonomic control of, 362
　electrical conduction of, 358, 359*f*
　great vessels and, 88–89, 88*f*
　hypoxia and, 498*b*
　Laplace's law in, 349
　layers of, 174
　receptors, 362
heart attack, atherosclerosis and, 541*b*
heart embryology, 233*f*
heart failure, 547–548
　pulmonary edema from, 549*b*
　signs and symptoms of, 548, 548*b*

heart murmurs, with valvular disease, 358
heart rate (HR)
　CO and, 353
　and contractility, 354
heart valves, 89
heat loss, ANS and, 308
heat regulation, ANS and, 308–309
heat transfer, ANS and, 309
heat-labile toxin, host tissue destruction
　　and, 451*t*
heavy polypeptide chains, 515
Heberden's nodes, osteoarthritis and, 593
heights of contour (HOC), teeth and, 640
helical amylose, starch, 259
helicase, DNA synthesis and, 296
helminths. *See* metazoa
hemagglutination, ABO blood typing and,
　522
hemagglutinin, influenza virus and, 473
hemangioma, 536
hematemesis, 559
　esophageal varices and, 563
hematocrit (HCT), 171, 347, 364
hematopoiesis, 169*f*, 172, 173*f*
hematopoietic cell damage, 571
hematuria, 565
heme, structure, 270, 270*f*
hemiazygos vein (inferior hemiazygos vein),
　95
hemidesmosome, 159
hemochromatosis, 501*t*
hemoglobin, 269, 373–378
　concentration, 365, 375
　myoglobin v., 270, 270*t*
　oxygen-binding curves of, 271
　types of, 270*t*
hemolytic anemias, 569, 569*b*–570*b*
hemolytic crisis, sickle-cell anemia and,
　570
hemopericardium, 543*b*
hemophilia, 577
　characterization, 577*b*
hemoptysis, 556*b*
hemorrhage
　baroreceptor reflex and, 363
　PUD and, 558
hemosiderin accumulation, 501, 501*t*
hemosiderosis, 501*t*
hemostasis, 366
Henderson–Hasselbalch equation, 387
hepadnavirus, 477*t*
hepatic artery, 103
hepatic fat synthesis, hyperlipidemia, 567*b*
hepatic sinusoids, 103, 184–185
hepatic veins, IVC and, 103
hepatitis, 564
　infections, serological profiles of, 479*f*,
　　479*t*
　viral, 564
　viruses, 478–479
　　comparison of, 478*t*
hepatitis B virus (HBV)
　serological findings, 479*f*, 479*t*
　vaccine, 479
　　preexposure protocol and, 448
hepatitis C virus (HCV), liver
　transplantation and, 479

hepatocellular carcinoma, cirrhosis, 562
hepatocytes, 184
hepatoduodenal ligament, 99
hepevirus, 473*t*
hereditary amyloidosis, cause and sites of,
　624
hereditary spherocytosis, 570
heredity, aplastic anemia and, 571
Hering–Breuer reflex, 363*b*, 381
herpesvirus, 477*t*
Hertwig's epithelial root sheath (HERS),
　　root formation and, 218, 218*f*
heterochromatin, 157
heterodont dentition, 632
heterolysis, enzymatic cellular degradation
　　and, 500
heterophile test, Burkitt's lymphoma and,
　　477*t*
heteropolymer chains, 260
heterozygote, sickle-cell anemia and, 570
hiatal hernia, 557
high altitude, respiration and, 382
high radiosensitive cells, 606
hindbrain, embryology of, 230
hindgut, 100, 105
hipbone (os coxa), 168
hippocampus, limbic system and, 309
His-Purkinje system, nodal/pacemaker
　　conduction system and, 360
histamine, 266
histidine, 266
histiocytes, 513, 625*b*
histiocytosis X, 625
histones, 295
HIV
　environmental surfaces and, 446
　RNA strands and, 472, 472*f*
hives, 534
HLA-B27
　ankylosing spondylitis, 587
　Reiter's syndrome and, 587
HOC (heights of contour), teeth and, 640
Hodgkin's lymphoma, 621–622, 621*b*
homodont dentition, 632
homozygote, sickle-cell anemia and, 570
horizontal fold, 22
hormone(s). *See also* parathyroid hormone
　calcium regulation and, 435
　endocrine glands and, 163
　kidney and, 389, 394–395, 436–437
　mechanisms, 416–417
　pancreas and, 426–427
　regulation, triacylglycerol lipase and,
　　triglyceride lipolysis and, 285
　second messengers and, 416
　smooth muscle and, 343
　teratogenesis and, 530
　types and classification, 415–416
Horner's syndrome, 124*t*
host defenses, evasion of, mediators of, 450
host tissue destruction, mediators of,
　　450–451
Hot T-Bone stEAk, 505*b*
Howship's lacunae, 167
HR. *See* heart rate
HTN. *See* hypertension
human choriogonadotropin (hCG), 425

inflammatory bowel disease, 559

inflammatory cytokines, 505–506, 505t–506t

inflammatory infiltrate, 201

inflammatory mediators, 505–507, 506t–507t

inflammatory reaction, leukemia and, 618

inflammatory stage of wound repair, 507

influenza virus, 473

infrahyoid muscles, 61, 62, 63f, 73, 670

infraorbital foramen, 9

infraspinatus, 81

infratemporal fossae, 15f
    boundaries of, 14t

inguinal canal, males v. female, 109–110

inhibitor concentration, reaction rate influencing factors, 254t

inhibitory neurotransmitters, 323

innate immunity, 510

inner ear, 138, 138f
    anatomy, 331, 331f

inner enamel epithelium (IEE), 216

inner medulla (of ovary), 190

innervation, dental, 635

inspiration, lung mechanics and, 371

inspiratory capacity (IC), lung volumes, 370, 370f

inspiratory reserve volume (IRV), lung volumes, 370, 370f

insulin, 426
    diabetes mellitus and, 579b

insulin clearance, 394

insulin deficiency, 578–579

integral proteins, 303

integument, 190–192

interalveolar septum, 210

intercalated disc, cardiac muscle and, 343

intercalated duct, 164

intercostal artery, 81

intercostal muscles
    orientation of, 82
    respiration and, 81

intercostal nerves, 81
    intercostal muscles and, 82

intercostal space, 81

intercostal vein, 81, 94

intercuspal relationship, 666

interdental papilla, 199

interdental spaces, 634

interferons (INF), 480, 505, 505t–506t

interglobular dentin, 203

interleukins (IL), 505, 505t–506t

intermediate filaments, 157

intermediate junction (zonula adherens), 158

intermediolateral horn, gray matter, 145

internal acoustic meatus, 9

internal basal lamina, 200

internal carotid artery (ICA), 27

internal cranial skull base, 10, 10f

internal jugular vein (IJV), 69
    brain, 24

internal oblique fibers, 84

internal skull, 10, 10f
    cranial base of, 11, 11f

internal thoracic artery, 93

interneurons, 169

internodal pathways, nodal/pacemaker conduction system and, 360

internuclear ophthalmoplegia, 124t

interoreceptors, CNS and, 315

interosseous membrane, 80

interphase, cell cycle and, 158

interproximal space, 634

interradicular septum, 210

interstitial fibrosis, 554b

interstitial growth, 165, 166

interstitial lamellae, 166

interstitial lung disease, sarcoidosis and, 553

interstitial pneumonia, 555

interstitial space, edema and, 386–387

intertubular dentin, 203

intestinal bacteria, vitamins synthesized by, 408b

intestinal glands, 182

intestinal lymphangiectasia, 559

intestinal secretions, pHs of, 403

intestinal villi, enzymes in, 105b

intraalveolar fluid, intrapleural fluid v., 550b

intracellular fluids (ICF), 384
    expansion, edema and, 386–387

intracranial circulation, 27–29

intracranial pressure, choroid plexus and, 25

intradental spaces, 635

intradermal nevi, 609

intrafusal fibers, 341

intramembranous growth, 6

intramembranous ossification, 166

intraperitoneal colon, 106b

intrapleural fluid, intraalveolar fluid v., 550b

intrapleural pressure, 371

intra-testicular duct system, 189

intrathoracic lymph nodes, eggshell calcification and, 501b

intrathoracic pressure, compliance, 355

intrinsic asthma, 549–550

intrinsic factor
    as gastric secretion, 399
    pernicious anemia and, 571

intrinsic muscles of tongue, 671

inulin, 260

invasion, metastasis and, 602

inverse myotatic (tendon reflex), 342

iodopsin, 194

IP3, hormones and, 416

ipsilateral motor loss, 320

ipsilateral tracts, 314b

iris, 192, 328

iron
    deficiency, 572
    transferrin and, 412

iron atom, heme, 270

irreversible cell injury, 499

irreversible inhibition, 255

irritant receptors, 381

IRV (inspiratory reserve volume), 370, 370f

ischemic heart disease, atherosclerosis and, 541b

ischemic injury, middle cerebral artery and, 29

Islets of Langerhans, 186

isoelectric point, 388

isograft, 518

isolated IgA deficiency, 522t

isomaltase, 259

isomerases, 251

isomerism, 258

isotonic solutions, membrane and, 387

isovolumetric contraction, cardiac cycle and, 356

isovolumetric relaxation, cardiac cycle and, 356

isozymes, 251

Ito cells, 185

ITP (idiopathic thrombocytopenic purpura), 576

IV drug users, tricuspid valve and, 544

IVC. See inferior vena cava

J

J (juxtacapillary) receptors, 381

jaundice, 563
    bilirubin levels and, 185
    causes, 405
    liver disease and, 563

jaw jerk reflex, 132

jejunum, 182
    blood supply and description of, 105

JG cells (juxtaglomerular cells), 187

JGA (juxtaglomerular apparatus), 187

Job's syndrome, 523t

joint receptors, types of, 315b

joints, 167–168. See also rheumatoid arthritis
    classification of, 167

jugular foramen, 9

jugular lymph trunk, 69
    venous emptying of, 70b

junctional complex, 158b, 159f

junctional epithelium, 199

junctional nevus, 609

juvenile periodontitis, 493

juxtacapillary receptors, 381

juxtaglomerular apparatus (JGA), 187

juxtaglomerular cells (JG cells), 187

K

K+ conductance, 322

K leak, 321

K+ permeability, repolarization and, 321

Kallmann syndrome, 335

karyokinesis, 158

karyolysis, cell death and, 502t

karyorrhexis, cell death and, 502t

keratinocytes, 196

keratoacanthoma, 612

keratohyalin granules, 196

kernicterus, 564, 570

ketoacidosis, 285, 579b

ketone bodies
    fatty acids and, 286
    ketoacidosis and, 579b

ketonuria, 565

ketoses, 259f

ketosis, 286

kidney(s), 96, 108–109
    components of, 187, 188f
    diseases, nephrotic syndrome and, 568
    embryology, stages of, 235f

medulla oblongata, 113, 310
medullary cystic disease, 566
medullary rays, cortex and, 187
medullary sponge kidney, 566
medulloblastoma, 609
meiosis, 158
meiosis II, fertilization and, 220
Meissner's corpuscles, 315
Meissner's plexus (submucous plexus), 398
melanocytes, 196
melanoma in situ, 610
membrane(s)
    capacitance, 323
    carbohydrates and, 303
    components, 302–303
    isotonic solutions and, 387
    phospholipids, 303f
    transport, 303
    type of substance movement, 304f
membrane-bound organelles, 156–157
membranous urethra, 189
meningeal veins, 24
meninges, 22–25, 145
    space and description of, 22
meningioma, 609
meningitis, 22
meniscus, 168
    articular disk of TMJ, 50–51
        damage, 50
    mandibular condyle and, 53f
menstruation, 424–425, 425f
mental foramen, 9, 21
mental nerve, 21
    distribution, 126
Merkel cells, 196
Merkel's disc, 315
mesencephalic nucleus, 128
mesencephalon. See midbrain
mesenchyme, thymus and, 91
mesentery, 98–99
mesiodens, 674
mesoderm, cardiovascular system from, 231
mesothelioma, 553b
mesothelium, 161
messenger RNA (mRNA), 294
metabolic acidosis, respiratory
        compensation for, 380
metabolic alkalosis, respiratory
        compensation for, 380
metabolic intermediates, 278, 279f
metabolic pathways, 277–290, 278f
metallic coenzymes, 251t
metalloproteinases (collagenases), host
        tissue destruction and, 450
metals, nonprotein enzyme components,
        251
metaphase, 158
metaplasia, 601
    cell injury, 499t
metastasis, 601
    bone, 628b
    breast cancer and, 607
    and invasion, 602
    routes of, 602
    squamous cell carcinoma and, 612
metastatic bone tumors, 626
metastatic cancer, to lungs, 614b

metazoa (helminths), 485
    human infection and, 487t
methemoglobinemia, 270
metronidazole, 465t, 467
MG (myasthenia gravis), 597
MI (myocardial infarction), 547
micelles, 402
Michaelis constant (K_m), 252
Michaelis–Menten equation, enzyme
        kinetics and, 252, 252f
microbodies, 515
microcytic anemia, macrocytic anemia v.,
        572
microdontia, 674
microfilaments, 157
microglia, 513
microorganisms, infectious diseases and,
        443, 443t
microtubules, 157
microvilli, 157, 182
midbrain (mesencephalon), 113, 310
    embryology of, 230
middle cerebral artery, 29
middle cranial fossa
    contents of, 8
    middle meningeal artery and, 7
middle ear, 137, 138f
    anatomy, 331
    muscles in, 138
middle meatus, sinus openings and, 19
middle meningeal artery, 67
    middle cranial fossa and, 7
midgut, 100
miliary tuberculosis, 556
milk, pasteurization of, 446
mineralization, plaque formation and, 491
mineralocorticoid. See aldosterone
minerals
    major, 411, 411t
    minor, 412, 412t
minor salivary glands, 44
minute ventilation, 372
miosis, eyeball and, 328
missense mutation, 299
mitochondria, 157
mitosis, 158
mitral valve, 89
mixed dentition, 658, 659
MO. See maximum opening
molar(s)
    extraction, lingual nerve damage and,
        128
    lobes, 641
    mandibular permanent teeth, 647–648,
        647f, 648f
    mandibular primary teeth, 652
    maxillary permanent teeth, 643–645,
        643f, 644f
    maxillary primary teeth, 650–651
molds, yeasts v., 483t
monoamine oxidase (MAO), monamines
        and, 313
monocytes, 172, 513
monoglycerides, triglycerides and, digestion
        and, 402
monophyodont dentition, 632
monosaccharides, 258, 258f–259f

mossy fibers, 112
motor branches, distribution, 126
motor control, and coordination, 309–310
motor innervation, skeletal muscle and,
        340
motor nerve, 125
motor nucleus, 128, 134
motor pathway, 310
motor units, 340b
mouth, formation, 240–246, 244f
mouth breathing, chronic, 196
mouthrinses, plaque control, 495
movement disorders, motor pathway, 310
MRI (magnetic resonance imaging), TMJ
        and, 51
mRNA (messenger RNA), 294
mucopolysaccharide storage diseases,
        260
mucous cells, conducting zone airways and,
        372
mucous membrane pemphigoid, 524t
mulberry molars, enamel and, 207
multiple myeloma, 623–624
multiple polyposis syndromes, 617
multiple sclerosis, 596b, 597
muscle(s), 338
    cellular components, 338
    controlling tongue, 33, 34f, 35
    exercise, 364
    innervation, 338
    of limbs
        arm movement, at elbow, 80
        functions by joint, 79–80
        hand movement, at elbow, 80
    of mastication, 48, 48f–49f, 670
    middle ear, 138
    receptors, 342
    spindles, 342
    tone, stretch reflex and, 342
    Trichinella spiralis and, 487t
    types of, comparison of, 338
muscle fiber, 341
muscle hypertrophy, 340
muscular arteries, 174
muscular triangle, of neck, 61
musculocutaneous nerve, 78, 80
musculoskeletal pathology, 585–595
mutagenesis, 605
mutagenic chemicals, mutations by,
        298–299
mutations, 298–299
    and carcinogenesis, 605–606
    change, 605
mutualism, 444
myasthenia crisis, 597
myasthenia gravis (MG), 597
mycobacteria, 462
    cell walls, mycolic acid and, 453
    comparison of, 462t
mycolic acid, mycobacteria cell walls and,
        453
mycosis fungoides, 623
mycotoxicosis, fungi and, 482
mydriasis, eyeball and, 328
myelin, 324
myelin sheath, 171
myelination, 170–171, 170t

nucleotides, 292
   biosynthesis of, 293
nucleus, 157
nucleus ambiguous, swallowing and, 41
NUG (necrotizing ulcerative gingivitis), 494
null cells, 620
NUP (necrotizing ulcerative periodontitis), 494
nutritional deficiency, enamel and, 207
nystagmus, 139

O

oat cell carcinoma, 614, 615
obligate aerobic, bacteria, 453
obligate anaerobic, bacteria, 454
obligate intracellular bacteria, 463*t*
oblique ridge, 634
obstructive jaundice, gallstones and, 561
obstructive lung diseases, 550
occipital artery, 65*f*, 66
occipital bone, 6
occipital lobe, 111, 111*f*, 307
occlusal adjustment, 662
occlusal contacts, 662–663
occlusal dimensions, 662
occlusal interferences, 668
occlusal ligaments, 671
occlusal musculature, 670–671
occlusal relationships, 663–664
   Angle's classification, 664, 664*f*–665*f*
   determinants of, 663
occlusal surface, 632
occlusal table, 632
occlusion, 662–666
Occupational Safety and Health
   Administration (OSHA), 447
ocular muscles, 122*f*
oculomotor nerve, 121–124, 122*f*
odontogenesis
   appositional stage, 217
   bell stage, 216*f*, 217
   bud stage, 216–219, 216*f*
   cap stage, 216–217, 216*f*
   initiation, 216, 216*f*
OEE (outer enamel epithelium), 216
Okazaki fragments, DNA synthesis and, 297, 297*f*
olfactory nerve (CN1), primary olfactory
   cortex and, 17
oligodendrocyte, 170*t*
oligodontia, 674
oligosaccharides, 258
olivospinal tract, 319
oncotic pressure (colloid osmotic pressure), 385
oocyte, maturation of, 221*f*
oogenesis, 425*b*
oogonia, 425–426
open bite, 663, 663*f*
ophthalmic artery
   ICA and, 28
   orbit and, 12
ophthalmic nerve (V1), 125, 126*f*
ophthalmic veins, retrograde flow and, 24*b*
ophthalmoplegia, 124*t*
opsonins, 514
opsonization, 514

optic canal, 9
optic disc, 194
optic nerve (CN II), 120–121, 121*f*
oral cavity, 29–41, 29*f*
   antifungal drugs and, 484
   origin, 240–246, 241*f*–242*f*
oral cavity proper, 29
oral microbiology, 490–491
oral mucosa
   layers, 196
   types of, 196, 198*t*
oral pathology, 491–494
oral vestibule, 29
orbicularis oculi (CN VII)
   eyelids and, 131*b*
   muscle, 135
orbicularis oris muscle, 135
orbit, 12, 13*f*
orbital septum, 13
organ of Corti, 332
organelles, 156, 156*f*
organogenesis, 229
oropharynx, 41*t*
orthomyxovirus, 475*t*
Osgood–Schlatter disease, 590
OSHA (occupational safety and health
   administration), 447
osmolality, 385
osmolarity, 385
osmoreceptors, pH levels and, 316
osmosis, 385, 386*f*
osmotic pressure, 385
osseous bone tumor, 626
osseous pathology, 587–592
osteitis fibrosa cystica, 589
osteoarthritis, 593
osteoblasts, 165
   alkaline phosphatase and, 589
osteochondroses, 590
osteoclasts, 167
osteocytes, 165
osteogenesis imperfecta, clinical findings, 590, 590*b*
osteoid bone matrix, 165
osteolytic lesions, multiple myeloma, 623
osteomalacia, 588
   blood chemistry values, 588
osteomyelitis, 591–592
   sickle-cell anemia and, 570
osteonecrosis of jaws, bisphosphonate drugs
   and, 592
osteopetrosis, 590–591
osteophytes, RA and, 594
osteoporosis, 587–588
   blood chemistry values, 588
osteosarcoma, 626–627
otitis externa, 138
otitis media, 138
outer cortex, of ovary, 190
outer enamel epithelium (OEE), 216
ovale foramina, of splenoid bone, 12
ovarian cancer, BRCA-1 and, 607
ovarian follicle development, 190
ovarian follicle, maturation of, 221*f*
ovary, 190
overbite, 663
overjet, 663, 663*f*

oviducts (fallopian tubes), 190
ovulation, 424, 424*b*
oxidative deamination, glutamate and, 288, 288*f*
oxidative phosphorylation
   ATP and, 279
   cyanide poisoning and, 548
oxidoreductases, 251
oxygen
   in blood, 375–376
   Laplace's law, 349
oxygen content, 375
   normal values for, 375
oxygen exchange, 350
oxygen saturation, 375
oxygen-hemoglobin dissociation curve, 373–374, 374*f*
oxyntic glands, 101
oxytalan fibers, blood vessels and, 213
oxytocin, 415
   breastfeeding and, 421
   smooth muscle and, 343

P

Pacinian corpuscles, 315
Paget's disease, 589
   blood chemistry, 588
pain
   CN V sensory distribution for, 129
   spinal lesions and, 320
palatal aponeurosis, tongue muscles and, 37
palatal foramen, 16
palatal salivary glands, location, 36
palate, 36–37. *See also specific types*
   blood supply, 36
   formation, 240–244, 244*f*
   formation defects, 244*f*
   innervation, 36
palate close, swallowing and, 41
palatine tonsils, 37
palatoglossus muscle, 34, 35
palmar digital nerves, 79
PALS (periarterial lymphatic sheath), of
   spleen, 176
pampiniform veins, 110
Pancoast tumor, 614*b*
pancreas, 107, 426–427
   amylases and, 259
   disorders, 560–562
   embryology, 236*f*
pancreatic acinar cells, triglycerides and,
   digestion and, 402
pancreatic acini, 186
pancreatic digestive enzymes, 186
   duodenum and, 107
   trypsin, 186
pancreatic ducts, 107
pancreatic hormones, 415
pancreatic islets, cells of, 186
pancreatic secretion, pHs of, 403
pancreatitis, 560–561
pandemic infection, 443
Panner's disease, 590
papillary cystadenoma, 604
papillary layer, of dermis, 191
papillary muscles, valve closure and, 89
papilloma, 604

phosphofructokinase (PFK), glycolysis and, 280, 281*f*

phospholamban (PLN), 354*b*

phospholipase A₂, corticosteroids and, 273

phospholipids
  membrane lipids and, 302, 303*f*
  types and structure, 272

phosphorus metabolism, 435–436

photophosphorylation, 280

photopigments, of eyeball, 329

photoreceptor, 316

phrenic nerve, 63, 64

physeal osteochondroses, 590

pia mater, 22

Pick's disease, 596

picornavirus, 473*t*

pigment epithelium, 192

pigmented nevi, 609

pineal gland, 177
  BBB and, 27

pitch
  sound wave and, 332

pituitary adenoma, 609

pituitary gland, 177, 418, 418*f*
  functional components of, 178*t*
  hormones, 177
  hypothalamus and, 417–424
  insulin and, 426
  surgical approach to, sphenoid sinus and, 19
  tumor, abducens nerve and, 25

placenta, immunoglobulins and, 515*t*

placentation, 224*f*

plane of occlusion, 662

plaque, 490–491, 490*t*
  chemical control of, 495, 495*t*
  formation, 490–491
  gingivitis induced by, 492
  mechanical control of, 495

plasma, body fluid and, 384

plasma cell membrane, 156, 302
  fluid mosaic model of, 302, 302*f*
  protein types, 303

plasma cells, multiple myeloma, 623

plasma proteins
  functions of, 268–269
  liver and, 268–269
  protein types, 303

plasmids, 449

platelets, 172, 575*b*

platysma muscle, 55, 55*f*

pleura, 98

pleural cavity, 87

plexuses, major, 148–149

plica fimbriata, 31

plicae circulares, 182

PLN (phospholamban), 354*b*

Plummer's disease, 434, 582

Plummer–Vinson syndrome, 572

PML (progressive multifocal leukoencephalopathy), 597

pneumoconioses, 552–553

pneumolysin, host tissue destruction and, 451

pneumonia, 554–555

PNS. *See* peripheral nervous system

point angle, 634

point mutations, 299

Poiseuille's law, resistance and, 347

poliomyelitis, 596

polyarthritis nodosa, 586

polycystic kidney disease (PCKD), 566

polycythemia, 573–574
  erythropoietin and, 366
  as myeloproliferative disorder, 574

polycythemia vera, 573–574

polydipsia, 420

polymerase chain reaction (PCR), clinical considerations in, 299

polymorphonuclear neutrophils, 513, 513*t*

polymyalgia, temporal arteritis v., 586

polymyxin B, 468

polyomavirus, 476*t*

polyphyodont dentition, 632

polysaccharide capsule, cell wall and, 449

polysaccharides, 258
  storage of, 259–260

polyuria, 420
  diabetes mellitus and, 427

Pompe disease (type II glycogenosis), 260

pons, 113, 310

portal blood, 97

portal circulation, 275

portal hypertension, 562–563
  splenomegaly and, 562

portal system, capillary beds of, 177

portal systemic anastomoses, 97*f*

portal triad, 97, 103, 184

portal vein, and branches, 96–97, 96*f*

portal venous blood, liver, 103

portocaval shunt, 97

Posselt's envelope of motion
  mandible and, 667, 668*f*
  planes of, 668*f*

postcentral gyrus (somatosensory cortex), 318, 318*f*

postconcussion syndrome, 595*b*

posterior abdominal muscles, innervation of, 107

posterior auricular artery, 65*f*, 66

posterior cord, nerves and, 79

posterior cranial fossa, contents of, 8

posterior cross-bite, 663

posterior deep temporal nerve, 51

posterior pituitary (diencephalon), 418
  hormones, 415, 420
  hypothalamic control of, 418

posterior rectus sheath, 84

posterior teeth, 632, 634

posterior triangle of neck, 59

posterior/dorsal horn, 145

postexposure protocol, 448

postganglionic autonomic fibers, 151

postganglionic autonomic systems, cholinergic effects, 312

postganglionic nerves, lacrimal gland and, 42

postganglionic neurons
  parasympathetic nervous system, 312
  sympathetic nervous system, 313

postganglionic receptors, nicotinic and muscarinic, 312

postsynaptic neurons, 325

Pott's disease, 556, 592

poxvirus, 478*t*

PPE (personal protective equipment), 448

preameloblasts, 217

precocious puberty, 424

predontoblasts, 217

preeclampsia, secondary hypertension and, 542, 542*b*

preexposure protocol, 448

preformed antibody vaccines, 480

preganglionic autonomic systems, cholinergic effects, 313

preganglionic neuron
  parasympathetic nervous system, 312
  sympathetic nervous system, 312–313

preganglionic parasympathetic nerve, 31
  cranial nerves and, 115

preganglionics, brainstem and, 115

pregnancy, preeclampsia and, 542*b*

preload, 354

premolars
  lobes, 641
  mandibular permanent teeth, 646–647, 646*f*
  maxillary permanent teeth, 642–643, 642*f*, 643*f*

presbycusis, 138–139, 332

presbyopia, 330

pressure, CN V sensory distribution for, 129, 130*f*

pressure-volume loop, cardiac cycle and, 356, 357*f*

presynaptic neurons, 325

pretracheal layer, of deep cervical fascia, 56, 56*f*

prevertebral layer, of deep cervical fascia, 56–57

Prevotella intermedia, plaque induced gingivitis and, 492

primary Addison's disease, 430
  secondary Addison's disease v., 584–585

primary amyloidosis, 624

primary bone tumors, 626

primary cusp triangle, first molar, 644

primary dentition, 658–659
  calcification of, 658*t*
  dental formula, 658
  development, 659, 659*t*
  eruption sequence and timing, 658
  number of teeth, 658
  permanent v., 656*t*
  primate space and, 650
  tooth labeling, 648–649, 649*f*

primary hemostasis
  bleeding problems and, 574
  disorders in, 575–577

primary hyperparathyroidism, 582–583

primary hypertension, 541–542
  clinical findings and complications, 542

primary nephrotic syndrome, 567

primary olfactory cortex, olfactory nerve and, 17

primary palate, formation, 242

primary polycythemia, 573–574

primary protein structure, 266

primary pulmonary hypertension, heart failure and, 548

primary response, immunoglobulins and, 515t

primary teeth, permanent teeth v., 649t

primary (deciduous) tooth form, 648–652, 649f, 651t

primary tuberculosis, 556

primate space, primary dentitions and, 650

prinzmetal angina, 547

prions, 481

productive cough, 552b

proelastin polypeptide chain, glycine-x-y and, 268

proenzyme, 256

profunda brachii artery, 76

progesterone
  hCG and, 425
  ovaries and, 422

progressive multifocal leukoencephalopathy (PML), 597

prokaryotic cells, 70s ribosomes and, 297

prolactin, breastfeeding and, 421

proline, collagen synthesis and, 268

prophage, 481

prophase, 158

proprioception, CN V sensory distribution for, 130f

proprioreceptors, CNS and, 315

prostaglandins, 273

prostate cancer, 608
  serum acid phosphatase level and, 589

prostate gland, 189

prostatic urethra, 189

protease, 256, 256f
  host tissue destruction and, 451t

protein A, 450

proteins, 264–271
  absorption, 402
  cirrhosis and, 367
  digestion and absorption, 401
  immunity and, 510
  kinases, 416
  metabolism, 286–289, 405
  peripheral, 303
  physiologically relevant, 267–271
  plasma membranes and, 303
  structure, 266–267

proteinuria, 565
  nephrotic syndrome, 567

proteoglycan aggrecan, 262f

proteoglycans (PGs), 261

prothrombin, coagulation and, 367, 367f

proton pump inhibitors, peptic ulcer disease, 558

protozoa, 485
  human infection and, 486t

protrusive contacts, 663

protrusive interference, 668

protrusive movement
  condylar movements as, 669
  mandible and, 667

proximal contacts of teeth, 639, 639f

proximal convoluted tubule, glomerular filtrate and, 390

proximal surfaces, shapes, 640, 640f

PSA testing, prostate cancer, 608

pseudogout, 594

pseudomembranous candidiasis (thrush), 494

pseudomembranous colitis, clindamycin and, 467

pseudostratified epithelial cell layer, 160

pterion, 7

pterygoid plexus of veins, 25, 67, 635
  connections, 25

pterygomandibular space, boundaries and contents, 47f

pterygopalatine artery, 67

pterygopalatine fossae
  boundaries of, 14t
  lateral scheme of, 16f
  major communications, 15

pterygopalatine ganglion, greater petrosal nerve and, 137

PTH. See parathyroid hormone

ptosis, lesions and, 124

puberty. See also precocious puberty
  in female, 422, 423f
  hormones and, 422–424
  in male, 422, 423f

PUD (peptic ulcer disease), 558

pulmonary artery, bronchus v., 87

pulmonary capillaries, ACE, 381

pulmonary chemoreflex, 381

pulmonary circulation, systemic circulation v., 351

pulmonary edema, 547, 548–549
  causes, 549b
  heart failure and, 549b
  left-side CHF and, 537

pulmonary embolism, 540b

pulmonary fibrosis, coal workers pneumoconiosis, 553

pulmonary function tests (PFTs), 551

pulmonary hypertension, 548

pulmonic valve, 88

pulp, 207–209
  aging and, 209
  classifications of, 208
  functions of, 208

pulp calcifications, 209

pulp chamber, 207, 656t

pulp horns, 656t

pulp morphology
  classification, 654
  permanent dentition, 654–655
  primary dentition, 656

pulp zones, 208–209, 208f

pulse pressure, narrow v. wide, 352

pupil, 192, 328

pupillary light reflex, 122, 123f

pure red cell aplasia, 573

purines, pyrimidines v., 293

Purkinje cells, 112

purpura, 576b

pus, 444

pyelonephritis, 565

pyknosis, cell death and, 502t

pyloric glands, 101

pyloric stenosis, 102

pylorus, gastric secretion and, 399

pyramidal system (corticospinal tract), 319, 320f

pyramids, medulla and, 187

pyriform recesses, food and, 41

pyrimidines, purines v., 293

pyruvate
  to alanine, transamination of, 286, 287
  metabolic fates, 281

pyruvate dehydrogenase, 282

Q

quantitative platelet deficiencies, 575–577

quaternary protein structure, 267

R

RA (rheumatoid arthritis), 594–595

radial nerve, 78, 79, 80

radiation, aplastic anemia and, 571

radiosensitivity, 606

rami, 20

rapidly progressive glomerulonephritis (RPGN), 568

rapidly progressive nephritic syndrome, 568

rate-limiting steps, metabolic pathway, 279t

Rathke's pouch (anterior pituitary), 418
  diencephalon and, 112

Raynaud's phenomenon, scleroderma and, 586

reabsorption, 391

reaction equilibrium, enzyme kinetics and, 253

reaction rate
  enzyme kinetics and, 253
  factors influencing, 254t

receptors
  CNS, 315
  of heart, 362
  by stimulus type, 316

recombinant DNA technology, clinical considerations and, 299

recombination, bacterial cell and, 449

rectum
  blood supply and description, 106
  GI cancer and, 616

rectus sheath, 84

recurrent caries, 491

recurrent laryngeal nerve, 74–75, 74f

recurrent periodontitis, 492

red marrow, 167

red pulp, of spleen, 176

reduced enamel epithelium (REE), appositional stage, 217

reducing sugars, 258

REE (reduced enamel epithelium), 217

Reed–Sternberg cells, HD and, 622

reflex arc, pathway, 123, 123f

reflexes, 86

refractory period, 321. See also relative refractory period
  heart and, electrical conduction of, 358, 359f
  skeletal muscle and, cardiac muscle v., 358b

refractory periodontitis, 492

regeneration
  acute inflammation and, 503
  wound healing and, 508

Reiter's syndrome, 587
  clinical triad with, 587

relative afferent pupil, 124t

relative polycythemia, 573

relative refractory period, 321
  heart and, 358, 359f
release, viral replication and, 471
remodeling stage of wound repair, 508
renal artery, 93, 96
renal blood
  flow, 393
  supply, 390, 390f
renal cell carcinoma, 617–618
renal clearance, 394
renal disease, secondary hypertension and,
  542
renal failure
  anemia and, 569b
  multiple myeloma and, 624
renal osteodystrophy, 588
renal sodium, edema and, 386
renal system, embryology of, 234–236, 235f,
  236f
renal vein, 96
renin
  JG cells and, 187
  kidney function and, 394
reovirus, 473t
repair, acute inflammation and, 503
reparative dentin, formation, 203
repeat mutation, 299
repolarization, 321, 322f
reproduction, 424–426
reproductive system, 189–190
rER (rough endoplasmic reticulum), 156
residual volume (EV), lung volumes, 370, 370f
resistance to blood flow, 347
  heart and, 89
  pulmonary circulation, systemic
    circulation v., 351
respiration
  accessory muscles of, 83
  intercostal muscles and, 81
  muscles of, 82–83
respiratory acidosis, status asthmaticus and,
  550b
respiratory arrest, 382
respiratory chemoreceptors, 379
respiratory compensation, anemia and, 365
respiratory conditions, 381
respiratory drive pathway, 379
respiratory rate, 372
respiratory regulation, 379–382
  function of, 379
respiratory system, 179–181
  components, 75
  divisions, 180
  functions, 179
  pathology, 549–556
  segments, 180t
respiratory zone, 373
rest position of mandible, 667
resting membrane potential,
  neurophysiology and, 320–321
restriction endonucleases, 299
restrictive lung diseases, 550, 551b
reticular lamina, 161
reticular layer, of dermis, 191
reticuloendothelial system, components of,
  513
reticulospinal tract, 319

retina, 192, 328–329
  layers of, 194
  vitamin A and, 194
retrograde flow
  infection and, 69
  ophthalmic veins and, 24b
retromandibular vein, 68
retroparapharyngeal space, 46
retroperitoneal structures, 106, 106b, 106f
retropharyngeal space, 57, 57f
retrovirus, 475t
reverse transcriptase
  clinical considerations and, 299
  retrovirus and, 471
reversible cell injury, 499
Reye's syndrome, aspirin and, 476
rhabdomyoma, 606b
rhabdomyosarcoma, 606
rhabdovirus, 475t
rheumatic carditis, rheumatic heart disease
  and, 546
rheumatic endocarditis, 545
rheumatic fever, 545–546
  diagnosis criteria for, 546
  mnemonics for, 545b
rheumatic heart disease, rheumatic carditis
  and, 546
rheumatoid arthritis (RA), 594–595
rhodopsin, 194
ribosomal RNA (rRNA), 294
ribosomes, 157
ribs, 81
  spleen injury and, 81
rickets, 588
  blood chemistry values, 588
ridges, 633–634, 633f
right atrium, 89
right auricle, 89
right gastric artery, 102
right gastroepiploic, 102
right heart failure, 548, 548b. See also heart
  failure
right lymphatic duct, 98
right vagus nerve, 141
  SA node and, 362
right ventricle, 89
  injury and, 81
right working movement, condylar
  movements as, 669, 669f
right-side CHF, peripheral edema and, 537
risorius muscle, 135
Rivian ducts, 31
RNA
  protein translation, 297–298, 298f
  transcription, 297, 298f
  types of, 294
  viruses and, 470, 474, 474t
RNA viruses, viral replication and, 471
roboviruses, 471
rods, 194, 329
Rokitansky–Aschoff sinuses, 186
root formation, 217–218, 218f
rootless teeth, 205
Rosenthal's syndrome, 577
rotator cuff, 81
rotundum foramina, of splenoid bone, 12
rough endoplasmic reticulum (rER), 156

RPGN (rapidly progressive
  glomerulonephritis), 568
rRNA (ribosomal RNA), 294
rubrospinal tract, 319
Ruffini's corpuscles, 315
rugae, 181

S
SA node. See sinuatrial node
sacral plexus, 149
saddle embolus, 540
saliva
  components of, 263
  secretions, 263
salivary control, 264
salivary fluid
  parotid gland and, 44
  submandibular gland and, 44
salivary glands, 43
  primary secretions of, 263
  structure of, 164
salmonella bone infections, sickle-cell
  anemia and, 570
saltatory conduction, 323–324
sanitization, 447
Santorini's duct, 107
sarcoidosis, 553–554
sarcolemma, 338
sarcoma, 603
sarcoma botryoides, 606b
sarcomere, skeletal muscle and, 339
sarcoplasm, 338
sarcoplasmic reticulum (SR), 338
satellite cells, 339
scalene muscles, 77
scalp, 21
  components of, mnemonic for, 21f
  venous drainage and, 68
scar, wound repair and, 508
Scheuermann's disease, 590
Schneiderian membrane, maxillary sinus
  and, 18
Schwann cell, 170t
SCID (severe combined immunodeficiency
  disease), 523t
sclera, 192
scleroderma, 586
  calcinosis and, 501b
sclerotic dentin, 203
sclerotome, derivatives, 227f
SCM (sternocleidomastoid muscle), 61
sebaceous glands, 192
seborrheic keratosis, 611
sebum, 192
second messenger, 416–417
second molar
  mandibular permanent teeth, 647–648,
    647f, 655t
  mandibular primary teeth, 652, 656t
  maxillary permanent teeth, 644, 644f, 655t
  maxillary primary teeth, 650–651, 656t
second premolar
  mandibular permanent teeth, 646–647,
    646f, 655t
  maxillary permanent teeth, 643, 643f, 655t
secondary Addison's disease, 430
  primary Addison's disease v., 584–585

squamous epithelial cells, 161
SR (sarcoplasmic reticulum), 338
stab wound, intercostal space and, 81
stable angina, 546–547
staging, malignant tumors and, 602
standing, sudden, 363
stannous fluoride, 495*t*
stapedius muscle, 135, 137
Staphylococci, 455, 457*t*
   comparison of, 457*t*
Staphylococcus aureus
   osteomyelitis and, 591
   sepsis and, 444
staphylokinase, host tissue destruction and, 451
starch, 259
starch hydrolysis, amylases in, 259
Starling forces, 384
Starling mechanism, 352
Starling's curve, 353*b*
statin and HMG-CoA reductase, 273
stationary phase, bacteria and, 449
status asthmaticus, 550*b*
steatorrhea, 559*b*
stellate reticulum, 217
Stephan curve, caries and, 491, 492*f*
stereocilia, 157
sterilization
   disinfection and, 444–448
   spores and, 454
   techniques, 445*t*
sternocleidomastoid muscle (SCM), 61
sternum, 81
steroids, 273
   asthma and, 550
   hormones, 415
Stevens–Johnson syndrome, 535
Still's disease, 594
stomach, 101–103, 101*f*, 181–182
   blood supply to, 102–103, 103*f*
   disorders of, 558–559
   gastric secretion and, 399
   glands of, 182*t*
   sphincters of, 102
stomodeum, 240
stone formation
   gallstones and, 561
   nephrolithiasis and, 565
stratified epithelial cell layer, 160
stratified squamous epithelium, 196
stratum basale, 191
stratum corneum, 191
stratum granulosum, 191
stratum intermedium, 217
stratum lucidum, 191
stratum spinosum, 191
strawberry gallbladder, 561
Streptococci, 455, 456*t*
   classification of, by hemolysis, 455, 455*b*, 456*t*
   comparison of, 456*t*
Streptococcus salivarius, 490
Streptococcus species, root caries and, 492*b*
streptodornase, host tissue destruction and, 450
streptokinase, host tissue destruction and, 451
streptolysin O, host tissue destruction and, 450

streptolysin S, host tissue destruction and, 450
stress, TSH secretion and, 432
stretch receptors, 363, 381
stretch reflexes, spine and, 342
striae of Retzius, 206
striated duct, 164
stroke, 29, 136
   atherosclerosis and, 541*b*
   lenticulostriate arteries and, 29
stroke volume (SV), 353, 353*b*
structural polysaccharides, 260–261
styloglossus muscle, 35
styloid process (of temporal bone), connections to, 62*b*
stylomandibular ligament, 671
stylomastoid foramen, 9
stylopharyngeus muscle, 41, 73
subarachnoid hemorrhage, 22*b*, 595*b*
subarachnoid space, communicating–obstruction in, 26*b*
subclavian arteries, 93
   branches of, 93
     upper extremities and, 76
     vertebral arteries and, 28
subclavius muscle, 83
subclinical infection, 444
subcondylar fracture, 47
subdural hematoma, 22*b*, 595
subepithelial connective tissue, oral mucosa and, 196
subgingival plaque, supragingival plaque v., 490*t*
sublingual gland, 43, 45*f*
sublingual space, boundaries and contents, 46, 47*f*
submandibular duct, 127
   relationships to, 35
submandibular gland, 60*f*
   innervation of, 43, 45*f*
   salivary fluid and, 44
submandibular space, boundaries and contents, 46, 47*f*
submandibular triangle, 59, 60*f*
submental space, boundaries and contents, 47*f*
submental triangle, of neck, 61
submucosa
   gallbladder and, 104
   oral mucosa and, 196
submucosal glands of Brunner, 182
submucous plexus (Meissner's plexus), 398
subscapularis, 81
substrate concentration, effect of, enzyme kinetics and, 252, 253*f*, 254*t*
substrate-level phosphorylation, 279
subunit vaccine, viruses and, 480
subunits, protein structures and, 266
succedaneous dental lamina, 217
succedaneous teeth, 658
sucrose, 258
   cariogenic bacteria, 262
sulcular epithelium, 199
sulcus, 634
sulcus terminalis, 89
sulfa drugs, polyarthritis nodosa, 586
sulfonamides, 465*t*
sun exposure, skin cancer and, 610

superantigen, 510
   host tissue destruction and, 451*t*
superficial spreading melanoma, 613
superficial temporal artery, 65*f*, 66
superficial temporal vein, 68
superficial thrombophlebitis, 540
superior epigastric artery, 93
superior hemiazygos vein (accesory hemiazygos vein), 95
superior labial artery, 18
superior laryngeal nerve, 75
superior mediastinum, 91
superior mesenteric artery (SMA), 94
superior mesenteric vein, 97
superior orbital fissure, 9
superior petrosal sinus, connections, 24
superior rectus, 122, 123*f*
superior salivatory nucleus, 42, 134
superior thyroid artery, 65*f*, 66
superior vena cava (SVC), 91, 95
superior vena cava (SVC) syndrome, 615, 615*b*
supernumerary teeth, 674
supplemental groove, 634
supporting alveolar bone, 211
supporting cells, 170
   of nervous tissue, 170*t*
supraclavicular nerves, 63
supragingival plaque, v. subgingival plaque, 490*t*
suprahyoid muscles, 62, 73, 670
supraorbital foramen, 9
supraspinatus, 81
suture, 167
SV (stroke volume), 353, 353*b*
SVC (superior vena cava), 91, 95
SVC (superior vena cava) syndrome, 615, 615*b*
swallowing, suprahyoid muscles, 670
swallowing center, sensory information and, 41
sweat chloride test, cystic fibrosis and, 532
sweat glands, 192
swinging flashlight test, 124*t*
symbiosis, 444
sympathetic ganglia of head and neck, 115, 313
sympathetic nervous system, 312–313
   compliance, 355
   exercise, 364
sympathetics, 137
symphysis, 167
synapses, 169–170, 325–326
synaptic cleft, 325
synaptic transmission, 326
synarthrosis, 167
synchondrosis, 167
syndesmosis, 167
syndrome of inappropriate ADH secretion (SIADH), 386*b*, 421
synovial cavity, 168
synovial fluid, 168
synovial joints, 167
   components of, 168
   types of, 168
synovial membrane, 168
synovium, 51

toxic shock syndrome toxin (TSST), host tissue destruction and, 451*t*

toxins
  aplastic anemia and, 571
  host tissue destruction and, 451, 451*t*
toxoid vaccine, 464
TPR (total peripheral resistance), 348, 351–352
trabeculae, 166
trabecular sinuses, lymph and, 175
trachea, branching pattern of, 75
transalveolar vessels, PDL and, 213
transaminases, medically relevant, 288*t*
transamination, protein metabolism and, 287
transcription, viral replication and, 471
transduction, DNA and, 450*t*
transfer RNA (tRNA), 294
transferases, 251
transferrin, blood plasma and, 412
transformation, DNA and, 450*t*
transition mutation, 299
transitional cell carcinoma, 603
transitional epithelial cells, 161
translation, viral replication and, 471
transplantation, 518
transport proteins, 303
transposons, 605
  bacterial cell and, 449, 450*t*
transudate, 504
transudate edema, 536–537
transverse cervical nerve, 63, 64
transverse groove, first molar, 644
transverse mutation, 299
transverse ridge, 634
trapezius muscles, 61
trauma. *See also* neurologic trauma
  DIC and, 576
trench mouth, 494
TRH-TSH-thyroid hormone axis (hypothalamic–pituitary–thyroid axis), 432
triacylglycerol lipase, hormone regulation and, triglyceride lipolysis and, 285
triacylglycerols (triglycerides), 272
  digestion and absorption, 402
  structure, 272
triangle of face, danger area, 69
triangles of neck, 58–61
triangular ridge, 634
triclosan, 495*t*
tricuspid valve, 89
  IV drug users and, 544
trigeminal nerve (CN V), 125–132, 635
  branches of, 126*f*
  divisions of, 125
  facial reflexes and, 132
  facial sensation from, 129, 130*f*, 131*f*
  lesions, type and findings, 131
trigeminal nuclei, 128
triglyceride lipolysis, 285, 285*f*
triglycerides. *See* triacylglycerols
triiodothyronine (T3), 71
tRNA (transfer RNA), 294
trochlear nerve, 121–124, 122*f*
tropical sprue, 560
tropocollagen, 268
tropoelastin, 268
tropomyosin, 338
  skeletal muscle contraction and, 341

troponin, 338
Trousseau's sign, tetany and, 584
true polycythemia, 573
trypsin, pancreatic digestive enzymes and, 186
tryptophan, 415
TSH (thyroid-stimulating hormone), 415, 432
TSH-secreting pituitary tumor, 434
TSST (toxic shock syndrome toxin), 451*t*
TTP (thrombotic thrombocytopenic purpura), 576
t-tubules in skeletal muscle contraction, 341
tubercle, 632
tuberculosis (TB), 556
  clinical presentation, 556*b*
  types of, 556
tuberculum impar, tongue and, 245, 245*f*
tuberous sclerosis, café au lait spots and, 589*b*
tubuloalveolar glands, 190
tumor markers, 603
tumor necrosis factors (TNF), 505, 505*t*–506*t*
tumors, 602. *See also* metastasis; neoplasia
  of adrenal medulla, 625
  of mesenchymal origin, benign v. malignant, 605
tunica adventitia, 174
tunica albuginea, 189
tunica intima, 173–174
tunica media, 174
turbulent flow, 348*f*
Turcot's syndrome, 617
Turner syndrome, 531
TV. *See* tidal volumes
twinning, 224*f*
twitch speed. *See* contraction speed
tympanum plexus, 140*f*
type 1 sensitivity, asthma and, 550
tyrosine, 415
tyrosine metabolism, pathway, 431
Tzanck cells, 535

U

ubiquinone, coenzyme Q as, 284
ulcerative colitis (UC), 559
  Crohn's disease v., comparison of, 559
ulnar nerve, 78
  hypothenar region and, 79
uncoating, viral replication and, 471
uncompetitive inhibition, 255
uniport, transport proteins and, 303
universal numbering system, dental, 638
universal precautions, 448
unstable angina, 547
upper digestive system, 181–184
  esophagus, 181
  functions, 181
  layers, 181
  stomach, 181–182
upper extremities, subclavian arteries and, 76
upper motor neurons, 319
  lesion of, 144
urea
  formation of, reactions and intermediates in, 286*f*
  nonprotein nitrogen and, 404

urea cycle, 289
  liver and, 404
  stoichiometry of, 289*f*
ureter, 109
urethra, 108, 109, 189
uric acid synthesis, 293
urinary bladder, 109
urinary infections, females and, 109
urinary system, 108, 187–189, 389–392
urine
  characteristics and contents, 389
  lipiduria and, 567
uronic acid, 260
uterine tube, fertilization and, 220
uterus, 190
UV light, mutations by, 298–299
uvea, 192
uveitis, 587
uvula, 37

V

V1 (ophthalmic) nerve, 125, 126*f*
V2 (maxillary) nerve, 125, 126*f*
V3 nerve. *See* mandibular nerve
vaccination, hepatitis B virus and, 479
vaccines. *See also specific types*
  bacterial, 464
  preexposure protocol and, 448
  viral, 480
vagal stimulation, asthma and, 550
vagina, 190
vagus nerve (CN X), 88
  cardiac branches of, 143
  course of, 141
  lesions, 143
vallate papillae, 333
vallecula recesses, food and, 41
valves, head and neck, 69
valves of Kerckring, 182
valvular disease, heart murmurs with, 358
valvular vegetations, 545*b*
vancomycin, 465*t*, 466–467
vascular compliance, 352
vascular-endothelial barrier, 27
vasoconstriction
  epinephrine and, 266
  serotonin and, 266
vasodilation
  histamine and, 266
  nitric oxide and, 266
vasopressin. *See* antidiuretic hormone
VC (vital capacity), 370
VDO. *See* vertical dimension of occlusion
VDR. *See* vertical dimension of rest
veins, 174, 351
veins of heart, 91
velopharyngeal incompetence, prevention of, 41
venous anastomoses, 97, 97*f*
venous drainage, from face, 68–69, 68*f*, 69*f*
venous return, 355, 355*f*
  CO and, 353
  dental, 635
  exercise, 364
venous sinuses, 23, 23*f*
venous thrombi, 539

CPSIA information can be obtained
at www.ICGtesting.com
Printed in the USA
JSHW021927300922
31119JS00007B/49